Transesophageal Echocardiography

Transesophageal Echocardiography

Edited by

William K. Freeman, M.D.
Consultant, Division of Cardiovascular Diseases and Internal Medicine,
Mayo Clinic and Mayo Foundation; Assistant Professor of Medicine, Mayo
Medical School, Rochester, Minnesota

James B. Seward, M.D.
Consultant, Division of Cardiovascular Diseases and Internal Medicine,
and Consultant, Section of Pediatric Cardiology, Mayo Clinic and Mayo
Foundation; Professor of Medicine and of Pediatrics, Mayo Medical
School, Rochester, Minnesota

Bijoy K. Khandheria, M.D.
Consultant, Division of Cardiovascular Diseases and Internal Medicine,
Mayo Clinic and Mayo Foundation; Assistant Professor of Medicine, Mayo
Medical School, Rochester, Minnesota

A. Jamil Tajik, M.D.
Chair, Division of Cardiovascular Diseases and Internal Medicine, and
Consultant, Section of Pediatric Cardiology, Mayo Clinic and Mayo
Foundation; Professor of Medicine and of Pediatrics, Mayo Medical
School, Rochester, Minnesota

Little, Brown and Company
Boston/New York/Toronto/London

Library of Congress Cataloging-in-Publication Data

Transesophageal echocardiography / edited by William K. Freeman . . . [et al.].
    p.   cm.
    Includes bibliographical references and index.
    ISBN 0-316-29293-1
    1. Transesophageal echocardiography. I. Freeman, William K.
    [DNLM: 1. Heart Diseases—diagnosis. 2. Echocardiography—methods. WG 141.5.E2 T7715 1994]
    RC683.5.T83T73   1994
    616.1′207543—dc20
    DNLM/DLC
    for Library of Congress   93-5357
                                                CIP

Printed in the United States of America

KP

Editorial: Nancy E. Chorpenning
Production Editor: Karen Feeney
Indexer: Dorothy Hoffman
Production Supervisor/Designer: Michael A. Granger
Cover Designer: Michael A. Granger

To our families

Contents

Contributing Authors

Martin D. Abel, M.D.
Consultant, Department of Anesthesiology, Mayo Clinic and Mayo Foundation; Associate Professor of Anesthesiology, Mayo Medical School, Rochester, Minnesota
  7. *Evaluation of Left Ventricular Function by Transesophageal Echocardiography*
 16. *Intraoperative Applications of Transesophageal Echocardiography*

Marek Belohlavek, M.D.
Research Associate in Cardiovascular Diseases, Mayo Graduate School of Medicine, Rochester, Minnesota
 18. *Three-Dimensional Reconstruction by Transesophageal Echocardiography*

Roger L. Click, M.D., Ph.D.
Consultant, Division of Cardiovascular Diseases and Internal Medicine, Mayo Clinic and Mayo Foundation; Assistant Professor of Medicine, Mayo Medical School, Rochester, Minnesota
  8. *Transesophageal Echocardiography in Ischemic Heart Disease*
 15. *Source of Embolism: Utility of Transesophageal Echocardiography*

Maurice Enriquez-Sarano, M.D.
Senior Associate Consultant, Division of Cardiovascular Diseases and Internal Medicine, Mayo Clinic and Mayo Foundation; Assistant Professor of Medicine, Mayo Medical School, Rochester, Minnesota
  9. *Transesophageal Echocardiographic Evaluation of NativeValvular Heart Disease*

Raúl Emilio Espinosa, M.D.
Senior Associate Consultant, Division of Cardiovascular Diseases and Internal Medicine, Mayo Clinic and Mayo Foundation; Instructor in Medicine, Mayo Medical School, Rochester, Minnesota
 15. *Source of Embolism: Utility of Transesophageal Echocardiography*

David A. Foley, M.D.
Senior Associate Consultant, Division of Cardiovascular Diseases and Internal Medicine, Mayo Clinic and Mayo Foundation; Assistant Professor of Medicine, Mayo Medical School, Rochester, Minnesota
 18. *Three-Dimensional Reconstruction by Transesophageal Echocardiography*

William K. Freeman, M.D.
Consultant, Division of Cardiovascular Diseases and Internal Medicine, Mayo Clinic and Mayo Foundation; Assistant Professor of Medicine, Mayo Medical School, Rochester, Minnesota
  3. *Transesophageal Echocardiographic Examination: Technique, Training, and Safety*
  9. *Transesophageal Echocardiographic Evaluation of Native Valvular Heart Disease*
 11. *Infective Endocarditis: Evaluation by Transesophageal Echocardiography*
 12. *Cardiac Neoplasms and Thrombi: Evaluation by Transesophageal Echocardiography*
 14. *Diseases of the Thoracic Aorta: Assessment by Transesophageal Echocardiography*
 16. *Intraoperative Applications of Transesophageal Echocardiography*
 17. *Transesophageal Echocardiography in Critically Ill Patients*

James F. Greenleaf, Ph.D.
Consultant, Department of Physiology and Biophysics, Mayo Clinic and Mayo Foundation; Professor of Biophysics and Associate Professor of Medicine, Mayo Medical School, Rochester, Minnesota
 18. *Three-Dimensional Reconstruction by Transesophageal Echocardiography*

Bijoy K. Khandheria, M.D.
Consultant, Division of Cardiovascular Diseases and Internal Medicine, Mayo Clinic and Mayo Foundation; Assistant Professor of Medicine, Mayo Medical School, Rochester, Minnesota
  2. *Organization of a Transesophageal Echocardiographic Laboratory and Role of the Sonographer-Assistant*
  3. *Transesophageal Echocardiographic Examination: Technique, Training, and Safety*
 10. *Echocardiographic Assessment of Prosthetic Heart Valves*
 11. *Infective Endocarditis: Evaluation by Transesophageal Echocardiography*
 15. *Source of Embolism: Utility of Transesophageal Echocardiography*

Thomas J. Losasso, M.D.
Consultant, Department of Anesthesiology, Mayo Clinic and Mayo Foundation; Assistant Professor of Anesthesiology, Mayo Medical School, Rochester, Minnesota
16. Intraoperative Applications of Transesophageal Echocardiography

Janel M. Mays, R.N., R.D.C.S.
Registered Nurse, Echocardiography Laboratory, Mayo Clinic and Mayo Foundation, Rochester, Minnesota
2. Organization of a Transesophageal Echocardiographic Laboratory and Role of the Sonographer-Assistant

Fletcher A. Miller, Jr., M.D.
Consultant, Division of Cardiovascular Diseases and Internal Medicine, Mayo Clinic and Mayo Foundation; Associate Professor of Medicine, Mayo Medical School, Rochester, Minnesota
10. Echocardiographic Assessment of Prosthetic Heart Valves

Donald A. Muzzi, M.D.
Consultant, Department of Anesthesiology, Mayo Clinic and Mayo Foundation; Assistant Professor of Anesthesiology, Mayo Medical School, Rochester, Minnesota
16. Intraoperative Applications of Transesophageal Echocardiography

Barbara A. Nichols, R.N., R.D.C.S.
Registered Nurse, Echocardiography Laboratory, Mayo Clinic and Mayo Foundation, Rochester, Minnesota
2. Organization of a Transesophageal Echocardiographic Laboratory and Role of the Sonographer-Assistant

Rick A. Nishimura, M.D.
Consultant, Division of Cardiovascular Diseases and Internal Medicine, Mayo Clinic and Mayo Foundation; Professor of Medicine, Mayo Medical School, Rochester, Minnesota
7. Evaluation of Left Ventricular Function by Transesophageal Echocardiography

Jae K. Oh, M.D.
Consultant, Division of Cardiovascular Diseases and Internal Medicine, Mayo Clinic and Mayo Foundation; Associate Professor of Medicine, Mayo Medical School, Rochester, Minnesota
8. Transesophageal Echocardiography in Ischemic Heart Disease
17. Transesophageal Echocardiography in Critically Ill Patients

Patrick W. O'Leary, M.D.
Senior Associate Consultant, Section of Pediatric Cardiology, Mayo Clinic and Mayo Foundation; Assistant Professor of Pediatrics, Mayo Medical School, Rochester, Minnesota
16. Intraoperative Applications of Transesophageal Echocardiography

Lyle J. Olson, M.D.
Consultant, Division of Cardiovascular Diseases and Internal Medicine, Mayo Clinic and Mayo Foundation; Assistant Professor of Medicine, Mayo Medical School, Rochester, Minnesota
9. Transesophageal Echocardiographic Evaluation of Native Valvular Heart Disease

Patricia A. Pellikka, M.D.
Consultant, Division of Cardiovascular Diseases and Internal Medicine, Mayo Clinic and Mayo Foundation; Assistant Professor of Medicine, Mayo Medical School, Rochester, Minnesota
8. Transesophageal Echocardiography in Ischemic Heart Disease

Guy S. Reeder, M.D.
Consultant, Division of Cardiovascular Diseases and Internal Medicine, Mayo Clinic and Mayo Foundation; Professor of Medicine, Mayo Medical School, Rochester, Minnesota
12. Cardiac Neoplasms and Thrombi: Evaluation by Transesophageal Echocardiography

James B. Seward, M.D.
Consultant, Division of Cardiovascular Diseases and Internal Medicine, and Consultant, Section of Pediatric Cardiology, Mayo Clinic and Mayo Foundation; Professor of Medicine and of Pediatrics, Mayo Medical School, Rochester, Minnesota
1. Transesophageal Echocardiography: Past, Present, and Future
4. Transesophageal Echocardiographic Anatomy
5. Multiplane Transesophageal Echocardiography
6. Critical Appraisal of Transesophageal Echocardiography: Limitations and Pitfalls
13. Congenital Heart Disease: Transesophageal Echocardiography
18. Three-Dimensional Reconstruction by Transesophageal Echocardiography

Lawrence J. Sinak, M.D.
Consultant, Division of Cardiovascular Diseases and Internal Medicine, Mayo Clinic and Mayo Foundation; Assistant Professor of Medicine, Mayo Medical School, Rochester, Minnesota
11. Infective Endocarditis: Evaluation by Transesophageal Echocardiography

A. Jamil Tajik, M.D.
Chair, Division of Cardiovascular Diseases and Internal
Medicine, and Consultant, Section of Pediatric
Cardiology, Mayo Clinic and Mayo Foundation;
Professor of Medicine and of Pediatrics, Mayo Medical
School, Rochester, Minnesota

Preface

The horizons of cardiac ultrasound have been greatly expanded by the development of transesophageal echocardiography (TEE). Through multiple unique windows within the esophagus and stomach, the heart and great vessels can be visualized by TEE in a myriad of high-resolution tomographic imaging planes. By overcoming many of the potential limitations of the transthoracic imaging approach, TEE has assumed an essential complementary role in the comprehensive echocardiographic evaluation of patients with a broad spectrum of cardiovascular disease.

Transesophageal Echocardiography begins with a description of the organization of a TEE laboratory, the role of the sonographer-assistant, and the fundamentals of TEE examination technique. Considerable emphasis is given to TEE imaging projections with anatomic correlation. An entire chapter is devoted to the limitations of TEE and potential pitfalls in interpretation. The next eight chapters focus on the utility of TEE in the evaluation of ventricular function, native and prosthetic valvular disease, intracardiac masses, congenital heart disease, and diseases of the thoracic aorta. Special attention is then given to applications of TEE in suspected source of embolism, in the operating room, and in critically ill patients. The text concludes with a look to the future through a discussion of three-dimensional imaging by TEE.

We are indebted to many people, without whom the completion of this book would not have been possible. We are very grateful for the efforts of the contributing authors, who submitted their chapters in timely fashion despite universally overcommitted schedules. The assistance of Dr. William D. Edwards of the Division of Anatomic Pathology in the preparation of anatomic sections is greatly appreciated. David T. Smyrk is to be congratulated for outstanding work in computer graphics and digital processing of photographs for nearly all the figures in this text. The ever-present technical support of Charlene R. Tri and Vernon P. Weber is also acknowledged. We especially recognize the tremendous efforts of the entire Section of Publications of the Mayo Clinic, particularly Roberta J. Schwartz for her constant vigilance and managerial expertise of this project since its conception, John L. Prickman for dedication and excellence in manuscript editing, Sharon L. Wadleigh for unrelenting industry in masterful manuscript preparation and organization, Dorothy L. Tienter for meticulous manuscript proofreading, and Jeanette Schlotthauer for expeditious coordination of the proofs. This textbook is a tribute to the magnificent work of all the involved personnel at Little, Brown and Company, and a special thanks is given to Nancy E. Chorpenning, Editor in Chief, who remained a perpetual source of encouragement and support. This book is recognized as a product of the dedicated efforts and ability of all echocardiologists, fellows, sonographers, and paramedical assistants of the Mayo Clinic Echocardiography Laboratory; our sincere esteem is extended to them all.

W.K.F.

Abbreviations

The following abbreviations are used in the figures:

A = anterior
ac = atrial contraction
AL = anterolateral
AML = anterior leaflet of the mitral valve
An = aneurysm
Ant = anterior
Ao = aorta
AP = aortic prosthesis
APEX, Apx = apex
APM = anterior papillary muscle
App = appendage
AR = aortic regurgitation
Arch = aortic arch
AS = atrial septum
ASD = atrial septal defect
AscAo = ascending aorta
Ath = atheroma
AV = aortic valve
AVR = aortic valve prosthesis
AW = anterior wall
Az = azygos

B = bronchus
BP = blood pressure

cath = catheterization
C = coarctation
CHD = congenital heart disease
CS = coronary sinus
CT = computed tomography
CXR = chest x-ray

DesAo = descending aorta
DT = deceleration time

E = esophagus
ECG = electrocardiogram
Exp = expiration
EV, ev = eustachian valve

FL = false lumen
FO = fossa ovalis
FU = follow-up

H = hematoma
HAz = hemiazygos
HR = heart rate
HTN = hypertension

I = inferior
IA = innominate artery
IAS = interatrial septum
IE = infective endocarditis
IL = inferolateral
Inf = inferior
Insp = inspiration
IS = inferoseptal
IV = innominate vein
IVC = inferior vena cava
IVS = interventricular septum
IW = inferior wall

LA = left atrium
LAA = left atrial appendage
LB = left bronchus
LC = left common carotid artery
LCA = left coronary artery
LL = left lower
LLPV = left lower pulmonary vein
LMCA = left main coronary artery
LPA = left pulmonary artery
LS = left subclavian artery
LSVC = left superior vena cava
LU = left upper
LUPV = left upper pulmonary vein
LV = left ventricle
LVO = left ventricular outflow
LVOT = left ventricular outflow tract

MG = mean gradient
MP = mitral prosthesis
MPA = main pulmonary artery
MR = mitral regurgitation
MV, mv = mitral valve
MVO, mvo = mitral valve opening
MVR = mitral valve prosthesis

NSVT = nonsustained ventricular tachycardia
NTG = nitroglycerin

OS = oblique sinus

P = posterior
Pap = papillary
PA = pulmonary artery
PE = pleural effusion

PHT = pressure half-time
PL = posterolateral
PM = papillary muscle
PPM = posterior papillary muscle
Post = posterior
PS = posterior septum
PsAn = pseudoaneurysm
PW = posterior wall

R = right
RA = right atrium
RAA = right atrial appendage
RB = right bronchus
RCA = right coronary artery
RL = right lower
RLPV = right lower pulmonary vein
RPA = right pulmonary artery
RU = right upper
RUPV = right upper pulmonary vein
RV = right ventricle
RVO = right ventricular outflow
RVOT = right ventricular outflow tract

S = apical septal
SEC = spontaneous echocardiographic contrast

SR = sewing ring
Sup = superior
SVC = superior vena cava
SVT = supraventricular tachycardia

T = trachea
$T\frac{1}{2}$ = half-time
TEE = transesophageal echocardiography
Th = thrombus
ThAo = thoracic aorta
TL = true lumen
TR = tricuspid regurgitation
TS = transverse sinus
TTE = transthoracic echocardiography
TV = tricuspid valve

u = ulcer

V = volume
VB = vertebral body
Vent = ventricular
VS = ventricular septum
VT = ventricular tachycardia

WMSI = wall motion score index

Transesophageal Echocardiography

Transesophageal Echocardiography

Past, Present, and Future

James B. Seward

HISTORY

The concept of transesophageal ultrasound dates back to the early 1970s and culminates with the active clinical application of two-dimensional transesophageal echocardiography (TEE) in the late 1980s. Transesophageal Doppler echocardiography was first reported by Side and Gosling [1] in 1971 and by Daigle et al. [2] in 1975. In 1976, Frazin et al. [3] reported on transesophageal M-mode echocardiography as a means of assessing ventricular function. The most dramatic breakthrough in transesophageal imaging occurred with the development of a rigid, mechanical, two-dimensional echocardiographic transesophageal endoscope in 1977 [4,5]. The initial transesophageal device was a mechanical rotating transducer mounted on a rigid endoscope. To overcome the logistical difficulties of introducing a rigid endoscope, transducers were subsequently mounted on flexible endoscopes, and linear and sector phased-array technology was incorporated. In 1980, DiMagno et al. [6] at the Mayo Clinic first reported the use of a linear phased-array flexible endoscope. This instrument, designed by the Stanford Research Institute, had a frequency of 10 MHz and was intended to be used for the ultrasonic detection of gastrointestinal disorders such as disease of the pancreas. Because of the limited field of view resulting from the high-frequency transducer (10

MHz), this endoscope received only limited cardiac application. Hisanaga et al. [7] reported in 1980 their experience with a flexible TEE probe with mechanical scanner that had a display angle of 180 to 260 degrees. In 1982, Souquet et al. [8], in conjunction with Varian Corporation, first produced a clinically usable flexible endoscope mounted with a sector phased-array, two-dimensional echocardiographic transducer. The initial frequency used was 2.25 MHz. These first prototype instruments were assessed by Dr. Peter Hanrath in Hamburg, Germany, and Dr. James B. Seward at the Mayo Clinic in the United States. An international conference held in Hamburg (1981) highlighted many of the potential and varied applications of TEE. Initial investigations in 1981 included monoplane and biplane transesophageal echocardiographic transducers, higher frequency transducers (3.5 and 5 MHz), intraoperative specialty transducers, and a proposed rotating multiplanar transesophageal transducer. These studies were very encouraging. Notable investigators in the early 1980s were Dr. Peter Hanrath, Hamburg, Germany [8]; Dr. James B. Seward, Mayo Clinic, Rochester, MN [9]; and Dr. Peter Kremer in association with Dr. Nelson Schiller, San Francisco, CA [10]. Three distinct applications were respectively studied by these groups: outpatient TEE [11], intraoperative monitoring of air embolism [12], and intraoperative monitoring of left ventricular function [13].

Broad clinical application of TEE remained relatively quiescent between 1981 and 1986 until a number of coincidental events occurred. The European Cooperative Study Group for Echocardiography experience with TEE assessment and diagnosis of aortic dissection showed a distinct clinical application [14,15]. It was suggested that TEE was comparable to angiography and computed tomography for the diagnosis and management of aortic dissection. Intraoperative monitoring of ventricular function and air embolism had become routine in the United States. Most important, Hewlett-Packard Corporation introduced a high-resolution (5 MHz) transesophageal probe with pulsed and color-flow Doppler capability. These events culminated in a heightened interest in clinical TEE.

Several manufacturers now have TEE capability. All devices have similar specifications, including standard endoscope without optics or suction, 5-MHz transducer, adult-sized shaft diameter (8 to 11 mm), 100-cm shaft length, four-way movable tip, pulsed and color-flow Doppler capability, and monoplane transverse imaging array [16]. Most manufacturers have incorporated continuous-wave Doppler and biplane transesophageal [16] echocardiographic capability. Newer devices include small (pediatric) shaft diameters down to 4 mm [17], transducers with higher (7 MHz) and lower (3.5 MHz) frequencies, variable-plane transducers typically allowing transducer rotation of 180 degrees [18], matrix transducers with simultaneous biplane imaging capability [19], and wide-field transducers with increased lateral field of view [20,21].

PRESENT TECHNOLOGY

Transesophageal echocardiographic endoscope technology is rapidly changing. There are three areas of active development:

1. *Smaller endoscope,* which is frequently referred to as a pediatric transesophageal device [17]. However, the smaller scope can be applied to the adult and has appeal as a long- or short-term monitoring probe for intraoperative use or for patients in intensive care units.

2. *Biplanar, multiplanar, and variable-planar imaging arrays.* Monoplane horizontal array is limited to short-axis and frontal views of the heart. Biplanar and variable-planar devices incorporate a longitudinal plane that completes the three-dimensional tomographic capability of an esophageal imaging device.

Two orthogonal planes permit a more nearly complete examination of cardiac anatomy from the confines of the esophagus. Newer variable-planar devices allow the transducer to be rotated along the long axis of the ultrasound beam [18]. The rotating transducer permits a sequence of images throughout a 180-degree rotation.

3. *Continuous-wave Doppler capability.* Now introduced into nearly all transesophageal devices, this capability permits a more comprehensive hemodynamic examination. However, the exact role of continuous-wave Doppler refinement in the transesophageal transducer has to date not been sufficiently investigated.

Transesophageal echocardiography has become a logical extension of a comprehensive echocardiographic examination [16,22]. If a precordial (transthoracic) examination is incomplete, TEE can become complementary in most circumstances. Currently, between 7% and 10% of all precordial examinations are complemented by TEE examination. Intraoperative TEE, also an expanding application, began as a technique for monitoring cardiac function and air embolism. At this time, however, intraoperative echocardiography is most frequently applied as a preoperative diagnostic technique and for intraoperative assessment of surgical result.

CURRENT APPLICATIONS

Awake Patient and Outpatient Examination (Fig. 1-1)

Source of Embolism

Transesophageal echocardiography has improved identification of systemic venous sources for systemic and pulmonary embolization [23,24]. The exact role of TEE in the evaluation of patients having an embolic event has not been fully established. Transesophageal echocardiography appears to be highly diagnostic for definite sources of systemic embolization, including atrial mass or thrombus, vegetation, and retained foreign body, such as a catheter or intra-aortic debris. Other definite sources for pulmonary embolism have been identified as thrombus in transit within the right atrial or right ventricular cavity, mural ventricular thrombus, and direct visualization of the proximal pulmonary emboli.

Indirect sources for embolization are more controversial but are easily diagnosed by TEE. They in-

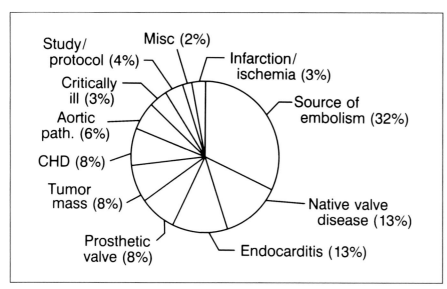

Fig. 1-1. Indications for TEE (3,827 procedures).

clude spontaneous echocardiographic contrast effect, patent foramen ovale with right-to-left shunt, mitral valve prolapse or other suspicious valve abnormality, and atrial septal aneurysm. Although these potential sources are easily diagnosed by TEE, their significance is currently being investigated.

Prosthetic Valves

Most prosthetic valve hemodynamic and pathophysiologic data can be obtained from a comprehensive transthoracic echocardiographic and Doppler examination [25–31]. However, because the prosthetic stent and mechanical components can produce acoustic shadows and obscure posterior or underlying structures, TEE has been used to extend a comprehensive surface echocardiographic examination. For assessment of the magnitude or cause of prosthetic mitral valve regurgitation, TEE has become the procedure of choice. Also, in patients with an obstructed prosthesis, recent embolism, or suspected endocarditis, TEE is considered a highly valuable adjunct.

Native Valvular Disease

An incomplete transthoracic echocardiographic examination for native valvular disease can be complemented by TEE [32,33]. A common lesion inadequately assessed by surface echocardiography is mitral valve regurgitation. Both causation and qualitative estimate of severity can be consistently determined by TEE. Because of the predictable high-quality examination from the esophageal window, TEE has become a routine extension of an incomplete or less than diagnostic transthoracic examination for valvular heart disease. Similarly, because of

the superior resolution of TEE, direct measurement of aortic valve area has been reported to be accurate [33].

Endocarditis

Because of the high incidence of serious complications associated with endocarditis, TEE has become a nearly mandatory examination in any patient with this clinical diagnosis [34–36]. Transesophageal echocardiography is a more sensitive examination for native or prosthetic valve vegetations, valve disruption, and abscess formation. Serial examination can be very helpful for guiding a more logical management of serious cardiac disease.

Tumors and Other Masses

Diagnostic and morphologic features of cardiac masses are markedly enhanced by TEE [37–39]. Transesophageal echocardiography is a significant adjunct to a complete transthoracic examination, particularly to detect masses located in the posterior cardiac chambers or embedded in the myocardium or to exclude malignant or infiltrative masses from benign lesions.

Thoracic Aorta

The entire thoracic aorta can be imaged with superb detail from the esophagus [14,15,27,40,41]. Monoplanar (horizontal plane only) imaging has difficulty visualizing a small portion of the upper ascending aorta. However, use of biplanar or variable-planar transducers nearly eliminates this problem [22]. Because the examination can be performed in any location (e.g., emergency room, bedside, trauma unit, intensive care unit), is of short duration (average,

15 to 18 minutes), and does not require contrast medium, TEE is rapidly becoming the diagnostic technique of choice for acute aortic dissection. The European Cooperative Study has shown that TEE is as diagnostic for aortic dissection as other conventional imaging modalities [15]. Transesophageal echocardiography will continue to make increasing inroads into the diagnostic workup of aortic pathologic conditions.

Critically Ill Patient

Because of its versatility and high-quality imaging capability, TEE has made a striking change in the management of the critically ill cardiac patient [42–44]. Patients with unexpected cardiovascular shock, hypotension, new murmur, or complicated myocardial infarction are ideal candidates for TEE. Transesophageal echocardiography can easily be brought to the patient, who may be on life support and cannot be transported without difficulty. Life support, including cardiac massage, tracheal intubation, and thoracic surgery or trauma, does not usually interfere with the TEE examination. The heart and mediastinal anatomy can be rapidly and confidently assessed at bedside.

Congenital Heart Disease

Anatomic and morphologic diagnoses can be rapidly and confidently made with TEE [45–53]. Atrial septal defect, anomalous pulmonary venous connections, left and right ventricular outflow obstructions, and intra-atrial membranes are confidently diagnosed by a TEE examination. Pediatric TEE usually is confined to intraoperative examination because a general anesthetic is necessary to accomplish esophageal intubation in children younger than about 10 years. As small diagnostic endoscopes become available, other applications will surely evolve. At present, outpatient TEE is most commonly used in the elucidation of adult congenital heart disease.

Intraoperative Applications

Three general uses of TEE have evolved in the operating room: monitoring of cardiac function, diagnosis of anatomic and functional abnormalities, and assessment of surgical result. Each application has brought the cardiologist, cardiovascular surgeon, and anesthesiologist into close collaboration.

Monitoring of Cardiac Function

One of the first applications of intraoperative TEE was monitoring cardiac function during high-risk surgery [54–58]. Patients with known ischemic heart disease or vascular complications such as aortic aneurysm repair are considered appropriate candidates for transesophageal cardiac monitoring. With time, the application of TEE monitoring has become more generally applied to cardiovascular surgery of almost any type.

Intraoperative Diagnosis

Transesophageal echocardiography has been applied in pediatric patients with congenital heart disease, in immediate assessment of mitral valve morphology in anticipation of mitral valve repair, and in rapid cardiovascular diagnosis in patients undergoing emergency surgery [59–62]. Increasingly in patients with mixed or complex anatomic and functional cardiovascular abnormalities, TEE is used to ensure a more complete assessment of preoperative and postoperative anatomy and function.

Assessment of Postoperative Result

The results of certain operative procedures can be difficult to assess by inspection. Mitral valve repair for mitral regurgitation and myectomy for hypertrophic obstructive cardiomyopathy are just two examples of lesions for which intraoperative TEE can rapidly recognize success or failure of the intended procedure. Complications can be more rapidly recognized and characterized in the immediate postoperative and perioperative period by TEE. Intraoperative TEE is one of the more rapidly expanding methods of ultrasound application that dramatically affects the outcome of certain surgical procedures.

Special Applications

Monitoring of Neurosurgical and Orthopedic Surgical Procedures

Transesophageal echocardiography is increasingly used to monitor neurologic and orthopedic surgical interventions. Air embolism is a serious complication of upright posterior fossa neurosurgery. In the upright position, air can be entrained in the veins of the skull and lead to unsuspected air embolism. Early recognition and use of corrective maneuvers can prevent serious embolic complications. Transesophageal echocardiographic monitoring of the cardiac chambers for air is an excellent means of recognizing air embolism and is considered a monitoring procedure of choice in patients undergoing upright neurosurgery [12].

Fat embolism during implantation of large bone prostheses is being monitored by TEE [63]. The exact role of this monitoring technique has not been established. However, fat embolism can easily be seen as it transits the cardiac chambers.

Esophageal Ultrasound Endoscopes

Gastroenterologists are increasingly interested in transesophageal ultrasound to diagnose lesions of the esophagus, such as carcinoma [64]. Multifrequency, 360-degree, rotating mechanical scanners are now available. A balloon offset and frequencies of 5, 7, and 12 MHz allow detailed ultrasonic imaging of the esophageal wall.

FUTURE DIRECTIONS

Transesophageal echocardiography, an exciting new imaging modality, heralds an era of invasive ultrasound techniques. Many of the applications of TEE will merge with other new ultrasound developments, in particular intravascular echocardiography. Small specialty devices will surely begin to appear in the next few years. Practical future innovations include some of the following.

Wide-Field Intraluminal Imaging

The esophageal as well as intravascular transducers can obtain images in a 360-degree tomographic format. Initial evaluation of transesophageal devices that can accommodate wide-field tomographic images is most encouraging [20,21]. Because of the proximity of the intrathoracic structures and the relatively limited field of view of conventional devices, wide-field imaging has considerable appeal. Rotating, tilting, and composite imagery are all feasible means of developing wide-field tomographic images.

Special Applications

Each function of a conventional transesophageal imaging system can be enhanced for special applications. *High-frequency transducers* (7 to 15 MHz) would assist in better resolution of near-field anatomy and may better permit tissue characterization of myocardial segments. *Transducer offsets* would allow imaging of the esophageal mucosa and near-

field structures. *Other devices,* including pacing endoscopes [62], multiple temperature probes, pressure channels, and capacity for recording other physiologic events, such as esophageal electrocardiography and respiration, may be incorporated. *Tissue characterization* [65] and *three-dimensional reconstruction* with use of a rotating transducer [66,67] are other possibilities.

SUMMARY

The introduction of TEE opened the era of invasive echocardiography. Numerous subspecialties will now begin to use innovative ultrasound devices that can probe the orifices and conduits of the body. Transesophageal echocardiography has been described as the ambassador of ultrasound because it has brought together many subspecialty disciplines, such as cardiology, anesthesiology, surgery (cardiovascular, neurologic, orthopedic, and vascular), radiology, and gastroenterology. Other disciplines will surely follow. Additional innovations will rapidly advance the application of ultrasound into other invasive environments.

REFERENCES

1. Side CG, Gosling RG. Non-surgical assessment of cardiac function (letter to the editor). *Nature* 1971;232:335–6.

2. Daigle RE, Miller CW, Histand MB, et al. Nontraumatic aortic blood flow sensing by use of an ultrasonic esophageal probe. *J Appl Physiol* 1975; 38:1153–60.

3. Frazin L, Talano JV, Stephanides L, et al. Esophageal echocardiography. *Circulation* 1976;54:102–8.

4. Hisanaga K, Hisanaga A, Nagata K, Yoshida S. A new transesophageal real-time two-dimensional echocardiographic system using a flexible tube and its clinical application. *Proc Jpn Soc Ultrasonics Med* 1977;32:43–4.

5. Hisanaga K, Hisanaga A, Ichie Y. A new transesophageal real-time linear scanner and initial clinical results. *Proc Jpn Soc Ultrasonics Med* 1978;35: 115–6.

6. DiMagno EP, Buxton JL, Regan PT, et al. Ultrasonic endoscope. *Lancet* 1980;1:629–31.

7. Hisanaga K, Hisanaga A, Hibi N, et al. High speed rotating scanner for transesophageal cross-sectional echocardiography. *Am J Cardiol* 1980;46:837–42.

8. Souquet J, Hanrath P, Zittelli L, et al. Transesophageal phased array for imaging the heart. *IEEE Trans Biomed Eng* 1982;29:707–12.

9. Seward JB, Tajik AJ, DiMagno EP. Esophageal phased-array sector echocardiography: an anatomic study. In: Hanrath P, Bleifeld W, Souquet J, eds. *Cardiovascular Diagnosis by Ultrasound*. The Hague: Martinus Nijhoff, 1982:270–9.

10. Schiller NB. Evaluation of cardiac function during surgery by transesophageal 2–dimensional echocardiography. In: Hanrath P, Bleifeld W, Souquet J, eds. *Cardiovascular Diagnosis by Ultrasound*. The Hague: Martinus Nijhoff, 1982:289–93.

11. Schlüter M, Langenstein BA, Polster J, et al. Transoesophageal cross-sectional echocardiography with a phased array transducer system: technique and initial clinical results. *Br Heart J* 1982;48:67–72.

12. Cucchiara RF, Nugent M, Seward JB, Messick JM. Air embolism in upright neurosurgical patients: detection and localization by two-dimensional transesophageal echocardiography. *Anesthesiology* 1984;60:353–5.

13. Kremer P, Schwartz L, Cahalan MK, et al. Intraoperative monitoring of left ventricular performance by transesophageal M-mode and 2–D echocardiography (abstract). *Am J Cardiol* 1982;49:956.

14. Erbel R, Börner N, Steller D, et al. Detection of aortic dissection by transesophageal echocardiography. *Br Heart J* 1987;58:45–51.

15. Erbel R, Engberding R, Daniel W, et al. Echocardiography in diagnosis of aortic dissection. *Lancet* 1989;1:457–61.

16. Seward JB, Khandheria BK, Oh JK, et al. Transesophageal echocardiography: technique, anatomic correlations, implementation, and clinical applications. *Mayo Clin Proc* 1988;63:649–80.

17. Omoto R, Kyo S, Matsumura M, et al. Recent technological progress in transesophageal color Doppler flow imaging with special reference to newly developed biplane and pediatric probes. In: Erbel R, Khandheria BK, Brennecke R, et al., eds. *Transesophageal Echocardiography: A New Window to the Heart*. Berlin: Springer-Verlag, 1989:21–6.

18. Flachskampf FA, Hoffmann R, Hanrath P. Experience with a transesophageal echotransducer allowing full rotation of the viewing plane: the omniplane probe (abstract). *J Am Coll Cardiol* 1991; 17:34A.

19. Omoto R, Kyo S, Matsumura M, et al. New direction of biplane transesophageal echocardiography with special emphasis on real-time biplane imaging and matrix phased-array biplane transducer. *Echocardiography* 1990;7:691–8.

20. Seward JB, Khandheria BK, Tajik AJ. Wide-field transesophageal echocardiographic tomography: feasibility study. *Mayo Clin Proc* 1990;65:31–7.

21. Hsu T-L, Weintraub AR, Ritter SB, Pandian NG. Panoramic transesophageal echocardiography: clinical application of real-time, wide-angle, transesophageal two-dimensional echocardiography and color flow imaging. *Echocardiography* 1991;8: 677–85.

22. Seward JB, Khandheria BK, Edwards WD, et al. Biplanar transesophageal echocardiography: anatomic correlations, image orientation, and clinical applications. *Mayo Clin Proc* 1990;65:1193–213.

23. Aschenberg W, Schlüter M, Kremer P, et al. Transesophageal two-dimensional echocardiography for the detection of left atrial appendage thrombus. *J Am Coll Cardiol* 1986;7:163–6.

24. Daniel WG, Angermann C, Engberding R, et al. Transesophageal echocardiography in patients with cerebral ischemic events and arterial embolism—a European Multicenter Study (abstract). *Circulation* 1989;80 Suppl 2:II–473.

25. Daniel LB, Grigg LE, Weisel RD, Rakowski H. Comparison of transthoracic and transesophageal assessment of prosthetic valve dysfunction. *Echocardiography* 1990;7:83–95.

26. Khandheria BK, Seward JB, Oh JK, et al. Value and limitations of transesophageal echocardiography in assessment of mitral valve prostheses. *Circulation* 1991;83:1956–68.

27. Karalis DG, Chandrasekaran K, Victor MF, et al. Recognition and embolic potential of intraaortic atherosclerotic debris. *J Am Coll Cardiol* 1991;17: 73–8.

28. Mohr-Kahaly S, Kupferwasser I, Erbel R, et al. Regurgitant flow in apparently normal valve prostheses: improved detection and semiquantitative analysis by transesophageal two-dimensional color-coded Doppler echocardiography. *J Am Soc Echocardiogr* 1990;3:187–95.

29. Nellessen U, Schnittger I, Appleton CP, et al. Transesophageal two-dimensional echocardiography and color Doppler flow velocity mapping in the evaluation of cardiac valve prostheses. *Circulation* 1988;78:848–55.

30. Pearson AC, Labovitz AJ, Tatineni S, Gomez CR. Superiority of transesophageal echocardiography in detecting cardiac source of embolism in patients with cerebral ischemia of uncertain etiology. *J Am Coll Cardiol* 1991;17:66–72.

31. van den Brink RBA, Visser CA, Basart DCG, et al. Comparison of transthoracic and transesophageal color Doppler flow imaging in patients with me-

chanical prostheses in the mitral valve position. *Am J Cardiol* 1989;63:1471–4.

32. Stoddard MF, Arce J, Liddell NE, et al. Two-dimensional transesophageal echocardiographic determination of aortic valve area in adults with aortic stenosis. *Am Heart J* 1991;122:1415–22.

33. Yoshida K, Yoshikawa J, Yamaura Y, et al. Assessment of mitral regurgitation by biplane transesophageal color Doppler flow imaging. *Circulation* 1990;82:1121–6.

34. Erbel R, Rohmann S, Drexler M, et al. Improved diagnostic value of echocardiography in patients with infective endocarditis by transoesophageal approach. A prospective study. *Eur Heart J* 1988;9:43–53.

35. Mügge A, Daniel WG, Frank G, Lichtlen PR. Echocardiography in infective endocarditis: reassessment of prognostic implications of vegetation size determined by the transthoracic and the transesophageal approach. *J Am Coll Cardiol* 1989;14:631–8.

36. Teskey RJ, Chan K-L, Beanlands DS. Diverticulum of the mitral valve complicating bacterial endocarditis: diagnosis by transesophageal echocardiography. *Am Heart J* 1989;118:1063–5.

37. Nellessen U, Daniel WG, Matheis G, et al. Impending paradoxical embolism from atrial thrombus: correct diagnosis by transesophageal echocardiography and prevention by surgery. *J Am Coll Cardiol* 1985;5:1002–4.

38. Reeder GS, Khandheria BK, Seward JB, Tajik AJ. Transesophageal echocardiography and cardiac masses. *Mayo Clin Proc* 1991;66:1101–9.

39. Seward JB. Cardiac tumors and thrombus: transesophageal echocardiographic experience. In: Erbel R, Khandheria BK, Brennecke R, et al., eds. *Transesophageal Echocardiography: A New Window to the Heart.* Berlin: Springer-Verlag, 1989:120–8.

40. Mohr-Kahaly S, Erbel R, Rennollet H, et al. Ambulatory follow-up of aortic dissection by transesophageal two-dimensional and color-coded Doppler echocardiography. *Circulation* 1989;80:24–33.

41. Mügge A, Daniel WG, Laas J, et al. False-negative diagnosis of proximal aortic dissection by computed tomography or angiography and possible explanations based on transesophageal echocardiographic findings. *Am J Cardiol* 1990;65:527–9.

42. Chan K-L. Transesophageal echocardiography for assessing cause of hypotension after cardiac surgery. *Am J Cardiol* 1988;62:1142–3.

43. Oh JK, Seward JB, Khandheria BK, et al. Transesophageal echocardiography in critically ill patients. *Am J Cardiol* 1990;66:1492–5.

44. Topol EJ, Weiss JL, Guzman PA, et al. Immediate improvement of dysfunctional myocardial segments after coronary revascularization: detection by intraoperative transesophageal echocardiography. *J Am Coll Cardiol* 1984;4:1123–34.

45. Calafiore PA, Raymond R, Schiavone WA, Rosenkranz ER. Precise evaluation of a complex coronary arteriovenous fistula: the utility of transesophageal color Doppler. *J Am Soc Echocardiogr* 1989;2:337–41.

46. Cyran SE, Kimball TR, Meyer RA, et al. Efficacy of intraoperative transesophageal echocardiography in children with congenital heart disease. *Am J Cardiol* 1989;63:594–8.

47. Goldfarb A, Weinreb J, Daniel WG, Kronzon I. A patient with right and left atrial membranes: the role of transesophageal echocardiography and magnetic resonance imaging in diagnosis. *J Am Soc Echocardiogr* 1989;2:350–3.

48. Kaulitz R, Stümper OFW, Geuskens R, et al. Comparative values of the precordial and transesophageal approaches in the echocardiographic evaluation of atrial baffle function after an atrial correction procedure. *J Am Coll Cardiol* 1990;16:686–94.

49. Muhiudeen IA, Roberson DA, Silverman NH, et al. Intraoperative echocardiography in infants and children with congenital cardiac shunt lesions: transesophageal versus epicardial echocardiography. *J Am Coll Cardiol* 1990;16:1687–95.

50. Oh JK, Seward JB, Khandheria BK, et al. Visualization of sinus venosus atrial septal defect by transesophageal echocardiography. *J Am Soc Echocardiogr* 1988;1:275–7.

51. Ritter SB. Transesophageal echocardiography in children: new peephole to the heart (editorial). *J Am Coll Cardiol* 1990;16:447–50.

52. Seward JB, Tajik AJ. Transesophageal echocardiography in congenital heart disease. *Am J Cardiac Imaging* 1990;4:215–22.

53. Stümper OFW, Elzenga NJ, Hess J, Sutherland GR. Transesophageal echocardiography in children with congenital heart disease: an initial experience. *J Am Coll Cardiol* 1990;16:433–41.

54. Currie PJ. Transesophageal echocardiography: intraoperative applications. *Echocardiography* 1989;6:403–14.

55. Meloni L, Abbruzzese PA, Cardu G, et al. Detection of microbubbles released by oxygenators during cardiopulmonary bypass by intraoperative transesophageal echocardiography. *Am J Cardiol* 1990;66:511–4.

56. Oka Y, Inoue T, Hong Y, et al. Retained intracardiac air: transesophageal echocardiography for defini-

tion of incidence and monitoring removal by improved techniques. *J Thorac Cardiovasc Surg* 1986;
91:329–37.

57. Pearce FB, Sheikh KN, deBruijn NP, Kisslo J. Imaging of the coronary arteries by transesophageal
echocardiography. *J Am Soc Echocardiogr* 1989;
2:276–83.

58. Smith JS, Cahalan MK, Benefiel DJ, et al. Intraoperative detection of myocardial ischemia in high-risk
patients: electrocardiography versus two-dimensional transesophageal echocardiography. *Circulation* 1985;72:1015–21.

59. Chan K-L, Marquis J-F, Ascah C, et al. Role of
transesophageal echocardiography in percutaneous
balloon mitral valvuloplasty. *Echocardiography*
1990;7:115–23.

60. Hellenbrand WE, Fahey JT, McGowan FX, et al.
Transesophageal echocardiographic guidance of
transcatheter closure of atrial septal defect. *Am J
Cardiol* 1990;66:207–13.

61. Kronzon I, Tunick PA, Schwinger ME, et al. Transesophageal echocardiography during percutaneous
mitral valvuloplasty. *J Am Soc Echocardiogr*
1989;2:380–5.

62. Lambertz H, Kreis A, Trümper H, Hanrath P. Simultaneous transesophageal atrial pacing and transesophageal two-dimensional echocardiography: a
new method of stress echocardiography. *J Am Coll
Cardiol* 1990;16:1143–53.

63. Ereth MH, Weber JG, Abel MD, et al. Cemented
versus noncemented total hip arthroplasty—embolism, hemodynamics, and intrapulmonary shunting.
Mayo Clin Proc 1992;67:1066–74.

64. Tytgat GNJ, Tio TL, eds. Endoscopic ultrasonography. *Scand J Gastroenterol Suppl* 1986;123:1–169.

65. Eaton MH, Lappas D, Waggoner AD, et al. Ultrasonic myocardial tissue characterization in the operating room: initial results using transesophageal
echocardiography. *J Am Soc Echocardiogr* 1991;4:
541–6.

66. Kuroda T, Kinter TM, Seward JB, et al. Accuracy
of three-dimensional volume measurement using
biplane transesophageal echocardiographic probe:
in vitro experiment. *J Am Soc Echocardiogr* 1991;
4:475–84.

67. Wollschläger H, Zeiher AM, Klein H-P, et al. Transesophageal echo computer tomography: a new
method for dynamic 3–D imaging of the heart (abstract). *J Am Coll Cardiol* 1989;13 Suppl A:68A.

2

Organization of a Transesophageal Echocardiographic Laboratory and Role of the Sonographer-Assistant

Janel M. Mays • *Barbara A. Nichols* • *Bijoy K. Khandheria*

Echocardiography provides the clinician with important information about cardiac anatomy, function, and hemodynamics. Transesophageal echocardiography (TEE) has become a valuable addition to the cardiovascular ultrasound imaging and hemodynamic laboratory because the more proximate and unobstructed esophageal window often markedly improves visualization of cardiovascular anatomy and a broad spectrum of lesions [1].

Incorporating TEE technology into the preexisting echocardiographic laboratory requires careful planning for space, equipment, and personnel. Because TEE is a semi-invasive examination, special considerations must be made to best accommodate the patient's comfort and safety during the procedure. Unless arrangements are made with another procedural area, such as the gastrointestinal endoscopy laboratory, the current echocardiographic laboratory must be properly organized to meet the special needs of TEE [1,2]. This chapter reviews how to incorporate TEE into the current echocardiographic laboratory.

ECHOCARDIOGRAPHIC LABORATORY FACILITY

When incorporating TEE into pre-existing laboratory facilities, allowances must be made for the space required for procedures and equipment that are in addition to those used for routine transthoracic echocardiography. There must be space for emergency resuscitation equipment, an area for cleaning and storing the transesophageal probe, and a patient preparation and recovery area.

Equipment directly used during the TEE procedure includes a standard ultrasound machine capable of performing transesophageal imaging, a TEE probe, a patient examination table, patient monitoring equipment, and a work station for the TEE support person (Fig. 2-1). Ultrasound machines and recording instruments may vary greatly among institutions, and individual preferences and machine size must be considered when a TEE procedure room is designed. The construct of the procedure room must take into account the electrical requirements of not only the ultrasound machine and recording instruments but also the monitoring and emergency equipment.

A comfortable examination table helps provide a relaxing environment for the patient. Although not essential, a table with special features is convenient for the TEE procedure. If the entire table can be raised and lowered, the patient can be brought to a working level comfortable to the physician performing the examination. Similarly, if the head of the table can be raised and lowered, the patient's comfort can be enhanced and special tests requiring

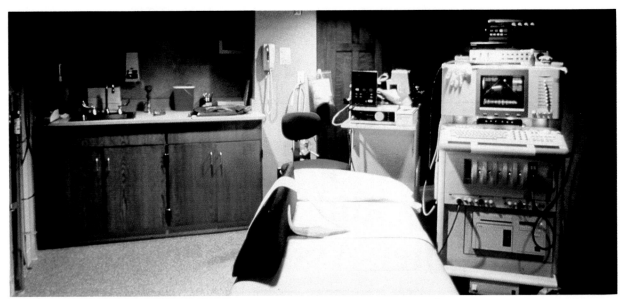

Fig. 2-1. Transesophageal echocardiography procedure room. Equipment and supplies are readily accessible to the assistant. Adequate space has been left near the patient should emergency intervention be needed.

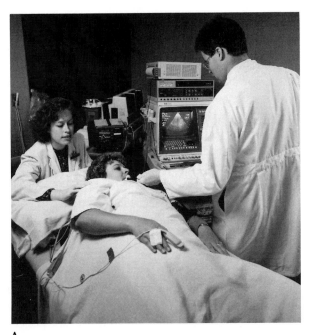

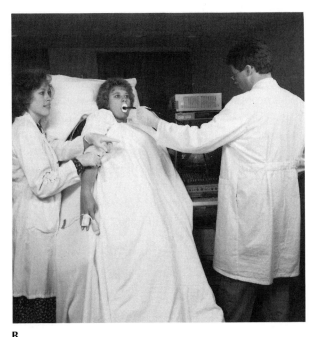

A   B

Fig. 2-2. Table positions for TEE examination. The head of the table can be raised from the horizontal position to nearly vertical positions. A. The patient is always secured with safety straps (beneath covers; see Figure 2-3) in the horizontal position. Mild degrees of head-up inclination may facilitate patient comfort; Trendelenburg positioning is also possible. B. Vertical positioning of the table is used during intravenous contrast evaluation for positional intracardiac shunting, such as with orthodeoxia. The patient is standing on a footrest at the far bottom of the photograph.

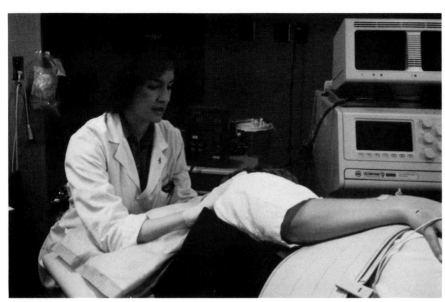

Fig. 2-3. Preparation for TEE examination. The patient lies in the left lateral decubitus position with a pillow wedge placed behind the back for support. Straps have been secured about the patient's hips and the wedge as a precautionary measure. The height-adjustable examination table is elevated to a comfortable working position for the TEE assistant (seated at the patient's head) and the physician.

specific positioning can be performed [3,4]. If a footrest is available on the table, the patient can be positioned nearly upright with the TEE probe in place (Fig. 2-2). This maneuver is used during intravenous contrast evaluation for positional intracardiac shunting, such as that observed when interatrial shunting causes orthodeoxia. The optimal examination table can place the patient in the Trendelenburg position if he or she becomes hypotensive during the procedure. For assurance that the patient is secure, especially after a sedative has been administered, safety straps should always be used to prevent rolling or falling. Safety straps are imperative when the patient is moved to any upright position on the examination table. A wedge support, held in place by the safety straps, helps prop the patient's back and maintain the correct left lateral position during the TEE procedure [4] (Fig. 2-3).

A work station located near the head of the examination table contains monitoring equipment and supplies such as disposable gloves, intravenous materials, saline flushes, and medications required during TEE. A lockable, secured cabinet or compartment should be available for the storage of controlled medications, such as midazolam and meperidine. The work station may also incorporate the oxygen, suction, and other emergency equipment for easy access to the TEE assistant caring for the patient [2–4]. A stool placed at the patient's head allows the TEE assistant to sit close to the patient and have ready access to the work station (Fig. 2-4). Support for hanging intravenous infusion bags, such as a sliding ceiling track apparatus or a moveable pole,

should be available close to the work station for administration of fluids, antibiotics, or emergency medications.

The patient's cardiac rhythm, blood pressure, pulse, and respiration should be monitored throughout the procedure. The patient's rhythm is continuously monitored by noting the electrocardiographic display on the ultrasound machine itself. Our practice is to monitor blood pressure, pulse, and oxygen saturation with an automated blood pressure monitor and pulse oximeter so that any potential patient instability during TEE can be immediately identified. If an automated blood pressure monitor is not available, a stethoscope and sphygmomanometer with the proper-sized cuff should always be on hand. The correct size of cuff should be selected according to the size and shape of the patient's upper arm.

In addition to the monitoring equipment, oxygen and suction should be readily available if required during the procedure. The most reliable method of oxygen delivery to the procedure area is through a central source from a wall- or ceiling-mounted adaptor. If this is not available, portable oxygen tanks may be used, but they must be periodically checked for oxygen capacity. Significant oxygen desaturation can most often be corrected by administration of oxygen through a nasal cannula. However, face masks and a bag-valve mask should be available for additional oxygen delivery if needed. An endotracheal intubation tray should also be available for the very rare case of respiratory difficulty approaching arrest.

An effective device for suctioning excess secre-

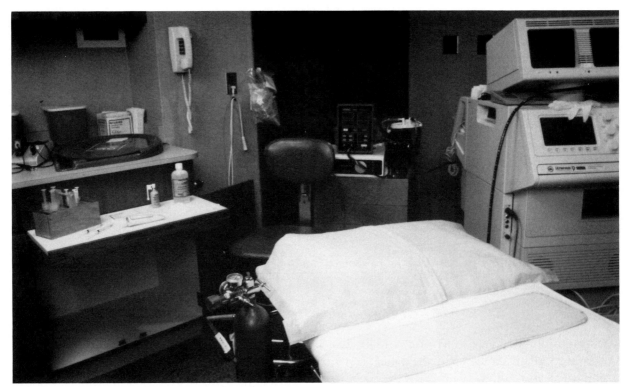

Fig. 2-4. The TEE work area incorporates many essentials close to the TEE assistant, who sits in the chair at the center. The retractable shelf can accommodate medications, contrast agents, anesthetic spray and gel, and other necessary supplies. A telephone and emergency call switch are within reach. Oxygen and suction equipment are always available. The pulse oximeter and automated blood pressure device are positioned so that the physician (who will operate the machine at the right) can also see their displays.

tions should always be present in the TEE procedure room. Portable units or central wall units may be used. A portable unit must provide adequate vacuum and flow for pharyngeal suctioning. Accessory supplies needed for suctioning include sterile suction catheters, a rigid pharyngeal suction tip (tonsil suction tip), plastic tubing, and a nonbreakable collection bottle. The oxygen and suction supplies must be readily accessible to the TEE assistant and must be located within an arm's reach of the patient's airway, regardless of the patient's position.

Because of the semi-invasiveness of TEE and the type of cardiopulmonary disease in some patients examined, the remote possibility of life-threatening complications always exists. It is imperative that emergency resuscitation equipment (Fig. 2-5) be immediately accessible. Attending personnel must be adequately trained in basic cardiac life support [5]. Examining physicians ideally should be certified in advanced cardiac life support [5]. Space should be reserved in the procedure room for storage of a mobile resuscitation cart. This cart (see Fig. 2-5) must contain all supplies, equipment, and drugs needed for cardiac emergencies and advanced cardiac life support and must be ready for use at all times. The defibrillator should be mounted on top of the resuscitation cart. As with all such resuscitation carts, periodic inventory of the medications and assessment of the working condition of the defibrillator are required. A telephone or emergency call light system (or both) should be installed in the procedure room to call for assistance should an emergency arise [2–4,6].

Another space requirement for a TEE procedure room is an area for cleaning and storage of the TEE probe (Fig. 2-6). A sink should be available for hand washing and cleaning of the probe. The equipment used for disinfecting the probe should be close to the sink because of the caustic properties of the disinfectant solutions. This area must also be well ventilated to dissipate potentially noxious fumes from disinfectant solutions. Many commercial containers, including a plastic soaking tray and a disinfectant column, are available to disinfect the TEE

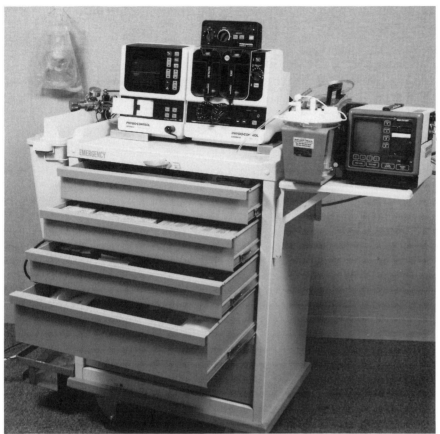

Fig. 2-5. A resuscitation cart containing all equipment and medications required for advanced cardiac life support should be immediately available during TEE procedures.

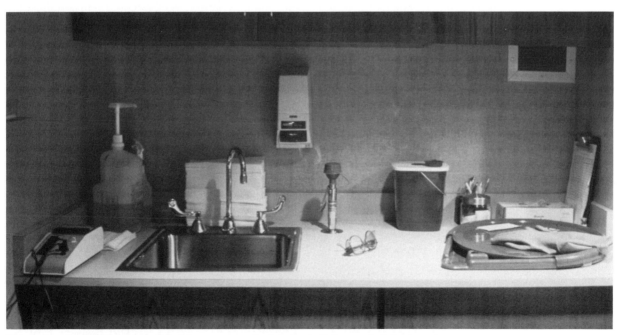

Fig. 2-6. The TEE probe disinfectant area. A sink (at left) is needed for hand washing and rinsing the probe after both enzymatic cleansing and disinfectant immersion. The tub (at right) containing the glutaraldehyde disinfectant should be located near an exhaust duct, with the area well ventilated. Skin and eye contact with glutaraldehyde disinfectant solution can be avoided with the use of heavy protective gloves and eyewear.

probe, and selection should be based on the disinfectant agent used and the space available. Proper storage of the TEE probe is essential to prevent damage and to maintain its integrity. It is recommended that when not in use, the TEE probe be maintained in a straight rather than a flexed (coiled) position. Commercially available wall-mounted racks are excellent for long-term storage because they securely hold and protect the TEE probe from damage. The wall rack holds the proximal control handle of the TEE probe securely while protecting the flexible shaft and distal transducer tip within a long, vertical, clear plastic tube. When a TEE procedure room is designed, these wall racks should be mounted away from extremes in temperature (such as heating or cooling vents) or direct sunlight to prevent damage to the probe from excessive temperature variation [2,4,7,8].

It is recommended that an area adjoining the TEE procedure room be available for patient preparation and recovery. A bed, reclining chair, or couch in this area promotes patient comfort and relaxation. A relaxed atmosphere provides an excellent environment for patient preparation, prophylactic administration of antibiotics, patient instruction, and patient recovery. Generally, patient recovery time is approximately 30 minutes. The recovery area adjoining the procedure room should be large enough for those accompanying patients to join them after the procedure and be involved in dismissal instructions.

ROLE OF THE SONOGRAPHER-ASSISTANT

Recommendations established by the American Society of Echocardiography and the policy followed at our institution state that TEE should be performed only by a physician properly trained in the technique, tomographic anatomy, and interpretation of TEE images [9]. Currently proposed physician training guidelines are described in Chapter 3.

With the physician assuming the responsibility of obtaining the TEE images, the function of the cardiac sonographer changes to one of patient support. Each echocardiographic laboratory must define what the sonographer or other TEE support person is to contribute to the TEE procedure. In addition, each laboratory must identify what resources and options are available to best meet the needs of the patient [5].

At our institution, only registered nurses who have been trained as cardiac sonographers assist during the TEE procedure. The skills of a registered nurse are ideally suited for monitoring the patient and vital signs closely, administering medications, obtaining and maintaining intravenous access, and being facile in the use of suction, oxygen, and other emergency equipment. All these functions, except administration of medications, may be done by an experienced paramedical person trained in basic cardiac life support [2–4]. If the TEE support sonographer is not a registered nurse, intravenous medications must be administered by the physician.

Many echocardiographic laboratories have registered nurses who have been trained as cardiac sonographers and are available to assist during the TEE procedure. Laboratories without such personnel may hire a registered nurse to assist with TEE procedures or make arrangements with other procedural laboratories, such as the gastrointestinal endoscopy laboratory, to time-share their nursing staff and facilities for the TEE procedure. If other staff are used, the cardiac sonographer is available to assist the physician performing the TEE procedure with the technical aspects of the ultrasound machine. Cardiac sonographers, because of their training and technical knowledge of ultrasound equipment, may assist the physician in optimizing the two-dimensional, Doppler, and color-flow images obtained by TEE.

Conduction of the entire TEE procedure is significantly expedited by qualified TEE support staff whether the responsibility is delegated to the sonographer, registered nurse-sonographer, or non-sonographer registered nurse. The sonographer or TEE support person carries out multiple functions necessary before, during, and after the TEE procedure. Although the physician performs the imaging portion of the examination, the TEE support person has the essential tasks of preparation of equipment and supplies, patient preparation and instruction, patient care during and after the TEE procedure, and care of the TEE probe [4,10] (Table 2-1).

PREPARATION OF TEE EQUIPMENT AND SUPPLIES

The TEE support person begins by providing an organized, friendly, and comfortable environment for the patient. Before the patient arrives, the equip-

Table 2-1. Duties of the sonographer-assistant during transesophageal echocardiography (TEE)

Before procedure
Preparation of equipment and supplies
  Assemble supplies
    Medications, isotonic saline for flushes, and agitated contrast injections
    Intravenous supplies (angiocatheter, three-way stopcock)
    Lidocaine spray and tongue blade
    Endoscope lubricant: lubricating jelly or viscous lidocaine, or both
    Gloves, safety glasses, TEE probe, and bite block
  Maintain and check suction, oxygen, and basic life support equipment
  Cover patient's pillow with absorbent material
Preparation of the patient
  Confirm that patient has had no oral intake for 4 hours before TEE
  Obtain brief history of drug allergies, asthma, glaucoma, and swallowing difficulties
  Explain procedure to patient
  Obtain baseline vital signs and monitor electrocardiogram
  Remove patient's dentures, oral prostheses, and eyeglasses
  Establish intravenous line for administration of medications
  Place patient in the left lateral decubitus position with wedge support and safety restraints
Drugs (administered by physician or registered nurse)
  Endocarditis prophylaxis: American Heart Association recommendations (high-risk patients only)
  Pharyngeal anesthesia: lidocaine 10% spray
  Drying agent: glycopyrrolate (Robinul)
  Sedative (anxiolytic): midazolam hydrochloride (Versed); reversed by flumazenil (Mazicon)
During procedure
Reinforce physician's instructions
Assist patient during esophageal intubation: head position, breathing, and reassurance
Position and maintain bite block stability
Monitor vital signs: electrocardiographic monitor, respiratory rate and pattern, blood pressure, and
  peripheral oxygen saturation
Comfort and reassure the patient
Use oral suction if necessary
Have basic life support equipment available
After procedure
Assist patient during recovery period; observe for 30 minutes if systemic sedation was used
Monitor vital signs and respiratory status
Remove intravenous access
Complete and reinforce instructions with patient and companion
Instruct patient not to drive for 12 hours if sedation was used
Record vital signs and patient's condition on dismissal
Clean TEE probe with enzymatic solution and glutaraldehyde disinfectant and secure in storage rack

Source: JM Mays, BA Nichols, RC Rubish, et al. Transesophageal echocardiography: a sonographer's perspective. *J Am Soc Echocardiogr* 1991; 4: 513–8. By permission of the American Society of Echocardiography.

ment and supplies needed during the TEE procedure (see Table 2-1) should be assembled and placed on the work station. The disinfected TEE probe should be checked for surface integrity and then connected to the ultrasound system to verify correct probe initialization. The probe should be placed unobtrusively on the ultrasound machine before the patient arrives so that additional anxiety about the procedure can be avoided. The suction, oxygen, and life support equipment should be checked to ensure that they are functioning properly. Because excess secretions are possible, we have found it helpful to cover the patient's pillow with an absorbent material. After these preliminary preparations have been completed, the patient is brought to the preparation area adjoining the TEE procedure room.

PREPARATION OF THE PATIENT

During the scheduling of a TEE examination, the patient is told to abstain from oral intake, except medications, for 4 hours before the procedure. If use of a sedative is anticipated, the patient should be accompanied by a relative or friend and should not operate a motor vehicle for at least 12 hours after the sedative has been administered. When the patient arrives for the TEE procedure, the TEE support person must confirm that the patient has been fasting for at least 4 hours and is not planning to drive for 12 hours after the procedure. At this time, a brief medical history of drug allergies, dentition, and swallowing difficulties should be elicited. A history of potential contraindications to sedative or

anticholinergic therapy should also be pursued. Patients at high risk for infectious endocarditis may receive antibiotic prophylaxis before the procedure begins according to the recommendations of the American Heart Association [11]. Time should be allotted to discuss the TEE procedure with the patient and address any questions or concerns. The patient who is well informed about the procedure and has had time to ask questions is most likely to tolerate TEE with minimal problems. Careful teaching about the procedure is essential in preparing the patient adequately for TEE [2,4].

Before the TEE procedure is begun, an automated blood pressure device and pulse oximeter are connected to the patient (Fig. 2-7). Baseline blood pressure, heart rate, and peripheral oxygen saturation

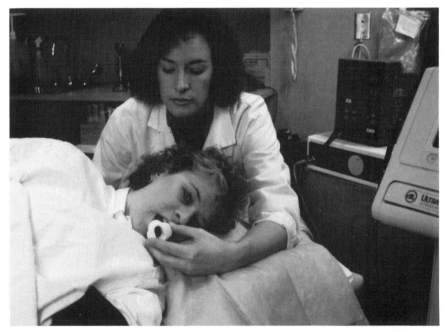

Fig. 2-7. A. Vital signs are monitored continuously so that the TEE assistant can perform other duties during the TEE procedure. B. An automated blood pressure device allows efficient serial measurement of blood pressure and heart rate. C. The patient's respiratory response to sedation is also continuously monitored by a pulse oximeter that measures peripheral oxygen saturation.

A

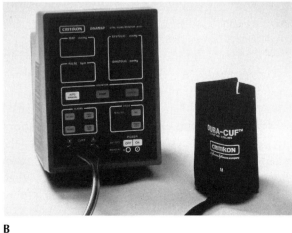

B

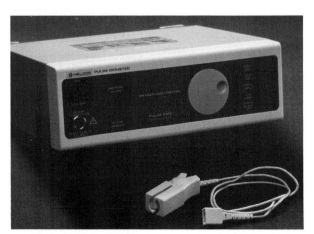

C

are obtained before any premedication is given. Electrocardiographic monitoring is continuously displayed on the monitor of the ultrasound machine. Proper attachment of the electrodes to the skin is essential for accurate rhythm monitoring. It may be necessary to prepare the skin before lead placement by shaving chest hair, cleansing with alcohol, or drying the skin thoroughly. The choice of electrode position is a matter of personal preference, but we most commonly use the modified chest lead (MCL_1) position.

Dentures and oral prostheses should be removed before the procedure begins to prevent damage and inadvertent migration into the esophagus or airway. If the patient has any teeth, a bite block should be used to prevent involuntary biting of the transesophageal probe, which may result in an electrically unsafe system for the patient and necessitate costly repairs. Eyeglasses are generally taken off unless the patient wants to observe the images.

A peripheral intravenous line is established according to the standards of each institution. A new intravenous line preferably is inserted in the right arm to allow easier accessibility and avoid the possibility of impaired venous return that occasionally occurs in the left arm when the patient is in the left lateral decubitus position. The intravenous line is used for administration of medications, injections of agitated saline for contrast echocardiography, and a ready access in the event of an emergency (Fig. 2-8).

The patient is placed in the left lateral decubitus position, facing the physician and the ultrasound machine. Placing the patient's right leg in front of the left helps maintain this position. A pillow between the knees often provides additional comfort. A wedge support is placed behind the patient's back, and both patient and wedge are enclosed within safety straps.

Certain clinical situations may require that the patient be examined in a position other than the left lateral decubitus. Patients with various orthopedic, neurologic, or postoperative conditions may not be able to lie on their left side. The TEE examination should then be conducted with the patient supine and the head of the table elevated to minimize the potential for aspiration. The extremely obese patient may also require an upright inclination of the examination table of 20 to 30 degrees to optimize the mechanics of respiration. Such patients must be positioned securely on the table, because the safety straps may not be large enough to confidently hold

the patient in place. As with all examinations done while the head of the table is elevated, the footrest must be in proper position to provide support and prevent the patient from sliding off the end of the table. In patients with significant cardiac displacement within the chest, such as those with dextrocardia or who have had pneumonectomy, placement in the right lateral decubitus position may be necessary to optimize TEE images.

Medications are administered by the physician or registered nurse [2,4]. The medications commonly used during TEE are reviewed in Chapter 3.

All personnel involved in the TEE procedure should wear disposable gloves. When performing the procedure on a patient with a known or suspected contagious infectious disease, protective eyewear, masks, and, in cases of strict isolation, gowns, in addition to gloves, should be worn. Any questions about isolation precautions should be pursued with the institution's infection control department.

THE TEE EXAMINATION

The esophageal intubation instructions to the patient during the examination are the responsibility of the physician. The TEE support person can help ease intubation by flexing the patient's head toward the chest to allow for better oropharyngeal entry and by reinforcing the physician's instructions. After insertion of the endoscope, the TEE assistant should carefully maintain the position of the bite block. It is not uncommon for the patient under sedation to unwittingly expel the bite block, exposing the TEE probe to potentially major damage from biting. The TEE assistant must always watch for this, and occasionally continuous stabilization of the bite block with one hand of the assistant is necessary. The TEE assistant may be asked to inform the physician of the depth of probe insertion, since the depth markers on the probe are often more easily seen from the assistant's vantage point at the head of the patient.

The patient's vital signs and pulse oximeter measurements should be closely monitored. Any significant change in vital signs should be reported to the physician immediately. In general, automated blood pressure measurements are quite accurate, although cardiac dysrhythmias may cause significant variation in blood pressure readings. With continuous monitoring of vital signs, most incipient problems can be recognized early, prompting intervention as needed to stabilize the patient. If problems develop,

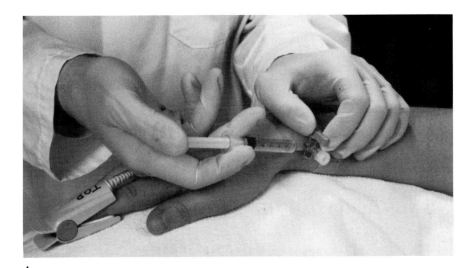

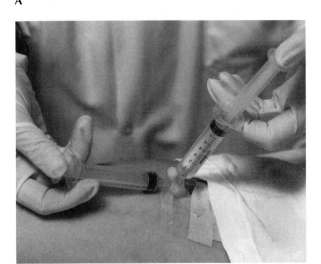
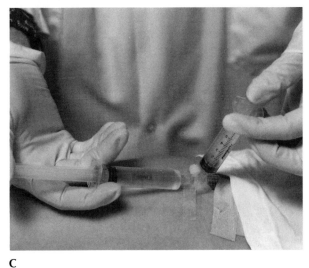

Fig. 2-8. A. Intravenous access is recommended for all TEE examinations. Also seen is a pulse oximeter probe attached to the patient's right index finger. A three-way stopcock connected to the intravenous catheter is useful for administration of both medications and contrast agent; saline flushes enhance peripheral venous transit. B, C. Two syringes connected to each other by the three-way stopcock, which is turned off to intravenous access, readily allow excellent agitation of saline for contrast injection. Saline is rapidly injected to and fro from one syringe to the other several times and then is quickly injected intravenously to produce generally excellent contrast opacification of the right heart.

the TEE support person must be prepared to use suction, oxygen, or other emergency equipment if necessary. Throughout the entire TEE procedure, the support person serves a vital function in reassuring and comforting the patient [2–4] (Fig. 2-9). It is also helpful to periodically inform the alert or anxious patient about the progress of the examination. Since the patient is unable to talk during TEE, the assistant should watch and respond to gestures that may indicate discomfort or distress.

In some situations, the patient's clinical status

precludes transportation to the echocardiography laboratory for TEE. Most bedside TEE examinations are performed in medical or surgical intensive care units. Before the bedside examination begins, the TEE assistant is responsible for coordinating plans with the patient's nurse, ensuring that monitoring and life support equipment is readily available, and setting up the patient's room for TEE. All standard supplies required for TEE should be available in a portable tray or bag to facilitate urgent bedside examinations. The TEE assistant serves the same

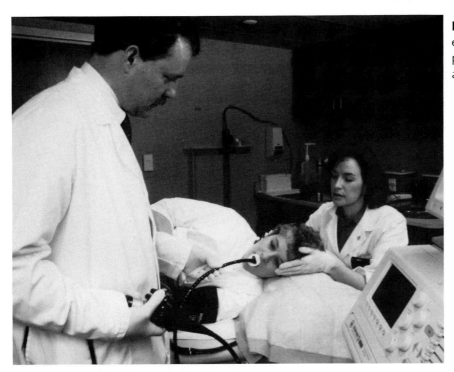

Fig. 2-9. During the TEE examination, the support person serves as both physician assistant and patient liaison.

functions at the bedside as in the echocardiography laboratory. However, if the patient is critically ill, it is best to have the nurse caring for the patient also assist in positioning the patient, monitoring vital signs and, particularly, life support equipment, and helping administer medications as needed. After the TEE procedure, follow-up care is reviewed with the patient's nurse. The TEE probe is transported back to the echocardiography laboratory in a disposable bag and disinfected.

AFTER THE TEE EXAMINATION

When the TEE procedure is over, the assistant continues to help the patient recover as comfortably as possible. The patient's vital signs should be monitored until they return to baseline values (Fig. 2-10), at which time the intravenous line may be removed. The teaching and dismissal instructions should not be given until the patient is fully aware of his or her surroundings and is ready to be dismissed. Recovery time after TEE with sedation varies with each patient, generally being less than 30 minutes and rarely up to 60 minutes. Whenever possible, precautions about residual medication side effects should be discussed with both the patient and the accompanying relative or companion. Predismissal instructions should include the following points.

1. Caution the patient not to drink any hot liquids until the oropharyngeal anesthesia has worn off (1 to 2 hours).
2. Caution the patient not to eat anything until the gag reflex returns (1 to 4 hours).
3. Caution the patient not to operate a motor vehicle for 12 hours after the procedure (if a sedative was given).
4. Alert patient and family to the possible short-term amnestic effect of sedation.
5. Review the symptoms of possible complications of the procedure (see Chapter 3) and whom to notify should they arise.

The patient's vital signs and condition at dismissal should be recorded on the appropriate form. If the patient is hospitalized, the attending nursing staff should be directly informed about the procedure and all medications administered should be recorded in the patient's chart.

CARE OF THE TEE PROBE

The sonographer and TEE support person are important in maintaining the integrity of the TEE probe. After each examination, the probe should be carefully inspected for defects with the transducer tip in the neutral position and all flexed directions. Defects that may be seen are metallic protrusions, perfora-

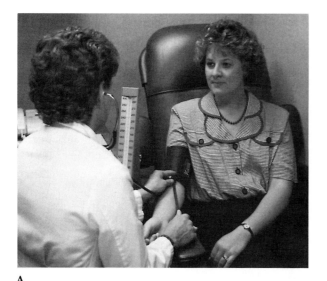

A

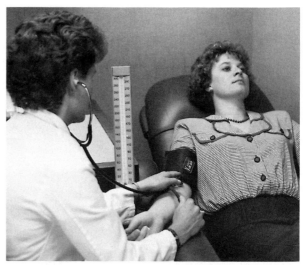

B

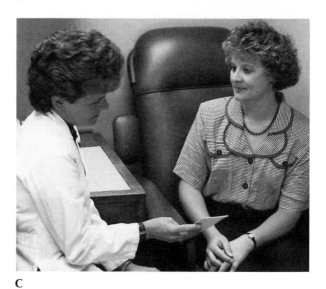

C

Fig. 2-10. A. During recovery, the patient's vital signs are monitored. B. The chair in this recovery area is a six-position recliner that can be adjusted into the supine position quickly if needed. C. Dismissal instructions are given when the patient is fully alert.

tions, abrasions, cracks, or dents in the insulating covering of the probe. These defects may cause trauma or expose the patient to infective, caustic, or electrical complications [4,7,8]. Whenever a defect is suspected, the endoscope should not be used until additional safety inspections and necessary repairs have been made by qualified personnel.

Visual inspection of the probe alone does not always guarantee that the outer insulating layer is intact. Commercial products are available to determine the electrical safety of the probe after each use. In addition to daily inspections of the probe, third-wire leakage current should be measured monthly by qualified technicians (Fig. 2-11). Quality control and malfunction guidelines are available from the manufacturer of the TEE probe.

The disinfected transesophageal probe should be placed in its carrying case for transfer from one area to another. After use in a patient outside the echocardiography laboratory, the probe should not be returned to the carrying case until it has been cleaned and disinfected, because the foam padding lining the case cannot be disinfected if contaminated by an unclean probe. For long-term storage, it is recommended that the TEE endoscope be kept in a straight position rather than in the flexed position required by the carrying case. Commercial racks that protect the flexible shaft in a clear plastic tube in the straight position are available for long-term storage.

After each procedure, the flexible shaft of the TEE probe and the bite guard must be cleaned and

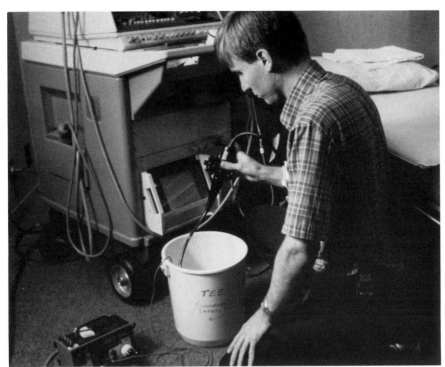

A

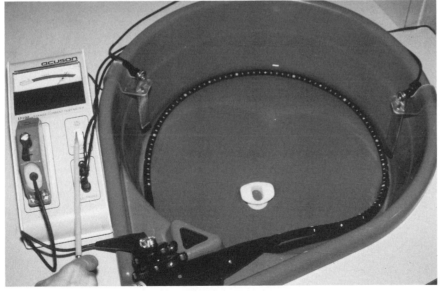

B

Fig. 2-11. The electrical safety of the TEE probe should be tested regularly by either (A) a qualified technician or (B) a commercially available meter to detect leakage current, with the disinfectant bath itself as a test solution. The applicability of a leakage current test meter may vary with individual TEE probes, and the manufacturer's specifications should be consulted.

disinfected. They are first washed in an enzymatic solution (such as Endozime or Protozyme) to remove any adherent mucus or secretions. The probe is then rinsed thoroughly with tap water and placed in a disinfectant. The enzymatic solution should be discarded after each use. Use of enzymatic solution is not mandatory but is routine in our laboratory.

Various commercial products are available to hold the disinfectant solution; which to use depends on the type of disinfectant and the amount of space in the TEE procedure area. The flexible shaft of the probe and the bite guard are soaked in a glutaraldehyde disinfectant solution (such as Metricide or Cidex) for 20 minutes. This period has been proved to be sufficient to destroy any viral contaminants or bacteria acquired from patients, including those under strict isolation. The disinfectant solutions are very caustic and should be handled with extreme care. The disinfectant area must be well ventilated. Anyone in contact with the solution should wear heavy-duty protective gloves and safety glasses at all times. After the disinfection process is complete, the probe and bite block are removed from the solution and rinsed thoroughly with tap water (Fig. 2-12). This is an ideal time to examine the probe shaft again for cracks, protrusions, or abrasions that may have occurred during the previous examination. After drying, the probe is ready to be stored in the

wall rack mentioned previously (Fig. 2-13). Before use on another patient, the probe should air dry for 20 minutes to allow any residual adherent glutaraldehyde to evaporate. The glutaraldehyde disinfectant solution should be changed according to package instructions or approximately every 2 weeks. Any questions about the disinfectant procedure should be directed to the institution's infection control department [4,7,8].

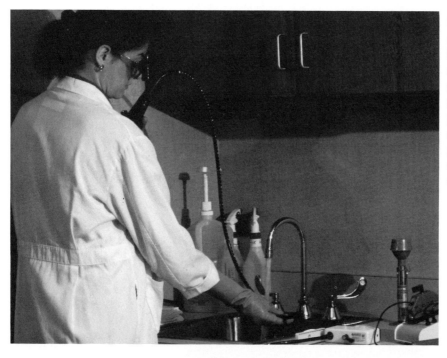

Fig. 2-12. The TEE assistant rinses the TEE probe after it has been immersed in disinfectant solution for 20 minutes. Heavy gloves and protective eyewear should be worn when the probe is in contact with the disinfectant. After rinsing, the probe is carefully inspected for defects in the outer protective covering and for misalignment.

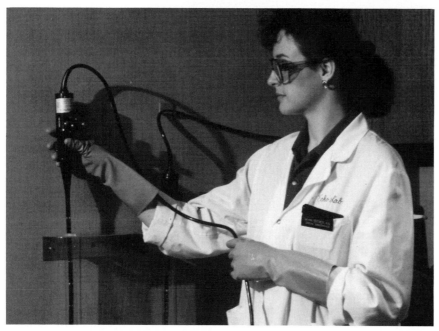

Fig. 2-13. After thorough rinsing of disinfectant from the TEE probe, it is allowed to air dry in a wall-mounted vertical storage tube. So that any residual disinfectant can completely evaporate, the probe is not used for at least 20 minutes after disinfection.

OPTIMAL TRAINING GUIDELINES FOR TEE SUPPORT PERSONNEL

Qualified TEE support personnel are essential in performing TEE. The selection and training of these persons must not be taken lightly. The cardiac sonographer with knowledge of TEE imaging who is also a registered nurse is ideally suited to assist during the TEE procedure. Optimal training guidelines must be developed by each institution to adequately prepare selected laboratory personnel to become able TEE assistants. These guidelines should include an instructional period in which these persons observe and assist in 30 to 40 TEE procedures under the guidance of a fully trained TEE assistant. Throughout this period, trainees should receive detailed instructions on care of the patient and the TEE probe (Table 2-2).

By reviewing current literature and attending inservice conferences and related extramural seminars, TEE support personnel receive basic training in ultrasound technology, the TEE procedure, TEE probe maintenance, patient care, and potential complications during TEE. Many of these guidelines are usually best instilled when the potential TEE assistant is in the observational period and is learning directly from trained TEE support personnel.

All personnel assisting with the TEE procedure must have successfully completed a course in basic cardiac life support according to the American Heart Association standards [5,6]. In addition, it is recommended that some TEE assistants and all physicians performing TEE be trained and remain certified in advanced cardiac life support. This advanced course trains one in the use of resuscitation equipment, the establishment of an intravenous line, the administra-

tion of fluids and drugs, cardiac monitoring, defibrillation, and other management of arrhythmias [5]. With a thorough knowledge of how to operate, maintain, and troubleshoot the monitoring and emergency equipment, TEE support personnel are best prepared to meet the needs of the patient if an emergency situation develops. Although few medications are given during the TEE procedure, TEE support personnel with a current knowledge of medication indications, dosages, contraindications, and side effects are most effective in preparing and observing the patient during and after the procedure [2–4].

Optimal training of TEE support personnel includes all the guidelines listed in Table 2-2. Well-trained TEE support staff are essential for the implementation of TEE in the echocardiographic laboratory and best meeting the needs of the patient undergoing TEE.

SUMMARY

Transesophageal echocardiography can be introduced into current echocardiographic laboratories by careful planning and knowledge of the support required to perform this procedure. Conscientious organization of the TEE procedure room and equipment optimizes not only the efficiency and safety of the examination but also patient comfort. The vital function of trained TEE support personnel from the first to the last steps of the procedure must be acknowledged and incorporated into the practice of TEE.

Table 2-2. Optimal training guidelines for transesophageal echocardiography (TEE) support personnel

Observation of TEE procedure
Basic training in ultrasound technology
Knowledge of TEE procedure, including complications
Knowledge of monitoring and emergency equipment use
Basic cardiac life support training
Ability to insert and care for intravenous access
Knowledge and administration of medications used
    (administered by physician or registered nurse)
Knowledge of how to care for TEE probe

REFERENCES

1. Seward JB. Cardiovascular ultrasound imaging and hemodynamic laboratory (echocardiography). *Curr Opin Cardiol* 1988;3:912–21.

2. Seward JB, Khandheria BK, Oh JK, et al. Transesophageal echocardiography: technique, anatomic correlations, implementation, and clinical applications. *Mayo Clin Proc* 1988;63:649–80.

3. Seward JB, Khandheria BK, Edwards WD, et al. Biplanar transesophageal echocardiography: anatomic correlations, image orientation, and clinical applications. *Mayo Clin Proc* 1990;65:1193–213.

4. Mays JM, Nichols BA, Rubish RC, et al. Transesophageal echocardiography: a sonographer's perspective. *J Am Soc Echocardiogr* 1991;4:513–8.

5. American Heart Association. 1985 National Conference on Standards and Guidelines for Cardiopulmo-

nary Resuscitation and Emergency Cardiac Care. *JAMA* 1986;255:2843–989.

6.   Mitchell MM, Sutherland GR, Gussenhoven EJ, et al. Transesophageal echocardiography. *J Am Soc Echocardiogr* 1988;1:362–77.

7.   *Phased Array Ultrasound Imaging Transducer for Transesophageal Echocardiography User's Guide.* Andover, MA: Hewlett-Packard Co., 1987.

8.   *Acuson 128XP Computed Sonography System User Manual for Cardiovascular Applications.* Mountain View, CA: Acuson Corp., 1991.

9.   Pearlman AS, Gardin JM, Martin RP, et al. Guidelines for physician training in transesophageal echocardiography: recommendations of the American Society of Echocardiography Committee for Physician Training in Echocardiography. *J Am Soc Echocardiogr* 1992;5:187–94.

10.   Philips J. Transesophageal echocardiography: the cardiac sonographer's role. *J Am Soc Echocardiogr* 1989;2:73–4.

11.   A statement for health professionals by the Committee on Rheumatic Fever and Infective Endocarditis of the Council on Cardiovascular Disease in the Young: Prevention of bacterial endocarditis. *Circulation* 1984;70:1123A–7A.

3

Transesophageal Echocardiographic Examination

Technique, Training, and Safety

Bijoy K. Khandheria • *A. Jamil Tajik* • *William K. Freeman*

The echocardiographic laboratory of the 1990s no longer serves the sole purpose of obtaining images but performs several important functions, including transthoracic echocardiographic evaluation of the structure and function of the heart, hemodynamic measurements, estimation of the severity of regurgitant lesions, and assessment of coronary artery disease with different forms of stress. Transesophageal echocardiography (TEE), a technology that has been accepted as an integral component of a comprehensive echocardiographic examination, has changed the hitherto noninvasive imaging laboratory into a semi-invasive one [1].

It is also important to recognize that TEE examinations constitute between 5% and 10% of all transthoracic examinations performed. This percentage has been consistently reflected at our institution over the past several years (Fig. 3-1) and appears to hold

Fig. 3-1. Patients undergoing transesophageal echocardiography (TEE) (5,441 procedures) as a percentage of those undergoing transthoracic echocardiography (TTE). Note that despite the increase in numbers of patients undergoing both TTE and TEE, the trend toward the percentage of patients undergoing TEE has been stationary.

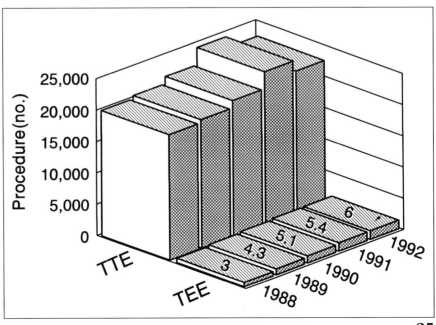

true at other major institutions [2]. Therefore, the number of TEE examinations can logically be expected to increase commensurately with the total number of echocardiographic examinations, but the percentage of transesophageal to transthoracic will remain around 5% to 10%.

Learning TEE and becoming aware of the associated risks and possible complications before using it in the day-to-day practice of echocardiography is important because it enables one to take the necessary precautions while performing the examination. A brief review of the anatomy of the esophagus is also in order before describing the technique of introduction of the TEE probe.

ANATOMY

The adult esophagus is a muscular tube from 23 to 28 cm long that passes through the mediastinum and connects the pharynx above and the stomach below. The esophagus begins in the neck at the inferior border of the cricoid cartilage at the level of the sixth cervical vertebra and continues downward to the gastroesophageal junction just below the diaphragm at the level of the eleventh thoracic vertebra (Fig. 3-2).

The esophageal length increases from 10 cm at birth to 24 to 28 cm in adulthood. The esophageal diameter increases from 5 mm at birth to approxi-

Fig. 3–2. A. Esophagus, cricopharyngeal constriction at level of sixth cervical vertebra (the level at which the upper esophageal sphincter lies), aortic constriction at level of fourth and fifth thoracic vertebrae, and lower esophageal sphincter located as shown. The approximate distance from the incisors is noted by the scale in centimeters at the left. Note that this is an adult esophagus, which is usually 24 to 28 cm in length. The esophagus extends from opposite the sixth cervical vertebra to the eleventh thoracic vertebra. B. Extent of the esophagus and its relationship with the heart, aortic arch, thoracic aorta, and vertebral bodies. The left bronchus has been removed for this diagram.

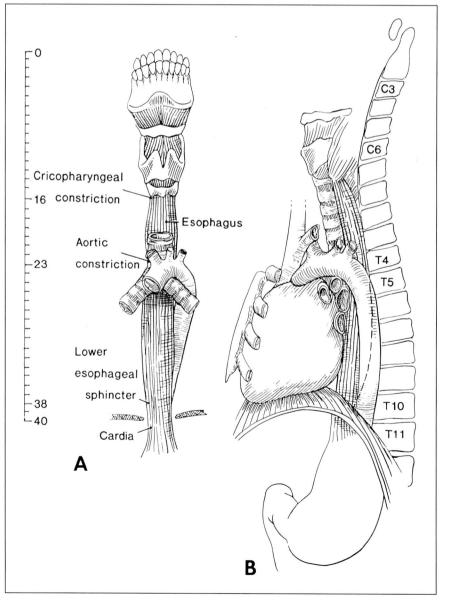

mately 26 mm in adulthood [3,4]. The lumen of the esophagus tends to be larger in the lower half, the largest portion being the most distal portion immediately above the diaphragm. This diameter of the esophagus is important to remember because larger-sized transducers are not amenable for use in children. It is also important to note that the esophagus is normally not uniform in diameter throughout its length but has three distinct narrowings: at its origin, where the cricopharyngeal part of the inferior pharyngeal constrictor muscle surrounds its orifice (cricopharyngeal constriction); at the level of the arch of the aorta or left main bronchus (aortic constriction); and at its distal end (diaphragmatic constriction) as it approaches and joins the cardia of the stomach.

The cricopharyngeal constriction is the narrowest portion of the esophagus and the point passed with the most caution by endoscopists because of the difficulty in negotiating the endoscope through it. This constriction is located approximately at the level of the sixth cervical vertebra. In adults, the average caliber at this level is 23 mm in the transverse diameter and 17 mm in the anteroposterior diameter. At this site the examiner must be gentle in negotiating the TEE probe into the esophagus. The aortic constriction is at the point of contact of the esophagus with the arch of the aorta and the left main bronchus, usually at the level of the fourth and fifth thoracic vertebrae. This juxtaposition is of some importance in patients with a dilated aortic arch, which may extrinsically compress the esophagus, causing some resistance as the probe is being advanced through this constriction.

The distal esophageal constriction is at the level of the tenth thoracic vertebra and is due to the esophagus passing through the diaphragm; this location coincides with that of the lower esophageal sphincter.

There are two sphincters: the upper esophageal sphincter, usually between 15 and 18 cm from the incisor teeth at the level of the cricopharyngeal constriction, and the lower esophageal sphincter, located between 30 and 50 cm from the incisors. These values are for adult men and women. Awareness of the sphincters is important, because they normally occlude the lumen of the esophagus except during the act of swallowing, and one can often expect minor resistance at these levels when introducing or advancing the TEE probe.

In the adult, mild resistance is usually encountered on introducing the probe at the level of the upper esophageal sphincter, and the patient may feel mild discomfort. This can easily be overcome with gentle pressure and by advancing the probe only while the patient swallows, an act that relaxes the upper sphincter. It is also important to note that Zenker's diverticulum may be near this level or somewhat superior to the cricopharyngeus muscle. If firm resistance to probe passage occurs at this level, the probe may have entered a diverticulum or caught on a ridge of cricopharyngeal muscle. In either event, the probe must never be forced beyond the point of resistance but should instead be withdrawn and repositioned. The risk of esophageal perforation is highest at this level of the esophagus.

Less commonly, at the level of the lower esophageal sphincter (between 30 and 40 cm from the incisors), the patient may again feel some discomfort and the examiner some resistance while the transducer is advanced beyond this sphincter. This effect can be overcome with maneuvers similar to those used at the level of the upper esophageal sphincter.

PHYSIOLOGY OF DEGLUTITION

Knowing the physiology of deglutition before learning how to introduce the TEE probe enables the examiner to determine when to advance the probe and when not to push. A good rule of thumb is that advancing the transducer during the phase of esophageal peristaltic relaxation that follows the peristaltic contraction wave enables easy introduction, even in patients who may otherwise be difficult to intubate. This approach clearly helps maximize patient comfort and tolerance.

Swallowing is traditionally divided into three phases: buccal, pharyngeal, and esophageal. During the buccal phase the front of the tongue is elevated against the surface of the hard palate. The tongue is retracted and depressed, displacing the food bolus into the pharynx. The pharyngeal phase occurs when the food bolus comes in contact with the pillars of the fauces, tonsils, soft palate, base of the tongue, and posterior wall of the pharynx. Contact triggers an involuntary reflex accomplished in less than 1 second. The pharyngeal muscles initiate a propulsive contraction over the pharynx. As a result, the food bolus is propelled toward the esophagus. At the same time, the soft palate presses against the posterior pharyngeal wall to seal off the nasopharynx and the larynx is protected by approximation of the epiglottis. These movements prevent food from entering the airway. The esophageal phase involves the relaxation of the upper esophageal sphincter and the beginning of the primary peristaltic wave, which traverses the entire esophagus. The act of swallowing, once the primary peristaltic wave is initiated, is independent of extrinsic innervation.

PREEXAMINATION MEASURES IN THE AWAKE PATIENT

Patient Preparation

First and foremost in the sequence of events before a TEE examination begins is a discussion of the goals, risks, and nature of the procedure with the patient and family members, if any (Table 3-1). Discussion serves to allay fear and anxiety and also establishes a rapport with the patient. This discussion should be undertaken by the physician performing the examination, with assistance from the sonographer or associate helping with the examination (see Chapter 2).

A brief history of symptoms related to the gastrointestinal tract needs to be obtained. Included is any record of dysphagia, odynophagia, hematemesis, upper gastrointestinal surgical procedures, esophageal varices, or results of previous x-ray or endoscopic examinations. Any instance of radiation therapy to the chest is also important to record, because the possibility of radiation-related changes in the esophagus always exists, and they may preclude TEE. Rheumatoid arthritis, especially if it involves the atlantoaxial joint or cervical spine in general, is important to elicit. During TEE the patient's neck is routinely flexed; if severe degenerative or rheumatoid arthritic disease is present, flexion may not be possible without significant pain or even potential harm to the patient.

A history of any drug allergies should always be elicited, and depending on the drugs used during TEE, contraindications should be determined.

For the elective TEE procedure, the patient should abstain from all oral intake other than medications for at least 4 hours before the examination. Dentures or other removable oral prostheses should be taken out before the examination. The positioning of the patient and role of the TEE assistant are reviewed in detaii in Chapter 2. Techniques of introduction

of the TEE probe and use of medications vary from institution to institution. Herein, the approaches used in our laboratory are described.

Intravenous access is established in all patients, usually by an intravenous catheter inserted into a dorsal hand vein or an antecubital vein. The patient is instructed to lie on his or her left side, facing the examiner. The left lateral decubitus position minimizes the risk of aspiration. The right knee is flexed and placed in front of the left leg to help ensure proper positioning and limit the tendency for the patient to roll to the right. The patient's head is comfortably flexed to facilitate oropharyngeal entry.

Table 3-1. Preprocedure checklist for transesophageal echocardiography

Explain procedure to patient and family
Take history
    Dysphagia
    Odynophagia
    Hematemesis
    Mediastinal radiation
    Problems related to cervical spine
    Chest trauma
    Operations on the gastrointestinal tract
    Recent endoscopic examination
    Drug allergy
    History of alcohol abuse
    History of urinary retention
    History of angle-closure glaucoma
    History of bronchial asthma
    Last oral intake
    Dentures, oral prosthesis (remove before procedure)
Check hemodynamics
    Blood pressure
    Pulse rate
    Oxygen saturation
Obtain intravenous access
Check TEE probe for breaks, cable tension
Keep probe in neutral position
Anesthetize patient
    Local spray
    Intravenous
Check gag reflex with tongue blade or fingers
Put patient in left lateral decubitis position
Fasten belt
Make sure that patient is comfortable
Lubricate probe

The usual patient position is shown in Figure 3-3.

Alternative positions for TEE examination are the supine and even the upright sitting. The supine position is used commonly in the critical care unit and almost always in the operating room. Gentle flexion of the neck by an assistant helps facilitate entry into the oropharynx even when the patient is supine or sitting. In rare, selected difficult introductions, some examiners have allowed the patient to attempt self-introduction of the transducer, which with encouragement often is successful in the sitting position. Neither the supine nor the sitting approach is recommended as the method of choice for intubation in the awake patient.

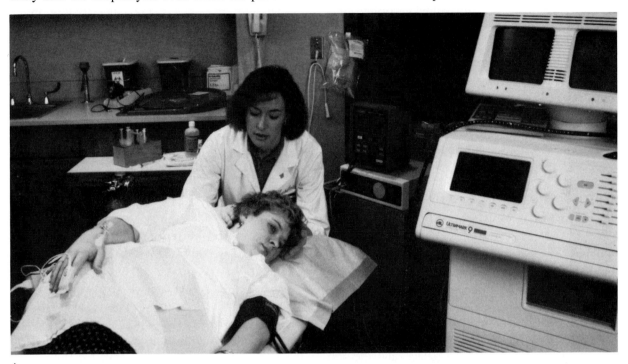

A

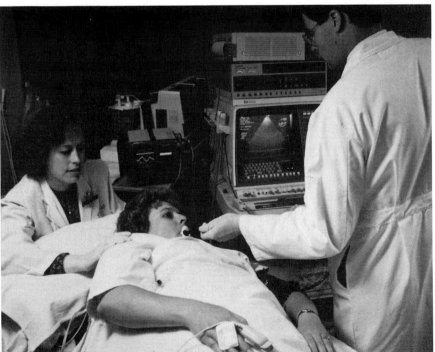

B

Fig. 3-3. A. Optimal position of the patient for TEE examination. The patient is left lateral decubitus, with the head gently flexed to facilitate entry of the TEE probe into the esophagus. Note the position of the assistant at the head of the examination table. The procedure room arrangement shown is fully described in Chapter 2. B. Patient, examiner, and assistant in the positions considered ideal for a TEE study.

Premedication

Awake patients scheduled to undergo TEE are premedicated for the following reasons: (1) Topical anesthesia of the oropharynx and hard and soft palates diminishes the gag reflex and reduces retching and possible laryngospasm during the procedure, (2) drying agents lessen salivary and gastrointestinal secretions, reducing the risk of aspiration, (3) sedatives and analgesics decrease anxiety and discomfort, promote cooperation, and often provide retrograde amnesia of the examination, and (4) antibiotic agents help prevent bacterial endocarditis in selected high-risk patients. Benzodiazepine and opioid-receptor antagonists should be available to reverse significant untoward effects of sedatives and analgesics given during TEE.

Topical Anesthesia

For anesthesia of the oropharynx, an aerosol local anesthetic solution of 10% lidocaine is used. It is preferable to spray the oropharynx, posterior tongue, and palate while the patient is sitting to minimize cough and aspiration into the trachea. Care should be taken to avoid spraying the anesthetic aerosol during deep inspiration, as aspiration of the spray may cause transient vocal cord paralysis. It is best to spray the tongue, the hard palate, and the soft palate and oropharynx in that order. Anesthetizing the tongue helps maintain the TEE probe in midline position and keeps the patient from moving it side to side during nondigital introduction. A tongue blade may be used to depress the tongue to get better visualization of the oropharynx. Liberal spraying of the soft palate and oropharynx provides significant, but usually not complete, relief from gagging and retching. The anesthetic effect begins within 2 to 3 minutes and may persist for 30 to 45 minutes. The effect is superficial and does not extend to the submucosal structures. The maximal safe total dose for topical lidocaine anesthesia in a healthy 70-kg adult is 750 mg, far less than that required for complete topical oropharyngeal anesthesia. To prevent potential mucosal injury after the TEE examination the patient should not eat or drink excessively hot or cold substances until the topical anesthesia has worn off.

Other agents used for topical anesthesia include viscous lidocaine, dyclonine, and tetracaine, which are local anesthetics belonging to the same family as lidocaine. Other topical anesthetic agents are 20% benzocaine (Hurricaine) or 14% benzocaine (Cetacaine), both of which are available for spray application. Alternatively, some laboratories have the patient gargle with lidocaine solution before the oropharyngeal mucosa is sprayed.

A superior laryngeal nerve block [5] can also be used to diminish and often abolish the gag reflex, although this is rarely, if ever, currently used in our laboratory.

Antisialagogic Agent

The use of a drying agent reduces oropharyngeal secretions, usually obviates oral suction, and minimizes the risk of aspiration. We use glycopyrrolate (Robinul) [6], a quaternary ammonium anticholinergic agent, to effectively control secretions. Glycopyrrolate is available in 1 ml (0.2 mg) single-dose vials. The desired antisialagogic effect in adults can be achieved with a dose of 0.2 mg administered intravenously a few minutes before the procedure. The peak effect of this drug is achieved within 1 to 3 minutes. The antisialagogic effect may persist up to 7 hours.

Glycopyrrolate was used in approximately 82% of the 5441 TEE procedures performed at our institution from November 1987 through November 1992. No significant complications were encountered with the use of this agent. In general, the amount of secretions was considerably less in patients receiving glycopyrrolate than in those not receiving the drug. In our practice, glycopyrrolate is not administered to patients who have resting sinus tachycardia or rapid atrial fibrillation. Occasionally, this drug causes an increase in the resting heart rate, but without detrimental effects [6].

Relative or absolute contraindications to administration of glycopyrrolate include tachycardia of any kind, closed-angle glaucoma, obstructive uropathy, paralytic ileus, toxic megacolon, and myasthenia gravis. This agent also should not be used in patients with bronchial asthma, because inspissation of secretions caused by glycopyrrolate may cause plugging of the bronchioles and severe respiratory compromise. Neostigmine, a quaternary ammonium anticholinesterase, can be used to reverse the side effects of glycopyrrolate if clinically indicated.

Ambulatory patients are cautioned against operating a motor vehicle or hazardous machinery because of the possibility of blurred vision or drowsiness resulting from anticholinergic premedication.

Sedation

In anxious patients, administration of a sedative belonging to the benzodiazepine group (such as midazolam or diazepam) greatly facilitates the procedure. We use midazolam hydrochloride (Versed) [7,8] intravenously in 0.5-mg to 1.0-mg increments, administered over a period of 1 to 2 minutes and supplemented as needed for adequate sedation. Benzodiazepines such as midazolam and diazepam are anxiolytic, cause short-term retrograde amnesia, produce mild to moderate sedation, and potentiate the effects of other anesthetic agents. However, benzodiazepines have only minimal analgesic effects. Hence, combination with a narcotic such as meperidine (Demerol) or fentanyl (Innovar, Sublimaze) is administered if needed for patient comfort. The dose of midazolam is titrated to the point at which the patient is adequately sedated but not asleep. Patients older than 50 years have a shorter induction time and require smaller doses of midazolam than do those younger than 50 years [9]. In the very elderly and infirm patient it may be prudent not to use this agent and to rely only on topical anesthesia. Sedation occurs in 3 to 5 minutes, and the half-life of the drug usually ranges from 1 to 4 hours [9]. In general, retrograde amnesia of events from introduction of the TEE probe to withdrawal occurs in 70% to 80% of patients premedicated with midazolam. The patient is observed for 25 to 30 minutes after the procedure. Reaction time under stress (such as operating machinery or driving a motor vehicle) may be prolonged well beyond gross recovery time; therefore, the patient should be cautioned against performing activities requiring full alertness for 12 to 24 hours.

Throughout the premedication, TEE examination, and immediate recovery, the patient's vital signs and peripheral oxygen saturation are monitored with an automated blood pressure device and pulse oximeter (see Chapter 2).

The major adverse reactions to midazolam are respiratory depression and hypotension. Cardiorespiratory depression is more pronounced when midazolam is combined with an opioid agent. Respiratory depression from midazolam may range from mild peripheral oxygen desaturation to apnea and respiratory arrest. The potential risk of such respiratory compromise is increased in the elderly and in patients with significant chronic obstructive lung disease.

Our experience with midazolam has been favorable, and we have not observed a statistically rele-

vant decrease from baseline in either the blood pressure or the oxygen saturation with general administration of this drug [6]. In our experience with 5441 procedures over 5 years, midazolam was used in 88% of these patients. The mean dose was 2.9 mg (range, 0.5 to 25 mg). In this series, only 0.4% of patients treated with midazolam experienced respiratory depression warranting any intervention [6].

Meperidine is a potent analgesic whose effects are detectable within 15 minutes of oral administration, reach a peak at about 2 hours, and subside gradually over several hours. The onset of action is quicker with parenteral injection. The onset of analgesic effect is noted within 5 to 10 minutes, peaking at 1 hour and lasting for 3 to 5 hours. Slow intravenous administration of 25 to 50 mg is commonly done in our laboratory and offers excellent analgesic effect. We use meperidine only in the occasional patient who is inadequately sedated and uncomfortable with full doses of midazolam. Meperidine also causes respiratory depression, and caution must be used when this agent is combined with midazolam or other benzodiazepines. Nausea, vomiting, and, uncommonly, hypotension are side effects that need to be noted.

Sufentanil and alfentanil are congeners of fentanyl and are also potent opioid analgesics with some properties of a sedative that act synergistically with midazolam. These agents can be combined with benzodiazepines and administered as premedication. Sufentanil induces profound analgesia and also, in adequate doses, anesthesia; cardiovascular stability is impressive with therapeutic doses of sufentanil.

Another category of sedatives that can be used is the butyrophenone group. They produce sedation, have antiemetic action, and can cause indifference to the procedure. Droperidol, an agent in this class of drugs, can be administered intravenously or intramuscularly in a dose of 0.625 to 10.0 mg. The onset of action is between 5 and 15 minutes, and the peak duration of action is approximately 6 hours. Uncommon side effects are dysphoria, extrapyramidal symptoms, and mild α-adrenergic antagonist action.

Benzodiazepine-Receptor Antagonist

Flumazenil, a recently introduced competitive benzodiazepine-receptor antagonist, can be used to reverse the effects of sedatives such as midazolam [10]. At pharmacologic doses it has little intrinsic pharmacologic activity and no effect on plasma benzodiazepine concentrations. Flumazenil induces potent antisedative and antiamnesic activity from the point of administration; no retrograde antiamnesic action is produced. Flumazenil does not reliably reverse significant respiratory depression occurring with benzodiazepine. This drug, however, is a safe and effective benzodiazepine antagonist for all other potential adverse reactions [10].

After intravenous administration of flumazenil, onset of reversal is rapid, occurring within 1 or 2 minutes. The initial dose is 0.2 mg, which is followed by 0.3 mg if required. The total dose should not exceed 1.0 mg over any period of 5 minutes or a cumulative dose of 3.0 mg over 60 minutes. Peak effects occur in 6 to 10 minutes, and a dose of 0.4 to 1.0 mg usually produces complete benzodiazepine antagonism. The duration of effect is dose-dependent, ranging from 15 minutes to 2.5 hours.

Clinical trials comparing flumazenil and placebo in subjects receiving benzodiazepine for anesthesia and endoscopic procedures have produced mixed results. In general, subjects receiving flumazenil recover more quickly, but after 60 to 120 minutes, differences between the drug and the control groups are insignificant. In studies comparing flumazenil and placebo in outpatient subjects receiving diazepam or midazolam for endoscopic procedures, flumazenil was effective in reversing the sedation induced by either benzodiazepine; however, all subjects had some degree of residual sedative effect at the time of dismissal. Patients receiving flumazenil after benzodiazepine sedation for outpatient procedures must be observed for loss of antagonist effect, resedation, or respiratory depression from a residual midazolam effect. The duration of observation depends on the benzodiazepine reversed and the dose of the agent used. Short-acting agents, such as midazolam in the doses commonly used for TEE, require shorter periods of observation than do longer acting benzodiazepines, such as diazepam and chlordiazepoxide. Seizures have been reported to complicate benzodiazepine reversal with flumazenil, but these usually occur in cases of benzodiazepine overdose or in patients receiving long-term benzodiazepine therapy.

Flumazenil should not be used as a substitute for close monitoring and care of benzodiazepine-induced respiratory depression, and the physician should always be prepared to manage the rare case of severe respiratory compromise induced by midazolam. Likewise, it should never be assumed that flumazenil totally reverses the depressant effects of benzodiazepines on the central nervous system, even if the patient appears fully awake. Such patients should still refrain from operating a motor vehicle or engaging in other precarious activities for at least 12 hours after the procedure.

Narcotic Antagonist

Naloxone (Narcan) administered in small doses (0.4–0.8 mg) intravenously can promptly reverse the effects of narcotics such as meperidine and fentanyl. Reversal of untoward narcotic side effects, including respiratory depression, usually occurs within 2 minutes after administration. Because the circulating half-life of naloxone is approximately 1 hour, repeat delayed doses are usually not required for the relatively small amounts of narcotics used during TEE. This drug must be kept available if narcotic agents are to be used as premedication for TEE.

Antibiotic Prophylaxis

The issue of endocarditis prophylaxis during TEE remains controversial. Because the procedure is similar to that of endoscopic examinations, there may be some merit to administering bacterial endocarditis prophylaxis based on the recommendations of the American Heart Association [11]. Factors that lead to endocarditis include duration of bacteremia, type of organism, underlying cardiac disease, number of colonies causing bacteremia, and host defense status. Obviously, this is not an all-inclusive list, and the issue of bacteremia and the true incidence of resultant infective endocarditis precipitated by TEE remains to be completely resolved.

The risk of bacteremia during TEE appears to be minimal, as shown by previously published prospective studies [12–14]. One case report in the literature suggests a temporal relationship between TEE and development of bacterial endocarditis [15]. Also, a report on a series of four patients seems to indicate a high risk of bacteremia during TEE [16]. However, the organisms isolated in the latter study were oral flora and not susceptible to the antimicrobial prophylaxis recommended by the American Heart Association [11].

Perhaps the most important issue regarding antibiotic prophylaxis for TEE is not whether endocarditis ever occurs after TEE but what the magnitude of the risk is relative to the well-known risks of widespread use of prophylactic antibiotics in both the individual patient and the general population. As

TEE use increases, undoubtedly there will be additional reports of patients who have had both TEE and subsequent endocarditis, whether the association is chance or causative. Current observations based on one documented case of TEE-related endocarditis and another four cases of bacteremia associated with TEE are insufficient to justify routine antibiotic endocarditis prophylaxis for all patients undergoing TEE, although it is entirely unknown how many such cases are not reported.

Final recommendations from the American Heart Association, however, are pending. Currently in our practice, we use antibiotic prophylaxis only in patients at the highest risk for development of infective endocarditis (i.e., patients with prosthetic heart valves or a past history of infective endocarditis) [11]. This is not necessarily the practice at all institutions, and the echocardiologist should exercise individual judgment in recommending prophylaxis or in forgoing it in patients potentially at high risk who are to have TEE. If infective endocarditis is the referral diagnosis, antibiotic prophylaxis is not given until blood culture specimens have been obtained.

INDICATIONS FOR TEE

Indications for a TEE examination encompass nearly all disease entities encountered in the practice of cardiovascular medicine.

In our experience with 5441 TEE procedures (excluding intraoperative TEE; see Chapter 16) over a period of 5 years, 36% of the patients had a clinically suspected embolic event, and TEE was performed to seek a potential intracardiac source of emboli (Fig. 3-4). Clearly, TEE is superior to transthoracic echocardiography for the visualization of the left atrial appendage, atrial septum, thoracic aorta, and prosthetic valves and generally affords superior resolution of cardiac and aortic anatomy and pathologic lesions, such as masses and thrombi, compared with the transthoracic approach. Since transthoracic echocardiography has been consistently shown to have a poor yield in patients with intracardiac sources of embolism, it is not surprising that many patients are referred for TEE to exclude an intracardiac source of embolism. The proportion of patients referred because of this diagnosis varies from institution to institution, but data from other tertiary care centers support the belief that TEE is being used with increasing frequency for evaluating suspected intracardiac source of embolism [17,18]. This issue is discussed in further detail in Chapter 15.

Patients with proven or suspected infective endocarditis represent the second most common referral (13% of patients) for TEE. Transesophageal echocardiography has been clearly shown to be superior to transthoracic in the diagnosis of vegetations and complications of endocarditis, such as abscess and fistula formation [19–21]. There is no debate about TEE being the procedure of choice in the evaluation

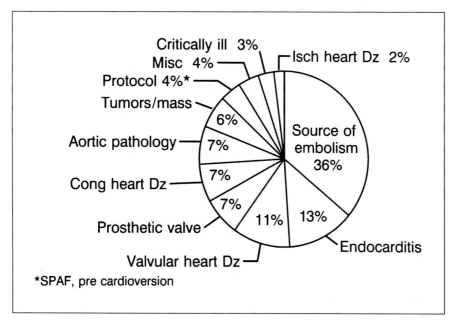

Fig. 3-4. Indications for TEE examination at the Mayo Clinic from November 1987 to November 1992 (5,441 procedures). Three major indications are source of embolism, native and prosthetic valve disease, and endocarditis (see text). (*SPAF*= Stroke Prevention in Atrial Fibrillation trial.)

of suspected endocarditis or its complications (see Chapter 11).

The next most common indications for TEE in our experience are native and prosthetic valvular disease (see Chapters 9 and 10). Use of TEE to evaluate valvular disease has proven to be very helpful, and ample data demonstrate that in a substantial number of patients, TEE provides clinically relevant information affecting patient management beyond that obtained by transthoracic echocardiography [22–24]. With the availability of steerable continuous-wave Doppler echocardiography in the newer biplane and multiplane TEE transducers, additional hemodynamic data can be obtained in patients with native or prosthetic valve disorders.

Transesophageal echocardiography has had a high degree of success in the evaluation of disease of the thoracic aorta, such as aortic dissection and atherosclerosis and its complications (see Chapter 14). At many institutions, TEE is the procedure of choice for diagnosis and follow-up of patients with aortic dissection and is superior to other imaging modalities in the assessment of atherosclerotic intra-aortic debris, a significant potential source of systemic emboli [25–28].

In addition, TEE has been found to be invaluable in the characterization and localization of intracardiac masses, such as thrombus, myxoma, and other neoplasms [29,30] (see Chapter 12). In our series, 6% of patients underwent TEE for this purpose.

Adult congenital heart disease is another source of referral for TEE (7% of patients in our experience). Conditions such as atrial septal defect, anomalous pulmonary venous connection, cor triatriatum, Ebstein's anomaly, and postoperative Fontan and conduit procedures are all readily characterized by TEE. Data suggest that TEE has a significant effect in clinical decision-making in the inpatient, outpatient [31–34], and intraoperative management of patients with congenital heart disease (see Chapters 13 and 16).

The utility of TEE in critically ill patients is now well recognized. In our practice, about 3% of patients undergoing TEE were critically ill in intensive care units. Transesophageal echocardiography can be performed safely in such patients, who are often too unstable or encumbered with life-support devices to permit other means of expeditious evaluation, and immediately provides a wealth of acutely relevant information for management [35] (see Chapter 17).

A wide variety of other indications for which TEE can be performed includes evaluation of the left atrium and appendage before cardioversion of atrial fibrillation, evaluation of pulmonary venous inflow for characterization of diastolic function in patients for whom transthoracic echocardiography is not feasible, visualization of the proximal coronary arteries, and even nonphysiologic stress testing. Transesophageal echocardiography can also facilitate multiple invasive interventional procedures, such as transseptal catheterization, balloon valvuloplasty [36], radiofrequency ablation of arrhythmogenic pathways [37], and myocardial biopsy. Any condition in which the transthoracic approach does not yield images of adequate quality is a potential indication for TEE [38,39]. The many intraoperative applications of TEE are reviewed in Chapter 16. The indications for TEE continue to expand, and the preceding discussion is meant not to be all-inclusive but rather to emphasize applications of TEE that are well established.

TECHNIQUE OF INTRODUCTION

The following descriptions of how to introduce the endoscope reflect commonly used techniques at our institution, which may vary from procedures used at other institutions. Whatever technique one uses, two guidelines must be remembered: (1) If the patient gives a history of significant dysphagia or odynophagia, it is best to pursue an upper gastrointestinal evaluation before proceeding with TEE; esophagogastroscopy may be indicated. (2) Any forceful introduction into the esophagus must be avoided. The main prerequisite to a safe procedure is knowing when and when not to advance the TEE probe. When in doubt, it is wise to seek the assistance of a more experienced colleague or gastroenterologist.

Preparation in the Awake Patient

The general approach for TEE examination is from the patient's left side, with the patient in the left lateral decubitus position (Fig. 3-3). The examiner faces the patient and the assistant sits or stands at the head of the patient. The machine is usually to the right of the examiner, within easy reach for manipulation of the controls. Some institutions have an additional sonographer assisting the cardiologist with the operation of the machine (making it a three-person procedure); this is unnecessary if the physician knows how to operate the controls.

To prevent the spread of communicable diseases, both operator and assistant should wear disposable gloves. They should be protected against bodily secretion by goggles, masks, and gowning procedures when examining patients infected with human immunodeficiency or hepatitis viruses. A condom sheath for the TEE probe is cumbersome and unnecessary, and it hinders the examination; it is not used at our institution. The standard methods of probe disinfection, described in Chapter 2, are fully adequate to eliminate the threat of cross infection with hepatitis viruses or human immunodeficiency virus.

The topical anesthetic spray ideally should be applied with the patient in the sitting rather than the supine position. Spraying the oropharynx, palate, and tongue while the patient is sitting is easier to accomplish and reduces the risk of aspiration. It is also advantageous to check the gag reflex once local anesthesia has been achieved. With a tongue blade, the buccal and oropharyngeal mucosa can be assessed for diminution of sensation to touch and decrease in gag reflex. The gag reflex cannot be completely eliminated, and it helps to tell the patient this before the examination so that the patient will know what to expect during introduction of the TEE probe. The examiner may also use a gloved finger to test the gag reflex. Intubation can be simulated with the gloved index finger substituting for the TEE probe tip to test the adequacy of the patient's premedication. This is also a good time to instruct the patient in how to perform the Valsalva maneuver if it will be required during contrast studies to rule out right-to-left interatrial shunt.

The distal portion of the probe is coated with lubricating jelly or a combination of lubricating jelly and viscous lidocaine. A bite guard is essential to allow manipulation and protection of the TEE probe if the patient is not completely edentulous. The probe must be introduced with the transducer tip in the unlocked position.

The different methods of introduction are (1) digital, or finger-guided, approach; (2) nondigital, or blind, tip manipulation; and (3) digital approach with guard in place. Each is described in detail below.

Digital Approach

In the digital approach (Fig. 3-5), the bite guard is placed over the distal part of the endoscope (unnecessary if the patient is edentulous). The assistant

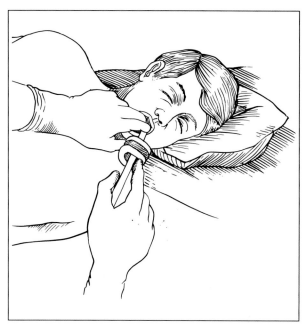

Fig. 3-5. Digital approach to the introduction of the TEE probe. Briefly, the examiner uses one or two fingers to depress the tongue and then introduces the transducer under the fingers, advancing it into the oropharynx. At this point, the patient is asked to simulate swallowing, or if the patient is unconscious, the tip is pushed gently along the movements caused by natural peristalsis. The bite guard is then placed between the teeth.

gently flexes the head of the patient. The physician holds the distal portion of the shaft in the right hand and makes sure that the transducer tip is unlocked. The proximal control handle and cable to the machine can be conveniently draped over the operator's shoulder or be placed alongside the patient so that both hands are free for probe introduction. After the patient's mouth is open, the left index finger or second and third fingers are inserted on top of the tongue, the tongue is depressed by the fingers, and the fingers are advanced to the posterior aspect of the tongue. At this time, the transducer tip is advanced into the mouth.

The transducer is then placed under the fingers, which are used to guide the tip to the midline of the oropharynx. With a gentle downward pressure, the partially flexed tip of the transducer is guided toward the esophageal orifice. When the tip is at the esophageal orifice (probe insertion of approximately 16 to 18 cm), the patient is told to swallow. This action not only relaxes the upper esophageal sphincter but also directs the transducer in the upper portion of the esophagus. The initiation of the swallowing reflex carries the transducer into the esophagus, beyond the upper esophageal sphincter. The transducer is advanced steadily but never with force. If resistance is encountered, the endoscope is simply withdrawn slightly, readjusted, and redirected centrally. Advancing the transducer into the esophagus about 25 cm from the incisors suppresses the gag reflex. The bite guard is slid into place between the teeth as the fingers are withdrawn.

This method of introduction is probably easier for physicians learning TEE, but it has some associated risks. Inadvertent biting of the fingers can result in painful injuries, and the possibility of resultant infection always exists. Bite damage to the instrument can require very expensive repairs. Passage of a transducer is a cooperative venture between the patient and the examiner; rapport and safety should never be compromised by undue persistence when the patient is distressed. If in doubt, the physician should remove the instrument and try again only when the patient is ready. Sometimes, one is unable to advance the transducer beyond 15 to 20 cm from the incisors, possibly because the tip is caught in a piriform fossa, one of two small recesses just inferior and lateral to the epiglottis. It is best to remove the probe and attempt reintroduction, making sure that the transducer is kept in the midline with the help of the fingers and using the same technique as outlined above.

Nondigital Approach

In the nondigital approach (Fig. 3-6), the operator stands facing the patient and holds the tip of the transducer and the distal end close to each other. The bite guard is first placed between the teeth, and the head is flexed slightly forward. The examiner passes the probe tip through the bite guard and over the tongue, maintaining the tip in the midline. Using the left hand over the control knob, the examiner anteflexes the tip gently to curve over the back of the tongue into the pharynx. The tip is advanced slightly while slight forward pressure is applied. The patient is asked to swallow to relax the cricopharyngeal sphincter. Constant words of reassurance and encouragement should accompany this phase to facilitate introduction beyond the level of the upper esophageal sphincter. At this point, one often feels the loss of resistance, an indication that the tip has

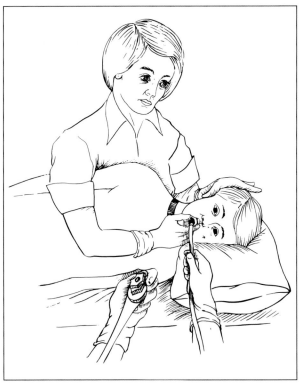

Fig. 3-6. Nondigital approach to the introduction of the TEE probe. The examiner does not use any fingers to depress the tongue but instead places the tip of the transducer in the midline with the bite guard already in place and secured by the assistant. The distal end of the probe is then mildly anteflexed and advanced. The next steps are similar to those in the digital technique.

passed beyond the upper esophageal sphincter. If the tip does not pass beyond this level after three to five simulated swallowing maneuvers, the examiner must withdraw the transducer and reintroduce it, keeping it in the midline. It is imperative not to force probe introduction against any significant resistance.

This approach works well for monoplane TEE probes, which have a relatively small transducer tip (and hence a small rigid distal portion). Biplane or omnidirectional transducer heads are considerably larger and have longer rigid distal tips. Most often, these probes require digital guidance to negotiate the curvature of the oropharynx. With the nondigital approach, the rigid tip often directly strikes the posterior wall of the oropharynx, causing discomfort to the patient.

Digital Approach With Bite Guard in Place

The digital approach with the bite guard in place (Fig. 3-7) is similar to the first technique, except that the bite guard is in place before the TEE probe is introduced. A finger is placed in the mouth alongside the guard. This method prevents accidental biting of the examiner's fingers or of the TEE probe. As in all approaches, the bite guard should be continuously monitored for secure position; it may be inadvertently expelled by a sedated patient, so that the examiner's fingers or the TEE probe is then at risk of being bitten.

Approach to the Unconscious or Anesthetized Patient

In the anesthetized or unconscious intubated patient, probe introduction is generally easier because the gag reflex is absent. The risk of accidental intubation of the trachea is minimal because of the endotracheal tube. Conversely, the patient is unable to simulate swallowing, and advancing the probe beyond the upper esophageal sphincter occasionally is difficult. Often, both endotracheal and nasogastric tubes are in place and may pose logistical problems during intubation of the esophagus. Usually, the patient is supine and need not be placed in the full left lateral decubitus position. The head should be in the midline with the neck slightly flexed. Flexion can be performed by an assistant. The endotracheal tube should be positioned to one side of the mouth, commonly the right side, to provide sufficient room for the TEE probe. The examiner should make sure that the endotracheal tube is firmly anchored and does not migrate during TEE probe introduction or during TEE examination. Nasogastric or feeding tubes may need to be removed if the TEE probe cannot be readily passed. There also may be some interference in TEE imaging if one chooses to leave such tubes within the esophagus. In most patients, however, TEE can be successfully performed with nasogastric and particularly smaller feeding tubes in place. Mobile monitoring devices, such as intraoperative esophageal temperature probes, should be removed to prevent migration into the stomach.

In the awake but intubated patient it is preferable to use sedation, drying agent, and topical spray. In the unconscious intubated patient, these premedic-

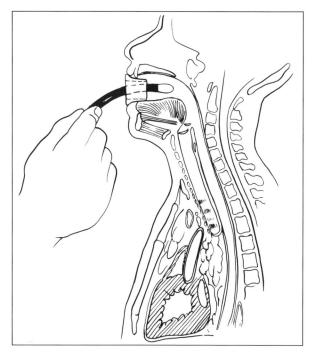

Fig. 3-7. Digital method of introducing the TEE probe with bite guard in place. This method is similar to the digital method except that the bite guard is in place and the fingers are then inserted from the side of the mouth along the bite guard.

ations and, usually, the bite guard are unnecessary. The transducer is introduced "blindly" by simply directing the tip into the posterior part of the pharynx, maintaining a midline position, and gently allowing the probe to flex passively. Frequently, the fingers must be used to guide the tip of the transducer into the esophagus or lift the laryngeal cartilage forward with additional neck flexion. Rarely, the laryngoscope is required for introduction of the probe under direct visualization. Again, it is important to remember not to use force. Because the patient is unable to complain of pain in the event of injury, one runs a greater risk of esophageal perforation if excessive force is used. It is important to note that the esophageal sphincter tends to relax during general anesthesia, and one may not encounter the same resistance at this level as in awake patients.

Examination technique, image orientation, and anatomic correlation of single plane, biplane, and multiplane TEE examinations are discussed below and in Chapters 4 and 5. Postprocedure patient care, dismissal instructions, and TEE probe disinfecting procedures are outlined in Chapter 2.

BIPLANE TEE EXAMINATION

When performing a comprehensive biplane TEE examination, the examiner must have a methodical approach consisting of a sequence of transducer positions and views. It is also important to remember that one may have to perform an abbreviated, goal-directed examination in some instances, obtaining only those images required to address the clinical questions prompting TEE referral. An example is exclusion of left atrial thrombus before percutaneous balloon mitral valvuloplasty in a patient with severe mitral stenosis already fully evaluated by transthoracic echocardiography. Some centers advocate a goal-directed examination in all patients, but our experience leads us to recommend and emphasize

a complete examination, even after the information that answers the referral question or questions has been obtained. We find that in 5% to 10% of cases, unsuspected findings are detected that could potentially alter the management of the patient.

Anatomic correlations and image orientation are described in detail in Chapters 4 and 5. The steps of biplane TEE examination, how to obtain various views (Figs. 3-8 and 3-9), and visualization of cardiac anatomy are described below. Potential pitfalls encountered with TEE are reviewed in Chapter 6, and a report has been published [40]. Newer instruments, such as the multiplane, or omniplane, device, have recently been introduced in the practice of TEE, and a description of how to perform a multiplane examination is detailed in Chapter 5.

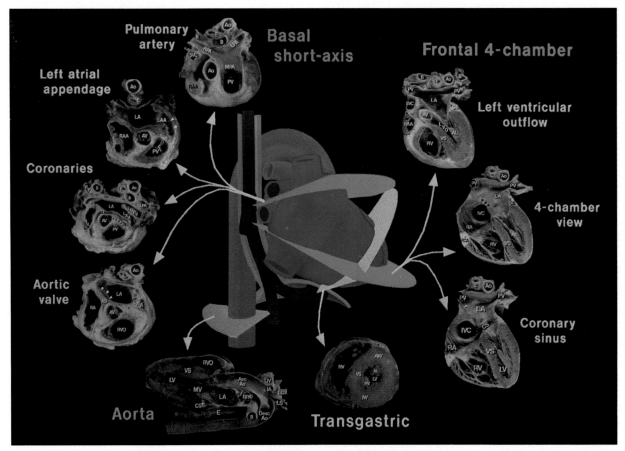

Fig. 3-8. Horizontal plane views. Common scan planes and structures that can be visualized at various levels are represented by anatomic specimens cut along these planes. These scan planes can be obtained in the horizontal plane with use of biplanar transducers. The four sets of views in this plane are basal short-axis, frontal four-chamber, transgastric, and, by turning transducer tip posteriorly, aortic.

There are two approaches to a comprehensive TEE study. One approach is to start imaging from the transgastric position (normally obtained when the transducer tip is about 40 to 45 cm from the incisors), sequentially pull the probe back to examine various sections of the heart from apex to base, and then view the aorta by rotating the transducer posteriorly. The second approach (our preference) is to start at the base of the heart (25 to 30 cm from the incisors), progress toward the transgastric views, and then examine the thoracic aorta during probe withdrawal. Either of these two methods is considered acceptable. One should try to minimize the number of probe excursions back and forth from the proximal esophagus to the gastric fundus. This practice helps optimize patient comfort and promotes a proficient, organized TEE examination.

HORIZONTAL TEE IMAGING

Basal Short-Axis Scan

For the basal short-axis scan (Fig. 3-10), the TEE transducer is advanced to within 25 to 30 cm from the incisor teeth, where it is posterior to the left atrium. With mild anteroflexion (tilting the tip superiorly) or slight withdrawal of the transducer, sequential basal short-axis scans are obtained that visualize the aortic valve, proximal ascending aorta, proximal coronary arteries, atrial appendages, superior vena cava, atrial septum, pulmonary veins, and proximal pulmonary arteries. Traditional orientation is to place anterior structures at the bottom of the sector and posterior structures at the apex; left-sided structures are to the viewer's right on the video display.

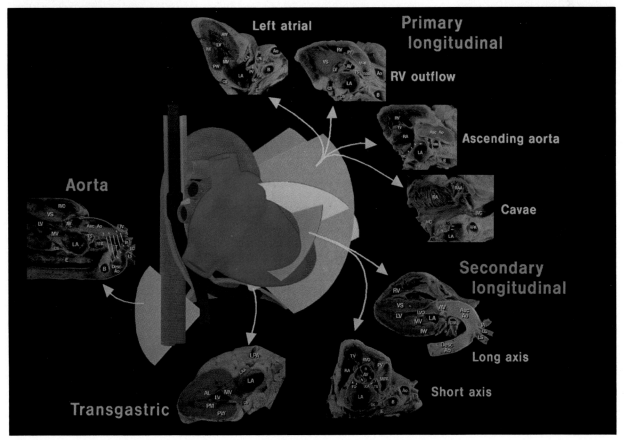

Fig. 3-9. Longitudinal plane views. Common scan planes and structures that can be visualized at various levels are represented by anatomic specimens cut along these planes. These scan planes can be obtained in the longitudinal plane with use of biplanar transducers. The four sets of views are primary longitudinal, secondary longitudinal, transgastric, and, by turning transducer tip posteriorly, aortic.

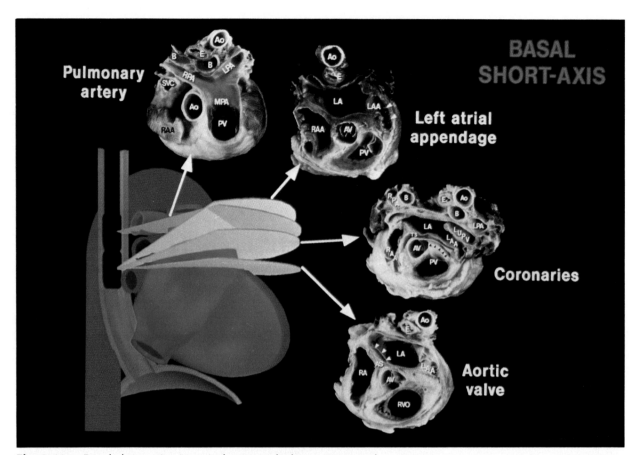

Fig. 3-10. Basal short-axis views in horizontal plane. *Aortic valve view:* Anatomic section of the basal short-axis view shows the aortic valve with its three cusps, atrial septum with the membrane of the fossa ovalis (*arrowheads*), left atrial appendage, left atrium, right atrium, and right ventricular outflow tract. Note the intimate relationship of the descending thoracic aorta to the esophagus. *Coronary artery view:* Anatomic section of the basal short-axis view shows the left coronary artery (*black arrowheads*), left upper pulmonary vein entering the left atrium, left atrial appendage, pulmonary valve *(PV),* and right atrial appendage. The transverse sinus, a pericardial reflection between the great arteries and left atrium, is seen. *Left atrial appendage view:* Anatomic section at the base of the heart shows the left atrial appendage with pectinate muscles (*arrowheads*), left atrium, aortic valve (a prosthesis in this specimen), and right atrial appendage. Once again, notice intimate relationship of the aorta to the esophagus. *Pulmonary artery view:* Anatomic section at the base of the heart shows the main pulmonary artery, left and right proximal pulmonary arteries, superior vena cava, and aortic root. This view is obtained with the transducer tip anteflexed and withdrawn slightly from the location at which the first three views were obtained.

The aortic root and the aortic valve cusps (left cusp to the right of the sector, right cusp inferiorly, and noncoronary cusp to the left of the image) are seen. The atrial septum, with its central thinned fossa ovalis membrane, separates the left and right atria (see Fig. 3-10, aortic valve view). Slight anteroflex-ion of the transducer superiorly allows visualization of the proximal coronary arteries (see Fig. 3-10, coronary artery view). The left coronary artery is visualized more often and more clearly than the right coronary. As noted in Chapter 8, reports in the literature describe the use of TEE to detect left main coronary stenosis and anomalous coronary arteries and to assess coronary blood flow [39,41–45]. However, complete TEE visualization of coronary arteries remains an elusive goal, even with the newest TEE transducers.

Further superior flexion of the transducer tip images the left atrial appendage, seen as a triangular extension of the left atrium (see Fig. 3-10, left atrial appendage view). Muscular ridges (pectinate muscles) within the appendage are often visible with high-resolution TEE transducers and should not be confused with thrombi. Also seen in this view is the left upper pulmonary vein, with a distinct ridgelike infolding of the common wall to the left atrial appendage, which often has a bulbous tip that could be misinterpreted as an abnormal mass. The right atrial appendage can also be partially seen anteriorly at this level. In addition, the transverse sinus, which usually is filled with fat or pericardial fluid, is seen in this view. If the tip of the transducer is tilted even more superiorly, one can image the transverse orifice of the superior vena cava and the aortic and pulmonary valves (see Fig. 3-10, left atrial appendage view). The right pulmonary veins are seen entering the left atrium at this level. The left and right atria, separated by the atrial septum, can also be seen in this view. On withdrawal of the transducer by 1 to 2 cm with concomitant anteflexion, one can visualize the main pulmonary artery and its bifurcation, proximal ascending aorta, and superior vena cava (see Fig. 3-10, pulmonary artery view). Clockwise rotation of the transducer enables the examiner to visualize the proximal portion of the right pulmonary artery. The very proximal portion of the left pulmonary artery can be seen by counterclockwise rotation of the TEE probe. The right pulmonary artery can be imaged distal to its first bifurcation; however, the more distal left pulmonary artery is obscured by air within the interposed left mainstem bronchus.

Frontal Four-Chamber Scan

In the frontal four-chamber scan (Fig. 3-11), the transducer is in the neutral position and the TEE probe is advanced farther into the esophagus to the midesophageal level (30 to 35 cm from the incisors). In the horizontal plane, four-chamber (frontal) scans are obtained. These scans image the atrioventricular valves, ventricles, and left ventricular outflow tract anteriorly and the coronary sinus posteriorly. The images are oriented with the apex down and the left ventricle to the right on the video screen. With multiplane imaging, however, this image orientation may change, as discussed in Chapter 5.

Sequential long-axis views of the heart can be obtained by retroflexion of the tip. The left ventricular outflow tract view and the conventional four-chamber views are readily obtained. These views are useful to visualize the morphologic characteristics of the cardiac crux, atrial septum, atrioventricular valves, and subvalvular support. The anterolateral papillary muscle is easily seen; posteromedial papillary muscle visualization requires extreme retroflexion, which could cause loss of contact between the transducer tip and the esophagus, resulting in inadequate images. Both papillary muscles can be seen on transgastric short-axis scans at the middle left ventricular level and particularly well with transgastric longitudinal scanning. Color-flow imaging for assessment of regurgitation of the atrioventricular valves is greatly facilitated with these views, as is pulsed-wave and continuous-wave Doppler interrogation of the native or prosthetic mitral valve. Doppler analysis of the tricuspid valve is somewhat difficult because of the angulation of the Doppler beam to the valve, which lies somewhat oblique to the transducer. Longitudinal plane scanning at the midesophageal level permits this evaluation.

Extreme retroflexion and further advancement of the tip by 1 or 2 cm allows visualization of the coronary sinus in its long axis. Anteflexion at this level or at the esophagogastric junction allows scanning of the entire mitral annulus in its short axis. This view is useful in localizing the site or sites of mitral regurgitation, visualizing the circumference of the sewing ring in patients with a prosthetic mitral valve, searching for abscess formation in the annular region, and visualizing the scallops of the posterior mitral leaflet.

LONGITUDINAL IMAGING

In the longitudinal plane, one can obtain primary and secondary longitudinal scans. Whereas anteflexion and retroflexion are the maneuvers used most often in the horizontal plane, axial rotation and lateral movement of the transducer are the most common maneuvers for optimizing anatomic delineation in the longitudinal plane.

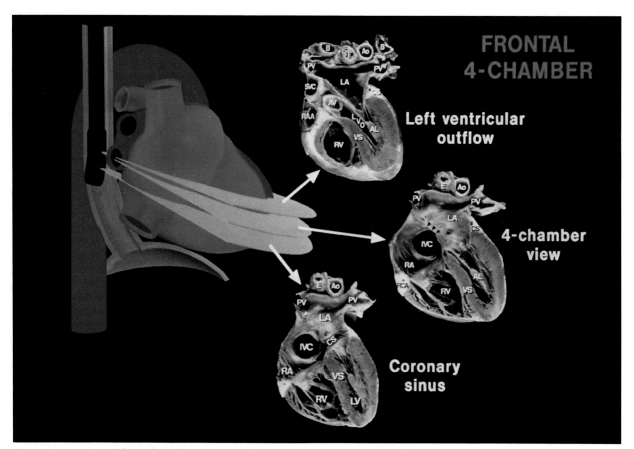

Fig. 3-11. Frontal four-chamber views in horizontal plane. These scans can be obtained with the transducer at 25 to 30 cm from the incisor teeth. Anteflexion provides the view with the left ventricular outflow tract. Retroflexion and extreme retroflexion provide the true four-chamber view and the view with coronary sinus, respectively. *Left ventricular outflow view:* Anatomic section cut along the frontal four-chamber plane shows the left ventricular outflow tract, left ventricle from base toward apex (note that the true apex may not be seen in all cases), anterolateral papillary muscle, aortic valve, left atrium, and mitral valve and its support structures. *Four-chamber view:* Anatomic specimen cut along the frontal four-chamber view shows the internal cardiac crux: atrial septum with membrane of the fossa ovalis *(black arrowheads),* ventricular septum, septal leaflet of the tricuspid valve, and the septal attachment of the anterior mitral leaflet. Note that the mitral valve inserts higher than the tricuspid valve. The anterolateral papillary muscle, coronary sinus, right atrium, right ventricle, right coronary artery in cross section, and inferior vena cava entering the right atrium are shown. *Coronary sinus view:* Anatomic section is cut along the plane of the four-chamber view but far posterior, which is why the left-sided chambers are largely excluded. The coronary sinus courses in the atrioventricular groove and enters the right atrium at the lower margin of the atrial septum. (*PV* = pulmonary vein.)

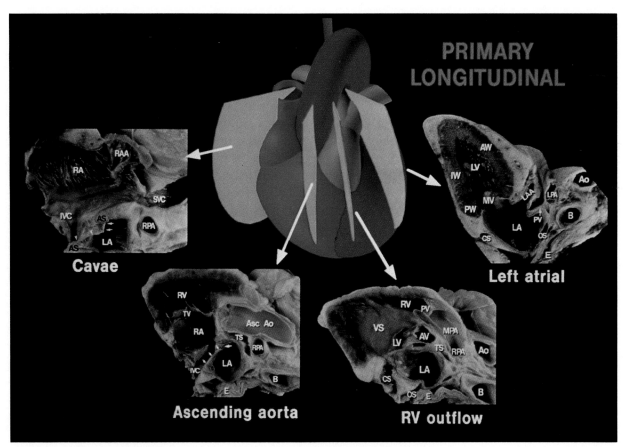

Fig. 3-12. Primary longitudinal views. Primary longitudinal views are obtained sequentially by rotating the transducer from the left to the right while maintaining gentle anteflexion. The corresponding anatomy is shown in this figure. The images generated from these views are comparable with those obtained by transthoracic echocardiography. *Left ventricular–left atrial two-chamber view:* Anatomic section is cut along the plane of the longitudinal left ventricular and left atrial chambers. The esophagus lies posterior to the left atrium. The left atrial appendage and entry of the left upper pulmonary vein *(PV, arrow)* into the left atrium are seen in this view. The mitral valve orifice is transected in the sagittal plane, as is the left ventricle. The posterior wall of the left ventricle is well seen. *Right ventricular outflow view:* The long axis of the right ventricular outflow tract is seen in this view. The right ventricle, pulmonary valve *(PV),* and main pulmonary artery are seen. Note the transverse sinus. *Ascending aorta view:* The proximal ascending aorta is partially visualized in this view. The atrial septum *(small arrows)* and valve of the fossa ovalis *(large arrow)* are also seen. Posterior to the ascending aorta is the right pulmonary artery in short axis. *Cavae view:* The posteriorly located esophagus is posterior to rightward component of the left atrium. The long axis of the superior vena cava, atrial septum, membrane of fossa ovalis *(arrowheads),* valve of fossa ovalis *(arrows),* and inferior vena cava are seen in this view. Also visualized is the right atrial appendage.

Primary Longitudinal Views

Primary longitudinal views (Fig. 3-12) can be obtained with the transducer tip 25 to 30 cm from the incisors. With the transducer in the neutral position, a sequence of tomographic sections can be obtained by rotation of the TEE transducer from the left side of the heart toward the right side. These images are in the sagittal plane of the thorax but are oblique to the heart. The TEE transducer needs to be advanced or withdrawn to image more inferior or superior structures lying in the same sagittal plane. The left ventricular and left atrial two-chamber view, right ventricular outflow long-axis view, ascending aorta and atrial septum view, and caval, right atrial, and atrial septal views are obtained in sequence on axial rotation of the transducer from the left to the right side of the heart. Aside from transducer rotation, usually only minor degrees of additional probe manipulation are required to obtain this series of imaging planes.

The left ventricular and left atrial view is ideal for longitudinal examination of the left atrial appendage, left pulmonary veins, and anterior and inferior walls of the left ventricle. This view is also very useful for assessment of abnormalities of the mitral leaflets and support apparatus; semiquantitative color Doppler estimation of mitral regurgitation when both planes are analyzed is significantly enhanced compared with single-plane imaging alone (see Chapter 9).

Rotating the TEE transducer to the right reveals the right ventricular outflow view, enabling full visualization of the right ventricular outflow tract, pulmonary valve, and main and proximal pulmonary arteries. This view is helpful in the assessment of congenital anomalies of the right ventricular outflow tract and for the detection of proximal pulmonary thromboembolism.

Further rotation of the TEE transducer to the right permits visualization of the ascending aorta view. Slight transducer manipulation can usually image the entire aortic root and ascending aorta in continuum (secondary longitudinal long-axis view). Withdrawal of the probe a short distance with slight anteflexion often brings the entire ascending arch into view (eliminating the "blind spot," previously a problem with monoplane horizontal imaging). Aortic dissection localized to the proximal portions of the aortic root is best delineated in this imaging plane. Posterior to the ascending aorta is the right pulmonary artery transected in short axis. This view also images the right atrium, right ventricle, and tricuspid valve. Tricuspid regurgitant jets are often directed medially toward the transducer in this view, allowing excellent angles of trajectory for steerable continuous-wave Doppler interrogation and, hence, calculation of right ventricular systolic pressures.

Rotation further to the right procures the caval and atrial septal view, showing the superior vena cava in long axis, which lies to the right of, and adjacent to, the ascending aorta. The left atrium is adjacent to the transducer. The fatty limbus of the atrial septum and fossa ovalis membrane separates the right and left atrial cavities. Anteriorly, the right atrium and the right atrial appendage are seen in sagittal cross section. The eustachian valve and the proximal portion of the inferior vena cava can be imaged adjacent to the sector apex by advancing the TEE probe a little farther in this plane. The superior vena cava view is commonly used during contrast echocardiography for detection of patent foramen ovale. Atrial septal defects are best delineated in this view. Small sinus venosus defects located in the posterosuperior atrial septum that may be missed on monoplane imaging are readily demonstrated on longitudinal examination in this view. This longitudinal plane also facilitates evaluation of atrial masses and thrombi (see Chapter 12).

Secondary Longitudinal Views

The longitudinal array can be reoriented from the sagittal plane of the thorax to planes that are in the long or short axis of the heart (Fig. 3-13). This manipulation necessitates some leftward or rightward flexion of the transducer tip. Leftward flexion results in the long-axis view of the heart, which permits visualization of the left ventricular outflow tract in the long axis. To optimize the view, one may need to concomitantly rotate the tip medially, keeping the leftward flexion (lateral rotation) knob in a held position and rotating the entire probe medially to avoid losing the image. The tip is then released from lateral flexion and from the neutral position; rightward flexion and lateral rotation bring out the short axis of the aortic valve. This view is analogous to a parasternal short-axis transthoracic imaging plane, and it is very important for the morphologic assessment of the aortic valve and semiquantitation of aortic regurgitation. This view also images the right ventricular outflow tract.

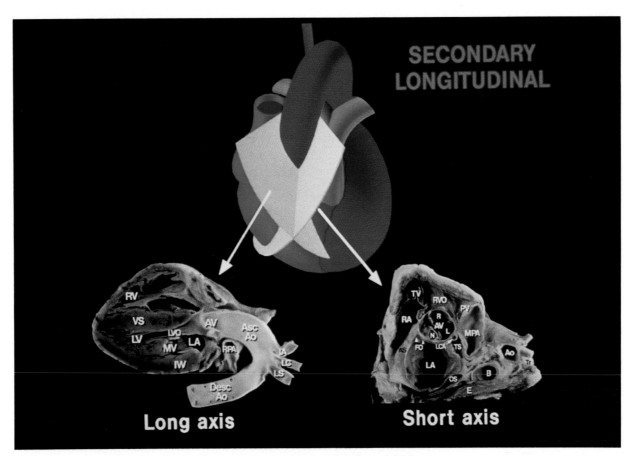

Fig. 3-13. Secondary longitudinal views are obtained with left or right flexion of the transducer tip at the mid-esophageal level. The corresponding anatomy is shown in this figure. *Long axis:* Leftward flexion of the tip of the TEE transducer places the longitudinal plane in the long axis of the left ventricular outflow. The left ventricle, aortic valve, and aortic root can be visualized in the long axis. This view is comparable to the parasternal long-axis view obtained from transthoracic echocardiography. *Short axis:* Rightward flexion of the tip of the TEE transducer places the longitudinal plane in the short axis relative to the aortic valve. This view is comparable to the conventional short-axis view obtained from transthoracic echocardiography. All three cusps of the aortic valve are well seen in this view. (*L* = left coronary cusp; *LCA* = left coronary artery; *N* = noncoronary cusp; *PV* = pulmonary valve; *R* = right coronary cusp.)

TRANSGASTRIC VIEWS

For transgastric views (Fig. 3-14), the transducer is advanced in the neutral position to approximately 40 cm from the incisors, at which point it is in the fundus of the stomach. By anteflexing the transducer, the examiner can scan in short axis from the apices of the left and right ventricles to the level of the atrioventricular valves in the horizontal plane. Images are oriented to show the anterior structures at the top and the left-sided structures toward the right of the screen. This orientation is similar to that obtained by transthoracic echocardiography, and it is our belief that the TEE learning curve for the echocardiologist is shorter when the images are oriented in this way. These views are useful for evaluation of left ventricular and right ventricular segmental and global systolic function. Evaluation of the mitral valve in short axis allows one to identify leaflet scallops that are prolapsing in patients undergoing mitral valve repair, aiding the surgeon in planning the type of repair procedure.

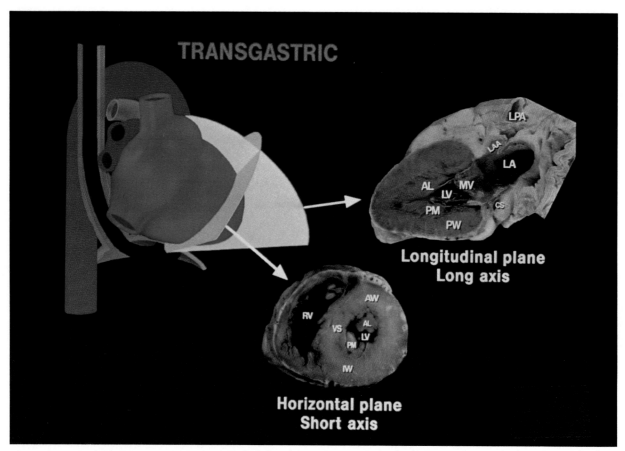

Fig. 3-14. Transgastric views. The TEE transducer is advanced into the fundus of the stomach in a neutral position. By anteflexing the transducer, one can obtain the short-axis view of the left ventricle and right ventricle. Degrees of anteflexion and return to almost neutral position allow imaging of the short axis at three or more levels. Shown in the figure is the anatomic specimen cut along the view that would be obtained at the level of the papillary muscles in the horizontal plane. The longitudinal plane permits evaluation of the heart in a format similar to that obtained by transthoracic echocardiography in the parasternal long-axis view. One such view is shown in this figure. Clockwise rotation brings into view the right ventricular outflow tract. (*AL* = anterolateral papillary muscle; *PM* = posteromedial papillary muscle.)

Switching to the longitudinal plane at the transgastric level yields a view similar to the parasternal long-axis view obtained from the transthoracic approach. This view permits evaluation of the inferior and anterior left ventricular walls, both papillary muscles, and the mitral valve. By clockwise rotation of the probe, the right ventricular inflow view can be obtained, permitting evaluation of the ventricular inflow tract, tricuspid valve, and chordae.

All the views mentioned above can be obtained in most patients whether they are supine or in the left lateral decubitus position. An unusual view that can be obtained about 50% of the time in the horizontal plane is achieved by advancing the transducer farther into the stomach and then anteflexing the transducer about 50 degrees. This view is akin to the four-chamber view with the left ventricular outflow tract visualized, the atria being at the top of the screen. This view allows anatomic visualization of the mitral apparatus, left ventricular outflow tract, aortic valve, and all four cardiac chambers. This same view permits the optimal continuous-wave Doppler interrogation of the left ventricular outflow tract and aortic valve by TEE.

EXAMINATION OF THE AORTA

Posterior rotation of the transducer enables visualization of the descending thoracic aorta. Detailed examination of the entire thoracic aorta is described in Chapter 14.

SAFETY OF TEE

Training Requirements

One of the most dangerous elements of performing any procedure is the error caused by misdiagnosis. This can be avoided if the procedure is undertaken by properly trained individuals. In 1987, the American Society of Echocardiography published recommendations for the training of physicians who take responsibility for the conduct and interpretation of echocardiographic studies [46]. That document recognized that echocardiography represents a family of rapidly evolving diagnostic techniques and that special expertise is likely to prove necessary for specialized applications. Recently, the American Society of Echocardiography published guidelines for training in TEE [47]. The minimal components believed necessary for developing and maintaining proficiency are listed in Table 3-2. They are intended to serve as guidelines and not to reflect a mandate to restrict or restrain growth or use of this technique. The cognitive and technical skills needed to perform TEE, also outlined in this position paper, are listed in Table 3-3.

There is no debate about who should perform TEE: only a trained echocardiologist. It is recommended that the cardiologist who wants to learn TEE should have at minimum completed level II training in transthoracic echocardiography [47].

Skills in introduction of the TEE probe are usually best acquired by first working with a gastroenterologist who is expert at endoscopic procedures. Alternatively, a fully trained echocardiologist could be the source of training in intubation techniques. Knowledge of oropharyngeal and esophageal anatomy, the physiology of deglutition, and the contraindications to performing a TEE examination is a prerequisite to beginning training.

Manipulation of the TEE transducer needs to be mastered in the learning phase of the procedure. One must practice with the actual transducer the maneuvers of flexion, extension, and lateral rotation and learn which knob movements control these motions before performing a patient examination. Videotapes, literature articles, and interactive computer-simulated programs help the trainee learn these skills before an examination is performed. Most of the available teaching material provide a comprehensive review of these skills [8,40,48].

Training requirements for anesthesiologists are currently being formulated, and they are likely to vary from institution to institution (see Chapter 16). As yet, no guidelines exist for training intensive care specialists, emergency and trauma physicians, and cardiovascular surgeons, but we believe that the requirements should be tailored to the use that the specific subspecialty intends to make of TEE in its practice. Essentially, to be fully trained to do diagnostic TEE studies, one must adhere to the guidelines proposed by the American Society of Echocardiography [47]. However, TEE training can be abbreviated for anesthesiologists if the only function to be carried out is intraoperative monitoring of left ventricular function without any additional diagnostic evaluation. It cannot be overemphasized that a team approach, including the anesthesiologist, echocardiologist, and surgeon, is essential when TEE is used in the operating room (see Chapter 16).

Contraindications

It is important to recognize patients in whom TEE is contraindicated either absolutely or relatively because of underlying conditions (Tables 3-4 and 3-5).

TEE examination is absolutely contraindicated in patients with an esophageal neoplasm, stricture, laceration, or perforation. Since TEE probe introduction and manipulation are not guided by direct esophageal visualization, patients with Zenker's diverticulum or other esophageal diverticula should not undergo TEE. Recent esophageal or gastric surgery may also be a relative or even an absolute contraindication to TEE, depending on the type of procedure and its proximity to the timing of TEE examination.

Esophageal varices and active but contained upper gastrointestinal bleeding from other lesions are only relative contraindications for TEE. To our knowledge, rupture of esophageal varices has not been reported as a complication of TEE examination. However, one should always be gentle, both with the insertion of the TEE probe and during probe

Table 3-2. Recommended training components for developing and maintaining skills in transesophageal echocardiography

Component	Objective	Duration	No. of cases (approx.)
General echocardiography, level II [46]	Background needed for performance and interpretation	6 months or equivalent	300
Esophageal intubation	TEE probe introduction	Variable	25
TEE examination	Skills in TEE performance and interpretation	Variable	50
Ongoing education	Maintenance of competence	Annual	50–75

Source: AS Pearlman, JM Gardin, RP Martin, et al. Guidelines for physician training in transesophageal echocardiography: recommendations of the American Society of Echocardiography Committee for Physician Training in Echocardiography. *J Am Soc Echocardiogr* 1992; 5: 187–94.

Table 3-3. Skills needed to perform transesophageal echocardiography

Cognitive skills

    Knowledge of appropriate indications, contraindications, and risks of TEE

    Understanding of differential diagnostic considerations in each clinical case

    Knowledge of physical principles of echocardiographic image formation and blood flow velocity measurement

    Familiarity with the operation of the ultrasonographic instrument, including the function of all controls affecting the quality of the data displayed

    Knowledge of normal cardiovascular anatomy, as visualized tomographically

    Knowledge of alterations in cardiovascular anatomy resulting from acquired and congenital heart diseases

    Knowledge of normal cardiovascular hemodynamics and fluid dynamics

    Knowledge of alterations in cardiovascular hemodynamics and blood flow resulting from acquired and congenital heart diseases

    Understanding of component techniques for general echocardiography and TEE, including when to use these methods to investigate specific clinical questions

    Ability to distinguish adequate from inadequate echocardiographic data and to distinguish an adequate from an inadequate TEE examination

    Knowledge of other cardiovascular diagnostic methods for correlation with TEE findings

    Ability to communicate examination results to patient, other health care professionals, and medical record

Technical skills

    Proficiency in performing a complete standard echocardiographic examination, using all echocardiographic modalities relevant to the case

    Proficiency in safely passing the TEE transducer into the esophagus and stomach and in adjusting probe position to obtain the necessary tomographic images and Doppler data

    Proficiency in correctly operating the ultrasonographic instrument, including all controls affecting the quality of the data displayed

    Proficiency in recognizing abnormalities of cardiac structure and function as detected from the transesophageal and transgastric windows, in distinguishing normal from abnormal findings, and in recognizing artifacts

    Proficiency in performing qualitative and quantitative analysis of the echocardiographic data

    Proficiency in producing a cogent written report of the echocardiographic findings and their clinical implications

Source: AS Pearlman, JM Gardin, RP Martin, et al. Guidelines for physician training in transesophageal echocardiography: recommendations of the American Society of Echocardiography Committee for Physician Training in Echocardiography. *J Am Soc Echocardiogr* 1992; 5:187–94.

Table 3-4. Absolute contraindications to transesophageal echocardiography

Esophageal obstruction (stricture, neoplasm)
Esophageal fistula, laceration, or perforation
Esophageal diverticulum
Cervical spine instability

Table 3-5. Relative contraindications to transesophageal echocardiography

Recent gastroesophageal operation
Esophageal varices
Upper gastrointestinal bleeding
Atlantoaxial disease
Severe cervical arthritis
Unexplained symptoms of dysphagia or odynophagia

manipulation, in patients with esophageal varices. A diaphragmatic hernia may significantly hinder TEE imaging because of lack of transducer mucosal approximation and if large enough may be a relative contraindication to TEE.

Relative contraindications also include atlantoaxial disease and severe generalized cervical arthritis; TEE should never be performed if there is any question about the stability of the cervical spine. Patients who have received extensive radiation to the mediastinum also have an increased likelihood of abnormal anatomic distortion. This can cause significant diffi-

culty in probe manipulation within the esophagus and is a relative contraindication if the anatomy of the esophagus is not known. Unexplained significant esophageal symptoms, such as dysphagia and odynophagia, are also at least a relative contraindication to TEE before further evaluation.

If TEE is essential to patient management, it can be undertaken in most patients (without esophageal obstruction or disruption) with appropriate caution, even if relative contraindications are present. One must inform such patients of the added risks and proceed cautiously and carefully.

Complications

Although TEE is "semi-invasive," it is generally very safe. In two recent large studies, major complications were unusual (0.18% to 0.5%), and two deaths were reported [2,49]. One must anticipate complications, however, to avert them or deal with potential consequences. Complications can be related to the probe itself, the procedure, or the medications used during the procedure (Fig. 3-15).

Probe-Related Complications
Probe-related complications include thermal or pressure injuries, mechanical problems of the TEE probe, and compression of structures adjacent to the esophagus due to large probes. Thermal injuries have not been reported in the literature. On the contrary, there is evidence of the safety of TEE probe intubation in animals for up to 48 hours [50]. Animal studies have also shown that no deleterious effects

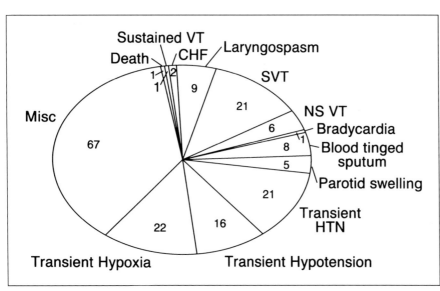

Fig. 3-15. Classification of 180 complications (3.3%) of TEE examinations encountered in the Mayo Clinic experience with 5,441 procedures between November 1987 and November 1992. Major complications included laryngospasm, sustained ventricular tachycardia, acute congestive heart failure (CHF), and one death.

or histologic abnormalities result from sustained pressure contact of the TEE probe with the esophagus [51]. However, one must view these results with reservation. Prolonged TEE probe intubation, such as that occurring during lengthy operations in patients who have gastroesophagitis or who are fully anticoagulated (such as during cardiopulmonary bypass procedures), rarely may lead to hemorrhage or Mallory-Weiss tears [52].

The most significant mechanical problem that has been reported with the TEE probe is buckling of the tip while the probe is in the esophagus. Four such cases have been reported in the literature [53]. All operators involved were experienced and noted uncomplicated initial probe introduction. In the course of the examination, however, the probe tip buckled over on itself, leading to difficulty in probe withdrawal. In these instances, the probe was safely removed after it was advanced into the stomach, where the buckled tip unfolded. The tips of the TEE probes in this report [53] were flaccid because of stretching and elongation of the steering cables. The examiner should be wary of signs that may indicate this malfunction, such as unusual mobility of the control knobs, imaging difficulty in the absence of a large diaphragmatic hernia, resistance to withdrawal of the probe, or finding a rotary control knob fixed in the maximally flexed position during examination. It is a good practice to routinely check the mechanism of the rotary controls after each examination, and if the tip is flaccid or the rotary controls are loose, the probe should be submitted for repair.

Probe-related compression of structures in the vicinity of the esophagus has been reported in children. In one such case, bronchial airway obstruction occurred in a 15-kg child studied with a 9-mm conventional echoscope [54]. This complication was noted during intraoperative TEE (see Chapter 16). Other complications believed to be due to the size of the TEE probe are pharyngeal pain, endoscopically confirmed esophageal erythema, and hypopharyngeal bleeding [55]. These problems occurred in children between the ages of 7 and 16 years during intraoperative applications of TEE with a probe 9 mm in diameter. No complications were reported in 25 children between the ages of 1 and 15 years when a smaller probe (5 mm in diameter) was used [56]. This observation serves to reinforce the belief that small probes are best suited for small-sized persons, and one should be cautious about using adult-sized transducers in small children (see Chapters 13 and

16). Transient vocal cord paralysis has also been reported as a complication of large TEE probes used in monitoring prolonged neurosurgical procedures with the patient in the upright position [57]. Most patients complain of a minor sore throat from probe irritation of the pharynx; administration of drying agents may increase the potential for such superficial mechanical irritation.

Procedure-Related Complications

Procedure-related complications include both ventricular and supraventricular arrhythmias, which are mainly brief, nonsustained, and self-limiting. However, infrequent episodes of hemodynamically significant ventricular or supraventricular tachycardia during TEE have been reported [2,40,49,58]. Supraventricular tachycardia can often be terminated by repositioning or removal of the TEE probe; antiarrhythmic agents are indicated only rarely. The rare event of ventricular tachycardia may also require pharmacologic intervention, but it is almost never sustained and usually ends once the probe is removed. A variety of bradyarrhythmias may occur because of vagal stimulation during TEE; these usually can be reversed with atropine or similar agents. In our experience, bradyarrhythmia complicating TEE has been quite rare. Perhaps the use of glycopyrrolate in approximately 82% of our patients may be acting as a deterrent to bradyarrhythmia because of the parasympatholytic properties of this agent.

Vomiting, nausea, and intolerance of the TEE probe are other minor complications related to the procedure. Generally, these problems do not preempt the examination. However, these symptoms often prompt a goal-directed examination rather than allowing a complete study. Blood-tinged oropharyngeal secretions are uncommon and are usually due to minor mucosal trauma. Pulmonary complications, such as bronchospasm, laryngospasm, and hypoxia, have also been reported in the literature [2,49]; they are largely related to the probe or the medication.

In our experience, transient hypotension, hypertension, and hypoxia have occurred in a small percentage (generally less than 0.5%) of patients undergoing TEE. None of these complications required the procedure to be aborted. However, supplemental oxygen via nasal cannula was necessary in patients with persistent hypoxia. The cumulative incidence of complications during TEE in our experience was 3.3%, including major and, in the vast majority of cases, minor complications (Fig. 3-15).

In the cooperative European experience involving 10,419 patients [49], the incidence of unsuccessful TEE probe introductions was 1.9%, whereas only 0.88% of examinations were interrupted before completion, primarily because of patient intolerance (72%). The incidence of significant respiratory compromise or arrhythmias was 0.07% for each of these complications.

Laryngospasm associated with TEE is caused by instillation and aspiration of topical anesthetic spray, inadvertent endotracheal intubation, or significant hypopharyngeal irritation by the TEE probe. The typical presentation is transient loss of speech, subjective sensation of inability to get a full breath, stridor, or laryngeal wheezing. Auscultatory findings are localized to the upper airway and are not those of typical bronchospasm. This complication is not life-threatening and resolves in 15 to 20 minutes with oxygen administration. It can be avoided by gently anesthetizing the posterior pharynx and by refraining from deep insertion of the tongue blade and voluminous spraying of the local anesthetic to the posterior pharynx, especially during inspiration. In our experience, laryngospasm occurred in 0.2% of procedures.

Congestive heart failure can occur rarely in patients with preexisting severe cardiovascular compromise. In our series, the two patients in whom acute exacerbation of heart failure developed during TEE had severely reduced systolic function, and the acute event most likely was precipitated by failure to take prescribed medications during fasting before the procedure. Additionally, endogenous catecholamine stimulation or sedation could have contributed to the symptoms of worsening heart failure. Both of these patients responded to intravenous diuretic therapy.

Ventricular tachycardia can be life-threatening, especially if sustained by hemodynamic compromise. We have had one patient in whom this occurred, and the rhythm returned to normal sinus after the TEE probe was removed.

There has been one death (0.02%) in our cumulative experience with TEE. The patient was a 64-year-old obese woman with diabetes mellitus and recurrent episodes of pulmonary edema. The cause was unclear, and an exercise thallium study did not reveal evidence of myocardial ischemia. The quality of transthoracic echocardiographic examination was inadequate for evaluation of mitral insufficiency; hence, TEE was undertaken. The only premedication was 1.5 mg of midazolam. The TEE procedure itself was entirely uneventful and uncomplicated. Approximately 10 minutes after the TEE probe was removed, the patient became acutely dyspneic while getting dressed. Pulse oximetry revealed severe hypoxia, and ventricular tachycardia soon developed and rapidly deteriorated into ventricular fibrillation. Prolonged resuscitation attempts were unsuccessful. At autopsy, the esophagus, lungs, and pulmonary and coronary arteries were normal. There was cardiomegaly with moderate left ventricular hypertrophy, mild left ventricular dilatation, and moderate right ventricular dilatation. There was also microscopic evidence of active lymphocytic myocarditis involving the left ventricle and sinus node, which likely contributed to her death.

The European multicenter study [49] also reported one death. The patient had a malignant lung tumor that had infiltrated into the esophagus, and during introduction of the probe, laceration of the tumor resulted in massive hematemesis and subsequent death.

SUMMARY

Transesophageal echocardiography is a low-risk procedure that yields an enormous amount of clinically relevant information when used appropriately. A well-organized approach to the TEE examination is essential, and an organized biplanar examination can generally provide a detailed three-dimensional tomographic reconstruction of cardiovascular anatomy and pathology in almost all patients. Transesophageal echocardiographic studies should be performed only by trained echocardiologists fully cognizant not only of diagnostic interpretation but also of technique, potential complications, and contraindications to TEE.

REFERENCES

1. Seward JB, Labovitz AJ, Lewis JF, et al. Transesophageal echocardiography. *J Am Coll Cardiol* 1992;20:506.

2. Khandheria BK, Oh J. Transesophageal echocardiography: state-of-the art and future directions. *Am J Cardiol* 1992;69:61H–75H.

3. Haase FR, Brenner A. Esophageal diameters at various ages. *Arch Otolaryngol* 1963;77:119–22.

4. Gray LP. The mole technique for dilatation of oesophageal strictures. *Med J Aust* 1957;2:573–7.

5. Reed AP. Successful transesophageal echocardiography in an unsedated critically ill patient with superior laryngeal nerve blocks. *Am Heart J* 1991;122: 1472–4.

6. Gilman AG, Rall TW, Nies AS, Taylor P, eds. *Goodman and Gilman's Pharmacological Basis of Therapeutics,* 8th ed. New York: Pergamon Press, 1990.

7. Khandheria BK, Seward JB, Oh JK, Tajik AJ. Transesophageal echocardiography: technique and training (letter to the editor). *J Am Soc Echocardiogr* 1990;3:177–8.

8. Seward JB, Khandheria BK, Oh JK, et al. Transesophageal echocardiography: technique, anatomic correlations, implementation, and clinical applications. *Mayo Clin Proc* 1988;63:649–80.

9. Dundee JW, Halliday NJ, Loughran PG, Harper KW. The influence of age on the onset of anaesthesia with midazolam. *Anaesthesia* 1985;40:441–3.

10. Amrein R, Hetzel W. Pharmacology of drugs frequently used in the ICUs: midazolam and flumazenil. *Intensive Care Med* 1991;17 Suppl 1:S1–S10.

11. Dajani AS, Bisno AL, Chung KJ, et al. Prevention of bacterial endocarditis: recommendations by the American Heart Association. *JAMA* 1990;264: 2919–22.

12. Steckelberg JM, Khandheria BK, Anhalt JP, et al. Prospective evaluation of the risk of bacteremia associated with transesophageal echocardiography. *Circulation* 1991;84:177–80.

13. Khandheria BK. Prophylaxis or no prophylaxis before transesophageal echocardiography? (Editorial.) *J Am Soc Echocardiogr* 1992;5:285–7.

14. Melendez LJ, Chan K-L, Cheung PK, Sochowski RA, Wong S, Austin TW. Incidence of bacteremia in transesophageal echocardiography: a prospective study of 140 consecutive patients. *J Am Coll Cardiol* 1991;18:1650–4.

15. Foster E, Kusumoto FM, Sobol SM, Schiller NB. Streptococcal endocarditis temporally related to transesophageal echocardiography. *J Am Soc Echocardiogr* 1990;3:424–7.

16. Görge G, Erbel R, Henrichs KJ, et al. Positive blood cultures during transesophageal echocardiography. *Am J Cardiol* 1990;65:1404–5.

17. Black IW, Hopkins AP, Lee LCL, et al. Role of transoesophageal echocardiography in evaluation of cardiogenic embolism. *Br Heart J* 1991;66:302–7.

18. Pearson AC, Labovitz AJ, Tatineni S, Gomez CR. Superiority of transesophageal echocardiography in detecting cardiac source of embolism in patients with cerebral ischemia of uncertain etiology. *J Am Coll Cardiol* 1991;17:66–72.

19. Daniel WG, Mügge A, Martin RP, et al. Improvement in the diagnosis of abscesses associated with endocarditis by transesophageal echocardiography. *N Engl J Med* 1991;324:795–800.

20. Klodas E, Edwards WD, Khandheria BK. Use of transesophageal echocardiography for improving detection of valvular vegetations in subacute bacterial endocarditis. *J Am Soc Echocardiogr* 1989; 2:386–9.

21. Mügge A, Daniel WG, Frank G, Lichtlen PR. Echocardiography in infective endocarditis: reassessment of prognostic implications of vegetation size determined by the transthoracic and the transesophageal approach. *J Am Coll Cardiol* 1989;14:631–8.

22. Khandheria BK, Seward JB, Oh JK, et al. Value and limitations of transesophageal echocardiography in assessment of mitral valve prostheses. *Circulation* 1991;83:1956–68.

23. Zamorano J, Erbel R, Mackowski T, et al. Usefulness of transesophageal echocardiography for diagnosis of mitral valve prolapse. *Am J Cardiol* 1992;69:419–22.

24. Castello R, Fagan L Jr, Lenzen P, et al. Comparison of transthoracic and transesophageal echocardiography for assessment of left-sided valvular regurgitation. *Am J Cardiol* 1991;68:1677–80.

25. Erbel R, Engberding R, Daniel W, et al. Echocardiography in diagnosis of aortic dissection. *Lancet* 1989;1:457–61.

26. Mohr-Kahaly S, Erbel R, Rennollet H, et al. Ambulatory followup of aortic dissection by transesophageal two-dimensional and color-coded Doppler echocardiography. *Circulation* 1989;80:24–33.

27. Karalis DG, Chandrasekaran K, Victor MF, et al. Recognition and embolic potential of intraaortic atherosclerotic debris. *J Am Coll Cardiol* 1991; 17:73–8.

28. Khandheria BK. Aortic dissection: the diagnostic dilemma resolved (editorial). *Chest* 1992;101: 303–4.

29. Mügge A, Daniel WG, Haverish A, Lichtlen PR. Diagnosis of noninfective cardiac mass lesions by two-dimensional echocardiography: comparison of the transthoracic and transesophageal approaches. *Circulation* 1991;83:70–8.

30. Reeder GS, Khandheria BK, Seward JB, Tajik AJ. Transesophageal echocardiography and cardiac masses. *Mayo Clin Proc* 1991;66:1101–9.

31. Stümper O, Sutherland GR, Geuskens R, et al. Transesophageal echocardiography in evaluation

and management after a Fontan procedure. *J Am Coll Cardiol* 1991;17:1152–60.

32. Stümper O, Witsenburg M, Sutherland GR et al. Transesophageal echocardiographic monitoring of interventional cardiac catheterization in children. *J Am Coll Cardiol* 1991;18:1506–14.

33. Stümper O. Transoesophageal echocardiography: a new diagnostic method in paediatric cardiology. *Arch Dis Child* 1991;66:1175–7.

34. Stümper O, Vargas-Barron J, Rijlaarsdam M, et al. Assessment of anomalous systemic and pulmonary venous connections by transoesophageal echocardiography in infants and children. *Br Heart J* 1991;66:411–8.

35. Oh JK, Seward JB, Khandheria BK, et al. Transesophageal echocardiography in critically ill patients. *Am J Cardiol* 1990;66:1492–5.

36. Jaarsma W, Visser CA, Suttorp MJ, et al. Transesophageal echocardiography during percutaneous balloon mitral valvuloplasty. *J Am Soc Echocardiogr* 1990;3:384–91.

37. Goldman AP, Irwin JM, Glover MU, Mick W, Penders J. Letter to the editor. *PACE* 1992;15:244.

38. Klein AL, Obarski TP, Stewart WJ, et al. Transesophageal Doppler echocardiography of pulmonary venous flow: a new marker of mitral regurgitation severity. *J Am Coll Cardiol* 1991; 18:518–26.

39. Iliceto S, Marangelli V, Memmola C, Rizzon P. Transesophageal Doppler echocardiography evaluation of coronary blood flow velocity in baseline conditions and during dipyridamole-induced coronary vasodilation. *Circulation* 1991;83:61–9.

40. Seward JB, Khandheria BK, Oh JK et al. Critical appraisal of transesophageal echocardiography: limitations, pitfalls, and complications. *J Am Soc Echocardiogr* 1992;5:288–305.

41. Smolin MR, Gorman PD, Gaither NS, Wortham DC. Origin of the right coronary artery from the left main coronary artery identified by transesophageal echocardiography. *Am Heart J* 1992;123:1062–5.

42. Yoshida K, Yoshikawa J, Hozumi T, et al. Detection of left main coronary artery stenosis by transesophageal color Doppler and two-dimensional echocardiography. *Circulation* 1990;81:1271–6.

43. Salloum JA, Thomas D, Evans J. Transoesophageal echocardiography in diagnosis of aberrant coronary artery. *Int J Cardiol* 1991;32:106–8.

44. Rubin DA, Zaki AM, Zaghlol S, et al. Visualization of coronary artery fistula with transesophageal echocardiography. *J Am Soc Echocardiogr* 1992;5: 173–5.

45. Pearce FB, Sheikh KH, deBruijn NP, Kisslo J. Imaging of the coronary arteries by transesophageal echocardiography. *J Am Soc Echocardiogr* 1989;2: 276–83.

46. Pearlman AS, Gardin JM, Martin RP, et al. Guidelines for optimal physician training in echocardiography: recommendations of the American Society of Echocardiography Committee for Physician Training in Echocardiography. *Am J Cardiol* 1987;60:158–63.

47. Pearlman AS, Gardin JM, Martin RP, et al. Guidelines for physician training in transesophageal echocardiography: recommendations of the American Society of Echocardiography Committee for Physician Training in Echocardiography. *J Am Soc Echocardiogr* 1992;5:187–94.

48. Seward JB, Khandheria BK, Edwards WD, et al. Biplanar transesophageal echocardiography: anatomic correlations, image orientation, and clinical applications. *Mayo Clin Proc* 1990;65:1193–213.

49. Daniel WG, Erbel R, Kasper W, et al. Safety of transesophageal echocardiography: a multicenter survey of 10,419 examinations. *Circulation* 1991; 83:817–21.

50. O'Shea JP, Southern JF, D'Ambra MN, et al. Effects of prolonged transesophageal echocardiographic imaging and probe manipulation on the esophagus—an echocardiographic-pathologic study. *J Am Coll Cardiol* 1991;17:1426–9.

51. Urbanowicz JH, Kernoff RS, Oppenheim G, et al. Transesophageal echocardiography and its potential for esophageal damage. *Anesthesiology* 1990;72: 40–3.

52. Dewhirst WE, Stragand JJ, Fleming BM. Mallory-Weiss tear complicating intraoperative transesophageal echocardiography in a patient undergoing aortic valve replacement. *Anesthesiology* 1990;73: 777–8.

53. Kronzon I, Cziner DG, Katz ES, et al. Buckling of the tip of the transesophageal echocardiography probe: a potentially dangerous technical malfunction. *J Am Soc Echocardiogr* 1992;5:176–7.

54. Gilbert TB, Panico FG, McGill WA, et al. Bronchial obstruction by transesophageal echocardiography probe in a pediatric cardiac patient. *Anesth Analg* 1992;74:156–8.

55. Cyran SE, Kimball TR, Schwartz DC, et al. Evaluation of balloon aortic valvuloplasty with transesophageal echocardiography. *Am Heart J* 1988;115: 460–2.

56. Stümper OFW, Elzenga NJ, Hess J, Sutherland GR. Transesophageal echocardiography in children with

congenital heart disease: an initial experience. *J Am Coll Cardiol* 1990;16:433–41.

57. Cucchiara RF, Nugent M, Seward JB, Messick JM. Air embolism in upright neurosurgical patients: detection and localization by two-dimensional transesophageal echocardiography. *Anesthesiology* 1984;60:353–5.

58. Chan K-L, Cohen GI, Sochowski RA, Baird MG. Complications of transesophageal echocardiography in ambulatory adult patients: analysis of 1500 consecutive examinations. *J Am Soc Echocardiogr* 1991;4:577–82.

Transesophageal Echocardiographic Anatomy

James B. Seward

IMAGE ORIENTATION

Ultrasound imaging is rapidly evolving toward more invasive applications [1] and three- and four-dimensional presentations [2–4]. The heart can be imaged from any direction and ultimately will be electronically extracted from the body for electronic vivisection [5]. Any recommendation for image orientation must be flexible enough to accommodate any technologic innovation. One should hold to the prerequisite that any anatomic presentation through imagery conform with prior standards and be corroborated by appropriate anatomic correlations.

Background

Standardization

Because ultrasound images are to be viewed by many users, including nonechocardiographers, the images obtained from the esophagus or, for that matter, from any transducer position must conform to familiar and established standards, such as those published by the American Society of Echocardiography (ASE) in 1980 [6] (Fig. 4-1). With each new technologic advance in echocardiography, including transesophageal echocardiography (TEE), one should not be tempted to create new image orientations. Echocardiographic images presented in unconventional orientations lead to spatial disorientation, lack of correlation, and inconsistency [7–19].

Anatomic Correlation

Anatomic correlations allow appreciation of out-of-plane as well as contiguous relationships. Any echocardiographic orientation must have *appropriate* anatomic corroborations [18,20–24]. Noncorresponding or mirror-image photography of cardiovascular anatomy only highlights the lack of anatomic understanding and validation [25] (Figs. 4-2 and 4-3). Artistic characterization of anatomy is also an unsuitable substitute unless it is faithfully drawn from the actual anatomic specimen and is not a reversed image of the specimen (Figs. 4-4 and 4-5).

Aesthetics

An aesthetic presentation of an image is also an important part of any image acquisition technique. Proper gain settings and optimal use of instrument controls are prerequisites. Likewise, the same image (e.g., long-axis view of the left ventricle), regardless of the transducer position from which it is obtained, should be displayed in a consistent orientation to maintain an aesthetically pleasing and familiar depiction of that anatomy [6]. The Standards Committee of the ASE in 1980 believed that "by adopting nomenclature and image orientation standards, the technique of two-dimensional imaging of the heart will be advanced and communication between laboratories improved"[6]. Therefore, our contention is

Several figures in this chapter are also in Seward JB, Khandheria BK, Freeman WK, et al. Multiplane transesophageal echocardiography: image orientation, examination technique, anatomic correlations, and clinical applications. *Mayo Clin Proc* 1993;68:523–51.

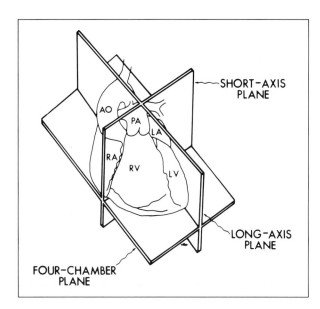

Fig. 4-1. Two-dimensional echocardiographic imaging planes: Diagram of the three orthogonal imaging planes of the heart used to visualize the heart with two-dimensional echocardiography. Note: In this original ASE document on standards (1980), designation of transducer position is not specified. The document only recommends tomographic presentation of cardiac structures, as follows: (1) the short axis is to be viewed from apex toward base, (2) the long axis is to be viewed from the left side toward the right, and (3) the four chambers can be viewed in two formats—option 1, apex down viewing from the anterior surface toward the posterior surface; and option 2, apex up viewing from the heart's posterior surface toward the anterior surface. Reproduced with permission from WL Henry, A DeMaria, R Gramiak, et al. Report of the American Society of Echocardiography Committee on Nomenclature and Standards in Two-Dimensional Echocardiography. *Circulation* 1980; 62:212–7. Copyright 1980 American Heart Association.)

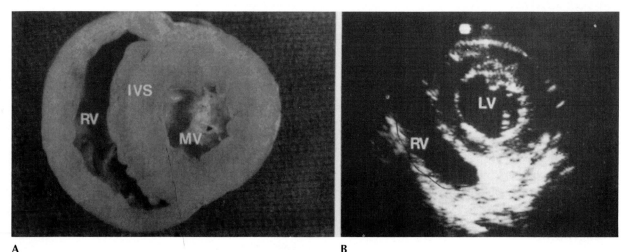

A   B

Fig. 4-2. Echocardiographic and anatomic correlation. An anatomic specimen and "corresponding echocardiographic image" are shown and imply a relationship. A. Note that the specimen is viewed from the ventricle looking toward the mitral valve and transected chordae. The right ventricle is to the viewer's left. As shown, the posterior wall of the heart would have to be at the bottom of the image. In the cardiac specimen thus cut, the specimen is looked at from apex toward base, corresponding to standards for short-axis echocardiographic views [6]. B. The "corresponding" TEE transgastric short-axis image places the posterior wall at the top of the image adjacent to the esophageal transducer. The right ventricle is to the viewer's left. Thus, in this "corresponding" echocardiogram, the heart is viewed from the base toward the apex, or just the opposite of the accompanying anatomy. The echocardiogram represents an orientation diametrically opposite to the previous anatomic standard. Additionally, there is no "corresponding" relationship of the anatomy and the image. (From SG Richardson, AR Weintraub, SL Schwartz, et al. Biplane transesophageal echocardiography utilizing transverse and sagittal imaging planes: technique, echo-anatomic correlations, and display approaches. *Echocardiography* 1991; 8:293–310. By permission of Futura Publishing Company.)

that a tomographic view, whether obtained from parasternal, suprasternal, subcostal, or esophageal transducer position, should be displayed in a similar manner to foster uniformity and communication among all persons requesting, performing, or interpreting echocardiograms.

An analogy is the presentation of posteroanterior and anteroposterior chest radiographs. Even though the x-ray beam (analogous to the echocardiographic transducer) is located posteriorly in the posteroanterior projection and anteriorly in the anteroposterior projection, by convention both images are presented with the same anatomic orientation (Fig. 4-6). It appears to be very inconsistent to view the heart during a surface echocardiogram in one orientation and then use the same ultrasound technology in TEE to view the heart in a totally different orientation (Figs. 4-7 and 4-8).

Comment

In the TEE literature, various arguments are advanced against the uniform approach to image orientation recommended in this text [26]. They include the following: (1) The electronic signal should always be at the top of the viewing screen; (2) with inverted electronics, the image appears out of focus; (3) "flip-flopping" the image requires additional concentration by the operator and slows performance of the examination; (4) basal heart structures should be placed to the right even if the heart is presented upside down; and (5) user preference. Each of these arguments falls far short of the primary objectives of uniform display of the image regardless of transducer position, multiuser understanding of images, and conformity to an accepted image format.

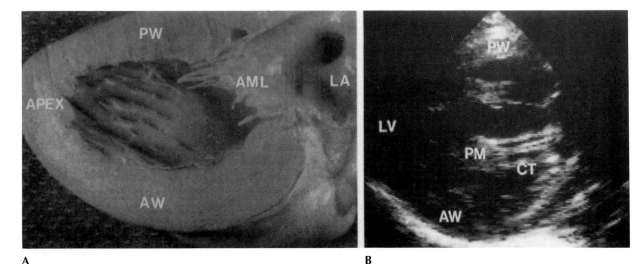

A   B

Fig. 4-3. "Sagittal plane imaging of the left heart from the transgastric window." A. The cardiac specimen is placed so that the posterior wall is at the top of the photograph and the anterior wall toward the bottom. The anterior leaflet of the mitral valve and transected chordae are also shown. Note at the bottom of the photograph that the bulk of the heart lies beyond the "anterior wall." (This portion of the heart, which is not labeled, is the right ventricular outflow tract.) Thus, the specimen is cut in such a way that the viewer is looking from the left side of the heart toward the right. To accomplish this impossibility (i.e., looking from the right side of the left ventricle and seeing the right heart), the authors have used negative reversal photography to portray the anatomy. B. The "corresponding" echocardiogram shows the same structures but represents a heart being viewed from the right side toward the left, a nonstandard presentation. The accompanying anatomy has no relationship to the echocardiogram except through the use of reversal photography. (From SG Richardson, AR Weintraub, SL Schwartz, et al. Biplane transesophageal echocardiography utilizing transverse and sagittal imaging planes: technique, echo-anatomic correlations, and display approaches. *Echocardiography* 1991; 8:293–310. By permission of Futura Publishing Company.)

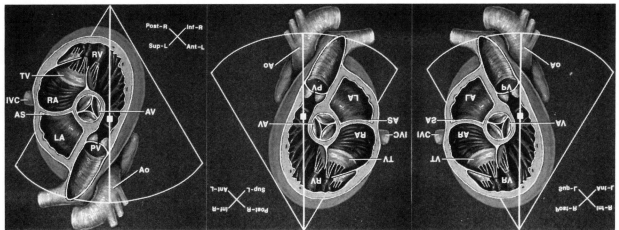

Fig. 4-4. ▲ Incorrect artistic characterization of anatomy. A common substitute for anatomic correlation is the drawing of anatomy to suit an intended correlation. If the anatomy is atypical, the artist may use composite images that result in anatomy that cannot exist in nature. Left: This anatomic drawing depicts a pulsed-wave Doppler sample volume in the right ventricular outflow tract. The illustration is shown as originally intended (courtesy of Advanced Technology Laboratories). Note: The aortic valve is depicted as though one were looking down on the valve (concave sinuses). However, the ascending aorta is in the far field as though one were looking from the cardiac apex toward the base. Center: The image has been rotated to place the apex downward. Now the aorta and pulmonary artery appear correct, and they suggest that the artist has simply drawn the aortic valve upside down. However, note that the right atrium is on the left side of the depiction (a reverse orientation of normal cardiac anatomy). Right: The illustration has been printed as a mirror-image reversal to show that the artist actually depicted the right atrium and right ventricle anatomy backward. However, note that the remaining anatomy now is incorrectly depicted. Thus, with each segment of the heart, the artist has used composite artistry in an attempt to illustrate an unfamiliar anatomic orientation. This type of anatomic depiction does not exist in nature and is not a substitute for faithful anatomic correlation. (*PV* = pulmonary valve.) (From an ATL Doppler exhibit. By permission of Advanced Technology Laboratories.)

Fig. 4-5. ▶ An anatomic drawing of the four-chamber view of the heart. Left: Note the position of the inferior vena cava in the floor of the right atrium and the pulmonary veins in the floor of the left atrium. However, if this were a correct depiction of the apex-up four-chamber view (option 2), in which the heart is viewed from the posterior surface toward the anterior surface, the vena cava and pulmonary veins should not exit from the anterior surface of the heart. Right: This is a negative reversal of the drawing, with the apex down, which shows that the artist had actually drawn the apex-down four-chamber view (option 1) [6]. Thus, the artist had drawn correct anatomy for a familiar anatomic orientation. The resultant drawing, however, was displayed in an orientation depicting the heart in a manner that does not exist in nature, namely, with the great veins arising from the anterior surface of the heart. This drawing represents the use of negative reversal artistry. (From PN Yu and JF Goodwin. *Progress in Cardiology.* 8. Philadelphia: Lea & Febiger, 1979:1–128. Used with permission of the publisher.)

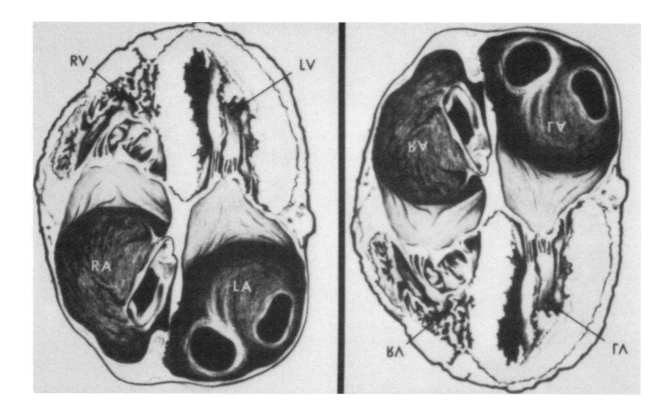

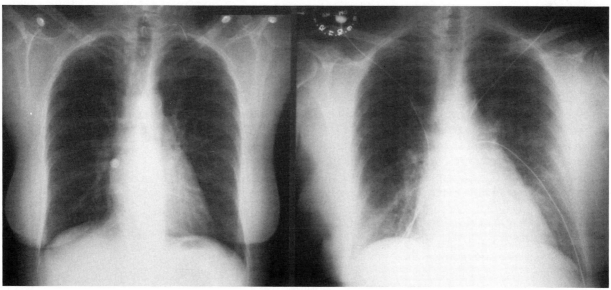

Fig. 4-6. Posteroanterior (left) and anteroposterior (right) chest radiographs. Even though the technique and image magnification of the near and far fields are different, the anatomic depiction of the chest radiograph is shown with the same orientation (i.e., the same anatomy is displayed in a similar manner regardless of the imaging beam direction). This is comparable to precordial (i.e., anteroposterior) and esophageal (i.e., posteroanterior) echocardiography.

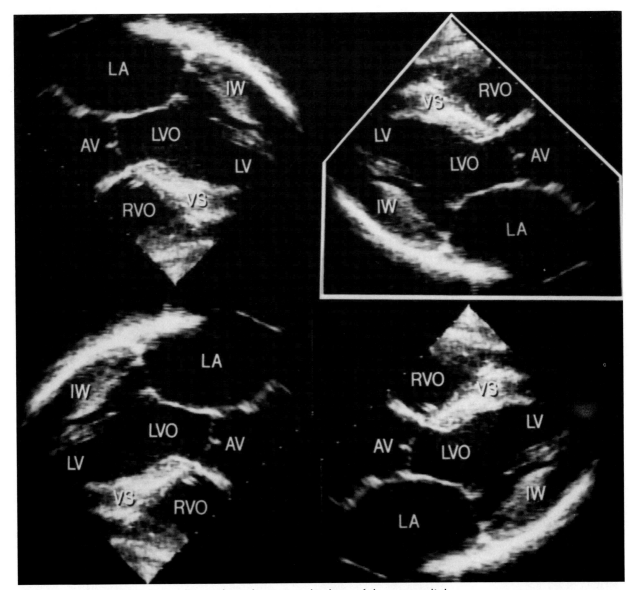

Fig. 4-7. Precordial echocardiography: Alternative displays of the precordial long-axis view of the left ventricle. Upper right: This highlighted image is the recommended display orientation [3] for a parasternal long-axis view. The heart is viewed as though one were looking from the left surface toward the right. All alternative views are described in relation to this familiar standard. Upper left: A 180-degree rotation of the standard long-axis view. This view has never been used in precordial echocardiography; however, some TEE laboratories prefer this orientation because it is "a more familiar surgical view of the heart" (i.e., the basal structures to the examiner's left) [5]. However, the patient would be lying face downward. Lower right: A mirror-image reversal of the standard long-axis view. The cardiac anatomy is thus viewed from its right surface toward the left. Early in the history of echocardiography, this view was used because it portrays the heart more like a right anterior oblique ventriculogram. This image orientation, however, has now been abandoned. Lower left: A mirror-image view of the standard precordial long axis (lower right illustration), which has been rotated 180 degrees. The heart is viewed from its right surface toward the left. This image orientation was not used before the advent of TEE. Many TEE investigators use this view because it retains the transducer artifact at the top of the image and orients the apex to the left and base to the right.

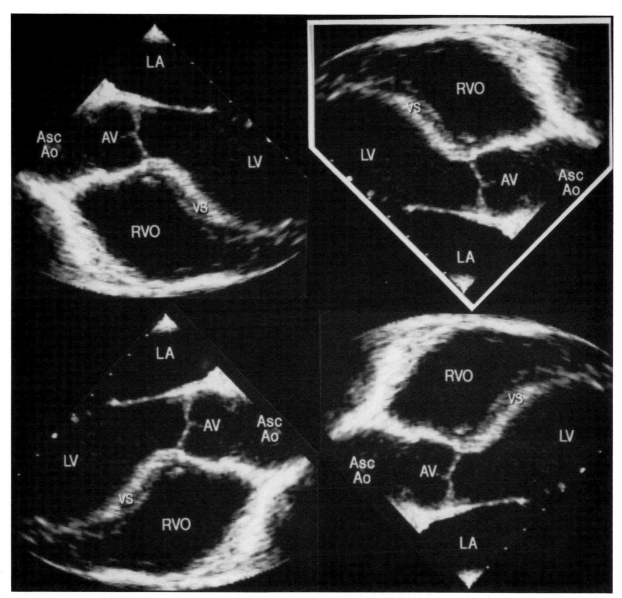

Fig. 4-8. Transesophageal echocardiography: Alternative displays of the transesophageal long-axis view of the left ventricle (135 degrees). This series of images is the same as that in Figure 4-7 except that the images are obtained from the esophagus. Upper right: This highlighted image orientation is identical to the precordial long-axis view in the upper right of Figure 4-7. This view corresponds to the original standards proposed by the ASE [3] for displaying a long-axis view of the left ventricle. Upper left and lower right: The alternative displays are identical to those of the precordial examination (see Fig. 4-7); however, these images were obtained from the esophagus. Lower left: A mirror image of a standard long-axis view rotated 180 degrees. Many echocardiographers use this image orientation when performing TEE. The heart is viewed from its right surface toward the left, and the posterior wall is at the top of the video image. This image orientation has no recognizable counterpart in the echocardiographic literature.

History

Society Recommendations

The original ASE recommendations on orientation of echocardiographic images [6] were largely based on the preferences of the recommending committee members, prevailing electronic constraints, and previous publications [27,28]. The intent, however, was to develop a standard approach to tomographic dissection of the heart. Anatomic correlations and validation had been presented for all major planes [27]. In the standards document [6], the cardiac planes presented did not designate a particular echocardiographic transducer position (see Fig. 4-1). The recommendations were flexible and were intended to be applied to all cardiac ultrasound tomographic imaging.

Long Axis

Views are imaged from the heart's left surface toward the right (Fig. 4-9). Basal structures are rightward, the cardiac apex is leftward, anterior structures are at the top of the video screen, and posterior structures are at the bottom of the video screen. The ASE Standards Committee elected to display the tomographic image of the heart with the patient in a recumbent position to better simulate the position of a cardiac examination, operation, or other procedure. Early ultrasound literature presented other approaches, but these options were ultimately dropped to conform to the ASE standard.

Four-Chamber View

In the original ASE document, there were two options for the frontal "four-chamber plane" (see Fig. 4-9). Option 1, apex-down, was perceived as aesthetically pleasing and corresponded more closely to the surgeon's view of the open thorax and to existing anatomic sections and drawings [29]. The option 1 format views the heart from its frontal surface toward the posterior surface. With apex down, left-sided structures are to the viewer's right and basal structures are at the top of the viewing screen.

A second option (option 2) was proposed because

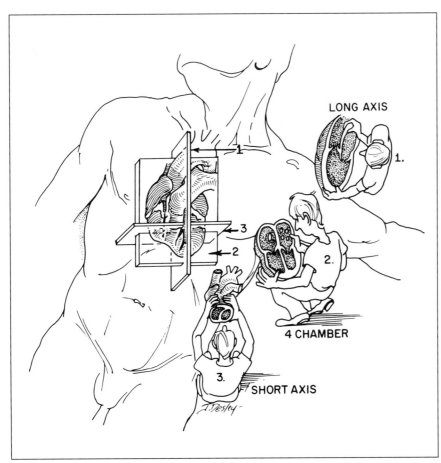

Fig. 4-9. Characterization of the recommended orientation for tomographic planes of the heart. The heart can be cut in three primary planes: (1) long-axis, (2) four-chamber, and (3) short-axis. Note that there is no designation of transducer position. Also note that the patient is depicted recumbent, as though lying on an examination table (e.g., for catheterization, physical examination, operation). 1. In the long-axis anatomy and accompanying tomographic image, the heart is viewed from left to right. 2. The four-chamber plane is easiest to appreciate with the apex down (i.e., ASE option 1). In option 2, apex up, the heart is viewed from the posterior of the patient's chest anteriorly. 3. Short-axis views are presented as though one were looking from the cardiac apex toward the base.

the ultrasound electronics could not be inverted in the two-dimensional ultrasound machines available at that time (1976–1980) [28]. This presentation views the heart from its posterior surface toward the anterior surface and puts the cardiac apex at the top of the viewing screen.

Once electronic image inversion became available, some laboratories and most congenital disease echocardiographers began to place the image consistently in the option 1 format with apex downward [23]. It is also interesting that an ASE paper on TEE states that "the four-chamber view should appear with the apex down and the left ventricle to the viewer's right" (i.e., option 1) [10]. This paper did not include an apex-up option.

Short Axis

The recommendation is to view the heart from the apex looking toward the base (see Fig. 4-9). Left-sided structures are to the viewer's right, right-sided structures are on the viewer's left, and anterior structures are oriented toward the top of the viewing screen. Tomographic anatomic cuts of the heart at the time sliced the heart opposite to the ultrasound recommendation and viewed the specimen from base toward apex. Now, however, pathologists [30,31], in deference to the echocardiographic community, orient the tomographic anatomic sections from the apex looking toward the base of the heart.

Heart or Electronic Orientation?

The electronics are a convenient marker designated by the transducer burst. Such an electronic signal at the upper portion of the video screen is often referred to as the top of the image. However, the electronics do not represent the orientation of the heart. With the evolution of a unique echocardiographic imaging technology such as TEE, it seems more appropriate to reemphasize the orientation of the heart and not the electronic signal. Consistency of cardiac presentation, as opposed to electronics, makes more sense for standardization and anatomic correlation.

Recommendation

The intent is to foster an organized and consistent orientation of the heart and not abdicate to the electronic constraints of technology. The anatomic planes of the heart should ideally be displayed in an identical manner regardless of transducer posi-

tion. In the correlations that follow, the displays of the three planes of the heart are identical to those recommended by the ASE [6] (see Fig. 4-1). The transducer artifact must be oriented at the bottom of the video screen (with the esophageal transducer being posterior to the heart) for all TEE views. The only exception is that if option 1, apex-down, four-chamber imaging is preferred, the image has to be inverted.

Consistency

When both precordial echocardiography and TEE are used, a far-field structure today may be a near-field structure tomorrow and, similarly, a transducer anterior to the heart can now be positioned posterior to the heart. Transducers are now also being placed within the cardiac chambers or vascular system. One should avoid temptations to create new tomographic orientations for each new technologic advancement. Any proposed image presentation should represent a consistent approach to image orientation. All techniques must go through a trial period, but the ultimate recommendation must be a critical and academic appraisal based on sound standards and anatomic references. Three-dimensional volume images electronically dissected in a tomographic format should also be displayed in a similar and consistent manner [5].

Future

Multiplane and three-dimensional imaging are innovations that will increasingly come into clinical practice in the near future. The object of these innovations is to image the heart. The specific imaging modality or immediate electronic constraint should not determine the presentation or dissection of the heart. The heart is the object to which standardization must be focused. If the heart is to be dissected by imaging in tomographic fashion, the presentation of the views should be consistent with previous dissections.

ANATOMIC CORRELATIONS

Depiction of Cardiovascular Anatomy

The first and most dominant application of ultrasound has been the acquisition of high-quality images without ionizing radiation, at comparatively low cost, and with portable instrumentation. Transesophageal echocardiography has greatly expanded the capability of echocardiography by obtaining high-quality, high-resolution images in nearly every circumstance. Transesophageal echocardiography images the heart from its posterior surface toward the anterior surface from a transducer positioned intimately adjacent to the posterior cardiac chambers.

In addition to being semi-invasive and requiring direct physician involvement, TEE has necessitated a major learning experience of the presentation of unusual and unfamiliar tomographic cardiovascular and thoracic anatomy. Because of this complex presentation, we have recommended an echocardiographic orientation format identical to that recommended by the ASE for transthoracic echocardiography [6]. Because the TEE transducer is posterior to the heart rather than anterior, the transducer artifact is routinely placed at the bottom of the viewing screen. This position maintains cardiac orientation identical to that of the precordial views, including an apex-up, four-chamber view that may be preferably reformatted in the apex-down orientation. We have found that a familiar imaging orientation fosters more rapid learning of TEE imaging planes.

In this chapter, we do not specifically distinguish among comparable images obtained by monoplane, biplane, and multiplane TEE. With each technology, there is an incremental increase in available tomographic planes. However, the basic planes for anatomic correlation remain the same: short (horizontal or transverse), long (longitudinal), and frontal (four-chamber).

Monoplane TEE can most easily obtain frontal (four-chamber) and short-axis views of the heart with a transverse array (perpendicular to the long axis or the endoscope) (Fig. 4-10). Only limited longitudinal views are obtainable and usually require considerable manipulation of the monoplane transducer tip. Biplanar imaging incorporates both transverse and longitudinal array transducers. Most biplane transducers are composed of two sets of elements stacked one above the other, with the horizontal array most distal on the endoscope shaft. The operator electronically switches from one plane to the other. A matrix biplane transducer allows simultaneous biplane image acquisition. Access to all three anatomic planes of the heart with biplane TEE increases available information by approximately 30% over that from a monoplane endoscope [12].

Because the biplane endoscope has a substantial advantage over the monoplane, it has rapidly supplanted the monoplane device in our TEE practice (Fig. 4-11).

Multiplane TEE involves a single transducer, either phased-array or mechanical, that can be rotated 180 degrees around the long axis of the ultrasound beam. The advantage is the ability to obtain all off-axis planes between the primary orthogonal tomographic planes of section (see Chapter 5).

Planes in TEE Imaging

The basics of the TEE imaging technique [9] have been described in Chapter 3. The sophistication of TEE has changed considerably since the introduction of this imaging modality. The emphasis of This presentation is anatomic correlation of tomographic echocardiographic views of the heart and great vessels as currently obtained during the TEE examination.

Primary Anatomic Planes of Body and Heart

All three-dimensional objects have three primary planes: (1) horizontal (short or transverse), (2) sagittal (longitudinal or long), and (3) frontal, or, in cardiac ultrasonography, four-chamber. A complete tomographic imaging device must be able to address all three primary planes of the object in question.

Individual parts of the body (e.g., the heart) are often spatially oriented differently to one another. The three primary planes of the heart do not lie in the same orientation as the body's three primary planes (Fig. 4-12). Thus, when describing the orientation of an imaging ultrasound array, one must mention not only the plane of orientation to the heart but also the plane to the body or other referenced organs (e.g., thoracic aorta and esophagus).

Transducer Plane

Current transducers are of two types, fixed and rotatable (see Fig. 4-10). The fixed arrays have two orientations to the long axis of the endoscope, transverse and longitudinal. Each fixed array can normally obtain two of the three primary planes of the heart or body. Only occasionally can the third plane be obtained with a single fixed array. The fixed array has an unchanging relationship to the endoscope. With the TEE endoscope in the esophagus, a fixed transverse or longitudinal array has its orientation aligned with that of the body and oblique to the primary planes of the heart.

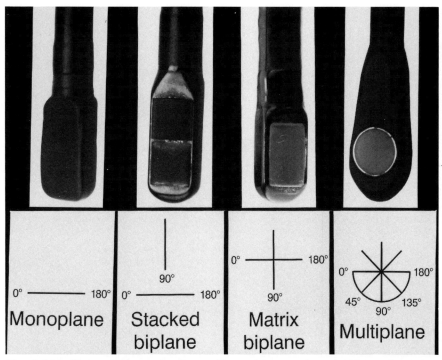

Fig. 4-10. Transesophageal echocardiographic transducers. *Monoplane:* A single plane (usually the transverse plane) is incorporated into the tip of an endoscope. A transverse plane can obtain short-axis and four-chamber views of the heart and only limited longitudinal projections. *Stacked biplane:* A distal transverse image plane is married to a more proximal longitudinal plane. The two sets of transducers are offset by approximately 1 cm. All the primary anatomic planes (short-axis, four-chamber, and longitudinal) can be obtained. *Matrix biplane:* Transverse and longitudinal image planes are interdigitated within a single transducer and simultaneous orthogonal imaging can be performed at the same anatomic level. *Multiplane:* A single array can be mechanically rotated around an arc of 180 degrees. A continuum of contiguous tomographic images is thus obtained without manipulation of the probe tip. All the primary anatomic planes of the heart and body are more easily obtained. In addition, off-axis images (those not in the primary plane) are much easier to obtain.

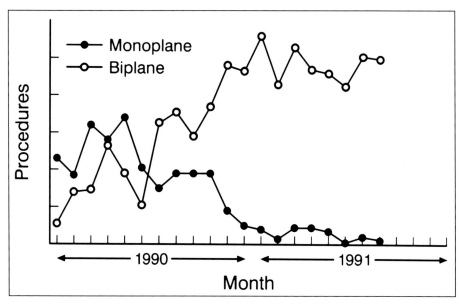

Fig. 4-11. In a span of approximately 2 years, biplane TEE has replaced the monoplane technique in our laboratory. It has been stated that there is approximately a 30% increase in diagnostic information with biplane TEE over monoplane TEE [12]. A similar study of multiplane TEE is not available.

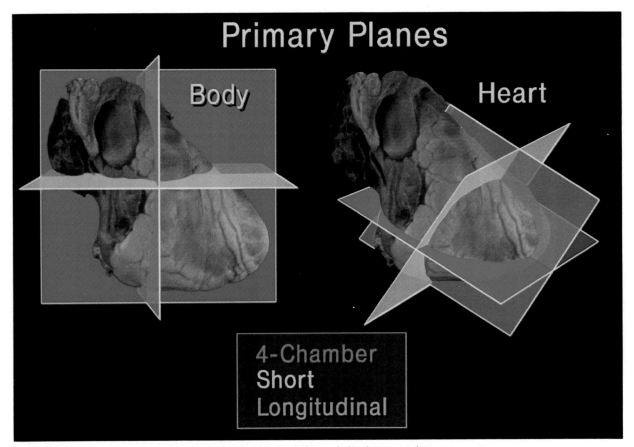

Fig. 4-12. The three primary planes of the body (left) and the heart (right). Note that the planes of the body are aligned with midline structures, such as the esophagus. The heart has its major axis oriented from right to left (i.e., right shoulder to left hip). The heart's long and short axes do not lie in the same plane as the body's long and short axes.

Off-axis image planes are obtained by changing the orientation of the transducer tip relative to the body or heart. This is accomplished by four-way flexion of the endoscope tip or incorporation of a rotatable array (i.e., multiplane) or both (see Fig. 4-10). Biplane and multiplane transesophageal transducers can be manipulated into all three primary planes of the body by flexion of the endoscope tip and the heart by rotation of the array. Some cardiac structures are aligned to the planes of the body (e.g., ascending aorta, right ventricular outflow, superior and inferior venae cavae), whereas other structures are best imaged in the primary planes of the heart (e.g., left ventricular outflow) and yet other structures are oblique to both the heart and the body (e.g., pulmonary veins).

Imaging the Primary Planes

The primary planes of the body are oriented differently from the primary planes of the heart (see Fig. 4-12). A brief description of each plane and the necessary endoscope or array manipulation to attain it highlights these differences.

Body Planes

With the endoscope tip in midesophagus, the planes of the body are obtained as follows:

Long axis

Biplane	Longitudinal plane without any tip flexion
Multiplane	90-degree array orientation

Short axis

Biplane	Transverse plane without tip flexion

Multiplane	0-degree array orientation
Frontal	
Biplane	Transverse plane with retroflexion of the endoscope tip; occasionally, slight withdrawal of the endoscope is necessary
Multiplane	0-degree array orientation with retroflexion of endoscope tip

Heart Planes

With the endoscope tip in the midesophagus, off-axis manipulations of either the endoscope or the image array must be performed to image the primary planes of the heart.

Long axis	
Biplane	Longitudinal plane with lateral flexion of the endoscope tip [12]
Multiplane	135-degree array orientation
Short axis	
Biplane	Transverse plane with lateral flexion of the endoscope tip or longitudinal plane with medial tip flexion [12]
Multiplane	45-degree array orientation
Four-chamber (frontal) plane	
Biplane	Transverse plane with retroflexion of the tip (often, slight withdrawal of the endoscope is necessary)
Multiplane	0-degree array orientation with retroflexion of the tip and slight withdrawal of the endoscope (same as biplane)

Introduction to Anatomic Correlation

Regardless of how an image is obtained, any resultant tomographic section can be viewed in only two ways. As in dividing a deck of cards, one can display only the front of one card or the back of the next card. Each card (front or back) can be rotated with various features up or down. The first discussion that follows deals with the confusing subject of "preferred" orientations of images. The remainder of the chapter deals with tomographic anatomic correlation with echocardiographic images. At no time is photographic negative reversal used. Considerable effort is made to explain how each image is obtained (i.e., transducer position and knob movement).

Various Image Displays and "Preferred" Orientations

Short-Axis Anatomy

For appropriate anatomic views, the heart is bisected along its short axis (Fig. 4-13). The cut surfaces can be viewed in two ways: looking from the apex toward the base and looking from the base toward the apex. The ASE in 1980 recommended the first option [6].

To retain the familiar short-axis projection, one views the specimen with the posteriorly located esophagus at the bottom of the image (Figs. 4-13 and 4-14). The right ventricle is to the viewer's left and left ventricle to the viewer's right.

With the advent of TEE, investigators initially displayed short-axis views with the transducer artifact (i.e., esophagus) and posterior cardiac wall at the top of the image (Figs. 4-13 and 4-15). The right ventricle was displayed to the viewer's left and left ventricle to the viewer's right. This arrangement appeared to simulate the familiar short-axis view obtained from the surface examination. However, the anterior and inferior walls are reversed, and the matching anatomic cut reveals that this orientation looks down the cardiac tube from base toward apex. This approach is not currently used in any other conventional tomographic imaging technique.

Long-Axis Anatomy

The heart is bisected along its anteroposterior (i.e., sagittal) long axis (Fig. 4-16). The cut surfaces can be viewed in two ways: looking from left toward right across the heart and looking from right toward left across the heart. The ASE has recommended looking from left toward right in this plane [6].

With TEE, three different orientations have been used [12,13,19] (Figs. 4-16, 4-17, and 4-18). One image presentation maintains a consistent image orientation comparable to the ASE recommendation (Figs. 4-16 and 4-17). The other two orientations retain the transducer artifact and posterior structures at the top of the image. One orients cardiac basal structures to the viewer's right, thus creating a totally new anatomic depiction of the heart (i.e., upside down and looking from right to left across the heart) (Figs. 4-16 and 4-18). The second places the cardiac base to the left, ostensibly to retain a "surgical" view of the heart (Figs. 4-16 and 4-19). Although the heart is viewed from left to right, it is presented

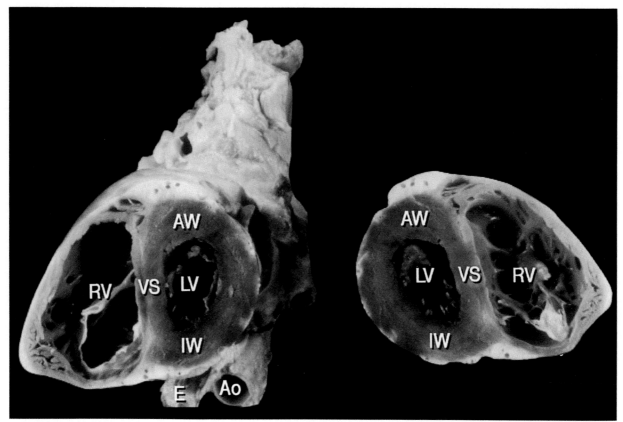

Fig. 4-13. Bisected cardiac specimen in the short axis. Left: The specimen is viewed from the apex toward the base. The esophagus is posterior and adjacent to both the thoracic aorta and inferior wall of the left ventricle. The right ventricular cavity is to the left. Right: The other half of the bisected specimen is viewed from the base toward the apex. With the inferior wall oriented downward, the right ventricle is to the viewer's right.

upside down as though the patient were lying face down.

Four-Chamber (Frontal) Anatomy

The heart is bisected along its frontal long axis (Fig. 4-20). This tomographic cut is commonly referred to as the four-chamber view, because a midheart frontal section simultaneously visualizes all four cardiac chambers. This cut can also be referred to as a frontal projection, as it results in a plane parallel to the anterior wall of the heart and chest wall. The ASE recommended two projections of this tomographic section [6]. Both from a precordial and from an esophageal transducer position, a consistent image orientation can be presented with the apex either up or down.

In the original standards document, apex down was considered more consistent with cardiac inspection (anteroposterior surgical dissection) and was considered preferable (option 1). However, instruments in 1978–1980 could not do an electronic inversion to achieve this, and thus this recommendation initially could not be implemented.

A second option (option 2) was proposed, primarily because it could be obtained easily during a precordial examination (i.e., from a short-axis orientation, the ultrasound beam is tilted upward while the transducer is moved downward on the chest wall). This identical view is obtained from the esophagus by a similar maneuver (i.e., from a short-axis view in midesophagus, the ultrasound beam is tilted downward while the transducer is slightly withdrawn) (Figs. 4-20 and 4-21). This view is historically preferred and familiar, yet with the advent of TEE is infrequently used because of the initial desire to keep the transducer artifact at the top of the image.

The transesophageal examination is confronted with the same dilemma encountered with the precordial examination (see Fig. 4-5). If apex-down four-chamber views are preferred, the image must be electronically inverted (Figs. 4-20 and 4-22).

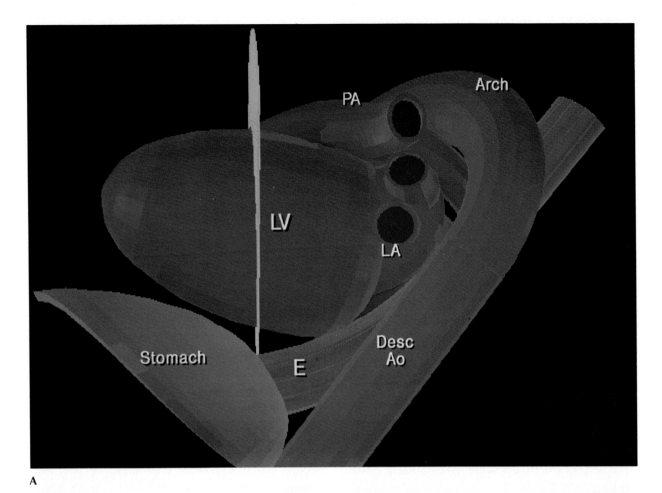

A

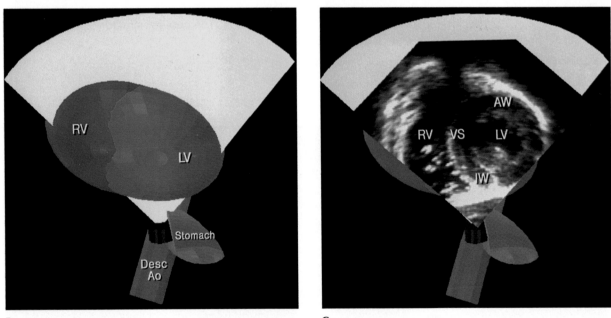

B   C

Fig. 4-14. Short-axis TEE. A. The TEE transducer is depicted in the lower esophagus transecting the left ventricle in the short axis. B. Relationship between heart and esophageal transducer when heart is viewed from apex toward base. C. The transesophageal echocardiogram is superimposed on the illustration. Note that the posteriorly located esophageal transducer lies adjacent to the left ventricular inferior wall. The heart is viewed from the apex toward the base with the right ventricle to the viewer's left and left ventricle to the right.

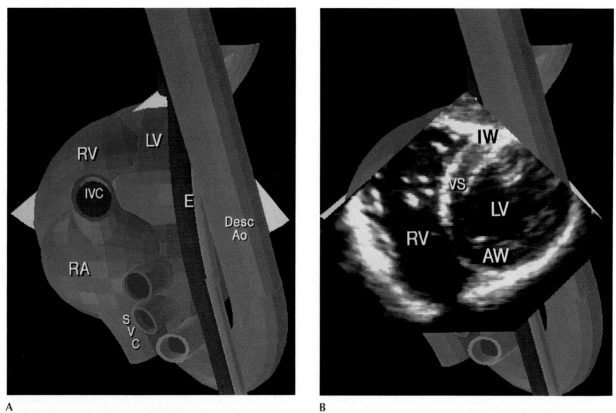

A   B

Fig. 4-15. Transesophageal short axis with the posterior structures at the top of the image and the right ventricle to the viewer's right. A. How the heart must be oriented to correspond to this tomographic echocardiogram. Note that the left ventricular posterior (inferior) wall is adjacent to the transducer. The right ventricle is to the viewer's left and the left ventricle to the viewer's right. Note that the heart is upside down and viewed from base toward apex. B. The transesophageal echocardiogram is superimposed on the illustration. The image is viewed from an unconventional base-to-apex projection. The anterior structures are located at the bottom of the image.

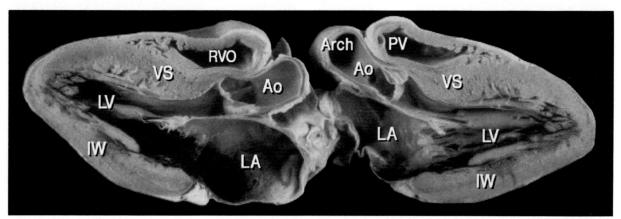

Fig. 4-16. Bisected cardiac specimen in the long axis. Left: The specimen is viewed from the left heart toward the right. The esophagus (not shown) is posterior to both the left atrium and the inferior wall of the left ventricle. Anteriorly, a portion of the right ventricular outflow is visualized. The aortic root *(Ao)* and basal heart are to the right and the apex to the left. This is the recognized standard for a longitudinal tomographic cut of the left ventricle. Right: The other half of the bisected specimen is viewed as though one were looking toward the free wall of the left ventricle. Note that the aorta, aortic arch, pulmonary valve *(PV)*, and main pulmonary artery are projected away from the viewer. With the inferior wall oriented downward, the cardiac apex is to the viewer's right.

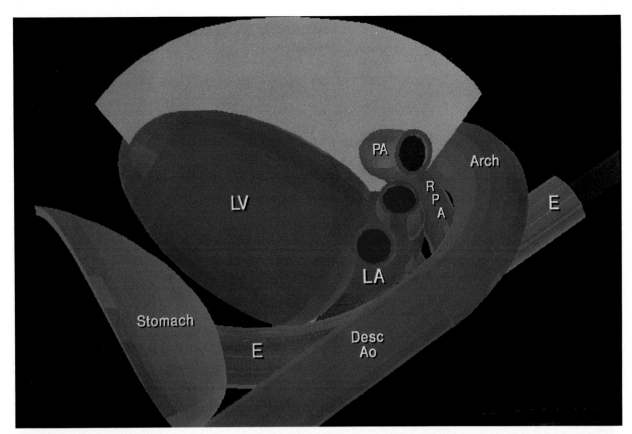

A

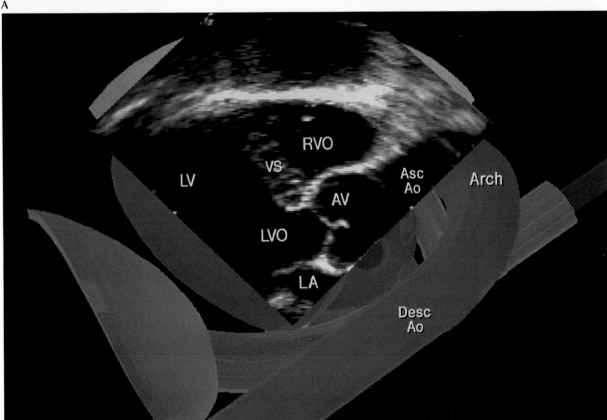

B

Fig. 4-17. Long-axis TEE. A. The transducer is posterior to the heart within the lumen of the esophagus. The left ventricle is cut in its anteroposterior (i.e., sagittal) long axis. B. The transesophageal echocardiogram is superimposed over the illustrated anatomy. Anterior structures, such as the right ventricular outflow tract, are at the top of the image, whereas the posterior left atrium is at the bottom, immediately adjacent to the transducer. The cardiac base is to the viewer's right and apex to the left.

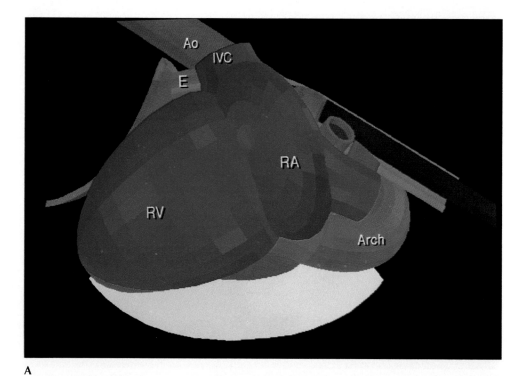

A

B

Fig. 4-18. Long-axis TEE with the transducer artifact at the top of the image and basal structures to the viewer's right. A. For imaging in this manner, the heart has to be viewed from an unconventional perspective (i.e., from the right heart toward the left). The posterior transducer is at the top of the image, and the basal structures are to the viewer's right. B. The transesophageal echocardiogram is superimposed on the illustration. The heart is presented upside down in an unconventional manner.

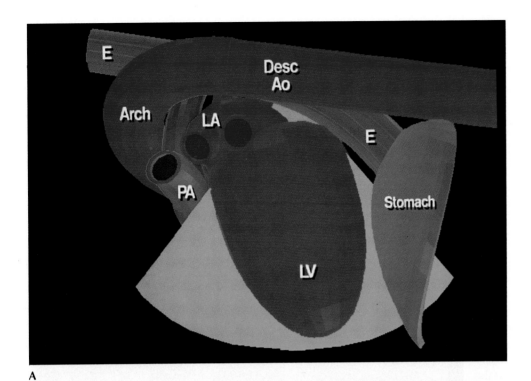

A

B

Fig. 4-19. Long-axis TEE with the transducer artifact at the top and the basal cardiac structures to the viewer's left. A. The posteriorly located transducer and cardiac structures are at the top of the image (patient lying face down in an unfamiliar surgical orientation). Basal structures are to the viewer's left. The heart is viewed from the left heart looking toward the right. B. Superimposed TEE long-axis view. The posteriorly located left atrium is at the top of the image, and the anteriorly located right ventricular outflow is at the bottom. This view of the heart is simply a top-to-bottom rotation of the anatomic depiction shown in Figure 4-17.

Fig. 4-20. Bisected cardiac specimen in the four-chamber, or frontal, view. Left: The bisected specimen (viewed from the heart's anterior surface toward the posterior) has been partially opened to show the relative relationships of the halves. Lower right: The apex-down format views the heart from its anterior surface toward the posterior. The left ventricle is to the examiner's right and right ventricle to the examiner's left. In the floor of the right atrium is the orifice of the inferior vena cava. Upper right: The apex-up format views the heart from its posterior surface toward the anterior. The orifices of the right atrial appendage and left atrial appendage are anterior in the roof of the right and left atrial cavities, respectively. (*AL* = anterolateral papillary muscle; *PM* = posteromedial papillary muscle; *PulV* = pulmonary vein; *PV* = pulmonary valve.)

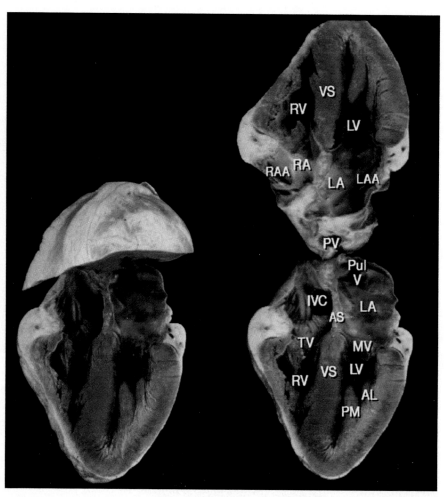

Fig. 4-21. ▶ Four-chamber anatomy. A. With the esophageal transducer in the midesophagus, the transverse plane is slightly retroflexed (i.e., the endoscope tip is flexed downward). The transducer is posterior and adjacent to the left atrium. Depending on how the image is displayed, an apex-down or apex-up presentation results. B. If the transducer artifact is retained at the bottom of the image throughout the examination, a four-chamber projection is displayed in an apex-up format familiar to transthoracic imaging. Note that this projection views the heart from its inferoposterior surface toward the anterior surface. The esophageal transducer is posterior and adjacent to the left atrium. C. The transesophageal four-chamber echocardiogram has been superimposed on the anatomic illustration. This view is obtained by retroflexion of the transverse image plane from midesophagus.

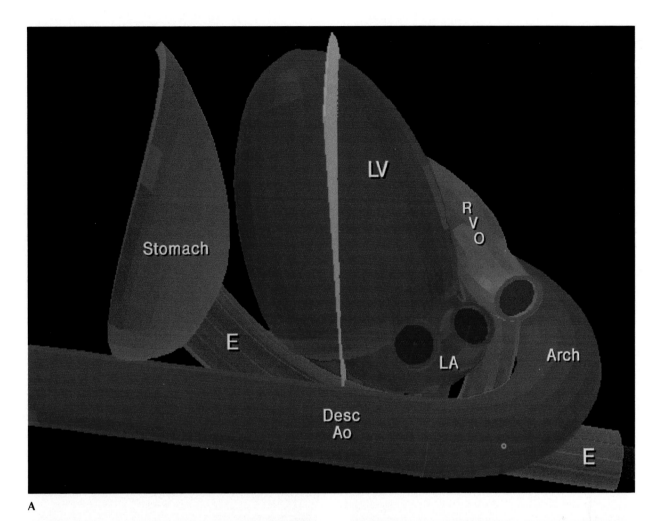

A

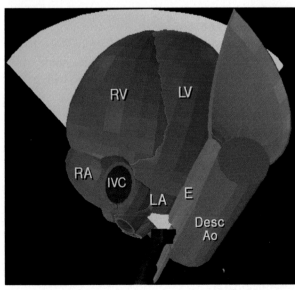

B

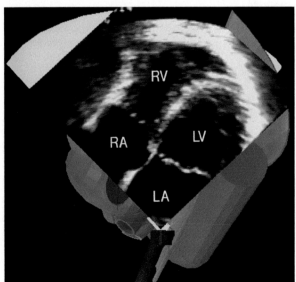

C

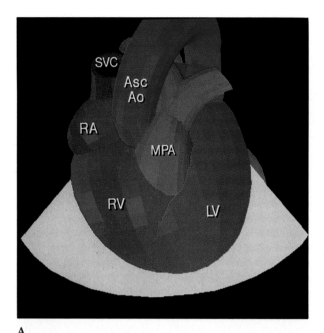 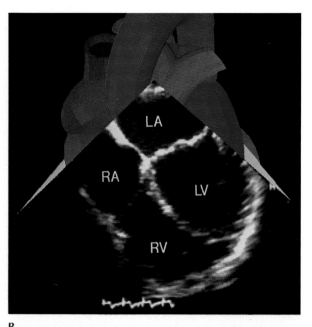

A   **B**

Fig. 4-22.   Apex-down four-chamber view. A. If apex-down four-chamber views are preferred, the transducer artifact must be reoriented at the top of the image (an electronic inversion of the image is required). The resultant view is from the anterior surface of the heart toward the posterior. The left-sided cardiac structures are to the viewer's right. B. The transesophageal image is superimposed on the illustration. Note that the esophageal transducer is posterior and adjacent to the left atrium.

Anatomic Correlation of the TEE Examination

General

The anatomic discussion that follows emphasizes an image orientation and display compatible with the previous document of standards by the ASE [6]. There are three primary planes of the body and three primary planes of the heart (see Fig. 4-12). A transesophageal transducer with two or more planes (biplane or multiplane) can image all three planes of the body or heart. The biplane transducer requires more dexterity to operate but usually can obtain the same planes as a multiplane (rotatable array) device with proper flexion maneuvers of the transducer tip.

The TEE examination is best discussed as a sequential examination similar to that with multiplane TEE (see Chapter 5). With each view, the transducer manipulations required to obtain that view are described. Additionally, any exception to a common image format is illustrated.

Multiplane TEE Anatomy

The word *multiplane* need not apply only to the newer TEE transducers that have a rotatable array. The multiplane concept can be achieved with a fixed monoplane or biplane transducer by use of four-way flexion of the endoscope tip. The following discussion of a multiplane approach to TEE anatomy describes how the same view can be obtained both with a fixed array biplane transducer and with a rotatable array "multiplane" transducer.

The multiplane approach describes tomographic planes as a sequence of orientations around a semi-circle (Fig. 4-23). A transducer oriented perpendicular to the endoscope shaft is in the *transverse orientation*. This has been designated 0 degrees in the imaging arc.

When the transducer is parallel to the long axis of the endoscope shaft, it is in the *longitudinal orientation*. This orientation has been designated 90 degrees, and a series of tomographic planes can be obtained.

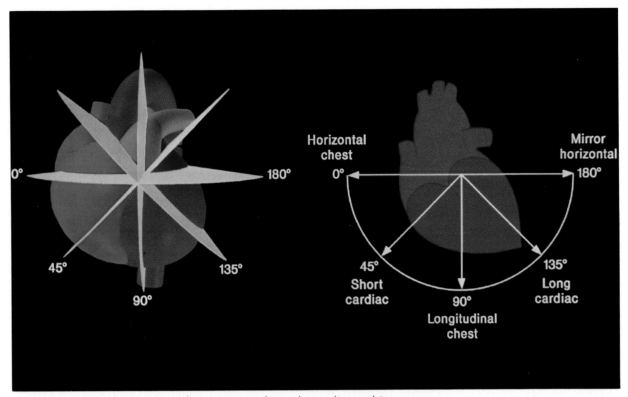

Fig. 4-23. Multiplane approach to tomographic echocardiographic anatomy. The acquisition of various tomographic views of the heart can be described in degrees around an arc. A plane is transverse at 0 degrees and longitudinal at 90 degrees to the shaft of the endoscope. In the midesophagus, 0 degrees is in the short axis of the body and 90 degrees is sagittal or longitudinal to the body. An array in midesophagus at 45 degrees is in the short axis of the heart and at 135 degrees in the long axis of the heart. A biplane endoscope can obtain the same off-axis views: 45 degrees short axis by medial flexion of the longitudinal plane or lateral flexion of the transverse plane; 135 degrees long axis by lateral flexion of the longitudinal plane or medial flexion of the transverse plane. A full 180-degree rotation of the transducer or a left-right electronic image reversal produces mirror-image tomographic anatomy.

Multiplane Examination With a Biplane Transducer

For a short-axis view of the basal cardiac structures, the imaging array must be at approximately 45 degrees (see Fig. 4-23). This position can be achieved with a multiplane device by array rotation or with a biplane transducer by medial flexion of the longitudinal plane or lateral flexion of the transverse plane (Fig. 4-24). The long axis of the heart lies at approximately 135 degrees (see Fig. 4-23). This projection of the heart can be obtained with a multiplane device by rotation of the array. With a biplane endoscope, the same orientation is gained by lateral flexion of the longitudinal plane or medial flexion of the transverse plane (Figs. 4-25 and 4-26). The angles for both the short-axis and long-axis planes vary depending on the degree of "horizontal" versus "vertical" orientation the heart has within the chest. The same primary and off-axis images can be obtained with both multiplane and biplane technologies. The fixed planes of a biplane endoscope, however, require added maneuvers (i.e., medial and lateral flexion of the endoscope tip).

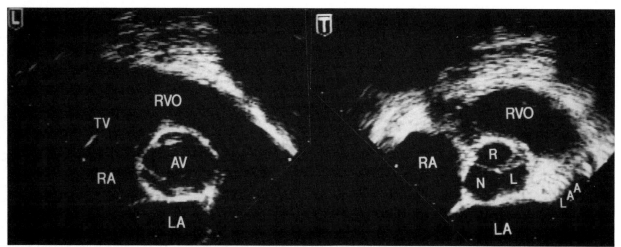

Fig. 4-24. Short-axis view of the aortic valve with the longitudinal *(L)* array and transverse *(T)* array of a biplane TEE endoscope in the same patient. Left: The short-axis view of the aortic valve is obtained by medial flexion of the longitudinal array. Right: The same view is obtained with the transverse array by lateral flexion of the endoscope tip. (*L* = left coronary cusp; *N* = noncoronary cusp; *R* = right coronary cusp.)

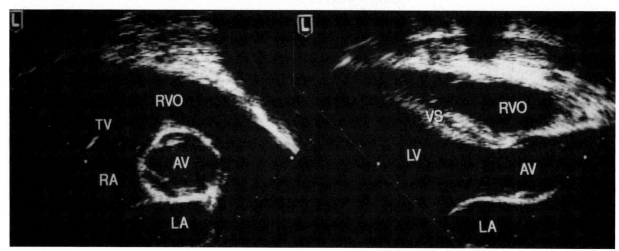

Fig. 4-25. Longitudinal array: off-axis biplane images. With the endoscope tip in the midesophagus, short- and long-axis images of the heart can be obtained by medial and lateral flexion of the tip. Left: Short-axis view of the aortic valve is obtained by medial flexion of the longitudinal *(L)* array. Right: In the same patient, long-axis view of the aortic valve and left ventricle is obtained by lateral flexion of the longitudinal array.

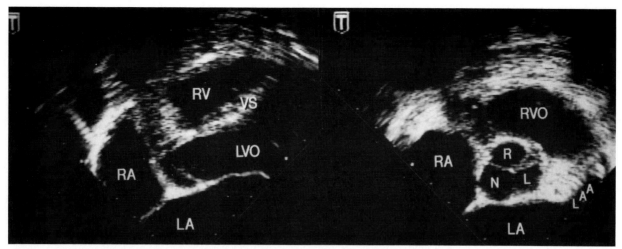

Fig. 4-26. Transverse array: off-axis biplane images. With the endoscope tip in the midesophagus, long- and short-axis images of the heart can be obtained by medial and lateral flexion of the tip. Note that the maneuver is just the opposite of that used in manipulating the longitudinal plane. Left: Long-axis view of the left ventricular outflow is obtained by medial flexion of the transverse *(T)* plane. A left-to-right reversal of the image would be necessary to obtain a more familiar image presentation. This maneuver is clinically useful but rarely necessary. Right: Short-axis view of the aortic valve obtained by lateral flexion of the transverse array. This maneuver is commonly used to optimally image the aortic cusps. *(L* = left coronary cusp; *N* = noncoronary cusp; *R* = right coronary cusp.)

Anatomic Correlations by a Sequential TEE Examination

Midesophageal Examination

Multiple Tomographic Planes
With biplane or multiplane TEE (Fig. 4-27), a series of short- and long-axis views can be obtained (Figs. 4-28 through 4-33). A uniform image presentation corresponding to all previous standard documents is emphasized. If a multiplane transducer is over-rotated (i.e., 180 degrees), a mirror image appears, which anatomically views the heart from the base toward the apex (Fig. 4-33). We no longer use non-standard views, preferring to keep the transducer artifact at the bottom of the image throughout the examination, as described earlier in this chapter.

Longitudinal Midesophagus Examination
With the biplane probe in the longitudinal plane or with the multiplane array at 90 degrees, the TEE endoscope shaft is rotated to produce a series of basal long-axis tomographic views (Fig. 4-34). A series of long-axis views (Figs. 4-35 through 4-39) is obtained, each identified by the basal anatomic structure cut in long axis: (1) mitral inflow (Fig. 4-36), (2) right ventricular outflow (Fig. 4-37), (3) ascending thoracic aorta (Fig. 4-38), and (4) superior and inferior venae cavae (Fig. 4-39). The anatomic correlations for these views have previously been described [12].

Four-Chamber and Related Apex-Up or Apex-Down Images
Various long-axis views obtained from the mideso-phagus have already been discussed (see Figs. 4-27 and 4-34). The four-chamber (long-axis) view is most consistently obtained from midesophagus. In the transverse plane (biplane or multiplane 0 degrees), the transducer tip is gently retroflexed. Retro-flexion moves the tip downward and reorients the scan plane from the short-axis to the more long-axis frontal view of the heart (see Fig. 4-21) and displays

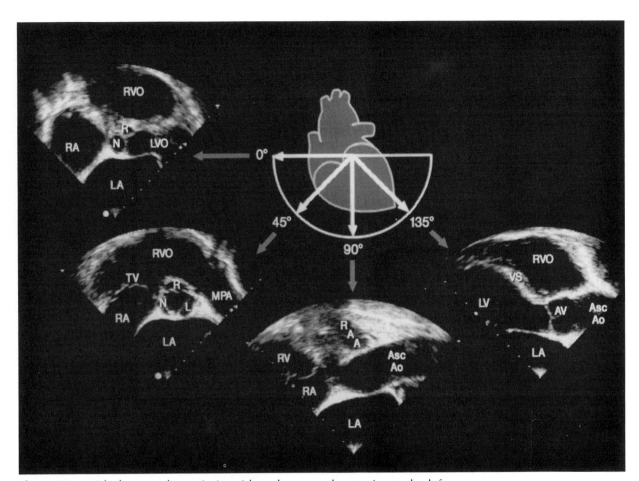

Fig. 4-27. With the transducer tip in midesophagus and posterior to the left atrium, a sequence of short- and long-axis views can be obtained (the ultrasound images are described from left to right). 0 degrees: The array is in a transverse (short-axis) orientation to the body (i.e., *biplane,* transverse plane without tip manipulation; *multiplane,* array set at 0 degrees). The heart (aortic valve) is cut obliquely. Only the right coronary *(R)* and noncoronary *(N)* cusps of the aortic valve are appreciated. 45 degrees: The array has been manipulated to lie in the basal short axis of the heart (i.e., *biplane,* medial flexion of the longitudinal plane or lateral flexion of the transverse plane; *multiplane,* rotation of the array to 45 degrees). The three cusps of the aortic valve are optimally visualized in short axis. 90 degrees: The array is in the longitudinal (long axis) orientation to the body (i.e., *biplane,* longitudinal plane without tip flexion; *multiplane,* array rotated to 90 degrees). The array is parallel to the long axis of the endoscope shaft. Note that the image is oblique to the long axis of the left ventricle but is in the long axis of the ascending aorta and other basal and upper mediastinal structures (see Fig. 4-34). 135 degrees: The array is in the long axis of the heart (i.e., *biplane,* lateral flexion of the longitudinal plane or, rarely, far medial flexion [and left-to-right image reversal] of the transverse plane; *multiplane,* array rotated to 135 degrees). The left ventricular outflow and mitral inflow are simultaneously imaged. This view is identical to a parasternal long-axis view of the left ventricle. (*L* = left coronary cusp.)

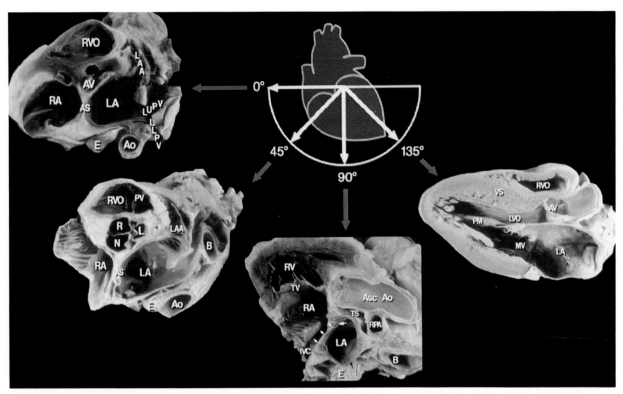

Fig. 4-28. Tomographic anatomy from midesophagus. Shown is a collage of anatomic specimens cut to correspond to the echocardiographic anatomy in Figure 4–27. The individual specimens are described in the next four figures. A fifth specimen (see Fig. 4-33) corresponds to basal images displayed with the transducer artifact at the top of the image.

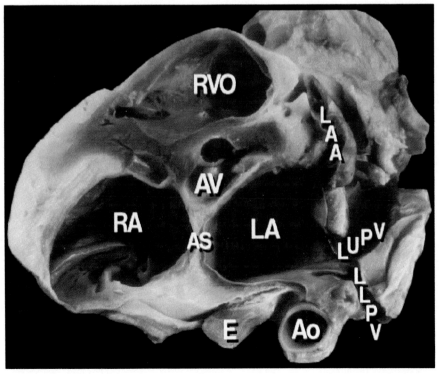

Fig. 4-29. An oblique short-axis cut at the base of the heart (0 degrees). The esophagus is posterior and adjacent to the left atrium. The image array is in the short axis of the body; consequently, the aortic valve cusps are cut obliquely. Often the left atrial appendage and left upper and lower pulmonary veins are best visualized in this short-axis view. The right atrium is to the viewer's left. The right ventricular outflow is anterior. (*Ao* = descending thoracic aorta.)

Fig. 4-30. Short-axis view of the aortic valve (45 degrees). Note that the three aortic valve cusps (*L* = left; *R* = right; and *N* = noncoronary) are more optimally displayed in the short axis. The descending thoracic aorta is cut obliquely. The right ventricular outflow is anterior, and the esophagus is posterior. (*PV* = pulmonary valve.)

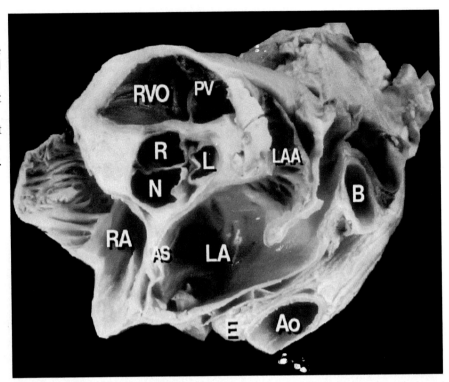

Fig. 4-31. Longitudinal scan (90 degrees). This view is longitudinal to the body. The basal cardiac structures of the cardiac specimen, including the proximal ascending aorta, lie in the long axis of the body. The esophagus is posterior. The membranous atrial septum *(small arrows)* and patent foramen ovale *(large arrow)* are seen in this view. The right pulmonary artery courses posterior to the ascending aorta. The transverse sinus is a pericardial space separating the left atrium, right pulmonary artery, ascending aorta, and right atrium.

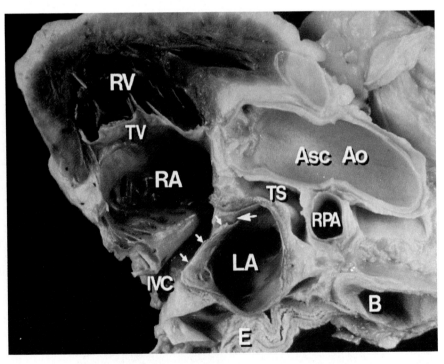

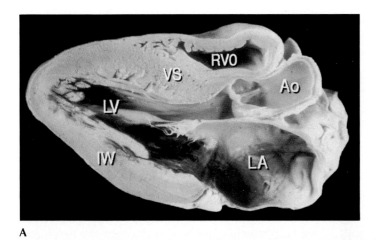

A

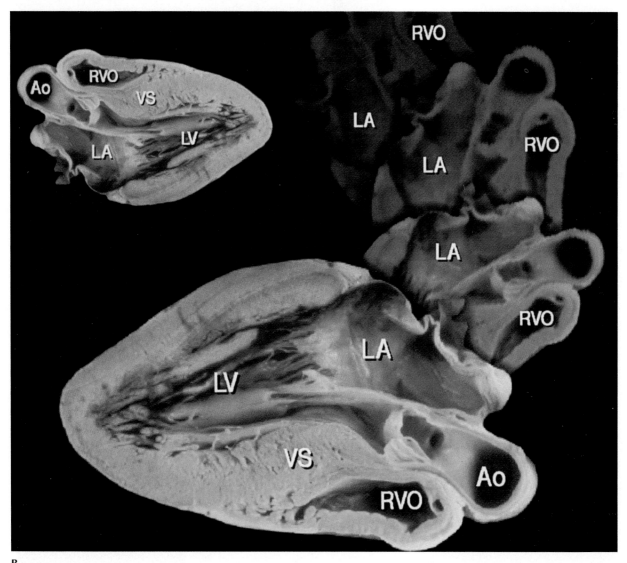

B

Fig. 4-32.   Long axis of the left ventricle (135 degrees). A. This view is identical to a parasternal long-axis view of the left ventricle. The esophagus is posterior and adjacent to the left atrium. The aortic valve, left ventricular outflow, and body of the left ventricle are viewed in the long axis. The right ventricular outflow is anterior. In this tomographic cut, the heart is viewed from the left ventricle toward the ventricular septum and right ventricle. B. The bisected half of this specimen (described in the legend for Figure 4-16 *right*) must be rotated 180 degrees to display the heart upside-down with the basal structures to the right. This heart is viewed as though one were looking toward the left ventricular free wall. This unconventional display of tomographic anatomy is not used in our laboratory.

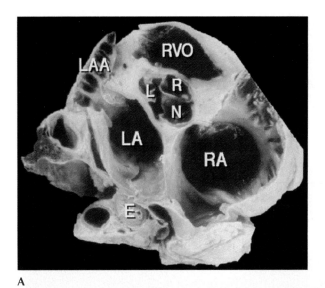

A

Fig. 4-33. Short-axis basal view with mirror-image orientation, a view commonly used when the transducer artifact is placed at the top of the image. A. This is the apical half of the bisected heart. This view looks down the cardiac tube. Note that the aortic cusps (*L* = left coronary; *N* = noncoronary; *R* = right coronary) are viewed from above. The esophagus is posterior. The left atrial appendage is to the viewer's left (looking from the base of the heart toward the apex). B. The specimen has been rotated 180 degrees, a commonly used TEE basal short-axis view that does not correspond to a standard image format (6) but places the esophagus at the top of the image and the left heart structures to the viewer's right. We have now abandoned this format for the more familiar convention shown in Figure 4-30.

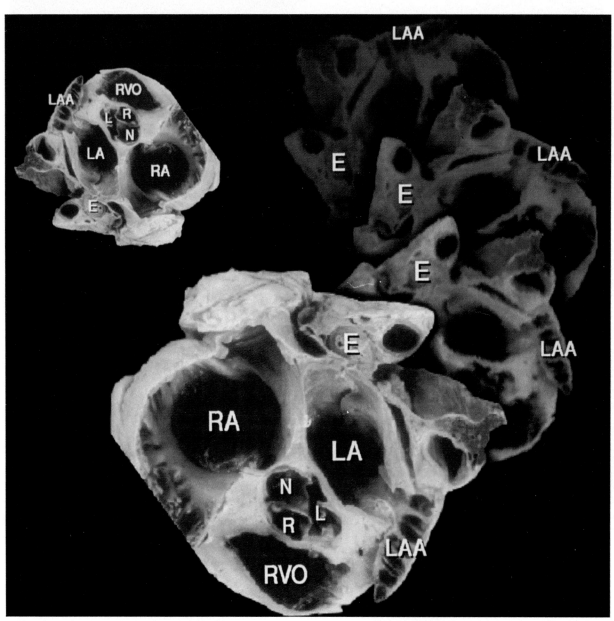

B

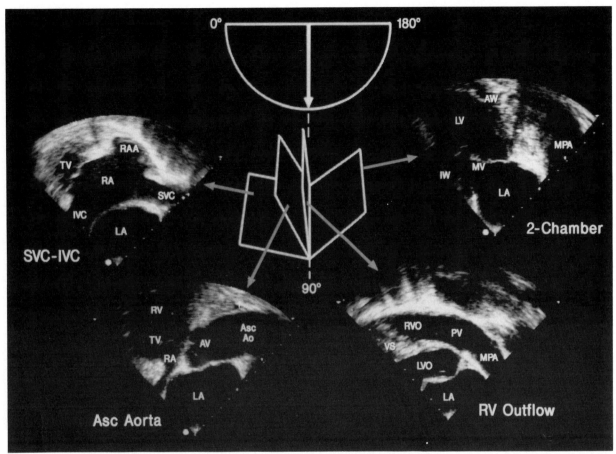

Fig. 4-34. Midesophageal longitudinal views. With the longitudinal plane of a biplane or multiplane array at 90 degrees, a sequence of longitudinal images is obtained [2]. This collage is described from the viewer's right to left, and each image is identified by a specific long-axis anatomic structure. *Two-chamber:* The longitudinal transducer is directed leftward to obtain the two-chamber view (i.e., left ventricle and left atrium). This view is frequently used to assess the mitral valve for regurgitation, stenosis, and so forth. *Right ventricular outflow:* By rotation of the endoscope shaft rightward, the next basal anatomic structures cut in long axis are the right ventricular outflow, pulmonary valve *(PV),* and proximal main pulmonary artery. *Ascending aorta:* Further rightward rotation of the endoscope shaft images the proximal ascending aorta in long axis. The aortic valve is cut obliquely. *Superior vena cava and inferior vena cava:* Further rightward shaft rotation visualizes the superior and inferior venae cavae in long axis. The atrial septum is also cut in long axis. The right atrial appendage and right atrium are anterior structures.

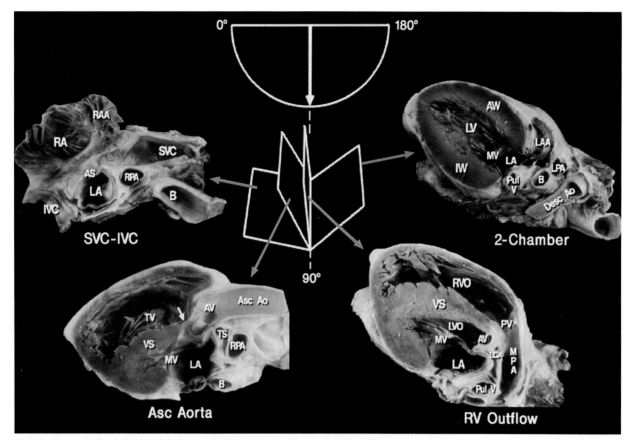

Fig. 4-35. Midesophageal longitudinal tomographic anatomy. This anatomic collage corresponds to the sequential echocardiographic anatomy shown in Figure 4-34. The individual specimens are described in the next four figures.

Fig. 4-36. Two-chamber view. In this tomographic cut, the esophagus is posterior to the left atrium. The two primary chambers visualized are the left atrium and the left ventricle. The mitral valve inflow is also well demonstrated. The left atrial appendage is imaged in the anterior left atrium. The specimen is viewed as though one were looking from the left ventricle toward the right heart chambers. (*PulV* = left lower pulmonary vein.)

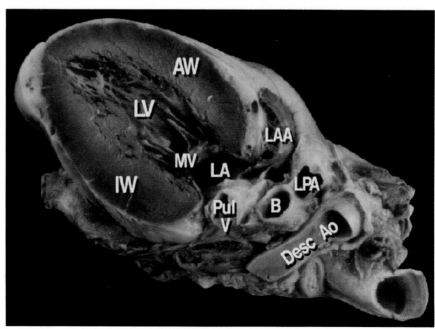

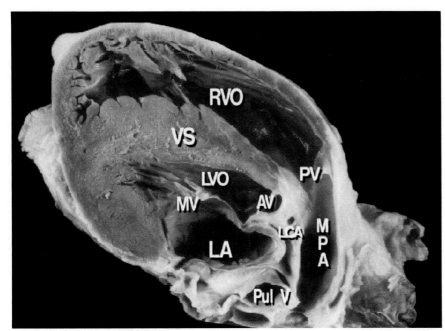

Fig. 4-37. Long-axis view of right ventricular outflow. This section is oblique to the body of the heart but in the long axis of the right ventricular outflow, pulmonary valve *(PV),* and proximal main pulmonary artery. The posteriorly located left atrium is adjacent to the esophagus. *(PulV =* left pulmonary vein.)

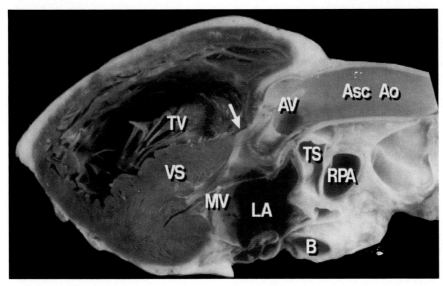

Fig. 4-38. Long axis to the proximal ascending aorta. The proximal ascending aorta is cut in long axis. The left ventricle and aortic valve are cut obliquely. This view also best visualizes the membranous ventricular septum *(arrow).* The right pulmonary artery is posterior to the ascending aorta. (This specimen is comparable with that shown in Fig. 4-31.)

the apex of the heart at the top of the video screen (Fig. 4-40). The maneuver of retroflexing the transducer tip in the midesophageal transducer position can actually produce a series of apex-up (Fig. 4-41) or, if one inverts the image, apex-down long-axis views. Apex display of multiple views is very helpful in mapping three-dimensional anatomy or pathophysiology, such as the jet of mitral regurgitation within the left atrium.

The apex-up four-chamber view displays cardiac anatomy as though one were looking from the posterior surface (Fig. 4-42). Conversely, if the apex-down format is preferred (an electronic inversion of the image is required), the anatomy is viewed as though one were looking from the anterior cardiac structures toward the posterior surface (Fig. 4-43).

Fig. 4-39. Long-axis view of the superior and inferior venae cavae. The specimen is viewed from the left looking toward the free wall of the right atrium. The right atrial appendage is anterior in the right atrial cavity. The right pulmonary artery, transected in short axis, courses posterior to the superior vena cava. The posteriorly located left atrium is adjacent to the esophagus.

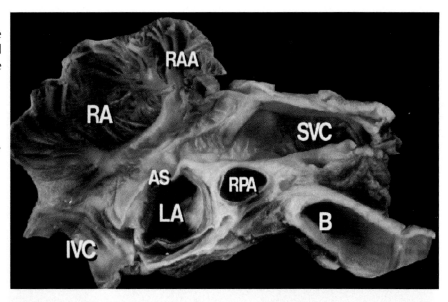

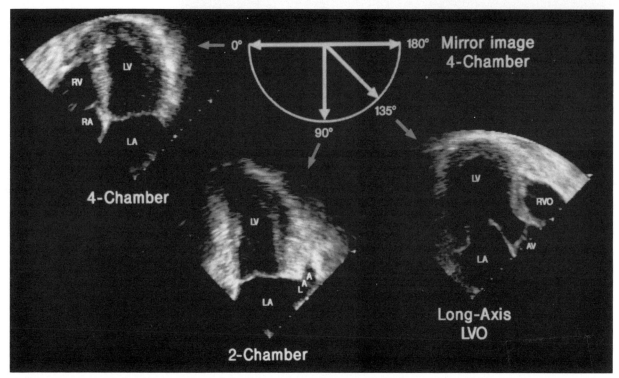

Fig. 4-40. Apex-up long-axis views of the heart. From the viewer's left to right in this collage, a series of images can be obtained with either biplane or multiplane TEE. *Four-chamber;* With the transverse plane of a biplane endoscope or a multiplane array at 0 degrees, the endoscope tip is retroflexed and usually slightly withdrawn. A conventional apex-up four-chamber view of the heart is obtained. *Two-chamber:* With the endoscope tip continuously retroflexed, the multiplane array is rotated to 90 degrees, or with a biplane endoscope, a switch is made to the longitudinal plane. When the biplane instrument is used, sometimes medial tip flexion is also required. (Image anatomy is the same as that in Fig. 4-36.) *Long-axis left ventricular outflow:* With the endoscope tip continuously retroflexed, the multiplane array is rotated to 135 degrees to obtain a long-axis view of the left ventricular outflow. If the biplane endoscope is used, retroflexion of the longitudinal plane is maintained during lateral flexion of the endoscope tip. (Image anatomy is comparable to that in Fig. 4-32.)

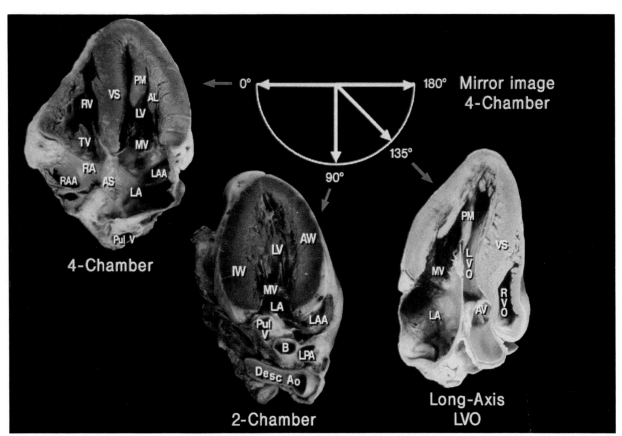

Fig. 4-41. Apex-up anatomic collage of images obtained from midesophagus with retroflexion of the transducer tip. The four-chamber view is discussed in Figure 4-42 and the alternative apex-down view in Figure 4-43. The two-chamber view is comparable to that in Figure 4-36 except for transducer retroflexion and display of the cardiac apex upward. The long-axis left ventricular outflow view is comparable to that in Figure 4-32 but with transducer retroflexion and upward display of the cardiac apex. (*AL* = anterolateral papillary muscle; *PM* = posteromedial papillary muscle; *PulV* = pulmonary vein.)

Transgastric Examination

From the transgastric transducer position, a grouping of short and long ventricular tomographic views can be obtained (Fig. 4-44). Off-axis views are usually easier to obtain with the multiplane rotatable transducer than with the fixed planes of the biplane transducer. The multiplane transducer can be held in a single position while off-axis views are obtained by mechanical rotation of the array. With the biplane endoscope, the transducer tip must be manipulated with each successive view, thus increasing the likelihood of having air or secretions interfere with good transducer contact with the stomach wall.

Short-axis views are obtained with the array in a transverse orientation (0 degrees for the multiplane device). Anteflexion tilts the ultrasound plane toward more basal views, and retroflexion of the endo-scope tip results in more apical short-axis views.

Longitudinal and off-axis views can be obtained with both biplane and multiplane transducers. In the longitudinal plane (biplane) or 90-degree array rotation (multiplane), a two-chamber view is obtained. Because the stomach is situated in variable positions posterior to the left ventricle, transducer orientation varies more when imaging is from the stomach.

The left ventricular outflow view is usually easier to obtain with the multiplane endoscope. Biplane transducers require lateral tip flexion, which often causes loss of transducer contact with the stomach wall.

From the transgastric transducer position, anatomic correlations (Figs. 4-45 through 4-50) are comparable to those obtained from the midesopha-

Fig. 4-42. Apex-up four-chamber view. The heart is viewed from the posterior surface looking toward the anterior surface. Thus, within the left atrium, the orifice of the left atrial appendage is visualized. Within the right atrium, the right atrial appendage is visualized anteriorly. In the left ventricular cavity are the posteromedial and anterolateral papillary muscles. The esophagus is located posteriorly adjacent to the left atrial wall. (*PV* = pulmonary vein.)

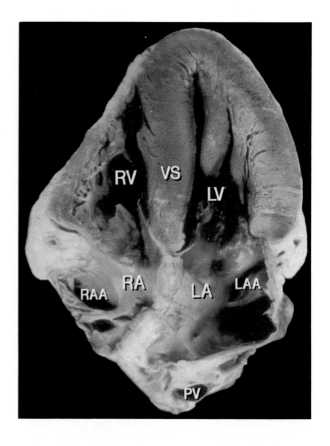

Fig. 4-43. Apex-down four-chamber view. The heart is viewed as though one were looking from the anterior surface toward the posterior surface. In the floor of the right atrium is the orifice of the inferior vena cava. The pulmonary veins *(PulV)* enter at the back of the left atrium. The heads of the anterolateral *(AL)* and posteromedial *(PM)* papillary muscles are seen in the left ventricular cavity.

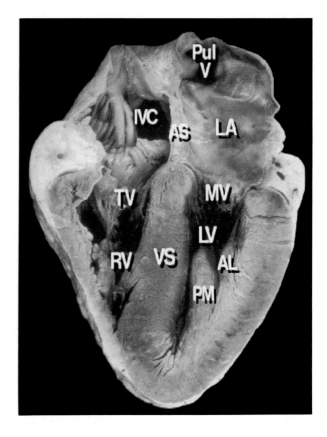

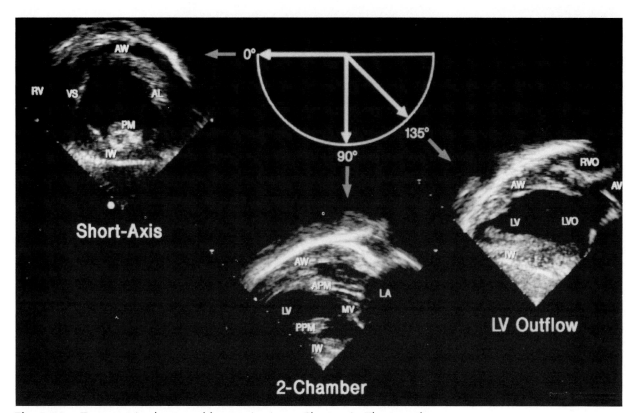

Fig. 4-44. Transgastric short- and long-axis views. *Short-axis:* The transducer tip is in the fundus of the stomach. The transverse plane of the biplane endoscope or 0 degrees rotation of the multiplane array is used to obtain this view. The transducer is posterior to the heart and adjacent to the left ventricular inferior wall. The anterior wall is at the top of the image. The posteromedial *(PM)* and anterolateral *(AL)* papillary muscles are visualized. The right ventricle is to the viewer's left. The heart is being viewed from apex toward base. *Two-chamber:* The longitudinal plane of the biplane endoscope or the multiplane array at 90 degrees rotation obtains this view. The left ventricle and left atrium are simultaneously viewed. This is an excellent view for assessing the mitral support apparatus. *Left ventricular outflow:* This view is obtained by lateral flexion of the biplane endoscope tip during imaging in the longitudinal plane. Alternatively, the multiplane array is rotated to approximately 135 degrees without endoscope tip manipulation. The aortic valve and left ventricular outflow are imaged from the left ventricle. The transducer is posterior to the inferior wall of the left ventricle.

gus. The only difference is that the transducer is posterior to the ventricles instead of the left atrium (Figs. 4-45, 4-46, and 4-47). Long-axis views are the same as those from midesophagus, except that they are imaged farther down the cardiac tube poste-

rior to the left ventricle (Figs. 4-45, 4-48, 4-49, and 4-50). The inferior wall of the left ventricle is the portion of the heart closest to the transducer when imaging is from the transgastric window.

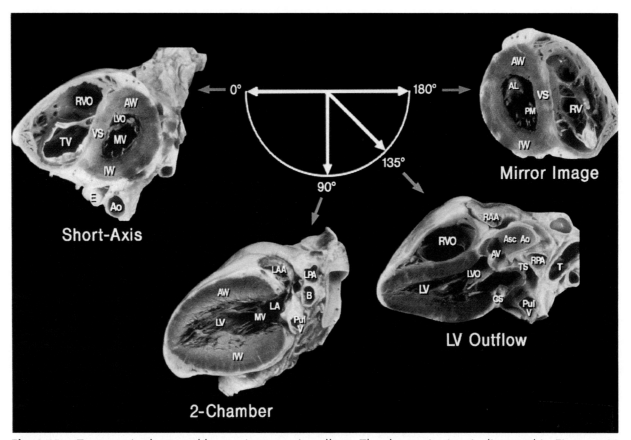

Fig. 4-45. Transgastric short- and long-axis anatomic collage. The short-axis view is discussed in Figure 4-46 and a mirror-image short-axis view (180 degrees) in Figure 4-47. The anatomic positions in the two-chamber view are comparable to the anatomy demonstrated in Figures 4-36 and 4-41. The only difference is that the view is obtained from the transgastric transducer position. The transgastric anatomy in the left ventricular outflow view is comparable to that in Figures 4-41 and 4-32. (*AL* = anterolateral papillary muscle; *PM* = posteromedial papillary muscle; *PulV* = pulmonary vein.)

Fig. 4-46. Transgastric short axis. This is a short-axis cut of the left and right ventricles with the specimen viewed from apex toward base. The esophagus is posterior and adjacent to the inferior wall of the left ventricle. The left ventricle is to the viewer's right and the right ventricle to the viewer's left. Anteriorly, the right ventricular outflow and left ventricular anterior wall are viewed. The thoracic aorta is posterior and to the left of the esophagus.

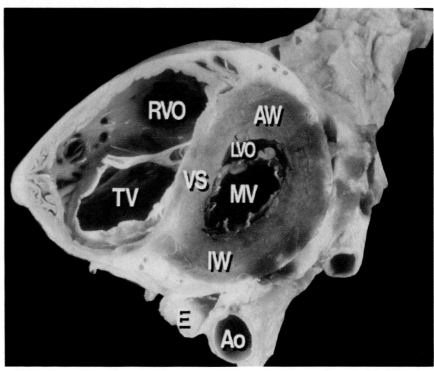

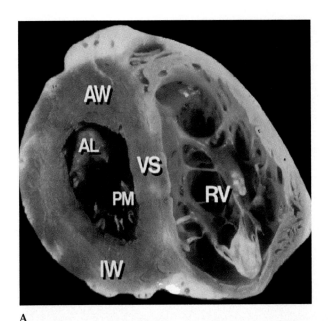

A

Fig. 4-47. Transgastric mirror-image short-axis view. Two ultrasound maneuvers result in this anatomic projection of the heart: a left-to-right image reversal and a 180-degree rotation of the multiplane array. This anatomic specimen is viewed as though one were looking from base toward apex (i.e., a nonstandard display). A. As displayed, the inferior wall of the specimen is posterior and the right ventricle is rightward. This is an unfamiliar anatomic view of the heart. B. This specimen has been rotated 180 degrees to represent an anatomic correlation to the short-axis transgastric image when the transducer artifact is at the top of the image and the right ventricle is to the viewer's left. The specimen is being viewed from the base toward the apex. In our laboratory, this viewing approach has been abandoned. (*AL* = anterolateral papillary muscle; *PM* = posteromedial papillary muscle.)

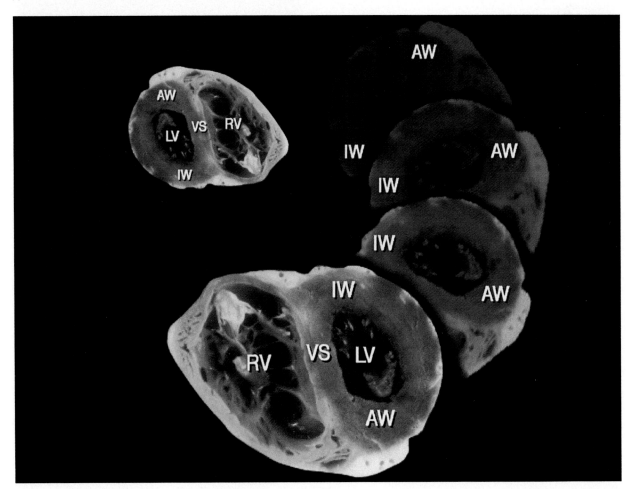

B

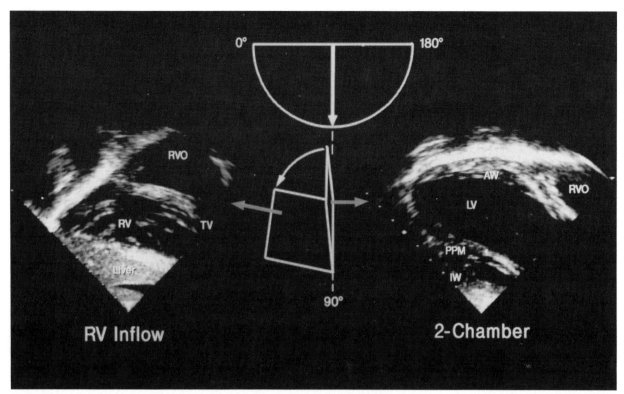

Fig. 4-48. Transgastric right ventricular inflow. Imaging begins with the longitudinal array of the biplane or the multiplane array at 90 degrees. Right: The starting image is a two-chamber transgastric view of the left ventricle (see Figs. 4-35, 4-41, and 4-45). Left: For the right ventricular inflow view, the shaft of the endoscope is rotated to the right. The tricuspid valve, right ventricular apex, and right ventricular outflow are consistently imaged with this maneuver.

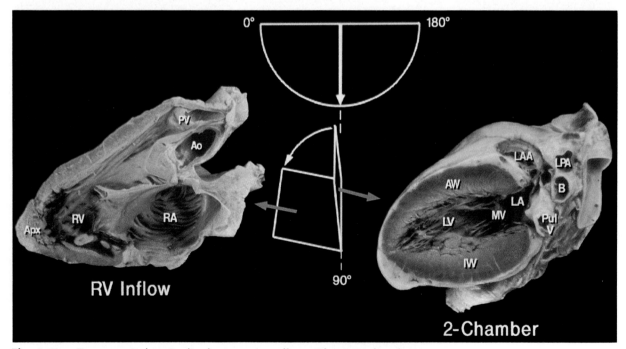

Fig. 4-49. Transgastric longitudinal anatomic collage. The two-chamber anatomy is described and shown in Figures 4-36, 4-41, and 4-45. The anatomy for right ventricular inflow is described in Figure 4-50. (*Ao* = proximal ascending aorta; *PulV* = pulmonary vein; *PV* = pulmonary valve.)

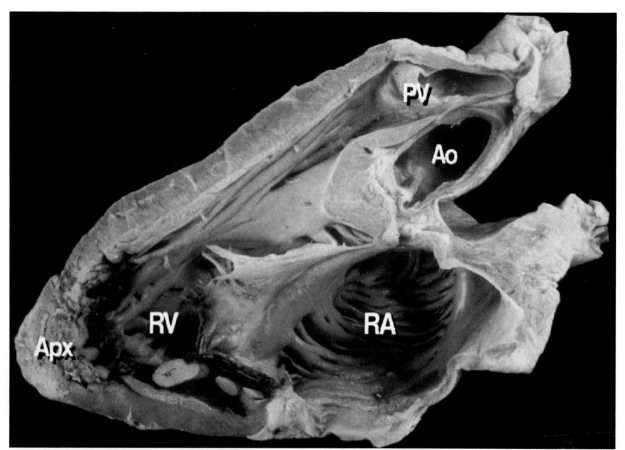

Fig. 4-50. Right ventricular inflow anatomic correlation. The specimen is viewed looking toward the right ventricular free wall. The transducer would be posterior and adjacent to the inferior wall of the right ventricle. The tricuspid valve leaflets are viewed from their ventricular surface. The apex of the right ventricle is to the left. Anteriorly, the right ventricular outflow and pulmonary valve *(PV)* are viewed. (*Ao* = proximal ascending aorta.)

Extracardiac Anatomy

The great veins and arteries of the heart and thorax (e.g., inferior and superior venae cavae, pulmonary artery, and aorta) can be consistently visualized by TEE [9,18].

Extracardiac Veins
Superior Vena Cava

The superior vena cava can be assessed in multiple tomographic views. One of the best examinations is the long-axis view obtained with the longitudinal plane in the midesophagus (see Figs. 4-34 and 4-39). The longitudinal image plane is directed rightward by rotation of the shaft of the endoscope. The superior vena cava enters the anterosuperior aspect of the right atrium.

One of the most helpful views for visualization of the superior vena cava is a basal short-axis cut at the level of the ascending aorta (Fig. 4-51). The superior vena cava lies rightward and courses parallel to the ascending aorta. The superior vena cava is anterior to the right pulmonary artery. The right upper pulmonary vein is adjacent and medial to the superior vena cava. An anomalous right upper pulmonary vein connected to the superior vena cava is best visualized in this tomographic section.

Inferior Vena Cava

The long-axis midesophageal view (see Fig. 4-39) is also excellent for visualizing the inferior vena cava and its entry into the right atrium. The four-chamber view with posterior tilt of the transverse image plane is also used to visualize the orifice of the inferior vena cava in the floor of the right atrium (see Fig. 4-43).

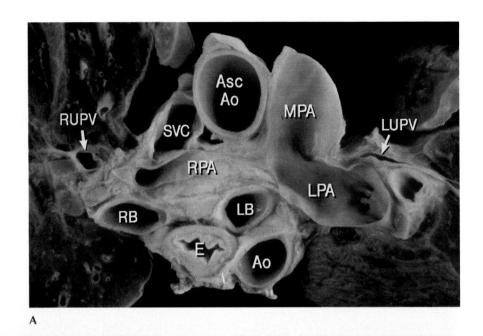

A

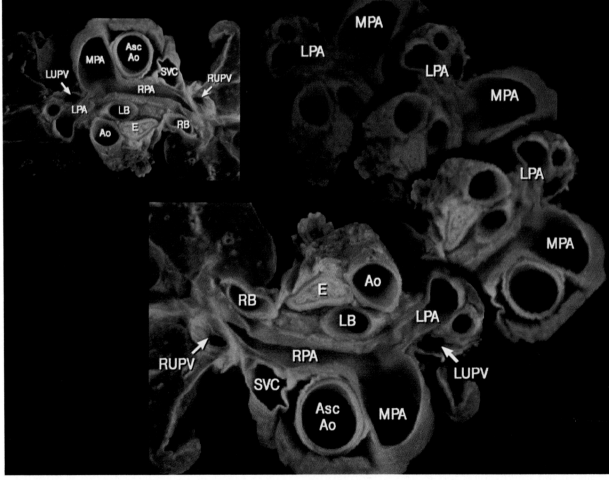

B

Fig. 4-51. ◀ Pulmonary bifurcation and short-axis view of the superior vena cava. A. The specimen is cut as viewed from the cardiac apex toward the basal structures. The esophagus is posterior to the right pulmonary artery and lies between the right and the left bronchi. The superior vena cava is anterior to the right pulmonary artery and adjacent to the ascending aorta. The right upper pulmonary vein is medial to the superior vena cava and anterior to the right pulmonary artery. When the right upper pulmonary vein is anomalously connected to the superior vena cava, this is the level at which these structures most typically communicate. The left pulmonary artery is usually difficult to see because of the intervening air-filled left bronchus. B. The other half of this bisected specimen (upper left segment of composite view) as seen from base toward apex. A 180-degree rotation is required to image the anatomy upside-down. The unconventional display of anatomy is not used in our laboratory but has commonly appeared in the TEE literature. (*Ao* = thoracic aorta.)

Pulmonary Veins

The pulmonary venous anatomy can be assessed in multiple tomographic sections (see Figs. 4-29, 4-30, 4-36, 4-37, 4-42, 4-43, and 4-45). The pulmonary vein orifices lie on the posterolateral (left pulmonary veins) and posteromedial (right pulmonary veins) aspects of the left atrial cavity. The upper pulmonary veins are directed anteriorly (see Fig. 4-30), whereas the lower veins enter the left atrium nearly perpendicular to the posterior atrial wall (Fig. 4-52). Using these anatomic features, one can consistently image the commitment of upper and lower pulmonary veins. For the left pulmonary veins, the longitudinal plane is used and the endoscope tip is slightly flexed laterally to an oblique long-axis view of the left ventricular outflow. For a multiple transducer, the array is set at approximately 110 degrees and the image plane is directed leftward by slow rotation of the endoscope shaft leftward. The Y-shaped configuration of the left upper and lower pulmonary veins (Fig. 4-53) is usually visualized. The main left pulmonary artery lies just anterosuperior to the left upper pulmonary vein. The Y relationship of the right pulmonary veins is obtained from the midesophageal longitudinal plane. The endoscope tip is slightly flexed medially to view a partial short axis of the aortic valve. When this off-axis longitudinal plane is rotated medially (i.e., the endoscope shaft is rotated), the right upper and lower pulmonary veins enter the left atrium in a Y relationship (Fig. 4-53).

Fig. 4-52. Left pulmonary veins. This tomographic specimen is viewed from the left lateral aspect of the left atrium. The courses of the left upper and left lower pulmonary veins are demonstrated. The course of the upper vein is anterior and slightly apical. The lower vein is nearly perpendicular to the left atrium. The esophagus is posterior to the pulmonary veins. A longitudinal image plane directed laterally (lateral tip flexion) simultaneously images the two veins in a Y configuration as they enter the left atrium. The right pulmonary veins have a similar relationship to the right side of the left atrium.

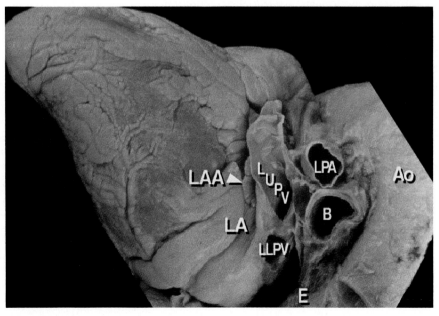

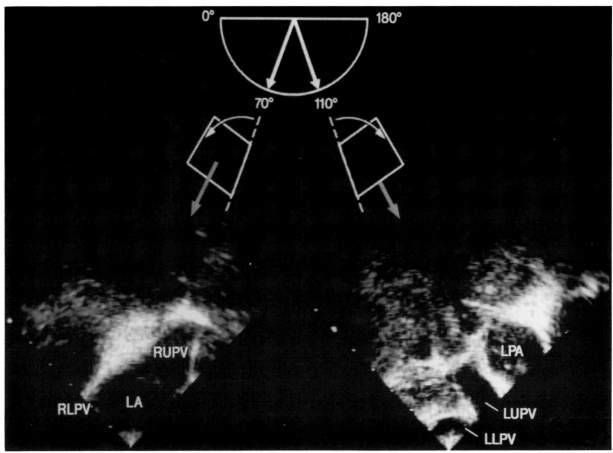

Fig. 4-53. Pulmonary vein visualization. Although not the only technique, the one described here is probably the most reproducible. Left: Right pulmonary veins: In the longitudinal plane of a biplane endoscope, the transducers are flexed medially to obtain an oblique short-axis view of the aortic valve (with the multiplane device, the array is rotated to approximately 70 degrees). The ultrasound plane is then directed medially by rotation of the endoscope shaft. The right upper and right lower pulmonary veins enter the medial aspect of the left atrium in a Y relationship. Right: Left pulmonary veins: In the longitudinal plane of the biplane endoscope, the transducer tip is flexed laterally to obtain an oblique long-axis view of the aortic valve (with the multiplane instrument, the array is rotated to approximately 110 degrees). The ultrasound plane is directed laterally by endoscope rotation. The left upper and left lower pulmonary veins enter the left atrium in a Y configuration. Note that the left pulmonary artery is visualized anteriorly and superiorly to the upper vein. See also Figure 4-52.

Extracardiac Arteries

Main Pulmonary Artery

The right ventricular outflow, pulmonary valve, and main pulmonary artery are usually examined in the same longitudinal tomographic plane. Longitudinal views best demonstrate the contiguous relationships of these structures (see Figs. 4-37 and 4-50). The main pulmonary artery and its branching into right and left pulmonary arteries is best visualized in a basal short-axis view in the transverse plane (see Fig. 4-51).

Right Pulmonary Artery

Both long (see Fig. 4-51) and short (see Figs. 4-31, 4-38, and 4-39) tomographic views of the right pulmonary artery can consistently be obtained. This combination of multiple planes often permits anatomic assessment beyond the first hilar bifurcation.

Left Pulmonary Artery

This vessel is less predictably imaged and only infrequently to the left hilum. Proximally, the left pulmonary artery is most consistently visualized with a basal short-axis view at the pulmonary bifurcation (see Fig. 4-51). More distal imaging of the left pulmonary artery is best accomplished with the longitudinal plane and laterally directed scan plane (see Figs. 4-36, 4-37, and 4-52).

Thoracic Aorta

The thoracic aorta (Fig. 4-54) can be completely assessed during a comprehensive tomographic TEE examination (see Chapter 14). The aorta and esophagus intertwine during their course through the upper abdomen and thorax. In the abdomen and lower thorax, the aorta is posterior to the stomach and esophagus [2]. In the midthorax, the esophagus and aorta lie side by side, with the aorta to the left (see Figs. 4-29 and 4-46). In the upper thorax, the esophagus is posterior to the aortic arch (see Figs. 4-51 and 4-54). Two anatomic features can interfere with a diagnostic aortic examination: (1) Air-filled lung surrounds the heart and mediastinal structures, causing reverberation artifacts, particularly in the midascending and mid-descending thoracic aorta. After recognition, these artifacts rarely cause a significant diagnostic problem [32]; and (2) The more significant problem is the air-filled left mainstem bronchus and distal trachea (Fig. 4-55). The longitudinal scan plane has greatly reduced this imaging problem [9] by allowing scanning over the bronchus from either below or above this air-filled structure. The brachiocephalic vessels are usually best imaged from the suprasternal transthoracic approach.

Fig. 4-54. Thoracic aorta. The entire thoracic aorta has been cut in a tomographic manner. The relationship of the esophagus and aorta is appreciated. (The esophagus is anterior to the aorta in the low thorax, medial in the middle thorax, and posterior in the upper thorax.) The aorta at the level of the right pulmonary artery is consistently visualized (see Figs. 4-31 and 4-38). The transverse and distal portions of the aortic arch are also consistently visualized [2]. Thus, potentially only a very small segment of the upper ascending aortic or proximal aortic arch may be obscured by the air-filled bronchial tree.

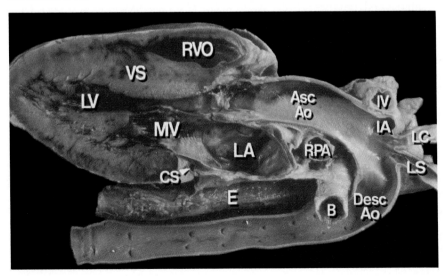

Fig. 4-55. Aortic arch. In an enlarged view of Figure 4-54, a segment of the upper ascending aorta is cut away *(arrowheads)* to simulate the potential blind spot *(white lines)* caused by tracheal and left bronchial air.

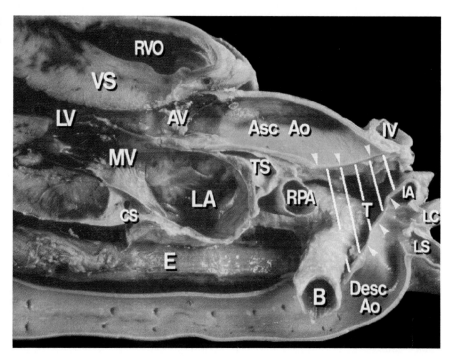

SUMMARY

Transesophageal echocardiography has advanced considerably since the early 1980s and has rapidly been clinically accepted. The concept of a uniform image presentation has matured and evolved with the increased clinical use of this tool. A difficult problem with TEE has been recognition of normal and abnormal anatomy, which often is presented in new and unfamiliar imaging formats [25,32].

Anatomic planes of section are unchanged, but the means of obtaining and displaying resulting images have changed considerably with TEE. It is indeed unfortunate when artistic and photographic techniques are erroneously reproduced and said to imply a correlation or anatomic conformation of echocardiographic images [25]. Only with an academic and critical approach can a consistent and user-friendly echocardiographic display of anatomy be achieved. The advent of TEE has, more than any other modality, emphasized the need for introspection into the whole question of faithful and consistent anatomic presentation through tomographic ultrasonography. We strongly advocate consistency of image presentation, adherence to time-tested standards of image presentation [6], and correct anatomic validation.

REFERENCES

1. Yock PG, Linker DT, White NW, et al. Clinical applications of intravascular ultrasound imaging in atherectomy. *Int J Card Imaging* 1989;4:117–25.

2. Kuroda T, Kinter TM, Seward JB, et al. Accuracy of three-dimensional volume measurement using biplane transesophageal echocardiographic probe: in vitro experiment. *J Am Soc Echocardiogr* 1991; 4:475–84.

3. Wollschläger H, Zeiher AM, Klein H-P, et al. Transesophageal echo computer tomography: a new method for dynamic 3–D imaging of the heart (abstract). *J Am Coll Cardiol* 1989;13 Suppl A:68A.

4. Rosenfield K, Losordo DW, Ramaswamy K, et al. Three-dimensional reconstruction of human coronary and peripheral arteries from images recorded during two-dimensional intravascular ultrasound examination. *Circulation* 1991;84:1938–56.

5. Belohlavek M, Foley DA, Gerber TC, et al. Three- and four-dimensional cardiovascular ultrasound imaging: a new era for echocardiography. *Mayo Clin Proc* 1993;68:221–40.

6. Henry WL, DeMaria A, Gramiak R, et al. Report of the American Society of Echocardiography Committee on Nomenclature and Standards in Two-Di-

mensional Echocardiography. *Circulation* 1980;62: 212–7.

7. Seward JB, Tajik AJ, DiMagno EP. Esophageal phased-array sector echocardiography: an anatomic study. In: Hanrath P, Bleifeld W, Souquet J, eds. *Cardiovascular Diagnosis by Ultrasound.* The Hague: Martinus Nijhoff, 1982:270–9.

8. Schlüter M, Hinrichs A, Thier W, et al. Transesophageal two-dimensional echocardiography: comparison of ultrasonic and anatomic sections. *Am J Cardiol* 1984;53:1173–8.

9. Seward JB, Khandheria BK, Oh JK, et al. Transesophageal echocardiography:technique, anatomic correlations, implementation, and clinical applications. *Mayo Clin Proc* 1988;63:649–80.

10. Schiller NB, Maurer G, Ritter SB, et al. Transesophageal echocardiography. *J Am Soc Echocardiogr* 1989;2:354-7.

11. Omoto R, Kyo S, Matsumura M, et al. Bi-plane color transesophageal Doppler echocardiography (color TEE): its advantages and limitations. *Int J Card Imaging* 1989;4:57–8.

12. Seward JB, Khandheria BK, Edwards WD, et al. Biplanar transesophageal echocardiography: anatomic correlations, image orientation, and clinical applications. *Mayo Clin Proc* 1990;65:1193–213.

13. Nanda NC, Pinheiro L, Sanyal RS, Storey O. Transesophageal biplane echocardiographic imaging: technique, planes, and clinical usefulness. *Echocardiography* 1990;7:771–8.

14. Bansal RC, Shakudo M, Shah PM, Shah PM. Biplane transesophageal echocardiography: technique, image orientation, and preliminary experience in 131 patients. *J Am Soc Echocardiogr* 1990; 3:348–66.

15. Cohen GI, Chan KL, Walley VM. Anatomic correlations of the long-axis views in biplane transesophageal echocardiography. *Am J Cardiol* 1990;66: 1007–12.

16. Stümper O, Fraser AG, Ho SY, et al. Transoesophageal echocardiography in the longitudinal axis: correlation between anatomy and images and its clinical implications. *Br Heart J* 1990;64:282–8.

17. Richardson SG, Weintraub AR, Schwartz SL, et al. Biplane transesophageal echocardiography utilizing transverse and sagittal imaging planes: technique, echo-anatomic correlations, and display approaches. *Echocardiography* 1991;8:293–310.

18. Wang X-F, Li Z-A, Cheng TO, et al. Biplane transesophageal echocardiography: an anatomic-ultrasonic-clinical correlative study. *Am Heart J* 1992; 123:1027–38.

19. Omoto R, Kyo S, Matsumura M, et al. Evaluation of biplane color Doppler transesophageal echocardiography in 200 consecutive patients. *Circulation* 1992;85:1237–47.

20. Silverman NH, Hunter S, Anderson RH, et al. Anatomical basis of cross sectional echocardiography. *Br Heart J* 1983;50:421–31.

21. Snider AR, Serwer GA. *Echocardiography in Pediatric Heart Disease.* Chicago: Year Book, 1990: 22–7.

22. Marino B, Thiene G. *Atlante di Anatomia Ecocardiografica Delle Cardiopatie Congenite.* Firenze: Uses Edizioni Scientifiche Firenze, 1990:19–37.

23. Seward JB, Tajik AJ, Edwards WD, Hagler DJ. *Two-Dimensional Echocardiographic Atlas, Vol 1: Congenital Heart Disease.* New York: Springer-Verlag, 1987:1–42.

24. Waller BF, Taliercio CP, Slack JD, et al. Tomographic views of normal and abnormal hearts: the anatomic basis for various cardiac imaging techniques. Part I. *Clin Cardiol* 1990;13:804–12.

25. Seward JB. "Nonanatomic" correlations of transesophageal echocardiography (editorial). *Echocardiography* 1991;8:669–70.

26. Richardson SG, Pandian NG. Echo-anatomic correlations and image display approaches in transesophageal echocardiography: purity with flip-flop or prudence without flip-flop? (editorial). *Echocardiography* 1991;8:671–4.

27. Tajik AJ, Seward JB, Hagler DJ, et al. Two-dimensional real-time ultrasonic imaging of the heart and great vessels: technique, image orientation, structure identification, and validation. *Mayo Clin Proc* 1978;53:271–303.

28. Silverman NH, Schiller NB. Apex echocardiography:a two-dimensional technique for evaluating congenital heart disease. *Circulation* 1978;57: 503–11.

29. McAlpine WA. *Heart and Coronary Arteries: An Anatomical Atlas for Clinical Diagnosis, Radiological Investigations, and Surgical Treatment.* New York: Springer-Verlag, 1978.

30. Edwards WD. Anatomic basis for tomographic analysis of the heart at autopsy. *Cardiol Clin* 1984 Nov;2:485–506.

31. Waller BF. Anatomic basis for newer cardiac imaging techniques. *Am J Card Imaging* 1987;1: 311–22.

32. Seward JB, Khandheria BK, Oh JK, et al. Critical appraisal of transesophageal echocardiography: limitations, pitfalls, and complications. *J Am Soc Echocardiogr* 1992;5:288–305.

5

Multiplane Transesophageal Echocardiography

James B. Seward

Transesophageal echocardiography (TEE) has become rapidly accepted in clinical cardiology practice despite its semi-invasive nature [1,2] and has had a major impact on decision making in patient management. In the relatively short period of approximately 5 years, multiple technologic advances have been incorporated in TEE probes, including higher frequency (7.0 MHz), frequency agility (3.5 to 5.0 to 7.0 MHz), a full complement of Doppler modalities (pulsed-wave, continuous-wave, and color-flow), smaller probes (4 to 7 mm in diameter), and biplane imaging capability. Most recently, a rotatable array, variously called *multiplane, variable plane (Varioplane),* and *Omniplane,* was introduced. This report describes this newest technologic innovation and its clinical application and impact. An image orientation consistent with familiar recommendations is used [3] (Fig. 5-1).

Multiplane, or variable plane, TEE was conceived in the early 1980s as a means of obtaining a larger number of imaging views from the confines of the esophagus [4].* Multiplane TEE consists of a single array of crystals or an imaging sector that can be electronically or mechanically rotated around the long axis of the ultrasound beam in an arc typically of 180 degrees. This capability produces a circular (conical) continuum of tomographic three-dimensional images.

COMPARISON OF MONOPLANE, BIPLANE, AND MULTIPLANE TEE

With each successive advance in TEE transducer technology, the number of available image planes has increased (Fig. 5-2). *Monoplane* devices are typically fitted with only the horizontal (transverse) imaging array. The monoplane device, therefore, can image only two primary planes of the heart, the short-axis and the four-chamber. The *biplane* TEE transducer has a second imaging array in the longitudinal orientation. The two arrays are orthogonal to each other and can image all three primary planes of the heart (short-axis, four-chamber, and long-axis). It has been noted that the biplane device adds at least 30% more diagnostic information to that derived from a monoplane device [2]. Biplane images are obtained with two different transducer technologies: stacked [2] and matrix [5]. The stacked biplane transducer places two imaging arrays at the endoscope tip, one above the other. This device does not allow simultaneous orthogonal images at the same level. The matrix system incorporates two arrays into a single transducer, thus permitting simultaneous orthogonal imaging. Off-axis and intermediate images with the biplane transducer are obtained by four-way flexion of the endoscope tip [2].

*N Harui, J Souquet. Transesophageal Echocardiography Scanhead, United States Patent No. 4,543,960, issued October 5, 1985.
Several figures in this chapter are also in Seward JB, Khandheria BK, Freeman WK, et al. Multiplane transesophageal echocardiography: image orientation, examination technique, anatomic correlations, and clinical applications. *Mayo Clin Proc* 1993;68:523–51.

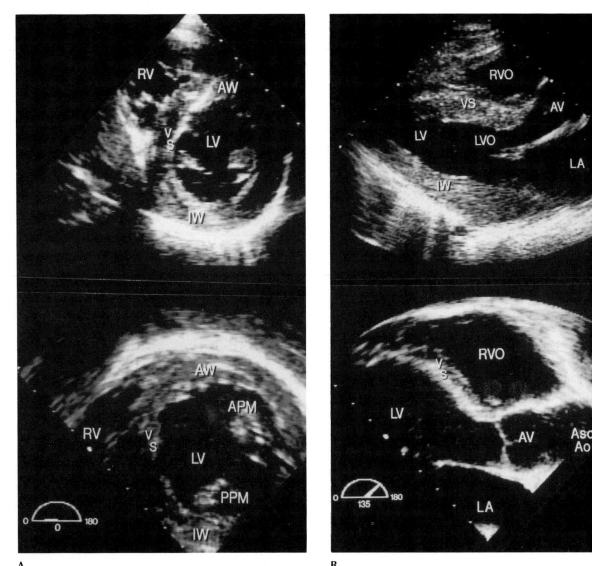

A   B

Fig. 5-1. Image orientation. In all four parts (A, B, C, and D), precordial images (top) and corresponding transesophageal images (bottom) are displayed in comparable orientations. A. *Short-axis* projections view the heart from the apex toward the base. Images are displayed with the right ventricle to the viewer's left and the left ventricle to the viewer's right. The inferior wall is at the bottom of the image and the anterior wall toward the top. The transesophageal image was obtained from the transgastric transducer position with the array at 0 degrees of rotation. B. *Long-axis* projections view the heart from the left side of the heart looking toward the right. Anterior structures (right ventricular outflow) are at the top of the image, and posterior structures (left atrium and inferior left ventricular wall) are at the bottom. Basal structures (ascending aorta and aortic valve) are to the viewer's right, and the ventricular apex (left ventricle) is to the viewer's left. The transesophageal image was obtained from the midesophageal transducer position with the array at 135 degrees of rotation.

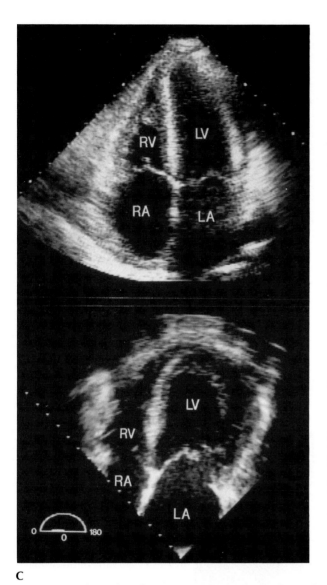

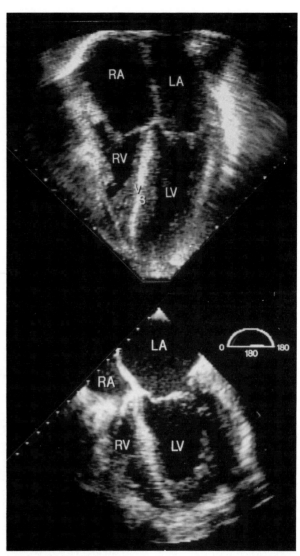

C   **D**

C. *Apex-up four-chamber* projections view the heart from its posterior surface toward the anterior surface. Left-sided structures (left ventricle and left atrium) are to the viewer's right, and right-sided structures (right ventricle and right atrium) are to the viewer's left. The apex is at the top of the image, and basal structures (left atrium and right atrium) are at the bottom. The transesophageal image was obtained from the midesophagus with the array at 0 degrees of rotation and the transducer tip retroflexed. D. *Apex-down four-chamber* projections view the heart from its anterior surface toward the posterior surface. The left-sided structures (left ventricle and left atrium) are to the viewer's right, and the right-sided structures (right ventricle and right atrium) are to the viewer's left. The cardiac apex is at the bottom of the image, and basal structures (left atrium and right atrium) are at the top of the image. The precordial apex-down four-chamber view was obtained from an electronic inversion of the image (C). Similarly, the transesophageal apex-down four-chamber view was obtained by electronic inversion of the image displayed in C.

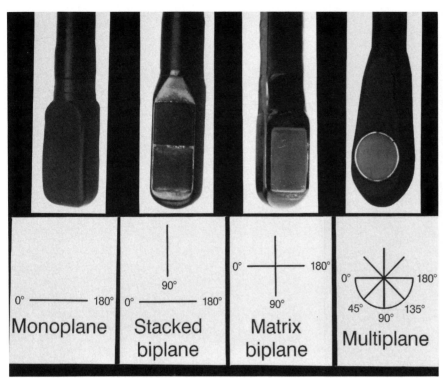

Fig. 5-2. Evolution of transesophageal ultrasound transducer technology. *Monoplane* (Hewlett-Packard) is typically a single transducer plane perpendicular (transverse) to the shaft of the endoscope. *Stacked biplane* (Hewlett-Packard) is a distal transverse plane complemented by a separate proximal longitudinal plane parallel to the long axis of the endoscope shaft. In the *matrix biplane* (Aloka), transverse and longitudinal plane arrays are interdigitated into a single transducer. *Multiplane* (Omniplane, Hewlett-Packard) uses a single array that can be rotated 180 degrees to produce a continuum of orientations relative to the endoscope shaft.

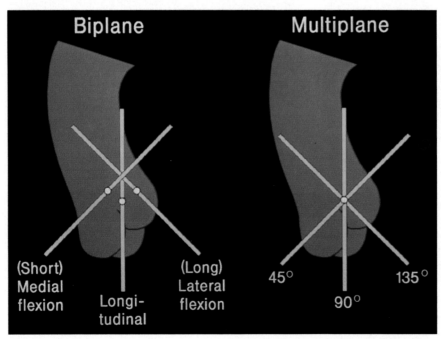

Fig. 5-3. Biplane and multiplane transducers obtain off-axis images in different manners. Left: The longitudinal plane of the biplane endoscope can be medially flexed to obtain the short-axis view of the aortic valve and laterally flexed to obtain the long-axis view. Right: The multiplane transducer rotates the array without transducer tip manipulation. Note that medial and lateral translation of the image plane with the biplane transducer when the tip is flexed does not occur with the multiplane transducer.

The *multiplane TEE* transducer produces a continuum of transverse and longitudinal images by rotation of the transducer array. In contrast to biplane technology, one can more easily visualize intermediate, transitional, and off-axis images between the primary planes. There is markedly less need to use lateral or medial tip flexion to obtain desired off-axis views than there is with biplane TEE. There is a small but significant increase in tomographic information gained with multiplane technology compared with biplane technology. Similar short-axis, long-axis, and four-chamber views are obtainable with both techniques [2] (Fig. 5-3). The primary advantages of multiplane TEE are the ability to obtain an uninterrupted series of adjacent images and the ease of accomplishing this task once the technique is mastered.

An analogy can be made by comparing the biplane and multiplane technologies with the two major techniques of coronary arteriography (Sones' and Judkins' techniques). Both angiographic techniques obtain images of the coronary arteries that are similar in quality and can be performed by a talented operator in about the same time. However, operator finesse and aptitude must be much greater for the Sones technique, whereas the preformed Judkins catheters (comparable to multiplane TEE) are designed for easier access to a specific coronary artery (analogous to a specific image).

Multiplane TEE can obtain specific views by predetermined degrees of rotation of the imaging array. The examination can be taught as a specific set of transducer orientations rather than as a particular set of more complex hand or endoscope manipulations. Biplane and multiplane TEE obtain comparable tomographic images; however, the multiplane technique allows greater versatility and more rapid understanding.

MULTIPLANE TEE IMAGES

Image Notation

Degrees of Array Rotation

Multiplane images are identified in degrees of rotation required to obtain a particular view (Fig. 5-4). Such a designation helps the examiner explain the transducer maneuver and record the position of the imaged structures relative to the esophagus, stomach, or thorax. In most circumstances, the examiner can preselect a specific tomographic plane based on degrees of array rotation and then optimize the image, if needed, with minor endoscope manipulations.

Array Orientation

The standard transverse array position is designated 0 degrees (i.e., the array lies transverse to the long axis of the endoscope) (see Fig. 5-4). A mirror image reversal of the array is a transverse transducer position of 180 degrees. The standard longitudinal array position is designated 90 degrees (i.e., the array is longitudinal to the long axis of the endoscope).

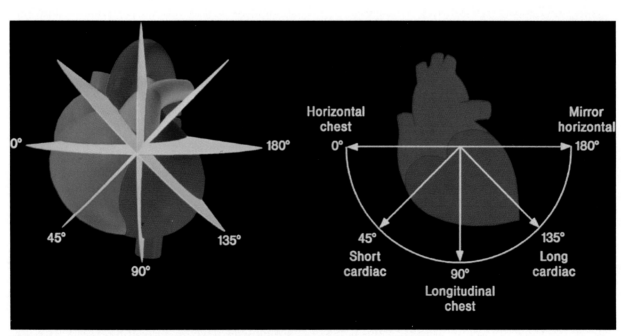

Fig. 5-4. Multiplane TEE. Selected degrees of array rotation (0, 45, 90, 135, and 180 degrees) permit a logical sequence of standard transducer orientations and resultant images. Such a display assists the examiner in acquisition of desired views. That is, 0 degrees is a transverse orientation horizontal to the chest at the midesophageal level, 45 degrees is a short-axis view of the base of the heart from midesophagus, 90 degrees is a longitudinal orientation in the sagittal plane of the body, 135 degrees is a long-axis view of the heart from the midesophagus, and 180 degrees is a mirror-image transverse plane.

Image Orientation

Anterior and Posterior Orientation

Multiplane imaging, more than any other modality, highlights the need for a consistent image presentation. Nearly all views obtained from the surface of the thorax can be duplicated by TEE (see Fig. 5-1). The ability to rotate the array allows smooth transition from one view to another without electronic image reorientation. The image orientation described herein eliminates the need to perform unnecessary electronic reversals to retain a consistent and familiar image presentation.

Analogy

Transthoracic echocardiography also is a multiplane examination. The examiner manually rotates a transducer from short-axis to long-axis view, four-chamber to two-chamber view, and so forth [6]. By convention, transthoracic tomographic images are displayed in a consistent and now very familiar orientation from examination to examination [3] (see Fig. 5-1). From any standard view, an orthogonal view is obtained by rotating the transducer approximately 90 degrees (e.g., short-axis view to long-axis view). Over-rotation of the transducer (e.g., 180 degrees) results in a right-left mirror image.

In multiplane TEE, an examination is made by mechanical rotation of the imaging array and, to a lesser extent, movements of the endoscope tip from the confines of the esophagus. The only difference between transthoracic echocardiography and TEE is that the TEE transducer is posterior to the heart instead of on the chest wall. Because of this location, one can display images identical to those obtained from the chest wall (see Fig. 5-1). This chapter presents the TEE image in a consistent and very familiar orientation identical to that obtained from the chest wall. A 180-degree rotation of the array results in a left-right mirror image for both the precordial and the TEE multiplane examinations.

Transducer Bang Artifact

The transducer is held against the anterior chest wall during a conventional transthoracic examination, and the electronic transducer artifact (bang) is oriented predominantly at the top of the displayed image. Conversely, when the transducer is introduced into the posterior esophagus and stomach during a TEE examination, for consistency the electronic transducer artifact is kept predominantly at the bottom of the display throughout the examination. A familiar image presentation is thus maintained throughout both examinations (see Fig. 5-1). Only if the cardiac *apex-down four-chamber view* is preferred for either a surface or a transesophageal examination is an electronic inversion of the image required [7] (see Fig. 5-1). Anatomic correlations and image orientations are thus preferably kept identical for both transthoracic echocardiography and TEE [3].

Right-Left Orientation

At 0 degrees, left-sided structures are displayed to the viewer's right and right-sided structures to the viewer's left, a presentation consistent with previous literature on standardized transthoracic image orientation [3]. Most manufacturers have a display mechanism (such as an icon alongside the displayed ultrasound array) for the depiction of left-right array orientation.

Multiplane Orientation

The primary intent of multiplane TEE is to make a smooth transition from one standard image orientation to another; for example, a transition from short axis to long axis should result in an appropriate orientation of both views without obligating operator intervention. Such a maneuver must retain consistent left-right, as well as anterior-posterior, relationships of the image. When the array is rotated from 0 to 90 degrees, it is realigned from a transverse to a longitudinal orientation. A consistent right-left, anterior-posterior, and basal-apical relationship must be retained (see Figs. 5-1 and 5-4). Similarly, a maneuver from a short-axis to a four-chamber view must retain familiar relationships.

INSTRUMENTATION

Most of the multiplane TEE experience described in this chapter is based on studies with the Hewlett-Packard Omniplane device. Other prototype devices, with which we have had limited experience, are the Advanced Technology Laboratory and Interspec multiplane TEE endoscopes. The Hewlett-Packard endoscope head (see Fig. 5-2) is larger than that of conventional devices, measuring 11.9 x 16.8 mm and diagonally, 18.8 mm. The endoscope shaft is 12.0 mm in diameter. The array is rotated by a motor-driven system controlled by a pressure-sensitive rocker switch on the handle (Fig. 5-5). The phased array in the endoscope head is rotated by a gear mechanism. Degrees of rotation are displayed on a video screen icon (Fig. 5-6).

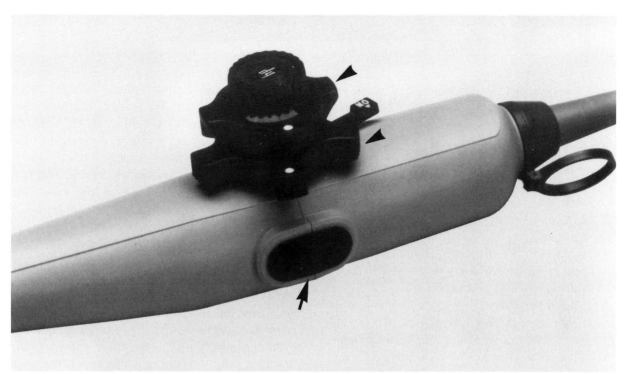

Fig. 5-5. The multiplane endoscope handle (Omniplane, Hewlett-Packard). A pressure-sensitive rocker switch *(arrow)* controls the movement of the rotatable transducer array. Conventional endoscope knobs *(arrowheads)* are used for four-way flexion of the endoscope tip.

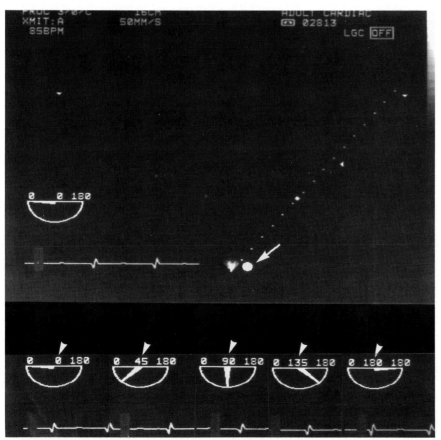

Fig. 5-6. Multiplane screen display. The transducer artifact (bang) is kept at the bottom of the image, and the right-left orientation is confirmed by the manufacturer's designation *(arrow)*. Left-sided structures are to the viewer's right and right-sided structures to the viewer's left. An icon on the endoscope is presented as a semicircle depicting the array rotation relative to the axis of the body and heart. At the bottom of this figure are the five standard array orientations as they appear on the endoscope. The degrees of rotation are displayed *(arrowheads)*, and a pointer shows the relative travel of the array through the semicircle. The transverse orientations, 0 and 180 degrees, are continuously displayed.

MAYO CLINIC EXPERIENCE

Of 300 consecutive patients studied with multiplane TEE at the Mayo Clinic, 178 were male and 122 female. Their ages ranged from 17 to 91 years, and the mean age was 60 years. After informed consent, the patients were prepared in the following manner:

1. A 20-gauge indwelling intravenous cannula was inserted for the administration of medications and contrast medium, if deemed necessary.
2. Lidocaine oral spray was applied for topical anesthesia.
3. Glycopyrrolate (Robinul), an anticholinergic, was given intravenously (0.2 mg) to reduce salivation (77% of patients).
4. Midazolam (Versed), a benzodiazepine, was given intravenously for sedation (0.5 to 15.0 mg; average dose, 3.5 mg) in 90% of patients.
5. Meperidine (Demerol) to reduce excessive gag (25 to 50 mg; average dose, 30 mg) was given intravenously to 15% of patients.

Indications for the TEE examination were similar to those previously described in patients undergoing biplane TEE [2].

In our initial experience with multiplane TEE, we found that our technique was slightly different from the examination protocol previously described [1,2]. Because of the larger endoscope head, great care was used in esophageal intubation. This introduction was exclusively performed by the digital technique. Furthermore, the mean dose of sedative was higher (3.5 mg) than in our previous experience with monoplane and biplane TEE (2.5 mg) [1,2]. Introduction of the endoscope was frequently more difficult even with the digital technique. Small patients (weight less than 35 kg) were excluded from any multiplane TEE study because of early recognition of consistent difficulty with introduction of the large endoscope head.

Intubation with the prototype multiplane transducer was unsuccessful in eight patients (2.6%). In all eight, intubation was achieved by the same examiner at the same time using a standard TEE endoscope (12 mm in diameter).

SYSTEMATIC MULTIPLANE TEE EXAMINATION

A step-by-step sequence results in a comprehensive multiplane TEE examination.

1. Setup

Before beginning the examination, set the image format so that the electronic artifact is at the *bottom* of the screen and the appropriate left-right image format is displayed (i.e., left-sided cardiac structures appear to the examiner's right) (see Fig. 5-6). In addition, set the image depth to accommodate the expected size of the heart, usually about 15 cm of depth. Before intubation, rotate the array to 0 degrees to place the transducer into a conventional transverse plane (i.e., array perpendicular to the long axis of the endoscope shaft).

2. Endoscope Insertion

Always use a bite guard unless the patient is adentulous. Place the imaging surface of the transducer toward the tongue so that the ultrasound beam is directed anteriorly toward the chest wall when the transducer is in the esophagus. Because of the large size of the multiplane transducer tip, we recommend using the digital technique [1] for esophageal intubation. Place the transducer tip beneath the left index finger and press downward toward the tongue. Slowly advance the endoscope tip with finger guidance while pressing downward and posteriorly. When the endoscope tip is in the posterior esophagus and hypopharynx, have the patient swallow. The endoscope tip should be advanced into the esophagus with only mild resistance. Great care must be taken in elderly patients, who may have hypertrophic cervical vertebral prominences, and in smaller adults. Advance the endoscope tip to approximately midesophagus (25 to 30 cm from the incisors) [1]. Flex the endoscope tip anteriorly (anteflex) toward the heart to optimize transducer contact. The first structures visualized are the left atrial cavity and, in an oblique short-axis view, the aortic valve (Fig. 5-7).

3. Multiplane Views

To image the primary multiplane views (Figs. 5-4 and 5-8), sequentially rotate the array: 0 degrees, transverse array orientation is in the horizontal plane of the body; 45 degrees, short-axis view of the aortic valve; 90 degrees, longitudinal transducer orientation, which is in the long axis of the body—from midesophagus, this plane best visualizes the long axis of the proximal ascending aorta; 135 degrees, from the midesophagus, the array is in the long axis

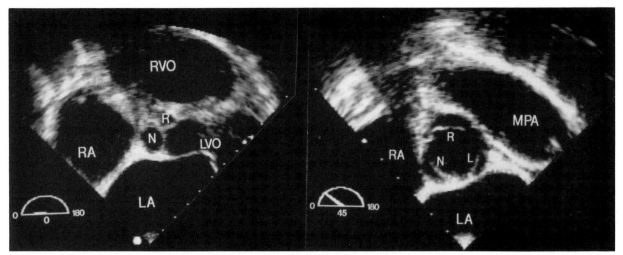

Fig. 5-7. Oblique short-axis view of the aortic valve. Left: The array is at 0 degrees rotation, which is a plane transverse to the body that cuts the basal cardiac structures slightly obliquely. Orientation of the image: Anterior structures are at the top of the image, posterior structures are at the bottom of the image, left structures are at the viewer's right, and right structures are at the viewer's left. The heart is projected as though one were looking from apex toward base. The transducer is within the esophagus posterior to and adjacent to the left atrium. Right: Rotation of the array from 0 to 45 degrees places the transducer in an optimal short-axis plane to the aortic valve. (L = left coronary cusp; N = noncoronary cusp; R = right coronary cusp.)

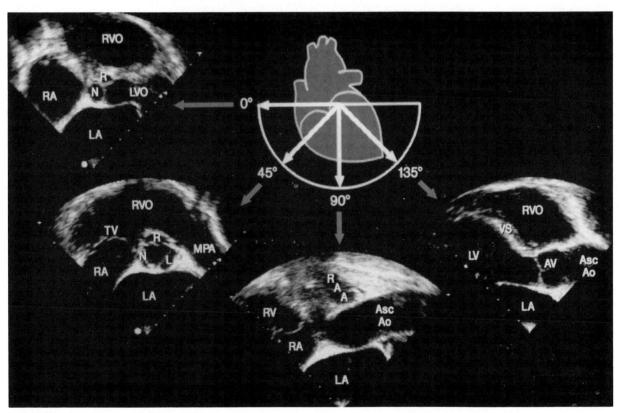

Fig. 5-8. Primary multiplane views are obtained by rotating the array from left to right as indicated on the icon. The transducer is in the midesophagus. At 0 degrees (transverse plane), an oblique view of the basal structures is visualized. At 45 degrees, a short-axis view of basal structures (e.g., aortic valve) is obtained. At 90 degrees (longitudinal plane), a long-axis view of the cardiac structures (e.g., ascending aorta) is visualized. At 135 degrees, the array is aligned with the long axis of the left ventricular outflow tract. (L = left coronary cusp; N = noncoronary cusp; R = right coronary cusp.)

of the left ventricular outflow tract; 180 degrees, a mirror image of the transverse plane (rarely used in clinical imaging).

4. Longitudinal Views

Rotate the array back to 90 degrees. This places the transducer in a longitudinal orientation (Fig. 5-9), which is in the sagittal plane of the body and slightly oblique to the long axis of the heart. Progressive leftward and rightward *rotation of the endoscope shaft* develops the four primary longitudinal views (remember that the array is 90 degrees throughout this maneuver). Leftward rotation of the endoscope shaft develops (1) the two-chamber left ventricular view. With progressive rightward rotation of the shaft, sequential longitudinal views are obtained: (2) right ventricular outflow, (3) long-axis view of the proximal ascending aorta, and (4) long-axis view of the superior and inferior venae cavae entering the right atrium.

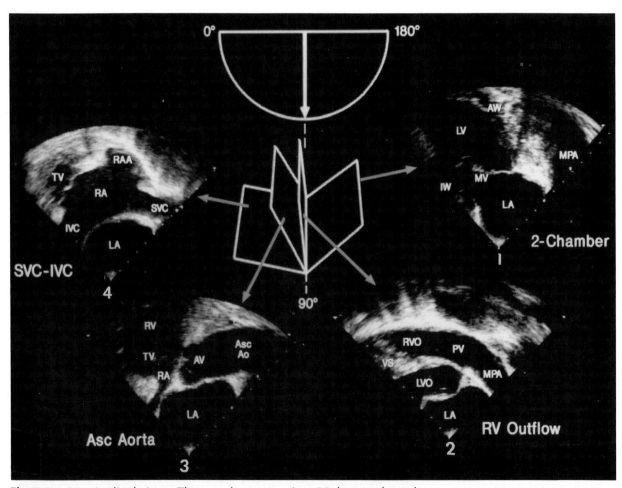

Fig. 5-9. Longitudinal views. The transducer array is at 90 degrees throughout this maneuver. The transducer tip is in the midesophagus. The shaft of the endoscope is rotated so that the image plane is to the patient's left and the mitral valve and left ventricular inflow are optimally imaged. A sequence of longitudinal views is obtained by progressive rotation of the endoscope shaft to the patient's right (remember that the array is at 90 degrees throughout). 1. Two-chamber left ventricular inflow view is obtained with the endoscope rotated to the left. 2. Right ventricular outflow is obtained by slight rightward scope rotation. 3. The next further rightward rotation results in a long-axis view of the proximal ascending aorta. 4. The long axis view of the venae cavae, atria, and atrial septum is obtained by further rightward endoscope rotation.

5. Four-Chamber Views

With the transducer tip in the midesophagus, rotate the array back to 0 degrees (transverse plane). Short-axis views are obtained by anteflexion of the endoscope tip, and retroflexion (posteriorly directed movement of the endoscope tip) develops the apex-up four-chamber view of the heart (Fig. 5-10). One can either image the more familiar apex-up four-chamber view or, if preferred, invert the electronic artifact to produce an apex-down presentation. This is the same electronic maneuver required during a transthoracic examination if apex-down is preferred. The left ventricle and left atrium are to the viewer's right.

6. Multiplane Apical Views

A unique feature of the variable plane (i.e., multiplane) transducer is the ability to visualize a continuum of images with the transducer tip in any fixed position. Beginning with a four-chamber view,

the rotatable array can be sequentially moved through the primary long-axis views of the heart (Fig. 5-11): (1) array at 0 degrees, four-chamber view; (2) array at 90 degrees, two-chamber longitudinal view; (3) array at 135 degrees, left ventricular outflow longitudinal view; (4) array at 180 degrees, mirror-image four-chamber view. This rotational maneuver permits a complete 360-degree sweep of the long axis of the heart. It is frequently used to completely visualize the mitral valve leaflets and support apparatus and fully delineate the extent of the mitral regurgitant jet by color Doppler mapping. All basal to middle left ventricular wall segments are also visualized with this scanning technique; complete visualization of the apical segments, however, is variable.

7. Transgastric Longitudinal Views

With the transducer tip in the midesophagus, rotate the array to 90 degrees and optimally visualize the longitudinal view of the proximal ascending aorta

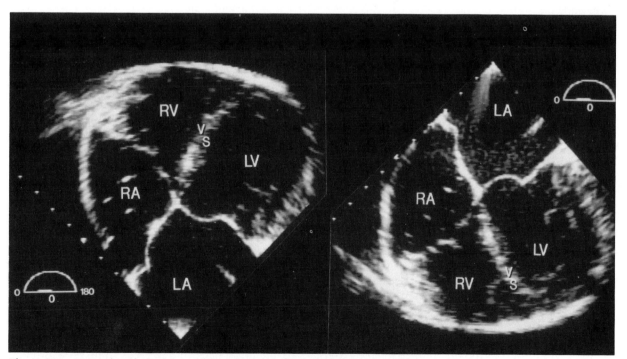

Fig. 5-10. Four-chamber views. The array is set at 0 degrees, a transverse plane. With the endoscope tip in the midesophagus, the transducer tip is retroflexed to generate an apex-up four-chamber view (left). This is comparable with the precordial apex-up four-chamber view and is referred to as the American Society of Echocardiography option 2. An electronic top-to-bottom inversion of the image is required if the apex-down, option 1 format is desired (right).

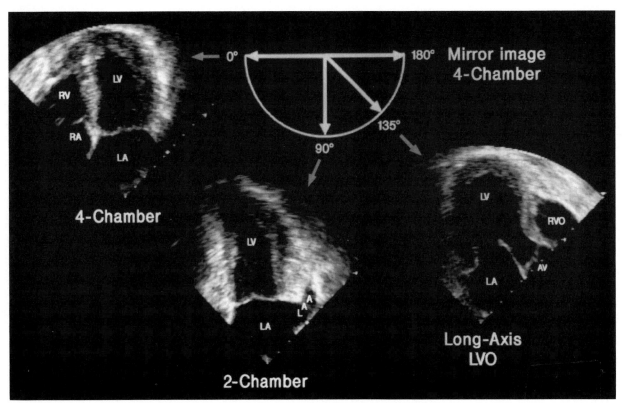

Fig. 5-11. Multiplane apical views. A sequence of apical views is obtained by rotating the array with the endoscope in a fixed position (e.g., midesophagus with retroflexed tip). Left: Array at 0 degrees, apex-up four-chamber view. Middle: Array rotated to 90 degrees, longitudinal two-chamber view of the left ventricle. Right: Rotation to 135 degrees, apical long-axis view of the left ventricular outflow. Rotation to 180 degrees would result in a mirror-image reversal of the four-chamber view (not shown).

(see Fig. 5-9). Slowly advance the transducer into the fundus of the stomach, with slight anteflexion of the endoscope tip. Slight leftward rotation of the endoscope shaft may be required to obtain a two-chamber long-axis view of the left ventricle (Fig. 5-12). Keep the array at 90 degrees and rotate the shaft of the transducer rightward to view the right ventricular inflow and outflow (Fig. 5-12).

8. Transgastric Multiplane Views

Rotate the array to 0 degrees to develop the short-axis view of the left and right ventricles. Anteflexion or slight withdrawal of the tip optimizes more basal views of the ventricles, whereas retroflexion of the transducer tip develops more apical views of the ventricles (Fig. 5-13). Sequential rotation of the multiplane array develops three primary transgastric views of the left ventricle (Fig. 5-14): (1) 0 degrees

array rotation, short-axis view of the ventricles; (2) 90 degrees rotation, longitudinal two-chamber view of the left ventricle; (3) 135 degrees rotation, transgastric left ventricular outflow view; visualization of the outflow tract ventricular aspects of the aortic valve is usually obtained. The third view also affords the optimal angle of incidence for steerable continuous-wave TEE Doppler interrogation of the left ventricular outflow tract and aortic valve.

9. Pulmonary Artery Bifurcation

With the transducer in the transgastric position, rotate the array back to 0 degrees (transverse orientation of the array). Slowly withdraw the transducer tip from the fundus of the stomach to the midesophagus adjacent and posterior to the left atrial cavity. To visualize the pulmonary artery bifurcation, continue the withdrawal of the transducer until the main pul-

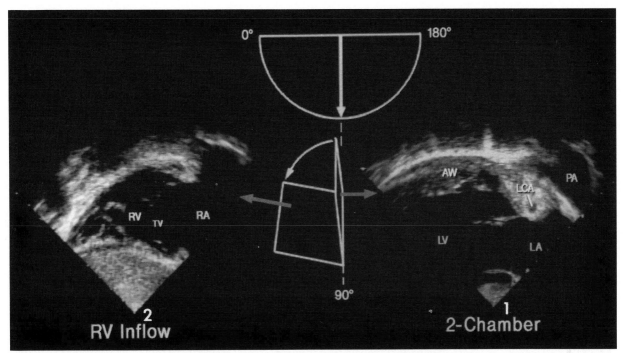

Fig. 5-12. Transgastric long-axis views of the left and right ventricles. The array is at 90 degrees (i.e., longitudinal), and the endoscope tip in the fundus of the stomach is anteflexed for optimal mucosal contact, usually with the shaft initially turned toward the left ventricle. 1. In the *two-chamber left ventricular view,* the transducer is posterior and adjacent to the left ventricular inferior wall. 2. With the array remaining at 90 degrees, the endoscope shaft is rotated rightward to the *right ventricular inflow view.* Fine adjustments in the array orientation may be necessary to optimize these views.

monary artery and the proximal bifurcation of left and right pulmonary arteries are visualized (Fig. 5-15). Rotate the shaft of the transducer to the patient's left to develop views of the proximal left pulmonary artery. Rotate the shaft of the transducer to the right to visualize the right pulmonary artery, short axis of the superior vena cava, and upper segment of the right pulmonary vein (Fig. 5-15B). Note: If the right upper pulmonary vein is anomalously connected to the superior vena cava, this view best demonstrates that congenital anomaly.

10. Left Atrial Appendage and Pulmonary Veins

Advance the imaging transducer to the midesophagus adjacent and posterior to the left atrium, with the image array at 0 degrees (transverse plane). Short-axis views of basal structures require an array orientation between 0 (transverse plane) and 45 degrees (short axis of aortic valve). Rotate the shaft

of the endoscope leftward to see the left upper pulmonary vein, left atrial appendage, and portions of the left lower pulmonary vein (Fig. 5-16). While visualizing the left upper pulmonary vein, slightly advance the endoscope to visualize more of the left lower pulmonary vein [2]. Rotate the endoscope shaft to the right to see the corresponding proximal left upper and lower pulmonary veins. The pulmonary veins can also be visualized in the longitudinal array orientation (i.e., 90 degrees) with corresponding right or left rotation of the endoscope shaft (Fig. 5-17).

The best means for visualizing the pulmonary veins is by the following two maneuvers:

1. For the *right pulmonary veins,* set the array at 70 to 80 degrees (an off-axis transverse view of the aortic valve). Rotate the shaft of the transducer to the patient's right to simultaneously visualize the Y configuration of the right upper and lower pulmonary veins [2] (Fig. 5-18).

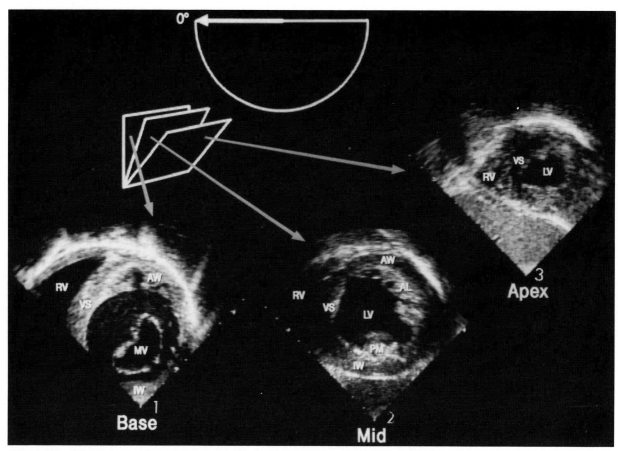

Fig. 5-13. Transgastric short-axis views. The array is maintained at 0 degrees (transverse plane). 1. Full anteflexion or slight withdrawal (or both) of the endoscope tip best visualizes the *basal short-axis view* at the level of the mitral valve orifice. 2. Mild anteflexion of the endoscope tip obtains the *midventricular short-axis view.* 3. Slight retroflexion of the endoscope tip produces the *apical short-axis view.*

2. For the *left pulmonary veins,* set the array at 100 to 110 degrees (an off-axis longitudinal view of the aortic valve). Rotate the transducer shaft to the patient's left to simultaneously visualize the Y configuration of the left upper and lower pulmonary veins (Fig. 5-18).

11. Thoracic Aorta

In the midesophagus, set the array at 0 degrees (transverse plane). The thoracic aorta is leftward and posterior to the esophagus. Thus, rotate the endoscope shaft to the patient's left. Because the aorta is posterior to the esophagus, the electronic artifact is usually inverted to give a more conventional presentation of aortic anatomy in the transverse plane [1]. Advance the endoscope to visualize the lower

thoracic and upper abdominal aorta. Withdraw the endoscope to visualize the upper thoracic aorta. In the upper thorax, the esophagus becomes posterior to the aorta. In the transverse plane, the electronic artifact is usually maintained at the top of the image; in the longitudinal plane, however, aortic anatomy is easier to understand if the artifact is at the bottom of the video screen [2] (Fig. 5-19).

CLINICAL APPLICATION OF MULTIPLANE TEE

The advantages of the variable plane array include ease of image acquisition. Specific planes can be obtained predominantly by four maneuvers: (1) multiplane rotation of the array, normally between 0 and 135 degrees; (2) rotation of the endoscope

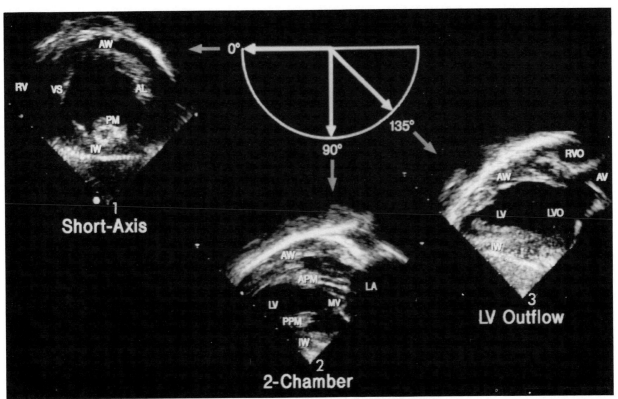

Fig. 5-14. Multiplane transgastric views. With the transducer tip in a stable position, the array can be rotated to obtain a sequence of short- and long-axis views. 1. *Short-axis view, left ventricle,* array at 0 degrees (transverse plane). 2. *Two-chamber view, left ventricle,* array at 90 degrees (longitudinal plane) with slight leftward endoscope rotation. 3. *Long-axis view, left ventricular outflow,* array at 110 to 135 degrees, which best visualizes the left ventricular outflow and aortic valve from the gastric transducer position.

shaft to visualize leftward or rightward anatomy; (3) advancement and withdrawal of the endoscope to see superior and inferior structures; and (4) tip anteflexion (transducer contact) and retroflexion (to develop four-chamber view). Lateral leftward and rightward tip flexions are infrequently used during the multiplane examination, unlike in biplane TEE, which often requires lateral flexion to obtain off-axis views.

Specific examples of clinical TEE applications facilitated by multiplane imaging are as follows:

Short- and Long-Axis Views of the Aortic Valve

Rotation of the multiplane array to 45 degrees (midesophagus) consistently results in an optimal short-axis view of the aortic valve (Figs. 5-20 and 5-21). The long axis is best with the array at 135 degrees, which places the transducer in the long axis of the

left ventricle. Oblique views obtained with the transverse plane (0 degrees) can create a pseudomass effect by obliquely cutting the aortic valve sinus [10]. This problem can be virtually eliminated by optimizing the multiplane short- and long-axis scans of the aortic valve. The number and structure of the aortic cusps can be more confidently assessed with the multiplane examination.

Long-Axis View of the Left Ventricular Outflow

Rotation of the multiplane array to 135 degrees consistently results in an optimal long-axis view of the left ventricular outflow (Fig. 5-22). Aortic and mitral valve regurgitation, vegetations, and other pathologic conditions are much more predictably appreciated with an optimized left ventricular long-axis view, which is more readily acquired with the multiplane technique.

Fig. 5-15. Pulmonary bifurcation. A. With the array at 0 degrees (transverse plane), the endoscope is withdrawn to the level of the pulmonary bifurcation (the image shown is a composite wide-field view [8] to better illustrate anatomy). The TEE transducer is posterior to the right pulmonary artery. Anteriorly, the ascending aorta and, rightward, the superior vena cava are visualized in their short axes. In this projection, only a small portion of the proximal left pulmonary artery is visualized. B. A similar projection at the pulmonary bifurcation with the transducer shaft rotated to the patient's right demonstrates the normal right upper pulmonary vein, which lies adjacent to the superior vena cava. Anomalous connection of the right upper pulmonary vein to the superior vena cava is best appreciated with this view.

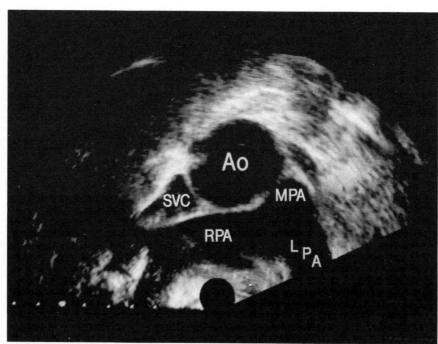

A

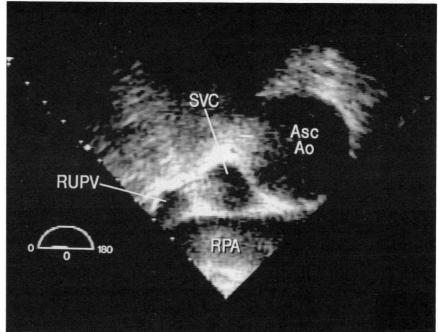

B

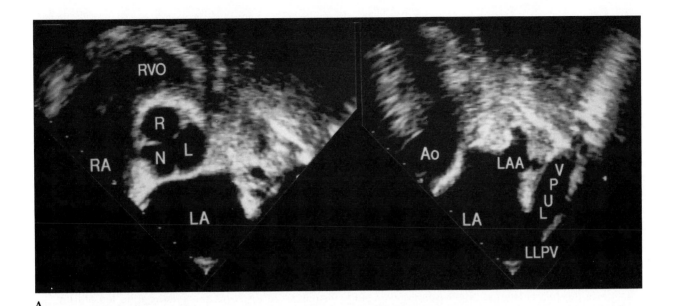

Fig. 5-16. A. Left upper pulmonary vein. Left: The array is at 45 degrees (short axis to the aortic valve). From this position, the endoscope must be rotated leftward and slightly withdrawn to visualize the left upper pulmonary vein. Right: The left upper pulmonary vein enters the left atrium just above the left lower pulmonary vein. For optimal visualization of the left lower pulmonary vein in this tomographic plane, slight advancement of the probe may be necessary. The left atrial appendage is transected obliquely. B. Left atrial appendage. Left: The array is at 0 degrees (transverse plane) in the midesophagus. The endoscope has been rotated to the left to visualize the left atrial appendage in the short axis. Right: The array is at 90 degrees (longitudinal plane). The endoscope has been rotated leftward to the two-chamber (left atrium and left ventricle) view. Anterior in the left atrial cavity is the long-axis projection of the left atrial appendage, which lies adjacent to the main pulmonary artery. (*L* = left coronary cusp; *N* = noncoronary cusp; *PV* = pulmonary valve; *R* = right coronary cusp.)

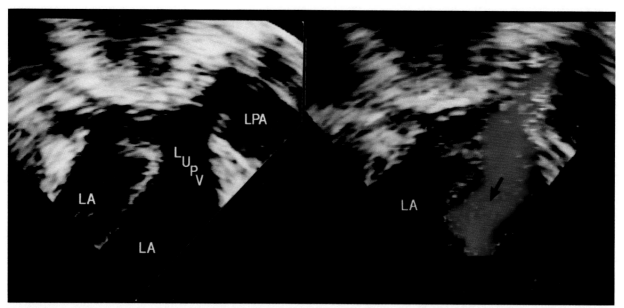

Fig. 5-17. Longitudinal scan to the left upper pulmonary vein. Left: The transducer is set at 90 degrees (longitudinal plane), the endoscope tip is in midesophagus, and the shaft of the endoscope is rotated to the left side of the heart. The left upper pulmonary vein is visualized in the long axis entering the left atrium. Right: Color-flow Doppler signal *(arrow)* confirms that blood is moving from the left upper pulmonary vein into the left atrium.

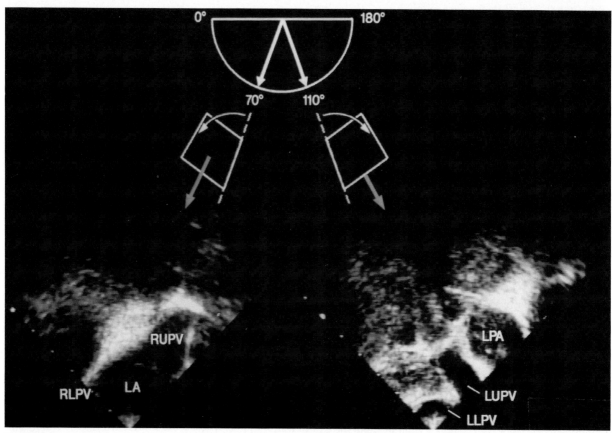

Fig. 5-18. Simultaneous visualization of upper and lower pulmonary veins. *Right pulmonary veins* (left on image): The array is set at 70 to 80 degrees (an off-axis transverse view of the aortic valve). The endoscope shaft is rotated rightward to view the Y configuration of the right upper and right lower pulmonary veins, which empty into the left atrium. *Left pulmonary veins* (right on image): The array is set at 100 to 110 degrees (an off-axis longitudinal view of the aortic valve). The endoscope shaft is rotated to view the Y configuration of the left upper and left lower pulmonary veins, which empty into the left atrium. Note that a more distal portion of the left pulmonary artery is also visualized with this maneuver.

120

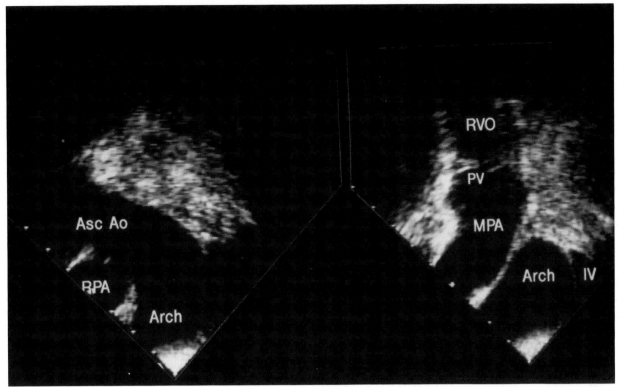

Fig. 5-19. Longitudinal view of the aortic arch. The transducer is very high in the esophagus and posterior to the aortic arch. The array is longitudinal (i.e., 90 degrees). Left: When the endoscope shaft is rotated to the patient's right, a longitudinal view of the ascending aorta can be visualized in about 30% of patients. The right pulmonary artery courses posterior to the aortic arch. Right: Leftward rotation of the endoscope shaft (array remains at 90 degrees) develops a longitudinal view of the main pulmonary artery, pulmonary valve *(PV)*, and right ventricular outflow. The left pulmonary artery courses over the left bronchus. The aortic arch and innominate vein are visualized in the short axis from this transducer position and array orientation.

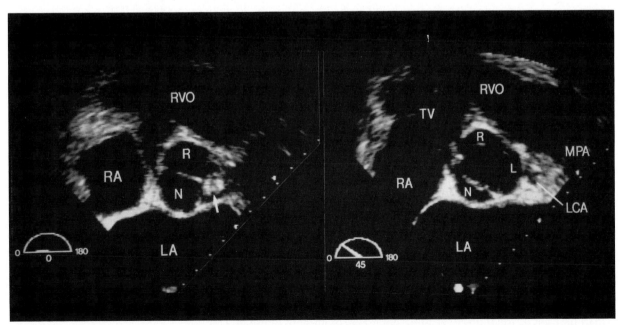

Fig. 5-20. Optimal short-axis view of the aortic valve. Left: At 0 degrees, the array is in a conventional transverse plane and is in the short axis of the thorax and slightly oblique to the aortic valve. This is an example of a common pitfall [9] observed in the left coronary sinus *(arrow)* of the aortic valve. A pseudomass is created by oblique transection of the belly of the left coronary sinus. Right: An optimized short-axis view of the aortic valve is obtained at 45 degrees rotation of the array. In a true short axis (45 degrees) or true long axis (135 degrees—not shown) to the aortic valve, such pitfalls can be easily recognized. (*L* = left coronary cusp; *N* = noncoronary cusp; *R* = right coronary cusp.)

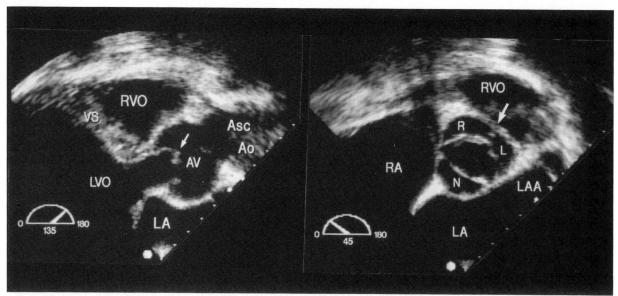

Fig. 5-21. Bicuspid aortic valve. Left: With the array at 135 degrees, an optimal long-axis view of the aortic valve is obtained. Note that the aortic cusps *(arrow)* are thickened with systolic doming, consistent with a congenitally stenotic aortic valve. Right: At 45 degrees, the array is in an optimal short axis to the aortic valve orifice. Note the fusion of the commissure between the left and the right aortic valve cusps *(arrow)*. The bicuspid valve orifice extends from 5 o'clock to 10 o'clock. Multiplane TEE allows easier assessment of aortic valve anatomy. (L = left coronary cusp; N = noncoronary cusp; R = right coronary cusp.)

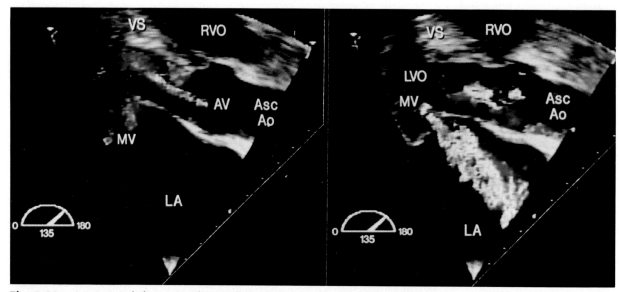

Fig. 5-22. Long-axis left ventricular outflow. The array is at 135 degrees, which best aligns the transducer in the long axis of the left ventricle. Left: (diastole): A narrow jet of aortic valve regurgitation is recorded. Right: (systole): Without a change in array orientation (135 degrees), systolic mitral valve regurgitation is also recorded. Optimal alignment of the valve orifices and flow jets is facilitated with the multiplane transducer.

Transgastric Multiplane Images

When the transducer tip is in the fundus of the stomach, frequently only a single optimal ultrasound window exists to visualize the heart. With a biplane transducer, the endoscope tip must be moved to obtain multiple off-axis images. Such transducer movement frequently results in less than optimal images, because air or gastric secretions become positioned between the transducer and the contact surface of the stomach wall. With multiplane TEE, the transducer can be placed and remain in the optimal imaging position; the imaging array is then rotated to obtain multiple off-axis views (see Fig. 5-14). This capability increases the likelihood of obtaining better, more diagnostic transgastric images (Fig. 5-23).

Short- to Long-Axis Scans

From both the esophageal and the transgastric transducer positions, the transition from one scan plane to another is much easier to comprehend with multiplane array rotation (Figs. 5-24, 5-25, and 5-26). The multiplane technique alleviates the abrupt transition from one plane to another and lateral tip flexion of the endoscope, which is obligatory with a stacked or matrix biplane transducer. Contiguous anatomy is much easier to appreciate with the multiplane examination.

360-Degree Rotation

A 180-degree rotation of a multiplane array actually permits a 360-degree tomographic scan of the underlying anatomy or color-flow Doppler signal (Fig. 5-27). This multiplane maneuver (360° visualization) is frequently used to determine the extent and distribution of a mitral regurgitant color-flow Doppler signal and to assess the seating ring of a prosthesis, the extent and distribution of aortic atherosclerosis, and the boundaries of cardiac masses. This rotational maneuver can also be used for three-dimensional reconstruction [11].

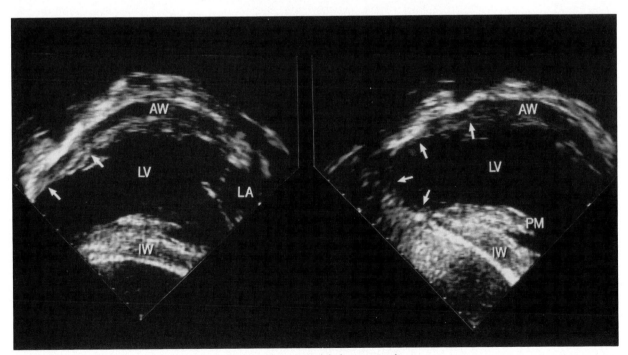

Fig. 5-23. Transgastric visualization of an anteroapical left ventricular infarction *(arrows)*. Left: Longitudinal view of the middle left ventricular cavity shows an anterior wall motion abnormality *(arrows)*. Right: With retroflexion of the endoscope tip, the longitudinal extent of the infarction *(arrows)* is best appreciated. Multiplane TEE allows better alignment of the transducer array with the anatomy in question.

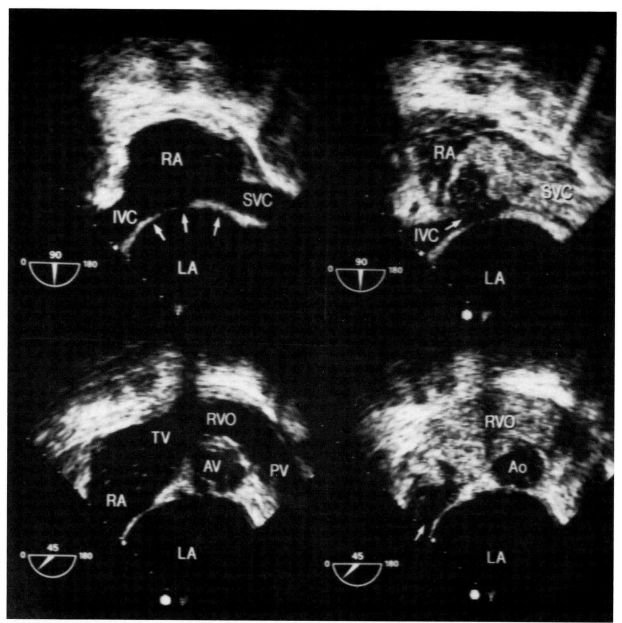

Fig. 5-24. Contrast echocardiography: Long- and short-axis scans of the atrial septum. Top: Long-axis view (90-degree array) of the inferior and superior venae cavae. The atrial septum and valve of the fossa ovalis *(arrows)* are viewed in long axis. After upper extremity injection of contrast medium *(right),* the superior vena cava and right atrium become opacified. Note the nonopacified blood originating from the inferior vena cava. Bottom: The array has been reoriented from 90 degrees (longitudinal) to 45 degrees to optimally view the short axis of the atrial septum and aortic valve. After echocontrast injection *(right)* the right atrium and right ventricular outflow become opacified. Note that nonopacified blood *(arrow)* from the inferior vena cava is appreciated in the posterior right atrial cavity. This patient did not have a right-to-left shunt. Transition from one axis to another is facilitated by multiplane TEE. *(PV = pulmonary valve)*

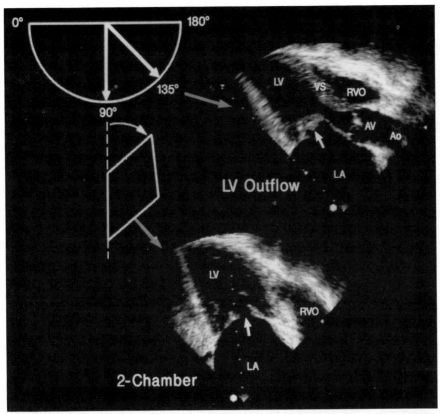

Fig. 5-25. Multiplane examination. Bottom: A *two-chamber left ventricular view* (90-degree array orientation with leftward rotation of the endoscope shaft). Note the thickened mitral valve leaflets *(arrow)*. Top right: A further reorientation of the multiplane array to 135 degrees develops the *long-axis view* of the *left ventricular outflow*. Note that rheumatic mitral valve stenosis is more evident with the array at 135 degrees.

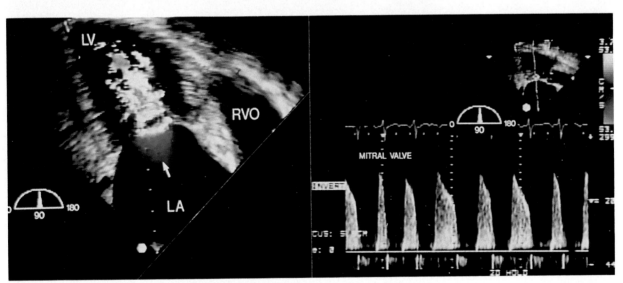

Fig. 5-26. Continuous-wave Doppler examination (same patient as that in Fig. 5-25). The optimal orientation of the array to assess Doppler hemodynamics of the stenotic mitral valve was the two-chamber view at 90 degrees array rotation. The Doppler signal has been inverted to show a more conventional presentation. Multiplane TEE permits fine adjustments of the transducer to optimize anatomy and Doppler signal for hemodynamic assessment.

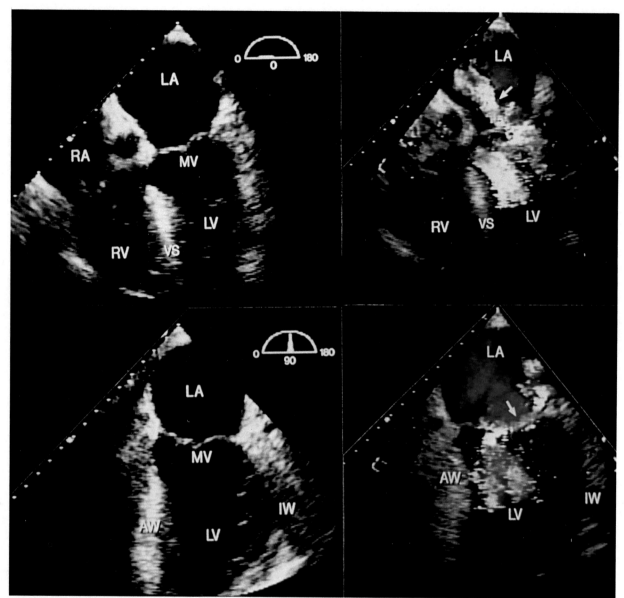

Fig. 5-27. Multiplane examination (360-degree visualization) of a mitral regurgitant jet by color Doppler signal. Top: Four-chamber apex-down format (0-degree array). The central mitral regurgitant jet *(arrow)* is visualized. Bottom: Apex-down, two-chamber long-axis view (90-degree array) shows that the mitral regurgitant jet *(arrow)* is, in fact, also directed posteriorly along the left atrial wall. Using a continuum of tomographic views (360-degree visualization), one can better appreciate contiguous anatomy and lesions such as a mitral regurgitant jet. The multiplane technique is unique for this type of examination.

Limitations of Multiplane Technology

The multiplane approach to clinical TEE increases the diagnostic power of this widely applied invasive technology. Features that may limit its optimal utilization include (1) large transducer size, (2) potentially higher maintenance costs, (3) cable hysteresis (unpredictable secondary rotation of the scan plane when the tip is flexed in endoscopes that incorporate a long cable linkage to the movable array), and (4) high unit cost (user-friendly but more expensive and intricate technology).

A very distracting limitation of this technology is the debate over image orientation. This technology obtains images identical to those of all previous tomographic techniques. However, we now have a tool that on one day can present the heart in one orientation and on the same day present it in a completely different manner. This change is most distracting and confusing to the physician unfamiliar with the available technology. To this author, it is absolutely imperative that all images of the same technology be oriented in the same manner.

Other clinical applications unique to multiplane will continually be realized with increasing use of this newest technologic advancement [10,12]. Multiplane transducer technology is the newest TEE innovation in a rapidly changing field of cardiovascular imaging. Any limitation today will likely be eliminated as expertise and technical advances progress.

SUMMARY

The primary advantage of multiplane TEE over biplane is the ease of moving the array from one orientation to another. An examiner very adept with a biplane device can obtain nearly all the same views, although considerably greater dexterity and manipulation are required. Multiplane TEE also has the advantage of moving sequentially through intervening anatomy rather than making an abrupt transition to an orthogonal plane or presenting the simultaneous orthogonal images of the biplane matrix probe. The distribution and contiguous nature of structures are better depicted. In most biplane endoscopes, the two arrays are separated by a distance of about 1 cm, so that orthogonal images are not at exactly the same anatomic location. Transducer contact and maneuverability also may differ between the two planes. These limitations are obviated by multiplane TEE.

Off-axis images (i.e., those not in the primary plane of the heart or body) are easier to obtain and recognize with a variable plane (multiplane) array. This advantage is particularly noticeable in the transgastric transducer position, in which manipulation of a standard monoplane or biplane endoscope often results in loss of contact with the mucosa of the stomach or interposition of distracting or impenetrable air. Conversely, the multiplane transducer array can be manipulated into a suitable position, and then the array can be rotated without concomitant manipulation of the endoscope tip.

Other advantageous clinical applications of multiplane imaging will come to light with more experience. At present, however, this newest TEE technology appears very promising and will potentiate the development of other transducer innovations.

In an initial prospective study, a trained TEE echocardiologist required from 30 to 50 additional multiplane examinations to master this newest technique. The TEE probe used was particularly large and required greater expertise to introduce. Once the technique was mastered, however, standard views were easier to obtain by the multiplane examination than by the biplane or monoplane examination. Although some current devices are comparatively large, the size has not precluded examining nearly all adult patients. A large endoscope head and transducer shaft may increase the incidence of complications. However, we have had no significant minor or major complications in our initial experience. We do not recommend use of these very large scan heads in patients less than 35 kg in weight.

The ultimate use of multiplane TEE will depend most importantly on (1) acquisition of added diagnostic information, (2) ease of use, and (3) future modifications of technology and endoscope size. With increased numbers of imaging planes, there should be an incremental increase in diagnostic capability. If this information is obtained with less effort and user adaptation, multiplane TEE will ultimately supersede biplanar TEE as the technique of choice.

REFERENCES

1. Seward JB, Khandheria BK, Oh JK, et al. Transesophageal echocardiography: technique, anatomic correlations, implementation, and clinical applications. *Mayo Clin Proc* 1988;63:649–80.

2. Seward JB, Khandheria BK, Edwards ED, et al. Biplanar transesophageal echocardiography: anatomic correlations, image orientation, and clinical applications. *Mayo Clin Proc* 1990;65:1193–213.

3. Henry WL, DeMaria A, Gramiak R, et al. Report of the American Society of Echocardiography Committee on Nomenclature and Standards in Two-Dimensional Echocardiography. *Circulation* 1980;62:212–7.

4. Schlüter M, Langenstein BA, Polster J, et al. Transesophageal cross-sectional echocardiography with a phased array system: technique and initial clinical results. *Br Heart J* 1982;48:67–72.

5. Omoto R, Kyo S, Matsumura M, et al. New direction of biplane transesophageal echocardiography with special emphasis on real-time biplane imaging and matrix phased-array biplane transducer. *Echocardiography* 1990;7:691–8.

6. Tajik AJ, Seward JB, Hagler DJ, et al. Two-dimensional real-time ultrasonic imaging of the heart and great vessels: technique, image orientation, structure identification, and validation. *Mayo Clin Proc* 1978;53:271–303.

7. Seward JB, Tajik AJ, Edwards WD, Hagler DJ. *Two-Dimensional Echocardiographic Atlas, Vol 1: Congenital Heart Disease.* New York: Springer-Verlag, 1987.

8. Seward JB, Khandheria BK, Tajik AJ. Wide-field transesophageal echocardiographic tomography: feasibility study. *Mayo Clin Proc* 1990;65:31–7.

9. Seward JB, Khandheria BK, Oh JK, et al. Critical appraisal of transesophageal echocardiography: limitations, pitfalls, and complications. *J Am Soc Echocardiogr* 1992;5:288–305.

10. Flachskampf FA, Hoffmann R, Hanrath P. Experience with a transesophageal echotransducer allowing full rotation of the viewing plane: the Omniplane probe (abstract). *J Am Coll Cardiol* 1991;17 Suppl A:34A.

11. Belohlavek M, Foley DA, Gerber TC, et al. Three- and four-dimensional cardiovascular ultrasound imaging: a new era for echocardiography. *Mayo Clin Proc* 1993;68:221–40.

12. Roelandt JRTC, Thomson IR, Vletter WB, et al. Multiplane transesophageal echocardiography: latest evolution in an imaging revolution. *J Am Soc Echocardiogr* 1992;5:361–7.

Critical Appraisal of Transesophageal Echocardiography

Limitations and Pitfalls

James B. Seward

Transesophageal echocardiography (TEE), the first widely used semi-invasive cardiovascular ultrasound examination, is considered a logical extension of a standard echocardiographic study in select groups of patients [1,2]. Although the images are of consistently superior quality and can be obtained in the great majority of patients, this technique has *limitations* because of the limited window within the confines of the esophagus and stomach and the inability to easily exchange transducers for special situations. *Pitfalls,* potential erroneous diagnoses resulting from misinterpretation of normal and abnormal anatomy, are prevalent because of the new tomographic presentation and the necessity of using transducers not optimized for all diagnostic situations. Complications of this technique (3–6) are discussed in detail in Chapter 3. This chapter critically reviews the current practice of TEE with particular emphasis on limitations and pitfalls.

This presentation comes from a prospective assessment of 3,827 TEE examinations (excluding intraoperative studies) performed in our echocardiographic laboratory. The patients were from 9 to 92 years old and had a mean age of 62 years; 2,152 were male (56%). The TEE technique and anatomic correlations have previously been reported [1,2] and are discussed in Chapters 3 and 4.

LIMITATIONS

Transesophageal echocardiography has introduced a new era of clinical invasive ultrasound [7,8]. The logistics and concerns of an invasive procedure are offset by diagnostic images of consistently high quality. However, in young and elderly patients, TEE has unique considerations and potential limitations. Children younger than 10 years usually require general anesthesia to undergo the examination [9–11]. Elderly patients are much more sensitive to systemic sedation [12] and have a higher incidence of esophageal and cervical spine disease that needs to be specifically addressed with each examination [13]. In our series of 3,827 consecutive examinations, the procedure was aborted in 42 patients (1.1%) because of unsuccessful intubation (36 patients [0.94%]), patient intolerance (5 patients), and esophageal disease (1 patient).

Imaging Limitations

New Tomographic Views

Transesophageal echocardiography is often referred to as a new window to the heart. The tomographic anatomy visualized is new and often initially strange and confusing. To the beginner, the examination is

This chapter originally appeared in different form in JB Seward, BK Khandheria, JK Oh, et al. Critical appraisal of transesophageal echocardiography: limitations, pitfalls, and complications. *J Am Soc Echocardiogr* 1992;5:288–305.

unfamiliar and consequently may pose limitations on interpretation, demonstration of anatomic relationships, and diagnostic application. It is important to relate this new echocardiographic examination to existing experience. A level II echocardiographer is very familiar with two-dimensional tomographic echocardiographic anatomy as visualized from a surface examination. The TEE examination obtains the identical images once the orientation techniques are mastered. Because the transducer is posterior to the heart, we recommend that all images be oriented in such a way that the transducer burst is at the bottom of the viewing screen. In this orientation, the short-axis, long-axis, and apex-up four-chamber views are identical to those obtained from the precordial examination. A uniform presentation of tomographic views regardless of transducer position or electronic burst fosters better understanding and reduces inherent limitations and pitfalls.

If we abandon established conventions and rules, we expose ourselves to multiple problems of image presentation, structure recognition and identification, and anatomic correlations. Images of familiar structures become difficult to intuitively recognize if they are presented in an unfamiliar format (for example, aortic valve and left ventricular short axis as mirror-image, upside-down presentations). Unconventional image orientations have produced, and will continue to lead to, potentially significant errors of interpretation. There is no logic in changing the entire image orientation just because the image transducer is in the esophagus rather than above the chest wall. Imaging planes that one obtains by TEE and transthoracic echocardiography are identical (long-axis plane, short-axis plane, and four-chamber plane). A series of views of the heart can be obtained along any of these primary planes by TEE. Therefore, it is to our advantage to uphold the American Society of Echocardiography standard of image orientation for the long-axis, short-axis, and four-chamber views irrespective of the position of the transducer or electronic burst. If we as echocardiographers have difficulty with our "own images," how can we effectively communicate with our nonechocardiographer colleagues?

Air

The walls of the esophagus and stomach are the portals through which the heart and great vessels of the thorax are visualized during the TEE examination. Although images are consistently superior to comparable surface images, maneuverability is limited within the lumen of the esophagus and fundus of the stomach. Entrapped air, because it is impervious to the transmission of ultrasound, may interfere with certain transducer maneuvers, particularly retroflexion of the endoscope tip in the midesophagus and imaging from the fundus of the stomach. Air within the upper gastrointestinal system rarely precludes a diagnostic examination. Biplanar [2] and multiplanar [14] transducers compensate for this limitation; however, in any particular examination, all areas of the heart may not be imaged with consistent predictability or quality.

Although no complete solution exists to the problem of interference by entrapped air, there are some helpful observations. First, there is more air in the esophagus at the beginning of the examination than at the end. Air is continually cleared out by esophageal and transducer action during the study. Early in the procedure, it is best to use views and endoscope manipulations that are not as likely to be affected by entrapped air. Anteflexion—movement of the transducer lens into apposition with the esophageal wall—is preferred over retroflexion, which moves the transducer away from the esophageal wall. Retroflexion more easily permits entrapped air to come in front of the transducer lens. Early in the examination, the longitudinal transducer or short-axis views with the transverse plane should be used because anteflexion produces the best images. Four-chamber views, which require retroflexion, should be obtained later in the examination. Passing the tip of the endoscope into the stomach also tends to clear air from the esophagus. Additionally, in the same-sized patient, larger endoscopes have greater esophageal mucosal contact and, hence, less air interference than probes with smaller endoscopic heads.

Trachea and Bronchi

The air-filled trachea and bronchi consistently interfere with certain tomographic planes of section. The basal cardiac and aortic arch examinations are particularly affected by these interposed portions of the respiratory tract. This problem can be largely circumvented with biplanar or multiplanar transducers, which allow off-axis imaging around interfering respiratory structures to areas of interest. Attempts to image the upper ascending aorta with the horizontal plane are limited by a "blind spot" caused by the interposed bronchus between the esophagus and the upper ascending aorta [1]. This limitation can be minimized by using an anteflexed longitudinal plane that directs the ultrasound beam around the left bronchus [2]. Similarly, the distal left pulmonary artery, which can be obscured by the left bronchus, is best imaged in the off-axis longitudinal plane.

Equipment

Current TEE systems consist of a two-dimensional echocardiographic instrument and an endoscope fitted with an ultrasound transducer. It is inconvenient and cumbersome to change transducers, alter frequency, or incorporate offset capability. Present transesophageal transducers are optimized only for midfield imaging. An ideal endoscope or family of endoscopes should be able to image near- and far-field extremes and incorporate multifrequency transducers, offset capability, and other innovations that would reduce these limitations. Newer esophageal endoscopes are smaller in diameter [15], incorporate steerable continuous-wave Doppler, and ultimately have wide-field imaging capability [16,17]. Tissue characterization [18–20], border recognition, and three- and four-dimensional scanning [21,22] remain elusive but potentially very useful innovations.

As with any technology in a state of evolution, certain limitations are inherent with the state of the art. Distinct advantages that have been the impetus of the clinical application of TEE are consistently superior images and low incidence of unacceptable examinations. Equipment limitations can be divided into those of transducer and of endoscope design.

Transducer Limitations

Scan Plane
The original monoplane (horizontal plane) transducer [1] is now largely being displaced by biplanar (horizontal and longitudinal planes) transducers [2]. Because the transducer is confined to the esophagus and fundus of the stomach, multiplanar [23] and ultimately omniplanar [14] endoscopes will become state of the art. New image presentation and inherent technologic constraints continue to press for more views because of the comparatively limited mobility of the esophageal transducer.

Near- and Far-Field Imaging
Most esophageal transducers are 5 MHz and are optimized for visualization of midfield cardiac structures, such as the atrial septum and mitral valve.

Far-field limitations include inability to optimally visualize the ventricular apices from the midesophageal region, acoustic shadowing of the anterior aortic

annulus and cardiac crux by the central fibrous body of the cardiac valves, and acoustic shadowing of more distant structures caused by interposed prosthetic material (for example, mitral prosthesis obscuring the left ventricular outflow tract and aortic prosthesis obscuring the anterior aortic root) (Fig. 6-1).

Near-field limitations include transducer burst artifact interfering with visualization of the lower pulmonary veins and poor visualization of the pediatric heart because of inappropriate transducer frequency and focal point. Multifrequency transducers, offset capability, and specialty endoscopes will ultimately reduce these limitations.

Image
Miniaturization or incorporation of multiple scan planes often requires a reduced number of imaging crystals per scan plane, and this degrades the quality of the resultant image. New transducers are being developed to optimize the relationship of transducer size and sophistication with the greatest image quality. This improvement is accomplished by multifrequency transducers, increased number of imaging crystals, and incorporation of multidirectional chains. Thus, limitations in image quality will directly depend on the current state-of-the-art technology.

Endoscope Limitations

General
The delivery device for TEE is a modified endoscope fitted with an ultrasound transducer. The endoscope length, depth markings, control knobs, lock mechanism, and handle design are, in most instances, optimized not for cardiologic application but for esophagogastroduodenoscopy. The shape of the transducer, obligatory electronics, and physiologic monitoring capability are unique to TEE. Depending on the application, any of the above features can be a potential limitation. Devices specifically suited for TEE application will reduce the annoying constraints of current technology.

Size
When first introduced, TEE used an adult endoscope (9-mm shaft) tipped with an ultrasound transducer. With increasing sophistication, many endoscope shafts have actually increased in size ($\pm$ 11 mm in diameter). (Note: An increase in shaft diameter from 9 to 11 mm increases the cross-sectional area of the

Fig. 6-1. Acoustic shadows. Far-field structures can be shadowed by interposed ultrasound reflectors. Prosthetic material, calcium, and the fibrous cardiac skeleton are common reflectors interfering with the far-field image. In this figure, a mitral bioprosthesis *(P)* and sewing ring *(white arrows)* produce linear shadows in the far field *(black arrows)*. Note that the upper ventricular septum, free wall of the right ventricle, and apex of the left ventricle are shadowed. (From JB Seward, BK Khandheria, JK Oh, et al. Critical appraisal of transesophageal echocardiography: limitations, pitfalls, and complications. *J Am Soc Echocardiogr* 1992;5:288–305. By permission of the American Society of Echocardiography.)

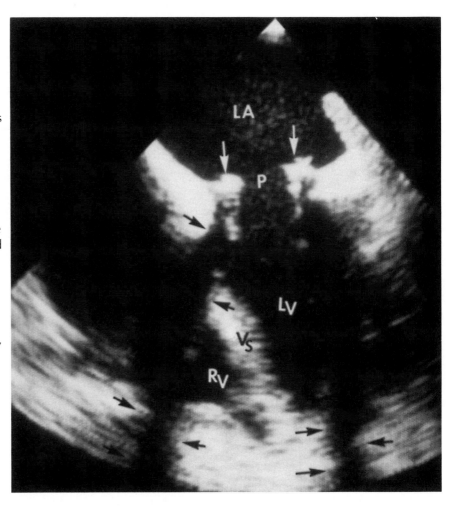

shaft by 50%, and a decrease in shaft diameter from 9 to 7 mm reduces the cross-sectional area by 40%. Additionally, the transducer tip usually has an even larger cross-sectional area.)

To our knowledge, no significant complications have been directly attributable to the size of the endoscope [24,25]. However, transient vocal cord paralysis has been reported in two patients after lengthy neurosurgical procedures in the upright position in which extreme anteflexion of the patient's head was required for the operative procedure while a large (9-mm shaft) transesophageal endoscope was positioned alongside an endotracheal tube [26]. This complication has not reoccurred with use of smaller diameter endoscopes. We have also experienced an increased incidence of inability to introduce larger endoscopes into some elderly patients, small adult or pediatric patients, and intubated patients. Extreme flexion of the transducer tip can injure or perforate the esophagus [27–29].

Smaller endoscopes are now commercially avail-able. However, smaller endoscopes currently incorporate fewer imaging crystals and have fewer controls and reduced planes of imaging. Concerns about inadequate transducer contact and a higher incidence of complications with smaller endoscopes have not been substantiated to date.

Maintenance

A number of poorly documented limitations have been encountered with endoscope maintenance. The cables that control the movement of the tip frequently stretch with time, significantly impairing maneuverability of the transducer head. Such stretching may allow the endoscope tip to become too flexible and may contribute to endoscope buckling within the esophagus [30]. Early devices had an unacceptably high incidence of excessive stretch and fracture of cable connections. These limitations have been substantially reduced. However, periodic readjustment of cable tension may still be necessary even with ideal maintenance of current instruments.

SAFETY CONSIDERATIONS

Transesophageal echocardiography is unique in many respects and has prompted concerns about probe safety and durability. The endoscope is manipulated predominantly within the esophagus. Resistance to motion may potentiate earlier fatigue of the cables or protective sheath. The electronic imaging system places a burden on the user to monitor electrical and thermal safety. The endoscope may carry pathogenic organisms or cause disruption of the mucosa, resulting in bacteremia.

Thermal Safety

Ultrasound transducers generate some heat. During the standard examination of about 20 minutes in the awake patient, transducer heat should not be a problem. Even longer periods of intubation have not resulted in detectable mucosal injury [25]. During cardiac surgery (see Chapter 16) using extracorporeal circulation, however, an endoscope is left in one place for an extended period while the patient undergoes systemic hypothermia. Continuous contact or a significant heat gradient (for example, if the patient is at 28°C and the probe at 38°C, a 10°C heat gradient results) may theoretically increase the chances of thermal injury to the esophagus.

Heat-sensing thermistors have been incorporated into all commercial endoscopes. However, two limitations are caused by current thermal-sensing circuitry. There is no manual reset, and the range of preset temperatures often does not match the clinical needs. Thus, very febrile patients occasionally cannot be adequately examined because the device senses the patient's temperature and repeatedly shuts down into the automatic cooling mode. Similarly, transducers used intraoperatively cease imaging function on sensing the heat of reperfused blood during rewarming after cardiopulmonary bypass. An override switch to be used at the discretion of the examining physician would be very useful in these annoying situations. Thermal gradient (that is, a significant difference between endoscope temperature and that of the patient) is not a standard function of commercially available thermal monitoring. The general contention is that current endoscope thermostats have done more to hinder patient evaluation than to avert very unlikely thermal complications.

During prolonged monitoring, the ultrasound device should be periodically shut down to allow cooling. In particular, during intraoperative monitoring, the ultrasound transducer should be inactivated when it is not being used (see Chapter 16). In febrile patients or situations when an inappropriate automatic cooling signal occurs, physicians have irrigated the esophagus with iced saline through a nasogastric tube or cooled the endoscope before introduction to facilitate an uninterrupted examination. More appropriate circuitry logic, comparison of patient and lens temperature, display of endoscope temperature, and the option for temporary operator override would reduce these limitations.

Electrical Safety

Perforation or near-perforation of the outer sheath of the endoscope results in a loss of "safe electrical grounding." The risk of electrical injury with currently available probes is extremely remote, because the endoscope is already electrically isolated from the ultrasound machine. Thus, the attendant electrical risks are minimal even with a poorly maintained endoscope.

An electrical leak, however, may indicate a small defect in the protective covering of the endoscope, a defect that may portend other safety problems. Infectious organisms or caustic cleaning solution may become entrapped beneath the sheath and potentially infect or injure the patient. Loss of electrical integrity also increases the chance of heat generation. Early endoscopes had a high incidence of electrical failure. With newer endoscopes, this problem has been considerably reduced but not totally eliminated. Continual monitoring of electrical integrity of the TEE probe is recommended. In our laboratory, electrical safety is checked after each examination, with the cleaning solution in which the endoscope is immersed used as the test bath (see Chapter 2).

Bacteriologic Safety

The endoscope should be cleaned after each use and immersed in a glutaraldehyde solution for 10 to 20 minutes [1]. Repeated prolonged immersions may accelerate deterioration of the instrument's protective sheath. Adherent glutaraldehyde solution should be washed off and the endoscope allowed to dry before reuse. Routine visual inspection and electrical checks are necessary to detect rents in the sheath of the endoscope that may retain caustic cleaning solution or potentially infective organisms.

Bacteremia and the risk of endocarditis with upper gastrointestinal endoscopy [31–35] or TEE [36–39] are considered negligible. Multiple studies suggest that routine prophylaxis is unnecessary; however, a few investigators have recommended prophylaxis for TEE examination [40,41]. As discussed in Chapter 3, there are small subsets of high-risk patients, such as those with prosthetic valves, previous endocarditis, or conduits, in whom administering prophylaxis may be clinically justified.

PITFALLS

False Masses

Transesophageal echocardiography vividly images structures previously inaccessible by transthoracic echocardiography. Thus, unfamiliar normal anatomy may be misinterpreted as abnormal (Figs. 6-2, 6-3, and 6-4).

Trabeculations of the Atria or Atrial Appendages

Muscular trabeculations (that is, pectinate muscles) and irregularities are seen in the walls of both atrial appendages, and the examiner should become well acquainted with the normal appearances (Fig. 6-5). These muscle ridges are usually small and refractile, move in concert with the atrial wall, and are typically multiple. However, thrombus is characteristically of different texture than the atrial wall and is more echo-refractile, is uniform in consistency, often is pedunculated, and typically occurs in conjunction with significant atrioventricular valve disease or low-output state (see Chapter 12). Tumors that extend into the atria or atrial appendage are also distinctly different in echo density from normal muscle ridges. We have found that multiplanar imaging is very helpful in recognizing atrial appendage pathologic conditions and differentiating them from normal muscle ridges.

Fig. 6-2. Spinal cord *(SC)*. If the transducer is rotated posteriorly, the spinal cord can be visualized at each neurointerspace of the thoracic spine. Spinal fluid *(SF)* and the spinal cord can produce a masslike appearance. This observation can be misinterpreted as an extracardiac mass or tumor. (From JB Seward, BK Khandheria, JK Oh, et al. Critical appraisal of transesophageal echocardiography: limitations, pitfalls, and complications. *J Am Soc Echocardiogr* 1992;5:288–305. By permission of the American Society of Echocardiography.)

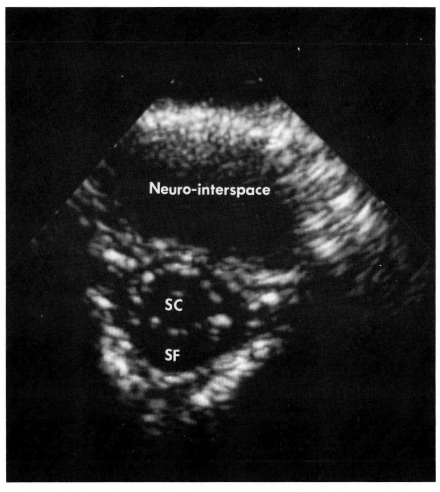

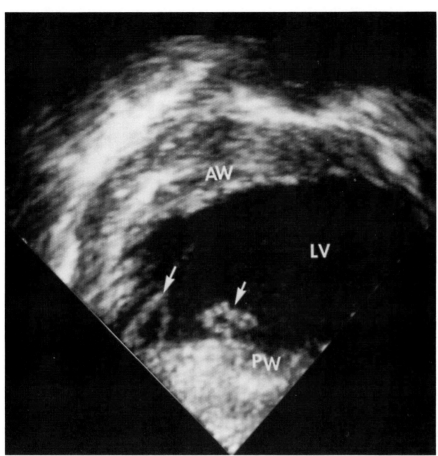

Fig. 6-3. Pseudomass. This transgastric long-axis view of the left ventricle is from a patient with a mitral prosthesis. Mobile transected chordae after mitral valve replacement within the left ventricle *(arrows)* give a mass effect. These transected chordae may appear multicentric, mobile, and pedunculated, features also associated with thrombus. However, there were no significant underlying left ventricular wall motion abnormalities, and the true identity as chordae could be discerned by long- and short-axis transgastric images. (From JB Seward, BK Khandheria, JK Oh, et al. Critical appraisal of transesophageal echocardiography: limitations, pitfalls, and complications. *J Am Soc Echocardiogr* 1992;5:288–305. By permission of the American Society of Echocardiography.)

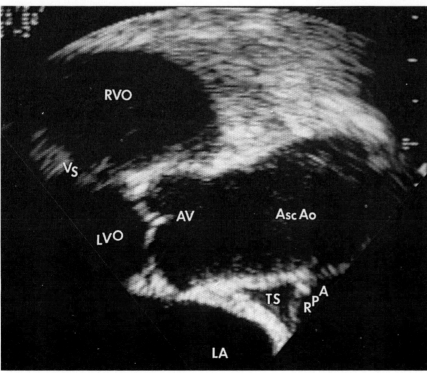

Fig. 6-4. Normal anatomic spaces that may be mistaken as pathologic cavities. A, B. Transverse sinus. A. Long-axis longitudinal scan of the proximal ascending aorta. The transverse sinus is surrounded anteriorly by the ascending aorta, superiorly by the right pulmonary artery, and posteriorly by the left atrium.

A

Fig. 6-4. (continued)
B. Short-axis longitudinal scan at the level of the aortic valve. The transverse sinus is bounded posteriorly by the left atrium, medially by the aortic valve, and anteriorly and internally by the main pulmonary artery. C, D. Membrane of the fossa ovalis.

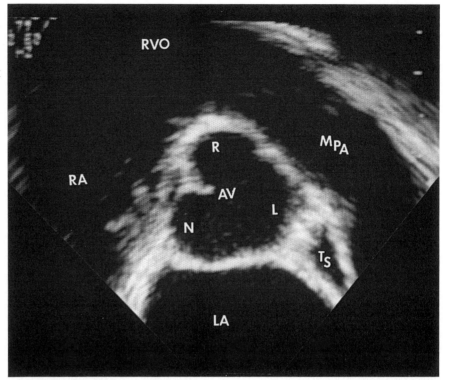

B

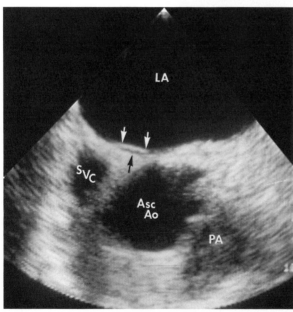

C

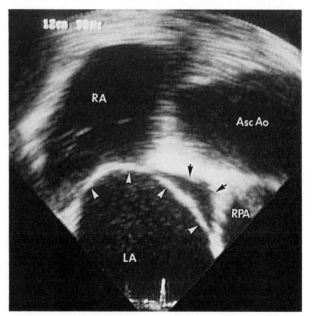

D

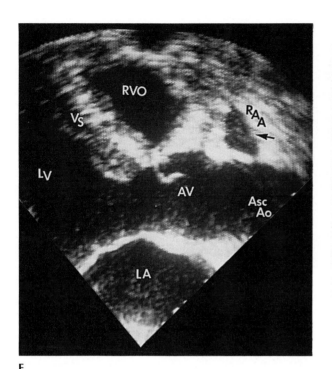
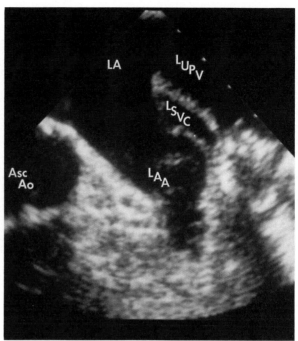

E   F

Fig. 6-4. (continued)   C. Horizontal scan at the level of the proximal ascending aorta. Overlapping of the membrane of the fossa ovalis *(white arrows)* with the posterosuperior limbus of the atrial septum produces an interposed cavity *(black arrow)*. When the foramen ovale is patent, the blood can cross between right atrium and left atrium through this potential orifice (valve of the fossa ovalis). D. Longitudinal scan of the membrane of the fossa ovalis *(white arrowheads)*. This membrane overlaps the superior margin of the atrial septum and posterior wall of the ascending aorta, producing an interposed space *(black arrows)*. E. Right atrial appendage *(black arrow)*. In a long-axis longitudinal scan of the ascending aorta, the right atrial appendage can be imaged anterior to the ascending aorta and should not be mistaken for a pathologic space, such as a para-aortic abscess. F. Persistent left superior vena cava. The partition between the left upper pulmonary vein and the left atrial appendage can appear as a space. Two circumstances typically cause this appearance: (1) There is a pericardial reflection within this partition that can become fluid-filled if pericardial effusion is present; usually, this is identified as fluid and associations such as fluid-filled transverse sinus and pericardial sac; or (2) persistent left superior vena cava (example shown), which courses within the common wall, is identified by color-flow Doppler blood flow and is associated with a significantly dilated coronary sinus. *(L = left coronary cusp; N = noncoronary cusp; R = right coronary cusp.)* (From JB Seward, BK Khandheria, JK Oh, et al. Critical appraisal of transesophageal echocardiography: limitations, pitfalls, and complications. *J Am Soc Echocardiogr* 1992;5:288–305. By permission of the American Society of Echocardiography.)

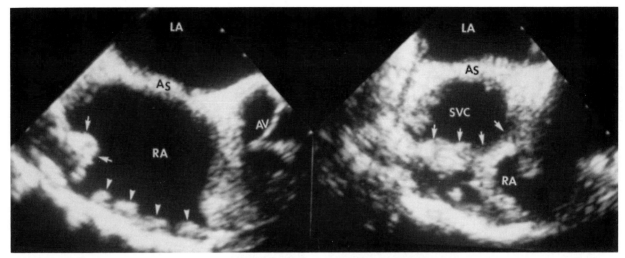

Fig. 6-5. Right atrial trabeculations or pectinate muscles *(arrowheads)* and muscular bands *(arrows)*. The right atrium is more trabeculated (that is, pectinate muscles) than the left atrium. A highly trabeculated atrial appendage may be difficult to clearly differentiate from thrombus. The example is from a patient with atrial septal defect (not seen in these views) in whom the atrial musculature is hypertrophied. Left: A larger muscle band *(arrows)* is commonly visualized at the orifice of the superior vena cava. Right: A normal atrial muscle bundle can be identified by slow withdrawal of the transesophageal endoscope in the transverse horizontal plane. Normal muscle *(arrows)* encircles the superior vena caval orifice, separating the superior vena cava and the right atrial appendage *(RA)*. (From JB Seward, BK Khandheria, JK Oh, et al. Critical appraisal of transesophageal echocardiography: limitations, pitfalls, and complications. *J Am Soc Echocardiogr* 1992;5:288–305. By permission of the American Society of Echocardiography.)

Within the left atrium, the orifices of the pulmonary veins are encircled by tissue that may appear masslike in some tomographic planes of section. One of the most frequent mass effects encountered is the common wall separating the left atrial appendage from the left upper pulmonary vein (Fig. 6-6). In a tomographic plane of section, the terminal portion of this partition appears globular and looks like a mass, especially as it undulates with cardiac motion. This common wall in its midportion is thin, and the globular end can sometimes be quite large, mimicking a left atrial tumor. Awareness of this common anatomic variant should prevent serious misinterpretation. A persistent left superior vena cava [42] and a potentially fluid-filled recess of the pericardial reflection course within this common wall and should not be misinterpreted as a cyst, abscess, or other abnormal structure (see Figs. 6-4A, 6-4B, and 6-4F). Notably, a persistent left superior vena cava is associated with a large coronary sinus, which normally enters the right atrium [1,42] and has color-flow–detectable blood movement within the space.

Pericardial fluid within the pericardial reflection does not generate a color-flow signal.

In the right atrium at the orifices of the superior and inferior venae cavae, muscle bundles can also appear masslike (see Fig. 6-5). In the horizontal plane, at the orifice of the right superior vena cava, an encircling muscle ridge appears ovoid and masslike. Slow withdrawal of the endoscope to the lumen of the superior vena cava completes visualization of the muscle ridge around the orifice of the superior vena cava and assures proper identification. Less commonly, a similar ridge of muscle is visualized at the orifice of the inferior vena cava. In the horizontal plane, advancing the endoscope completes imaging of the encircling eustachian valve. Biplane or multiplane imaging consistently eliminates confusion.

Atrial Septum

The atrial septum surrounding the centrally located membrane of the fossa ovalis is fat-laden and in older patients normally can be up to 1 cm thick (Fig. 6-7). In certain tomographic planes, the limbus of the

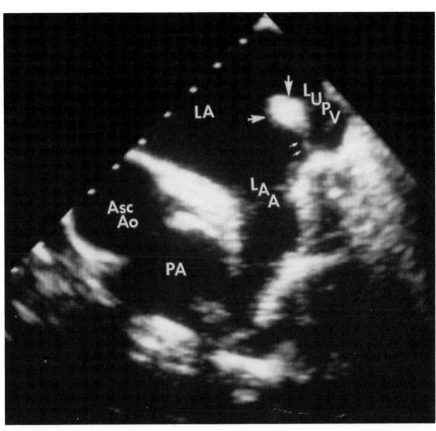

Fig. 6-6. Left atrial pseudomass. The normal partition between the left upper pulmonary vein and left atrial appendage can be fat-laden and appear masslike *(large arrows)*. The proximal portion of the common wall is usually thin *(small arrows)* and the distal portion bulbous *(large arrows)*, features adding to the mass effect. (From JB Seward, BK Khandheria, JK Oh, et al. Critical appraisal of transesophageal echocardiography: limitations, pitfalls, and complications. *J Am Soc Echocardiogr* 1992;5:288–305. By permission of the American Society of Echocardiography.)

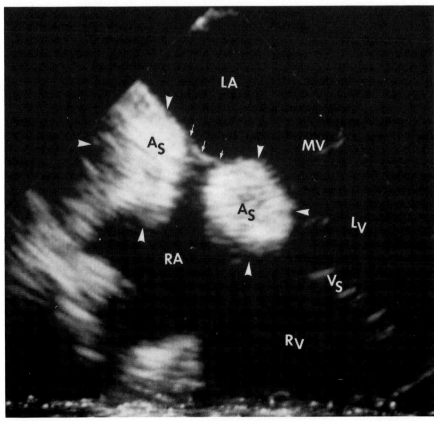

Fig. 6-7. Lipomatous atrial septum. The atrial septum frequently becomes inundated with fatty tissue (lipomatous hypertrophy). A characteristic mass effect is observed. The membrane of the fossa ovalis *(small arrows)* is spared, but the fatty atrial septum is thickened with hyperechoic fat *(large arrowheads)*. A pathognomonic dumbbell shape of the atrial septum is observed. The amount of fatty infiltrate varies but can be impressive. This condition is usually considered benign. (From JB Seward, BK Khandheria, JK Oh, et al. Critical appraisal of transesophageal echocardiography: limitations, pitfalls, and complications. *J Am Soc Echocardiogr* 1992;5:288–305. By permission of the American Society of Echocardiography.)

fossa ovalis can appear masslike. When excessively thick, it is referred to as *lipomatous hypertrophy* or *atrial septal lipoma* [43]. This usually appears as an echo-dense mass of variable size and consistency and occasionally may reach large proportions. Confusion arises particularly when the lipomatous hypertrophy of the atrial septum is asymmetrical. This pitfall is more common with a monoplane TEE examination, and a biplane examination clarifies the appearance. The condition is benign but can easily be misinterpreted by an inexperienced examiner.

Tricuspid Annulus

The tricuspid annular sulcus at the free wall of the right ventricle can be filled with various amounts of fatty tissue (Fig. 6-8). This can produce a mass effect in the tricuspid atrioventricular groove, particularly when viewed obliquely in the horizontal tomographic plane. This common observation should not be misinterpreted as a tumor or ring abscess. Magnetic resonance imaging has been diagnostic when the observation remains in doubt.

Mitral Valve Annulus

The mitral valve annulus usually causes fewer problems; however, annular calcification and, occasionally, fat can be very impressive and appear masslike. Because of the near-field location, calcium occasion-

ally may not be as dense-appearing and may be mistaken as a tumor. However, the characteristic location and reflectance of calcium usually allow easy recognition.

Aortic Valve

A frequently observed mass effect occurs when a cusp of the aortic valve is cut obliquely in the short axis or in transitional views from the left ventricular outflow tract. The ovoid appearance of the aortic cusp is often mistaken for an aortic valve vegetation or tumor (Fig. 6-9). Similarly, the aortic valve can be incorrectly interpreted as either bicuspid or tricuspid when cut obliquely. These phenomena most often occur with horizontal planar imaging and when incomplete tomographic analysis is performed. Biplane and multiplane views of the aortic valve eliminate these potential pitfalls and emphasize the importance of examination within true orthogonal short-axis planes and confirmation of the analysis in other imaging planes.

Sutures and Other Materials

Surgical sutures can be visualized at the sewing ring of prosthetic valves or at the margins of prosthetic patch material (Fig. 6-10). Redundant sutures can appear filamentous or pedunculated and undulate

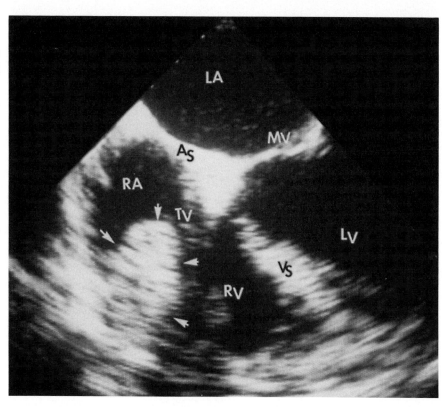

Fig. 6-8. Pseudomass of the tricuspid valve annulus *(arrows).* The tricuspid annulus at the right ventricular and right atrial junction normally contains fat, which can give a mass effect *(arrows).* This is particularly noticeable in oblique horizontal imaging planes. (From JB Seward, BK Khandheria, JK Oh, et al. Critical appraisal of transesophageal echocardiography: limitations, pitfalls, and complications. *J Am Soc Echocardiogr* 1992;5:288–305. By permission of the American Society of Echocardiography.)

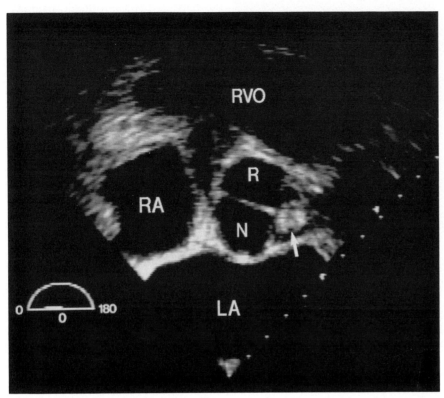

Fig. 6-9. Aortic valve pseudomass; off-axis longitudinal plane. The left coronary cusp of the aortic valve is imaged obliquely *en face* and has the appearance of a mass *(arrow)*, which may be incorrectly identified as a tumor or vegetation. This finding was not present in standard short-axis imaging planes of the aortic valve. *(N = noncoronary cusp; R = right coronary cusp.)*

with the cardiac motion. The regular spacing and highly refractile appearance of sutures help one make a correct interpretation. Although redundant suture material moves with the cardiac cycle, these structures should not appear multicentric, irregularly spaced, independently mobile, elongated, or bulbous—features that are more consistent with adherent thrombus or vegetation.

Other intracardiac structures that in an off-axis tomographic plane may appear like a mass are pacing wires, prosthetic patch material, artificial valves, and sewing rings.

Membranes

Membrane of the Fossa Ovalis

This membranous portion of the atrial septum can be redundant or aneurysmal and show variable undulating motion with each cardiac and respiratory cycle [44]. Occasionally, if the membrane has a large excursion, it can produce a mass effect in the left atrium, particularly with a monoplane examination. Biplane imaging easily elucidates the true identity of this structure.

Valve of the Fossa Ovalis

The posterosuperior margin of the fossa membrane overlaps the superior fatty limbus of the atrial septum (that is, the valve of the fossa ovalis). Nonfusion of these structures results in a patent valve of the fossa ovalis. The overlap between the fatty atrial septum and the fossal membrane in certain tomographic planes (particularly the horizontal plane) appears as a cavity [42] (see Figs. 6-4C and 6-4D). If the valve of the fossa ovalis is patent, shunting from one atrium to the other can be observed within this space. Longitudinal planar images best delineate this potentially confusing anatomy.

Left Atrial Membrane

A thin membrane or partial form of cor triatriatum extends from the common wall separating the left upper pulmonary vein and left atrial appendage and crosses the atrial cavity to the superior limbus of the foramen ovale [42,45,46] (Fig. 6-11). This membrane varies in extent but is usually incomplete and nonrestrictive to blood flow within the left atrium when imaged by color-flow Doppler study.

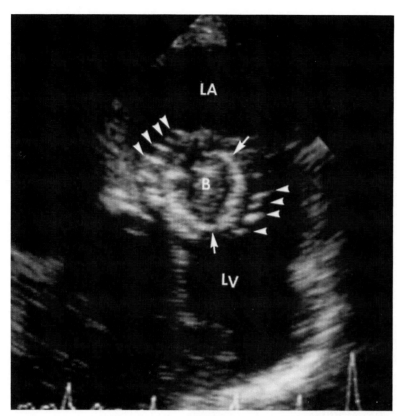

Fig. 6-10. Sutures. Off-axis horizontal plane image of the sewing ring of a Starr-Edwards mitral prosthesis *(arrows)*. Prosthetic material is usually hyper-refractile and causes far-field shadowing. Sutures pose a special problem because they may appear elongated and multicentric. Along a prosthetic sewing ring, sutures appear as regular, immobile hyper-refractile structures *(arrowheads)*. They may act as a nidus for thrombus and vegetation. Suture material is not pedunculated or bulbous and does not undulate or appear as multiple shaggy and irregular filaments. These features are more typical of pathologic vegetation or thrombus. *(B = ball.)* (From JB Seward, BK Khandheria, JK Oh, et al. Critical appraisal of transesophageal echocardiography: limitations, pitfalls, and complications. *J Am Soc Echocardiogr* 1992;5:288–305. By permission of the American Society of Echocardiography.)

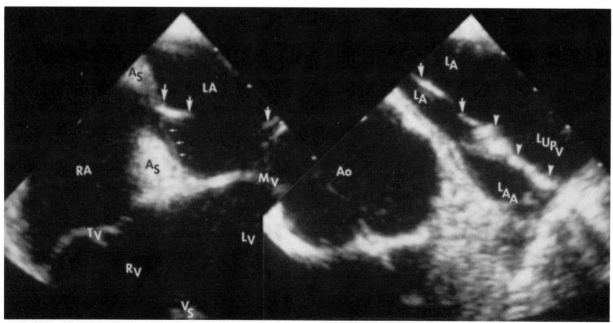

Fig. 6-11. Left atrial membrane. A forme fruste of cor triatriatum appears as an incomplete membrane in the left atrial cavity. Left: Horizontal four-chamber view. Medially at the atrial septum, the membrane *(large arrows)* originates from the posterior margin of the membrane of the fossa ovalis *(small arrows)*. Right: Basal view at aortic valve; horizontal plane. Laterally, the membrane *(arrows)* inserts into the common wall *(arrowheads)* separating the left upper pulmonary vein and left atrial appendage. (From JB Seward, BK Khandheria, JK Oh, et al. Critical appraisal of transesophageal echocardiography: limitations, pitfalls, and complications. *J Am Soc Echocardiogr* 1992;5:288–305. By permission of the American Society of Echocardiography.)

Eustachian Valve

In the right atrium at the orifice of the inferior vena cava, the eustachian valve often appears as a mobile, undulating membrane or mass partially encircling the orifice of the inferior vena cava as it enters the floor of the atrium [46] (Fig. 6-12). Accurate identification is readily accomplished with biplane or multiplane imaging.

Echo-Free Spaces

Transverse Sinus

The transverse sinus, a pericardial reflection between the left atrium and the great vessels at the base of the heart, typically contains a small amount of pericardial fluid that produces a small crescent-like, echo-free space between the left atrium and the aorta when visualized in the horizontal plane and a triangular space in the longitudinal planes [2]

(see Figs. 6-4A and 6-4B). When filled with larger amounts of fluid, this space can be misinterpreted as a pathologic finding and confused with a cyst or abscess cavity. Within the fluid-filled space, the left atrial appendage, its outpouchings, and attached epicardial fat may appear as mobile cystic or solid masses (Fig. 6-13). Biplanar imaging and careful sweeps of the ultrasound beam across the sinus and atrial appendages permit proper identification.

Oblique Sinus

The oblique sinus, a posterior pericardial reflection between the pulmonary veins, can appear as a fluid-filled space interposed between the left atrium and the esophagus. A pericardial cyst can also appear in the same position (see Chapter 12). Recognition of the pericardial layers usually permits proper identification of the pericardial cyst or the fluid-filled oblique sinus.

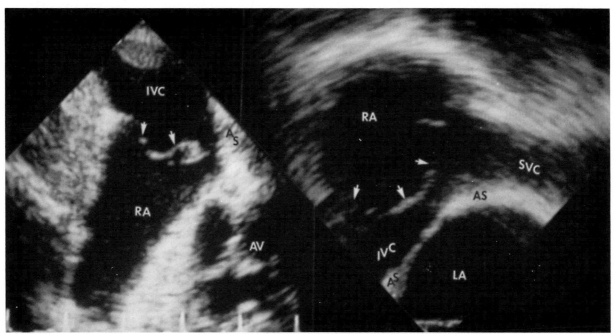

Fig. 6-12. Eustachian valve. Left: In the horizontal plane with the transducer at the gastroesophageal junction, the orifice of the inferior vena cava can be visualized. Surrounding the anterior orifice and interposed between the inferior vena cava and the body of the right atrium is the eustachian valve *(arrows)*. This structure usually is membranous and undulates throughout the cardiac cycle. Right: In the longitudinal plane, the eustachian membrane *(arrows)* originates from the anterior lip of the inferior vena cava orifice and partially separates the body of the right atrium and atrial septum. This undulating membrane can be mistaken for a mass or thrombus or even a catheter. (From JB Seward, BK Khandheria, JK Oh, et al. Critical appraisal of transesophageal echocardiography: limitations, pitfalls, and complications. *J Am Soc Echocardiogr* 1992;5:288–305. By permission of the American Society of Echocardiography.)

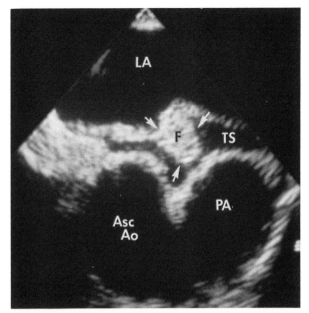

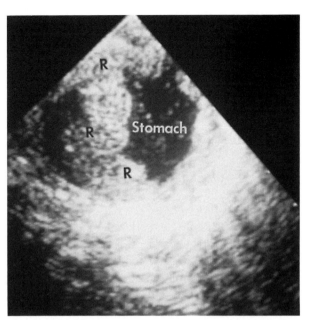

Fig. 6-13. Pseudomass in the transverse sinus. Within this pericardial reflection (transverse sinus) between the left atrium and the ascending aorta and pulmonary artery, there is epicardial fat *(F, arrows).* When the transverse sinus contains fluid, epicardial fat or the atrial appendage can appear masslike. (From JB Seward, BK Khandheria, JK Oh, et al. Critical appraisal of transesophageal echocardiography: limitations, pitfalls, and complications. *J Am Soc Echocardiogr* 1992;5:288–305. By permission of the American Society of Echocardiography.)

Fig. 6-14. Hiatal hernia. Stomach or bowel can herniate into the thorax and become interposed between the normal esophagus and the heart. Rugal folds *(R)* within the stomach can be mistaken for a tumor or mass. The heart can be obscured from visualization, as in this example. (From JB Seward, BK Khandheria, JK Oh, et al. Critical appraisal of transesophageal echocardiography: limitations, pitfalls, and complications. *J Am Soc Echocardiogr* 1992;5:288–305. By permission of the American Society of Echocardiography.)

Other Pericardial Reflections

Because of the high-resolution tomographic presentation of anatomy, pericardial reflections and recesses are easily visualized and are potentially confusing. A pericardial reflection between the wall separating the left atrial appendage and the left upper pulmonary vein can also appear as a cystic space or mass.

Hiatal Hernia

A large hiatal hernia can markedly inferfere with a complete TEE examination [47] (Fig. 6-14). Occasionally, however, a large fluid- or gas-filled hernia becomes interposed between the heart and the esophageal lumen. When fluid-filled, the hiatal hernia can appear as a thick-walled cystic mass posterior to the left atrium. When filled with gas, the hernia produces the expected problem of interference with ultrasound transmission causing shadowing of more anterior structures and resulting in a technically difficult TEE examination.

Color-Flow Doppler Imaging

Because of the close proximity of cardiac chambers and use of higher frequency transducers, color-flow Doppler signals are more exquisitely visualized and overlap at low Nyquist velocities. The increased sensitivity makes the color signals appear more extensive, so that they cannot be directly compared with those of a surface color Doppler examination. With experience, however, reliable semiquantitation of the severity of valvular regurgitation can be obtained, making TEE superior to the transthoracic examination in most patients. Experience and knowledge of the technology are important prerequisites for proper interpretation. Timing of rapid diastolic and systolic events is best accomplished with color-flow Doppler M-mode display or by pulsed-wave Doppler analysis. Quantitative techniques have not received sufficient validation.

Regurgitant Jets

Systolic flow reversal into pulmonary veins, extent of flow disturbance in the receiving chamber, size of the regurgitant orifice, and hemodynamic and anatomic associations usually allow accurate semi-quantitation of color-flow jets [48,49] (see Chapter 9). Mitral and tricuspid valve regurgitation is best evaluated with biplanar examinations, whereas aortic and pulmonic valve regurgitation is best imaged with the longitudinal plane. With the increased sensitivity of TEE, trivial "physiologic" regurgitation, particularly of the mitral and tricuspid valves, is frequently recognized [1]. Similarly, the "closing volume" of mechanical prostheses (see Chapter 10) is uniformly observed and must be recognized as a normal observation [50]. The "normal" color-flow jets seen in native valves and mechanical prostheses are small and of brief duration. These jets usually represent trivial regurgitant events, are not appreciated on physical examination, and do not in themselves prompt endocarditis prophylaxis or further investigation.

Off-Axis Regurgitant Jets

Two-dimensional echocardiographic color-flow imaging is a tomographic examination that allows imaging of blood flow. Because of limited transducer mobility within the confines of the esophagus, eccentric regurgitant jets may be incompletely delineated and appear spuriously small. Misinterpretation of the source or amount of regurgitation can occur with limited tomographic views. It is important to visually confirm the source of any regurgitant jet. The regurgitant source is appreciated as flow convergence and color overlapping of the color signal. Multiplanar imaging, slow sweeping of the color-flow image, and confident identification of the source eliminate the potential misinterpretations (see Chapter 9).

Atrial Septal Defects

Atrial septal defects are more confidently diagnosed by TEE with color-flow imaging [42]. The degree of shunting must be adjusted to the increased sensitivity and not equated with the transthoracic examination. Accurate measurement of the defect size and recognition of right-sided volume overload are equally important clinically relevant observations.

Phenomena

Spontaneous Contrast Effect

Because of the proximity of the transducer to the atrial cavities and the higher frequency transducers used, visualization of blood movement within the cardiac chambers is more commonly observed [51,52] (Fig. 6-15). The phenomenon is associated with reduced blood flow and poor clearance of blood from the cardiac chamber. It is reported that the risk of systemic embolism is significantly increased when this phenomenon is observed (see Chapter 15). This phenomenon, commonly ascribed to erythrocyte rouleau formation, is equated with stagnation of blood and a prethrombotic state.

Reverberations and Ghosting

The esophagus is surrounded by air-filled lung. Reverberation signals or ghost artifacts are common because of the strong ultrasonic reflection from impedance mismatch between tissue and air. Linear artifacts most frequently occur within the upper ascending aorta and mid-descending thoracic aorta, which have air-filled lung in the immediate far-field image (Fig. 6-16). Imaging the thoracic aorta is one of the highly diagnostic examinations of TEE [53,54] (see Chapter 14). Linear artifacts often lie in nonanatomic planes, cross normal anatomy, have artifactual motion, do not alter Doppler-depicted blood flow, and may disappear with change in imaging depth. Nearly perfect duplication of Doppler signals and structures can be obtained in certain imaging planes, consistently so when the descending thoracic aorta is imaged (Fig. 6-17). Duplication of the aorta and Doppler signal occurs if the field of view is expanded to accommodate a second signal. The only way to avoid misinterpretation is to be aware of these phenomena and to be cautious not to misinterpret atypical anatomy, such as a double thoracic aorta or Doppler signal lying outside the blood-filled aorta or cardiac chambers.

Extracardiac Fluid

Accumulations of pleural fluid are easily visualized by TEE. However, loculated fluid may appear ovoid or suspiciously like a normal or abnormal structure (Fig. 6-18). Fibrous bands within the fluid-filled space may give the false appearance of dissection or rupture of the thoracic aorta [55]. It is imperative to track all fluid-filled spaces to their source—for

Fig. 6-15. Spontaneous contrast effect. A. In a patient with mitral stenosis and spontaneous contrast effect in the left atrium, the mitral valve is thickened and the left atrium enlarged. Spontaneous contrast is visualized within the left atrium. B. A more subtle contrast effect *(arrows)* is noted in the left atrial appendage of a patient with less severe mitral valve disease. In extreme cases, spontaneous contrast phenomenon may have the appearance of a thrombus or mass. There is an association between spontaneous contrast effect and a higher incidence of thromboembolic events. Close observation distinguishes the immobility and unchanging margins of thrombus, whereas the spontaneous contrast effect is recognized by slow, swirling blood movement. (From JB Seward, BK Khandheria, JK Oh, et al. Critical appraisal of transesophageal echocardiography: limitations, pitfalls, and complications. *J Am Soc Echocardiogr* 1992;5:288–305. By permission of the American Society of Echocardiography.)

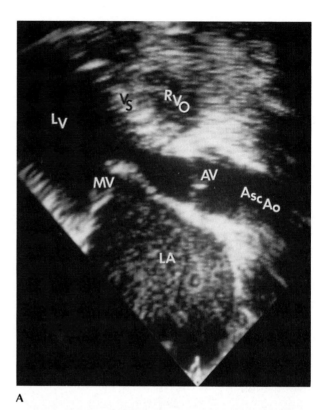

A

B

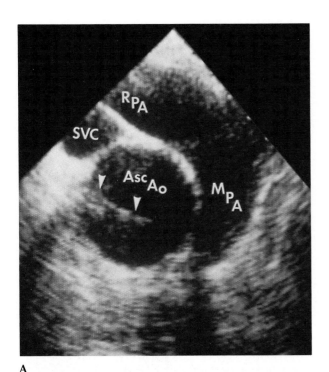

A

Fig. 6-16.   Linear reverberations. Horizontal scan (A) and longitudinal scan (B) of the ascending aorta. Frequently in the upper ascending aorta and less commonly in the mid-descending thoracic aorta, linear reverberations *(arrowheads, arrows)* are observed. These are thought to occur because of acoustic reflection from overlying lung. These linear shadows can be confused with pathologic dissecting membranes. Change in transducer frequency, alternation of the depth of image, nonanatomic appearance, and undisturbed color flow patterns can distinguish the artifactual nature of this observation in most situations. Rarely, linear artifacts cannot be adequately differentiated from aortic dissection. (From JB Seward, BK Khandheria, JK Oh, et al. Critical appraisal of transesophageal echocardiography: limitations, pitfalls, and complications. *J Am Soc Echocardiogr* 1992;5:288–305. By permission of the American Society of Echocardiography.)

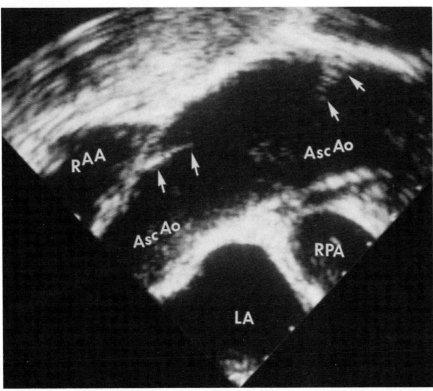

B

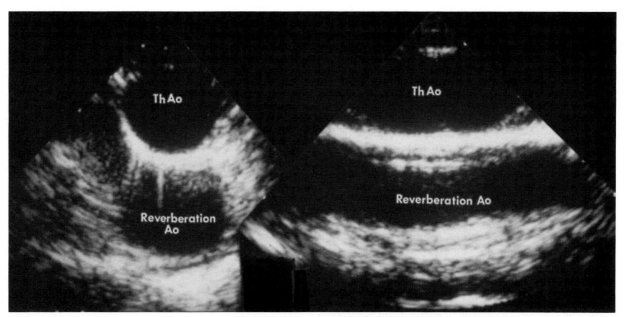

Fig. 6-17. Reverberation artifact; descending thoracic aorta, horizontal plane (left) and longitudinal plane (right). A common reverberation artifact occurs when the ultrasound beam is directed toward air-filled lung, which acts as an ultrasound reflector. Near-field structures are duplicated in the far field as a reverberation artifact. All signals are duplicated, including color-flow Doppler. This artifactual duplication of anatomy and Doppler signal should not be mistaken as a true structure. This example depicts reverberation artifact of the descending thoracic aorta. In the far field, a reverberation artifactual aorta is imaged when the ultrasound beam is directed toward the left lung. (From JB Seward, BK Khandheria, JK Oh, et al. Critical appraisal of transesophageal echocardiography: limitations, pitfalls, and complications. *J Am Soc Echocardiogr* 1992;5:288–305. By permission of the American Society of Echocardiography.)

example, a ventricular aneurysm to the ventricle or aortic dissection to the thoracic aorta. Biplanar and multiplanar imaging usually permit proper diagnosis. Difficulty in correct identification may be compounded by color-flow artifacts or ghosting phenomena within the fluid-filled space. These artifacts are usually of low velocity and should not be confused with pathologic blood movement within the fluid-filled space. Because of the proximity of structures and use of higher frequency transducers, Doppler artifacts are frequently observed within any fluid-filled space. To avoid misinterpretation, one should be cautious of interpreting very low-velocity signals and always search for a source of communication. Motion artifacts are very common, whereas pathologic communication from aneurysm or aortic dissection is much less frequently observed.

COMMENT

The limitations and pitfalls of TEE can best be minimized by experience. Initial training should not be circumvented, and maintenance of competency should be strictly monitored. Physicians with less than level II echocardiographic training should work in close collaboration with an active echocardiographic laboratory and have appropriate review of current examinations. Both individual and laboratory standards for maintenance of competency should be established.

Transesophageal endoscopes are being continuously modified and refined to address current limitations. Multiple imaging planes, continuous-wave Doppler imaging, and small tip and shaft size are now being introduced. Display and safety features

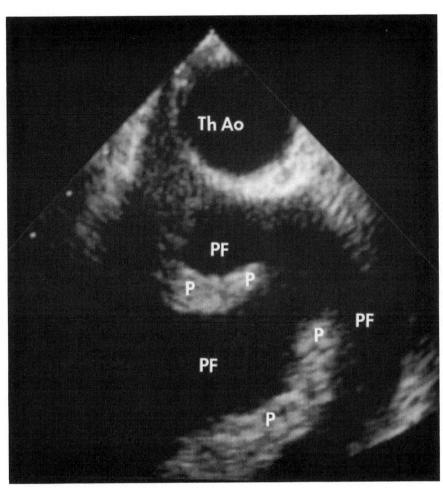

Fig. 6-18.   Pleural fluid *(PF)*; horizontal plane. Fluid accumulation in the thorax, particularly around the thoracic aorta, can be confused with aortic dissection, extravascular mass, or tumor. Bands of filamentous stranding *(P)* or even portions of lung tissue can be mistaken for pathologic structures such as tumor or dissecting membrane. Wide field of view and careful delineation of underlying anatomy and pathologic conditions avoid mistaken diagnoses. (From JB Seward, BK Khandheria, JK Oh, et al. Critical appraisal of transesophageal echocardiography: limitations, pitfalls, and complications. *J Am Soc Echocardiogr* 1992;5:288–305. By permission of the American Society of Echocardiography.)

continue to improve. An ideal TEE endoscope should incorporate all the functions of currently available transthoracic transducers and have a wider field of view and smaller diameter.

SUMMARY

As with any imaging technology, there are limitations and pitfalls. The semi-invasive nature of TEE also has potential for serious complications. Because of the new presentation of cardiac and extracardiac anatomy, unfamiliar but normal anatomy may initially be confused as abnormal. Additionally, certain structures are viewed in a manner that may mimic pathologic conditions. Because of the superior resolution afforded by TEE, phenomena such as spontaneous contrast and ghosting are much more commonly observed than they are with transthoracic imaging. Highly detailed anatomic structures, such

as atrial muscle bundles, sutures, and adipose tissue, are to be recognized and differentiated from thrombi, vegetations, and masses.

Although TEE has been a dramatic step forward in diagnostic imaging, there is potential for serious misinterpretation. This chapter discusses most of these potential problems; however, there will always be unique situations in which the findings must be consistently addressed and differentiated as normal, artifact, new observation, or misinterpretation.

REFERENCES

1. Seward JB, Khandheria BK, Oh JK, et al. Transesophageal echocardiography: technique, anatomic correlations, implementation, and clinical applications. *Mayo Clin Proc* 1988;63:649–80.

2. Seward JB, Khandheria BK, Edwards WD, et al. Biplanar transesophageal echocardiography: ana-

tomic correlations, image orientation, and clinical applications. *Mayo Clin Proc* 1990;65:1193–213.

3. Daniel WG, Erbel R, Kasper W, et al. Safety of transesophageal echocardiography: a multicenter survey of 10,419 examinations. *Circulation* 1991; 83:817–21.

4. Khandheria BK, Seward JB, Bailey K, et al. Safety of transesophageal echocardiography: experience with 2070 consecutive procedures (abstract). *J Am Coll Cardiol* 1991;17 Suppl A:20A.

5. Geibel A, Kasper W, Behroz A, et al. Risk of transesophageal echocardiography in awake patients with cardiac diseases. *Am J Cardiol* 1988;62:337–9.

6. Savino JS, Weiss S. Safety of transesophageal echocardiography is still unclear (letter to the editor). *Anesthesiology* 1990;73:366.

7. Hanrath P, Bleifeld W, Souquet J, eds. *Cardiovascular Diagnosis by Ultrasound; Transesophageal, Computerized, Contrast, Doppler Echocardiography.* The Hague: Martinus Nijhoff, 1982.

8. Erbel R, Khandheria BK, Brennecke R, et al., eds. *Transesophageal Echocardiography: A New Window to the Heart.* Berlin: Springer-Verlag, 1989.

9. Cyran SE, Kimball TR, Meyer RA, et al. Efficacy of intraoperative transesophageal echocardiography in children with congenital heart disease. *Am J Cardiol* 1989;63:594–8.

10. Cyran SE, Myers JL, Gleason MM, et al. Application of intraoperative transesophageal echocardiography in infants and small children. *J Cardiovasc Surg (Torino)* 1991;32:318–21.

11. Ritter SB. Transesophageal real-time echocardiography in infants and children with congenital heart disease. *J Am Coll Cardiol* 1991;18:569–80.

12. Dundee JW, Halliday NJ, Loughran PG, Harper KW. The influence of age on the onset of anaesthesia with midazolam. *Anaesthesia* 1985;40:441–3.

13. Ofili EO, Rich MW. Safety and usefulness of transesophageal echocardiography in persons aged ≥ 70 years. *Am J Cardiol* 1990;66:1279–80.

14. Flachskampf FA, Hoffmann R, Hanrath P. Experience with a transesophageal echotransducer allowing full rotation of the viewing plane: the omniplane probe (abstract). *J Am Coll Cardiol* 1991 17 Suppl A:34A.

15. Omoto R, Kyo S, Matsumura M, et al. Recent technological progress in transesophageal color Doppler flow imaging with special reference to newly developed biplane and pediatric probes. In: Erbel R, Khandheria BK, Brennecke R, et al., eds. *Transesophageal Echocardiography: A New Window to the Heart.* Berlin: Springer-Verlag, 1989;21–6.

16. Seward JB, Khandheria BK, Tajik AJ. Wide-field transesophageal echocardiographic tomography: feasibility study. *Mayo Clin Proc* 1990;65:31–7.

17. Hsu TL, Weintraub AR, Ritter SB, Pandian NG. Panoramic transesophageal echocardiography: clinical application of real-time, wide-angle, transesophageal two-dimensional echocardiography and color flow imaging. *Echocardiography* 1991;8: 677–85.

18. Skorton DJ, Melton HE Jr, Pandian NG, et al. Detection of acute myocardial infarction in closed-chest dogs by analysis of regional two-dimensional echocardiographic gray-level distributions. *Circ Res* 1983;52:36–44.

19. Chandrasekaran K, Chu A, Greenleaf JF, et al. 2D echo quantitative texture analysis of acutely ischemic myocardium (abstract). *Circulation* 1986;74 Suppl 2:II–271.

20. Fitzgerald PJ, McDaniel MD, Rolett EL, et al. Two-dimensional ultrasonic tissue characterization: backscatter power, endocardial wall motion, and their phase relationship for normal, ischemic, and infarcted myocardium. *Circulation* 1987;76:850–9.

21. Kuroda T, Kinter TM, Seward JB, et al. Accuracy of three-dimensional volume measurement using biplane transesophageal echocardiographic probe: in vitro experiment. *J Am Soc Echocardiogr* 1991;4: 475–84.

22. Wollschläger H, Zeiher AM, Klein H-P, et al. Transesophageal echo computer tomography: a new method for dynamic 3–D imaging of the heart (abstract). *J Am Coll Cardiol* 1989;13 Suppl A:68A.

23. Omoto R, Kyo S, Matsumura M, et al. New direction of biplane transesophageal echocardiography with special emphasis on real-time biplane imaging and matrix phased-array biplane transducer. *Echocardiography* 1990;7:691–8.

24. Urbanowicz JH, Kernoff RS, Oppenheim G, et al. Transesophageal echocardiography and its potential for esophageal damage. *Anesthesiology* 1990;72: 40–3.

25. O'Shea JP, Southern JF, D'Ambra MN, et al. Effects of prolonged transesophageal echocardiographic imaging and probe manipulation on the esophagus—an echocardiographic-pathologic study. *J Am Coll Cardiol* 1991;17:1426–9.

26. Cucchiara RF, Nugent M, Seward JB, Messick JM. Air embolism in upright neurosurgical patients: detection and localization by two-dimensional transesophageal echocardiography. *Anesthesiology* 1984;60:353–5.

27. Dewhirst WE, Stragand JJ, Fleming BM. Mallory-Weiss tear complicating intraoperative transesophageal echocardiography in a patient undergoing aortic valve replacement. *Anesthesiology* 1990;73: 777–8.

28. Watts HD. Mallory-Weiss syndrome occurring as a complication of endoscopy. *Gastrointest Endosc* 1976;22:171–2.

29. Knauer CM. Mallory-Weiss syndrome: characterization of 75 Mallory-Weiss lacerations in 528 patients with upper gastrointestinal hemorrhage. *Gastroenterology* 1976;71:5–8.

30. Kronzon I, Cziner DG, Katz ES, et al. Buckling of the tip of the transesophageal echocardiography probe: a potentially dangerous technical malfunction. *J Am Soc Echocardiogr* 1992;5:176–7.

31. Botoman VA, Surawicz CM. Bacteremia with gastrointestinal endoscopic procedures. *Gastrointest Endosc* 1986;32:342–6.

32. Leitch DG, Collins JSA, Radhakrishnan S, et al. Bacteraemia following endoscopy. *Br J Clin Pract* 1986;40:341–2.

33. Norfleet RG, Mitchell PD, Mulholland DD, Philo J. Does bacteremia follow upper gastrointestinal endoscopy? *Am J Gastroenterol* 1981;76:420–2.

34. Perucca PJ, Meyer GW. Who should have endocarditis prophylaxis for upper gastrointestinal procedures? (editorial). *Gastrointest Endosc* 1985;31:285–7.

35. Shorvon PJ, Eykyn SJ, Cotton PB. Gastrointestinal instrumentation, bacteremia, and endocarditis. *Gut* 1983;24:1078–93.

36. Steckelberg JM, Khandheria BK, Anhalt JP, et al. Prospective evaluation of the risk of bacteremia associated with transesophageal echocardiography. *Circulation* 1991;84:177–80.

37. Melendez LJ, Chan K-L, Cheung PK, et al. Incidence of bacteremia in transesophageal echocardiography: A prospective study of 140 consecutive patients. *J Am Coll Cardiol* 1991;18:1650–4.

38. Völler H, Schröder KM, Gast D, et al. Does the incidence of positive blood cultures during transesophageal echocardiography necessitate antibiotic prophylaxis? (abstract). *Circulation* 1990;82 Suppl 3:III–244.

39. Nikutta P, Mantey-Stiers F, Becht I, et al. Risk of bacteremia induced by transesophageal echocardiography: analysis of 100 consecutive procedures. *J Am Soc Echocardiogr* 1992;5:168–72.

40. Görge G, Erbel R, Henrichs KJ, et al. Positive blood cultures during transesophageal echocardiography. *Am J Cardiol* 1990;65:1404–5.

41. Foster E, Kusumoto FM, Sobol SM, Schiller NB. Streptococcal endocarditis temporally related to transesophageal echocardiography. *J Am Soc Echocardiogr* 1990;3:424–7.

42. Seward JB, Tajik AJ. Transesophageal echocardiography in congenital heart disease. *Am J Card Imaging* 1990;4:215–22.

43. Fyke FE III, Tajik AJ, Edwards WD, Seward JB. Diagnosis of lipomatous hypertrophy of the atrial septum by two-dimensional echocardiography. *J Am Coll Cardiol* 1983;1:1352–7.

44. Hanley PC, Tajik AJ, Hynes JK, et al. Diagnosis and classification of atrial septal aneurysm by two-dimensional echocardiography: report of 80 consecutive cases. *J Am Coll Cardiol* 1985;6:1370–82.

45. Schlüter M, Langenstein BA, Thier W, et al. Transesophageal two-dimensional echocardiography in the diagnosis of cor triatriatum in the adult. *J Am Coll Cardiol* 1983;2:1011–5.

46. Goldfarb A, Weinreb J, Daniel WG, Kronzon I. A patient with right and left atrial membranes: the role of transesophageal echocardiography and magnetic resonance imaging in diagnosis. *J Am Soc Echocardiogr* 1989;2:350–3.

47. Freedberg RS, Weinreb J, Gluck M, Kronzon I. Paraesophageal hernia may prevent cardiac imaging by transesophageal echocardiography. *J Am Soc Echocardiogr* 1989;2:202–3.

48. Yoshida K, Yoshikawa J, Yamaura Y, et al. Assessment of mitral regurgitation by biplane transesophageal color Doppler flow mapping. *Circulation* 1990;82:1121–6.

49. Castello R, Pearson AC, Lenzen P, Labovitz AJ. Effect of mitral regurgitation on pulmonary venous velocities derived from transesophageal echocardiography color-guided pulsed Doppler imaging. *J Am Coll Cardiol* 1991;17:1499–506.

50. Khandheria BK, Seward JB, Oh JK, et al. Value and limitations of transesophageal echocardiography in assessment of mitral valve prostheses. *Circulation* 1991;83:1956–68.

51. Daniel WG, Nellessen U, Schröder E, et al. Left atrial spontaneous echo contrast in mitral valve disease: an indicator for an increased thromboembolic risk. *J Am Coll Cardiol* 1988;11:1204–11.

52. Black IW, Hopkins AP, Lee LCL, Walsh WF. Left atrial spontaneous echo contrast: a clinical and echocardiographic analysis. *J Am Coll Cardiol* 1991;18:398–404.

53. Erbel R, Engberding R, Daniel W, et al. Echocardiography in diagnosis of aortic dissection. *Lancet* 1989;1:457–61.

54. Karalis DG, Chandrasekaran K, Victor MF, et al. Recognition and embolic potential of intraaortic atherosclerotic debris. *J Am Coll Cardiol* 1991;17:73–8.

55. Kronzon I, Demopoulos L, Schrem SS, et al. Pitfalls in the diagnosis of thoracic aortic aneurysm by transesophageal echocardiography. *J Am Soc Echocardiogr* 1990;3:145–8.

7

Evaluation of Left Ventricular Function by Transesophageal Echocardiography

Rick A. Nishimura • *Martin D. Abel*

Echocardiography has emerged as an excellent modality for determining the status of the left ventricle [1]. Direct visualization of the myocardium allows analysis of cavity size, wall thickness, regional wall motion, and systolic function. Doppler echocardiography provides accurate measurement of blood flow velocity and has been used to calculate volumetric flow and to assess diastolic filling of the left ventricle [2]. All of these variables have been assessed by transthoracic echocardiography.

The major clinical usefulness of transesophageal echocardiography (TEE) in the past has been in evaluation of cardiac structures and valve function, because high-resolution images of the heart are consistently obtainable in nearly all patients [3]. However, TEE may also be used for examining the status of the left ventricle. Transesophageal echocardiography has several advantages over transthoracic echocardiography: (1) it provides high-resolution two-dimensional echocardiographic images in nearly all patients; (2) it can be used for continuous monitoring; and (3) Doppler velocities not readily detectable on most transthoracic examinations, such as those from the pulmonary veins, can be obtained.

The ability of TEE to assess both systolic and diastolic properties of the left ventricle makes it a promising modality for use in the operating room and in the critically ill patient. Information about regional wall motion, left ventricular volume, and overall contractility of the left ventricle is attainable by TEE. In addition, cardiac output measurements and left ventricular filling pressures can be obtained. This chapter describes the methods by which TEE can provide this type of information.

SYSTOLIC FUNCTION

Assessment of Global Systolic Function (Semiquantitative Approach)

The left ventricular myocardium can be imaged from multiple planes with a monoplane transesophageal probe [3]. The short-axis view from the transgastric approach allows segmental analysis of the short axis of the heart at different levels along the long axis of the heart. The four-chamber view provides images of the inferoseptal and lateral walls. Because of the position of the long axis of the heart in relation to the echocardiographic beam, the true apex of the left ventricle may be difficult to visualize in some patients, specifically when monoplane short-axis imaging is used. This deficiency has been mostly overcome by use of longitudinal plane imaging. Biplane TEE has also provided additional information, because a two-chamber view allows assessment of inferior and anterior walls. Multiplane imaging has the potential to display all regions of the myocardium in one sequential scan.

Both global and regional systolic function can be assessed by a subjective visual approach. Overall cavity size and a visual estimate of ejection fraction can be rapidly obtained. The visual estimate of ejection fraction is accurate and reproducible when performed by experienced echocardiographers [4]. Regional wall motion abnormalities can be detected by incorporating endocardial motion and wall thickening of individual segments. The basal and middle left ventricular segments can be assessed by longitudinal and short-axis transesophageal imaging nearly always. In 20% to 30% of patients, however, analysis of the distal apical segmental contraction may be limited. Improved visualization of the left ventricular apex may be achieved with left lateral angulation of the transesophageal probe from the transgastric window in either the transverse or the longitudinal imaging plane.

For a semiquantitative assessment of regional wall motion, a wall motion score index has been derived. In this analysis, the left ventricle is divided into 16 segments (Fig. 7-1). Each segment is given a score: 1, normal; 2, hypokinetic; 3, akinetic; 4, dyskinetic; and 5, aneurysm. The sum of the scores for the individual segments is divided by the number of segments visualized to derive a wall motion score index (WMSI): WMSI = sum of segmental wall scores divided by number of segments analyzed. In this particular approach, which has been proposed by the American Society of Echocardiography [5], a score of $\geq$ 2.0 is compatible with a poorly contracting ventricle and low ejection fraction (< 30%), whereas a score of $\leq$ 1.5 describes a near-normal ventricle.

The use of cine-loop digitization has greatly enhanced the accuracy of visual assessment in depicting changes in global contractility and wall motion. It has been particularly useful intraoperatively, because a baseline short-axis view can be stored and compared directly on line side-by-side with the current image.

Indirect clues about the status of overall left ventricular function can be obtained by TEE examination of the base of the heart. In the past, left ventricular function was indirectly assessed on M-mode echocardiography by separation of the mitral valve E point from the septum. This measurement is influenced by the volume of the left ventricle as well as the cardiac output. It is larger in patients with dilated left ventricles and poor systolic func-

tion. This concept has been applied to two-dimensional echocardiography by measurement of the angle between the mitral valve leaflets and the septum in diastole [6] (Fig. 7-2 A). An inverse correlation between this angle and ejection fraction provides a simple method for a quick analysis of global systolic function (Fig. 7-2 B).

Mitral annular motion during systole also provides an indirect measure of systolic function of the left ventricle [7]. During myocardial contraction, shortening of the long axis of the heart brings the apex closer to the base of the heart. Visualizing the descent of the mitral annulus relative to the cardiac apex provides information about this shortening of the long axis, which is less in patients with poor global systolic function. Regional systolic dysfunction can be assessed by examining the annulus descent from different areas of the myocardium. The lateral and septal walls are represented in the four-chamber view and the anterior and inferior walls in the longitudinal two-chamber view.

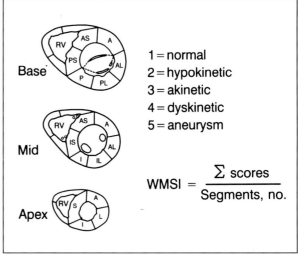

Fig. 7-1. American Society of Echocardiography recommendations for a 16-segment analysis of left ventricular function for transthoracic parasternal short-axis imaging. (*AS* = anterior septum; *IS* = inferior septum; *L* = lateral apical) (Modified from NB Schiller et al. Recommendations for quantitation of the left ventricle by two-dimensional echocardiography. *J Am Soc Echocardiogr* 1989;2:358–67)

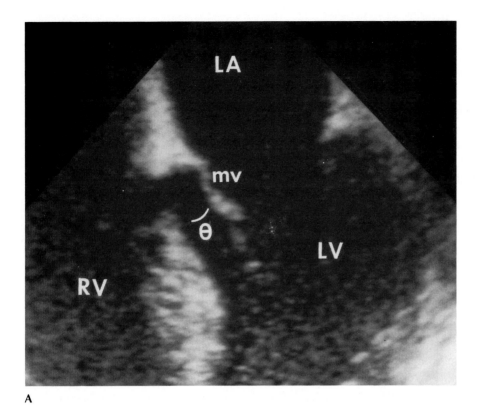

A

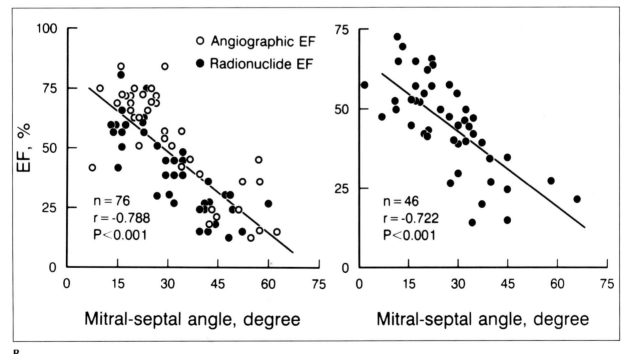

B

Fig. 7-2.   A. Four-chamber view shows angle of incidence *(θ)* between anterior leaflet of mitral valve and ventricular septum. B. Correlation of the mitral septal angle with ejection fraction *(EF)* by angiography and radionuclide studies. (With permission from EG Abinader et al. Mitral-septal angle: a new two-dimensional echocardiographic index of left ventricular performance. *Am Heart J* 1985;110:381. By permission of Mosby-Year Book.)

Assessment of Global Systolic Function (Quantitative Approach)

Objective measurements of the left ventricle—measuring the cavity area of a short-axis view at midventricular level—have been made in the operating room [8]. With the advent of cine-loop formats and direct transfer of video images to digital images, diastolic and systolic areas can be readily measured (Fig. 7-3). A fractional area change (FAC) can be calculated from Equation 7-1.

$$FAC = \frac{EDA - ESA}{EDA} \qquad [7\text{-}1]$$

in which EDA is the end-diastolic area and ESA is the end-systolic area. The end-diastolic area provides a relative index of the preload of the heart, and the fractional area change provides a relative index of global systolic function. Although these measurements examine only a portion of the myocardium, they are useful for determining sequential changes in preload and contractility. When multiple regional wall motion abnormalities are present, a three-level evaluation may be performed, attaining the end-diastolic area and end-systolic area at base level, midventricular level, and apical level. A more accurate fractional area change can then be provided by the mean value obtained from these three levels.

These values may change dramatically throughout cardiac surgery, and they provide a basis for therapeutic maneuvers by the anesthesiologist [8]. For example, a hypotensive patient who has had a decrease in end-diastolic area and an increase in fractional area change most likely has hypovolemia as the cause for the hypotension, and the therapy is

volume replacement. Conversely, an increase in end-diastolic area with reduction of fractional area change indicates deterioration in myocardial contractility and should prompt inotropic and preload reduction therapy. As shown in Figure 7-4, dramatic changes occur in diastolic area and fractional area throughout an operation. These changes in loading conditions and contractility may not always be evident by other monitoring modalities, such as right heart catheterization.

Intrinsic Myocardial Contractility

The most commonly used measures of systolic function in clinical practice involve the ejection phase indices, that is, ejection fraction, fractional shortening, and cardiac output. However, these measures are highly dependent on the loading conditions of the left ventricle. A decrease in a variable such as ejection fraction may be due to a decrease in intrinsic myocardial contractility but may also occur as a result of an increase in afterload or decrease in preload. For clinical investigation, it may become important to establish the effect of a drug or an intervention on the intrinsic myocardial contractility independent of the changes that may occur on the loading conditions.

The relation of end-systolic pressure to volume has been proposed as a method to measure intrinsic myocardial contractility [9]. This concept is based on the observation that for a given myocardial contraction, the pressure and volume at end-systole under different loading conditions form a linear relationship when pressure is plotted against volume. The slope of this linear relationship is termed *maxi-*

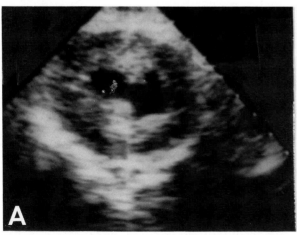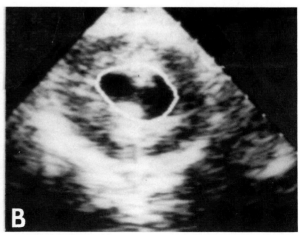

Fig. 7-3. Measurement of end-systolic area by digitization. A. Video image before digitization. B. Image after digitization; area has been outlined by computer format.

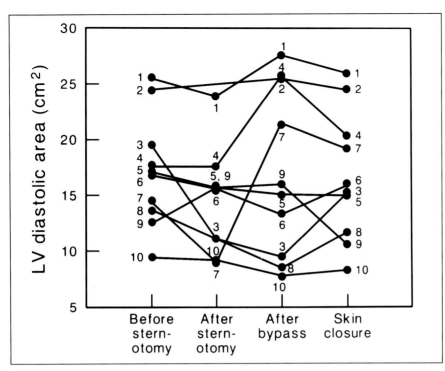

A

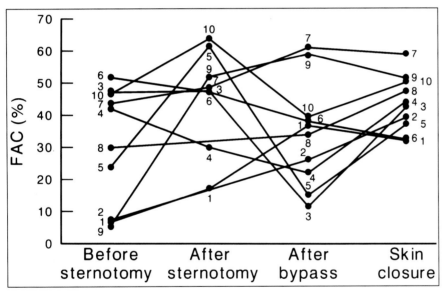

B

Fig. 7-4. A. Changes in diastolic area during coronary artery bypass grafting. B. Changes in fractional area change *(FAC)* during coronary artery bypass grafting.

mal elastance, or E-max, and represents the degree of myocardial contraction. With a decrease in intrinsic contractility of the heart, the E-max slope will be less steep and shifted downward and to the right (Fig. 7-5).

It has been proposed that TEE can provide an indirect measurement of E-max. This proposal is based on the concept of measuring end-systolic pressures and relative volumes at different preloads. One such technique has been used during open-heart surgery to evaluate the effects of different anesthetic agents on the heart [10]. Short-axis imaging of the left ventricle from the transgastric approach provides a stable format to evaluate end-systolic area during systolic pressure monitoring and preload manipula-

tion, such as occlusion of the inferior vena cava. The slope of the linear relationship between the end-systolic area and systolic pressure represents the intrinsic contractility of the left ventricle. As contractility is increased, the slope is shifted leftward and upward. This phenomenon has been used to assess the effect of an anesthetic agent on the myocardium by construction of an E-max slope. An anesthetic agent such as isoflurane may not change the ejection phase indices, such as ejection fraction and cardiac output, because of its effect on lowering afterload. However, with this technique of examining the relation of end-systolic pressure to area, it has been shown that isoflurane is a true myocardial depressant [10].

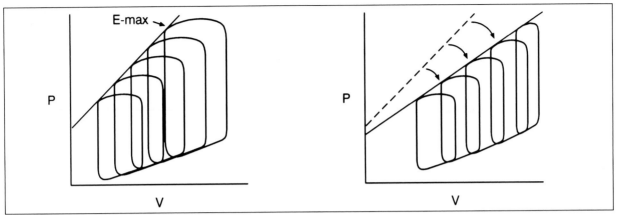

Fig. 7-5. Left. Schematic diagram of left ventricular pressure *(P)* and volume *(V)* of multiple cardiac cycles during different loading conditions. The end-systolic pressure-volume points lie on a straight line termed "maximal elastance," or "E-max." The slope of this line represents the intrinsic myocardial contractility. Right. With a decrease in intrinsic myocardial contractility, there is a shift of the E-max line downward and toward the right with a less steep slope *(arrows)*.

Cardiac Output

Cardiac output can be accurately and reproducibly measured by Doppler echocardiography [11,12]. The calculation of cardiac output uses the concept of volumetric flow through a rigid tube, as shown in Equation 7-2.

$$Q = V \times A \qquad [7\text{-}2]$$

in which Q is volumetric flow, V is velocity of flow through the tube, and A is cross-sectional area of the tube. Extrapolating this equation to the clinical setting, one can obtain volumetric flow by Doppler echocardiographic measurement of the time velocity integral (TVI) of flow through a valve or orifice. The area of the orifice is then obtained by measurement of the orifice diameter on a two-dimensional frame and conversion of this figure to area, with the assumption that the cross-sectional area is fixed and circular. The product of the TVI and the area equals stroke volume, which multiplied by heart rate gives cardiac output.

Using transthoracic echocardiography, the left ventricular outflow tract has been the most accurate location for measuring cardiac output, since the velocity profile is relatively flat [11]. The imaging planes available from TEE are not suitable for this approach, however, because of a significant angle of incidence of the pulsed-wave Doppler sample volume to the left ventricular outflow tract. Occa-

sionally, adequate pulsed-wave Doppler sample volume of the left ventricular outflow tract can be obtained by apex-down longitudinal imaging from the transgastric window. The left ventricular outflow tract diameter is readily obtained from longitudinal long-axis imaging. Previous investigators have used the pulmonary outflow tract for measuring volumetric flow with monoplane TEE [13].

We have found that interrogation of the mitral annulus provides a relatively accurate reproducible measurement of cardiac output, since the flow of blood through the annulus is directly parallel to the Doppler beam in the four-chamber view (Abel MD, Nishimura RA, unpublished data). The technique of this measurement is shown in Figure 7-6 A. Measurement of mitral annulus diameter is made from a still frame of the four-chamber view in diastole. A pulsed-wave sample volume is then placed at the level of the mitral annulus, and the laminar velocity curve is integrated to provide a TVI (Fig. 7-6 B). Multiplication of the cross-sectional area (πr^2) by the TVI gives a measure of stroke volume. Multiplying the stroke volume by heart rate gives a measurement of cardiac output.

Several assumptions go into calculation of cardiac output by this technique. The cross-sectional area is assumed to be circular and to remain constant throughout diastole. Also, it is assumed that there is laminar flow through the mitral valve orifice. The sample volume is assumed to stay at a constant

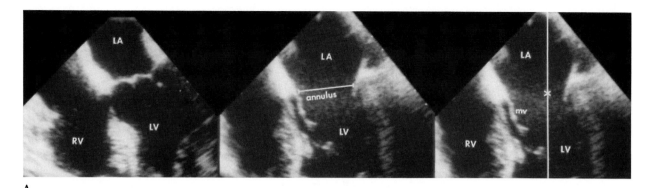

A

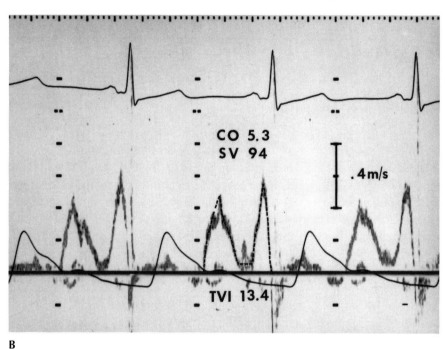

B

Fig. 7-6. A. Four-chamber view of the heart shows measurements required for calculation of cardiac output through the mitral valve annulus. Diameter of the annulus is measured during diastole. Pulsed-wave sample volume *(X)* is placed at level of the mitral valve annulus. B. Time velocity integral *(TVI)* of mitral flow velocity. Cardiac output *(CO)* and stroke volume *(SV)* are calculated.

location relative to the heart throughout the entire diastolic period. Despite these assumptions, measuring cardiac output from TEE correlates well with measurements obtained by thermodilution (Fig. 7-7). This method is not applicable to patients with significant mitral regurgitation or mitral stenosis. In patients with irregular rhythms, such as atrial fibrillation or multiple premature contractions, ten or more cycles must be averaged to provide an accurate measurement of cardiac output.

DIASTOLIC FUNCTION

Diastolic Filling of the Left Ventricle

In recent years, there has been great interest in evaluating diastolic filling of the heart by Doppler echocardiography [14–16]. There has not been a

clinically available method to assess diastolic function because of the complexity of the multiple interrelated processes involved. These include myocardial relaxation, erectile coronary effect, diastolic suction, viscoelastic forces of the myocardium, ventricular interaction, pericardial constraint, and atrial contribution [17–19]. It has recently been proposed that Doppler echocardiography may provide insight into diastolic filling of the left ventricle [14–16]. Although simple measurements of flow velocity may not provide an absolute measurement of the diastolic properties of the left ventricle, the mitral and pulmonary venous flow velocity curves provide valuable information pertaining to the overall state of diastolic filling of the left ventricle at any one time. These measurements can then be extrapolated to provide information about the left heart filling pressures.

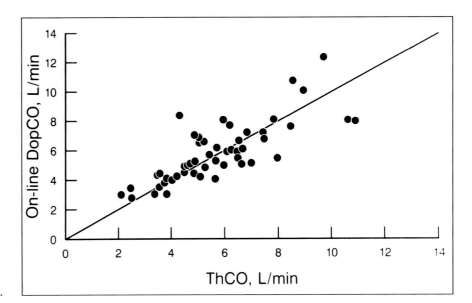

Fig. 7-7. Correlation of cardiac output by thermodilution *(ThCO)* with cardiac output by Doppler echocardiography *(DopCO)*.

Mitral Flow Velocity Curves

Mitral flow velocity curves are measured by placing a pulsed-wave sample volume at the tip of the mitral valve leaflets as they open into the left ventricle. These velocity curves provide information regarding the diastolic filling of the left ventricle. To understand these mitral flow velocities, they must be regarded as the "driving pressure" across the mitral valve, representing the instantaneous relationship between left atrial pressure and left ventricular pressure [14] (Fig. 7-8). During myocardial relaxation, the decrease in left ventricular pressure below left atrial pressure opens the mitral valve. A "driving force" is created across the mitral valve, and, thus, flow velocity accelerates on the mitral flow velocity curve. As relaxation continues throughout the first one-third to one-half of diastole, the effect of the viscoelastic forces of the myocardium, ventricular interaction, and pericardial restraint then come into play. The left ventricular pressure increases to meet, or even exceed, the left atrial pressure, and the result is a deceleration of mitral flow velocity. During mid-diastole, left atrial and left ventricular pressures equalize but very low forward velocity continues because of inertial effects. Finally, at atrial contraction, left atrial pressure increases above left ventricular pressure and blood flow reaccelerates across the mitral valve. Simple measurements of the mitral flow velocity curve can be performed for clinical use (E velocity, A velocity, deceleration time).

The changes that occur in the mitral flow velocity curves during different loading conditions of the heart are governed by the relationship between the left atrial pressure and the left ventricular pressure [14,20–23]. An explanation of these changes allows the development of a conceptual framework through which the various mitral flow velocity curves can be interpreted (Fig. 7-9). If preload is high, left atrial pressure is increased at mitral valve opening. The result is a high driving pressure across the valve that causes the mitral flow velocity curve to display rapid initial acceleration and high E velocity. Since the diastolic pressure volume loop is curvilinear, left ventricular pressure rises rapidly during early diastole. This increase causes rapid deceleration of the mitral flow velocity as the left ventricular pressure approximates and exceeds the left atrial pressure. Therefore, the major effects of increasing the preload of the heart are an increase in the E velocity and a shortening of the deceleration time. Conversely, a reduction in preload causes a lower left atrial pressure at mitral valve opening and a slower increase of left ventricular pressure during the rapid filling phase. The result is a decrease in the E velocity and prolongation of deceleration time. Because forward output is less, the velocity at atrial contraction is decreased. If afterload is high, the rate of relaxation of the decrease in left ventricular pressure is prolonged. This results in a lower E velocity, prolongation of deceleration time, and a high velocity at atrial contraction.

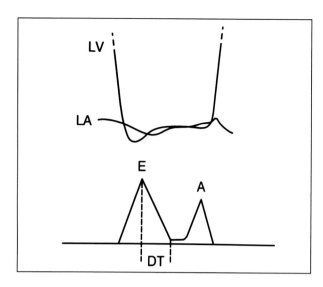

Fig. 7-8. Bottom. Mitral flow velocity curve with early *(E)* filling, deceleration time, and atrial *(A)* contribution. Top. Diastolic left atrial and left ventricular pressures (see text). (From RA Nishimura et al. Assessment of diastolic function of the heart: background and current applications of Doppler echocardiography. Part II. Clinical studies. *Mayo Clin Proc* 1989;64;181–204. By permission of Mayo Foundation.)

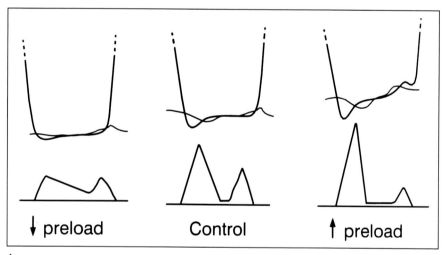

A

Fig. 7-9. Changes in mitral flow velocity and left atrial and left ventricular curves during different preloads. A. Left atrial and left ventricular curves with mitral flow velocities. (From RA Nishimura et al. Assessment of diastolic function of the heart: background and current applications of Doppler echocardiography. Part II. Clinical studies. *Mayo Clin Proc* 1989;64:181–204. By permission of Mayo Foundation.) B. Actual mitral flow velocities from a patient during different preloads. (*W* = pulmonary capillary wedge pressure)

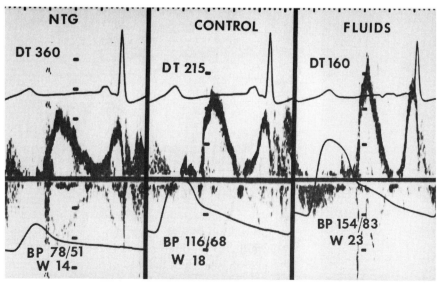

B

Because of the multiplicity of various factors governing diastolic filling of the heart, the findings of single mitral flow velocity curve are difficult to interpret at one point in time. Sequential analysis of these curves is of great value, however, in following the patient's course through an operation. An increase in the E velocity and a shortening of the deceleration time are indicative of an increase in preload of the heart and higher left atrial filling pressures. Conversely, a decrease in the E velocity and prolongation of the deceleration time with preservation of the E-to-A ratio indicate that the preload has been significantly reduced, with lower left atrial filling pressures. If the E velocity is decreased, the deceleration time is prolonged, and the A velocity is higher, the major effect is due to either an increase in afterload or prolongation of relaxation, such as may occur with ischemia.

Pulmonary Vein Velocities

Further information about diastolic filling of the left ventricle can be gained by an examination of pulmonary vein velocities [24,25]. The left upper pulmonary vein can be easily interrogated by monoplane TEE in basal short-axis imaging (Fig. 7-10). The right upper pulmonary vein is less often accessi-

ble by monoplane imaging but can be easily identified and interrogated in the longitudinal two-chamber imaging plane (see Chapter 4). The normal pulmonary vein velocity consists of systolic forward flow, diastolic forward flow, and velocity reversal at atrial contraction (Fig. 7-11). The systolic forward flow depends on atrial relaxation, descent of the mitral annulus, left atrial pressure, and coexistent mitral regurgitation. Systolic flow velocities are lower if atrial fibrillation is present, cardiac output is low, and left atrial pressure is high [25]. With severe mitral regurgitation, systolic forward flow is reversed [26]. The diastolic forward flow reflects the early transmitral filling pattern.

The most useful variable in the pulmonary vein velocity curve for determination of filling pressures is the velocity at atrial contraction. During atrial contraction the mitral valve is fully open and there is forward flow into the left ventricle and reverse flow into the pulmonary veins. If left ventricular end-diastolic pressure is high, the velocity of flow into the pulmonary vein is greater and forward flow through the mitral valve is less. Conversely, if preload is low, velocity at atrial reversal into the pulmonary veins is lower and forward flow into the left ventricle is higher

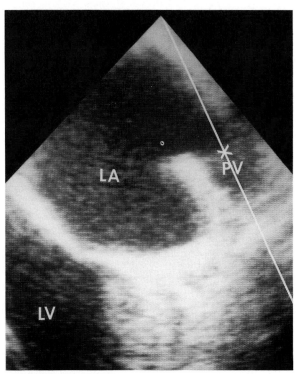

Fig. 7-10. Two-dimensional view from transesophageal approach shows placement of sample volume *(X)* in pulmonary vein *(PV)*.

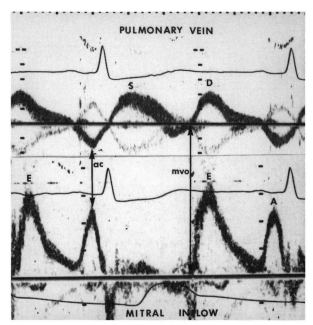

Fig. 7-11. Pulmonary vein velocity superimposed on mitral flow velocities (see text). (*A* = atrial filling; *D* = diastolic filling; *E* = early filling; *S* = systolic filling.) (Modified from RA Nishimura et al. Relation of pulmonary vein to mitral flow velocities by transesophageal Doppler echocardiography: effect of different loading conditions. *Circulation* 1990;81:1488–97.)

(Fig. 7-12). Figure 7-13 demonstrates the direct relationship between changes in the reversal at atrial contraction and the pulmonary capillary wedge pressure.

Preliminary investigation utilizing transthoracic pulsed-wave Doppler echocardiography has found a good correlation of pulmonary venous atrial reversal velocities (PV-ar) and the absolute left ventricular end-diastolic pressure (LVEDP) measured at catheterization [27]. No significant correlations of peak E or A velocities with left ventricular end-diastolic pressure were found. In the absence of significant left atrial enlargement or atrial fibrillation, an estimation of left ventricular end-diastolic pressure could be obtained by Equation 7-3 [27]:

$$LVEDP = (0.48) (PV\text{-}ar) - 1.6. \qquad \textbf{[7-3]}$$

Normally, systolic forward flow in the pulmonary vein consists of a single velocity signal. In the presence of low filling pressures there is biphasic systolic forward flow as the contribution from atrial relaxation separates from that of the mitral annulus descent (see Fig. 7-12).

Combined Use of Mitral and Pulmonary Vein Velocities

Direct information about the filling pressures of the left ventricle can be extrapolated from the combined use of the mitral and pulmonary vein velocity curves. As stated previously, the *changes* in the loading conditions of the heart can be assessed by examining the sequential changes in mitral flow velocity curves, assuming that the intrinsic myocardial function has not been affected. However, certain patterns allow determination of absolute filling pressures when both the mitral and the pulmonary vein velocities are examined. If a high E velocity (> 1.5 m/sec) and a short deceleration time (< 150 msec) are found in conjunction with a high velocity at atrial reversal (> 0.3 m/sec) and loss of systolic forward flow (without severe mitral regurgitation or atrial fibrillation) on the pulmonary vein velocity, the pulmonary capillary wedge pressure will be high (> 25 mm Hg). Conversely, if E velocity is low (< 0.6 m/sec), deceleration time is prolonged (> 250 msec), and A veloc-

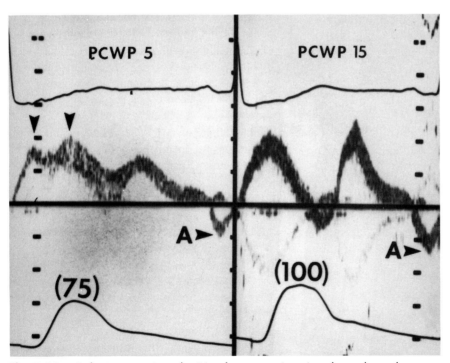

Fig. 7-12. Pulmonary vein velocities from a patient in whom the pulmonary capillary wedge pressure *(PCWP)* was raised from 5 to 15 mm Hg. Reversal of atrial contraction *(A)* is significantly increased. The biphasic systolic forward flow on the left *(arrowheads)* is seen with low filling pressures because the contribution of atrial relaxation is separated from that of mitral annulus descent. (From RA Nishimura et al. Relation of pulmonary vein to mitral flow velocities by transesophageal Doppler echocardiography: effect of different loading conditions. *Circulation* 1990;81:1488–97. By permission of the American Heart Association.)

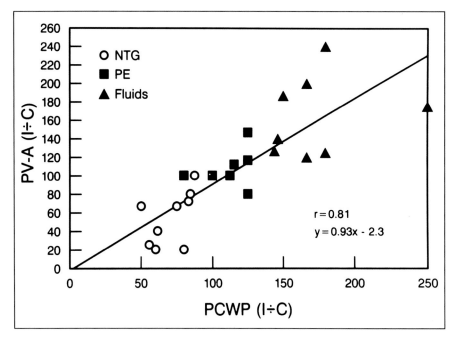

Fig. 7-13. Changes in pulmonary capillary wedge pressure *(PCWP)* plotted against velocity at atrial contraction *(PV-A)*. *(C =* control state; *I =* intervention state; NTG = nitroglycerin; *PE* = phenylephrine. (Modified from RA Nishimura et al. Relation of pulmonary vein to mitral flow velocities by transesophageal Doppler echocardiography: effect of different loading conditions. *Circulation* 1990;81:1488–97.)

ity is low (< 0.4 m/sec) on the mitral velocity curve and velocity at atrial reversal is low (< 0.1 m/sec) on the pulmonary vein velocity curve, the pulmonary capillary wedge pressure will be low (< 8 mm Hg).

SUMMARY

Transesophageal echocardiography can provide valuable clinical information about the function of the left ventricle. Information about both the systolic properties and the diastolic properties can be readily obtainable in nearly all patients. Left ventricular volumes, systolic contractility, cardiac output, and diastolic filling parameters of the left ventricle can be accurately and reproducibly determined.

REFERENCES

1. Tajik AJ, Seward JB, Hagler DJ, et al. Two-dimensional real-time ultrasonic imaging of the heart and great vessels: technique, image orientation, structure identification, and validation. *Mayo Clin Proc* 1978;53:271–303.

2. Hatle L, Angelsen B. *Doppler Ultrasound in Cardiology: Physical Principles and Clinical Applications.* Philadelphia: Lea & Febiger, 1982.

3. Seward JB, Khandheria BK, Oh JK, et al. Transesophageal echocardiography: technique, anatomic correlations, implementation, and clinical applications. *Mayo Clin Proc* 1988;63:649–80.

4. Stamm RB, Carabello BA, Mayers DL, Martin RP. Two-dimensional echocardiographic measurement of left ventricular ejection fraction: prospective analysis of what constitutes an adequate determination. *Am Heart J* 1982;104:136–44.

5. Schiller NB, Shah PM, Crawford M, et al. Recommendations for quantitation of the left ventricle by two-dimensional echocardiography. *J Am Soc Echocardiogr* 1989;2:358–67.

6. Abinader EG, Kuo LC, Rokey R, Quinones MA. Mitral-septal angle: a new two-dimensional echocardiographic index of left ventricular performance. *Am Heart J* 1985;110:381–5.

7. Simonson JS, Schiller NB. Descent of the base of the left ventricle: an echocardiographic index of left ventricular function. *J Am Soc Echocardiogr* 1989;2:25–35.

8. Abel MD, Nishimura RA, Callahan MJ, et al. Evaluation of intraoperative transesophageal two-dimensional echocardiography. *Anesthesiology* 1987;66:64–8.

9. Suga H, Sagawa H, Shoukas AA. Load independence of the instantaneous pressure-volume ratio of the canine left ventricle and effects of epinephrine and heart rate on the ratio. *Circ Res* 1973;32:314–22.

10. Weinlander CM, Abel MD, Piehler JM, Nishimura RA. Isoflurane is a potent myocardial depressant in patients with ischemic heart disease (abstract). *Anesthesiology* 1986;65 Suppl A4.

11. Zoghbi WA, Quinones MA. Determination of cardiac output by Doppler echocardiography: a critical appraisal. *Herz* 1986;11:258–68.

12. Huntsman LL, Stewart DK, Barnes SR, et al. Noninvasive Doppler determination of cardiac output in man: clinical validation. *Circulation* 1983;67:593–602.

13. Muhiudeen IA, Kuecherer HF, Lee E, et al. Intraoperative estimation of cardiac output by transesophageal pulsed Doppler echocardiography. *Anesthesiology* 1991;74:9–14.

14. Nishimura RA, Abel MD, Hatle LK, Tajik AJ. Assessment of diastolic function of the heart: background and current applications of Doppler echocardiography. Part II. Clinical studies. *Mayo Clin Proc* 1989;64:181–204.

15. DeMaria AN, Wisenbaugh T. Identification and treatment of diastolic dysfunction: role of transmitral Doppler recordings (editorial). *J Am Coll Cardiol* 1987;9:1106–7.

16. Labovitz AJ, Pearson AC. Evaluation of left ventricular diastolic function: clinical relevance and recent Doppler echocardiographic insights. *Am Heart J* 1987;114:836–51.

17. Nishimura RA, Housmans PR, Hatle LK, Tajik AJ. Assessment of diastolic function of the heart: background and current applications of Doppler echocardiography. Part I. Physiologic and pathophysiologic features. *Mayo Clin Proc* 1989;64: 71–81.

18. Gaasch WH, Levine HJ, Quinones MA, Alexander JK. Left ventricular compliance: mechanisms and clinical implications. *Am J Cardiol* 1976;38: 645–53.

19. Grossman W, McLaurin LP. Diastolic properties of the left ventricle. *Ann Intern Med* 1976;84:316–26.

20. Choong CY, Herrmann HC, Weyman AE, Fifer MA. Preload dependence of Doppler-derived indexes of left ventricular diastolic function in humans. *J Am Coll Cardiol* 1987;10:800–8.

21. Courtois M, Vered Z, Barzilai B, et al. The transmitral pressure-flow velocity relation: effect of abrupt preload reduction. *Circulation* 1988;78:1459–68.

22. Choong CY, Abascal VM, Thomas JD, et al. Combined influence of ventricular loading and relaxation on the transmitral flow velocity profile in dogs measured by Doppler echocardiography. *Circulation* 1988;78:672–83.

23. Nishimura RA, Abel MD, Housmans PR, et al. Mitral flow velocity curves as a function of different loading conditions: evaluation by intraoperative transesophageal Doppler echocardiography. *J Am Soc Echocardiogr* 1989;2:79–87.

24. Nishimura RA, Abel MD, Hatle LK, Tajik AJ. Relation of pulmonary vein to mitral flow velocities by transesophageal Doppler echocardiography: effect of different loading conditions. *Circulation* 1990; 81:1488–97.

25. Kuecherer HF, Muhiudeen IA, Kusumoto FM, et al. Estimation of mean left atrial pressure from transesophageal pulsed Doppler echocardiography of pulmonary venous flow. *Circulation* 1990;82:1127–39.

26. Klein AL, Obarski TP, Stewart WJ, et al. Transesophageal Doppler echocardiography of pulmonary venous flow: a new marker of mitral regurgitation severity. *J Am Coll Cardiol* 1991;18:518–26.

27. Nakatani S, Yoshitomi H, Tamai J, et al. Noninvasive estimation of left ventricular end-diastolic pressure using transthoracic Doppler-determined pulmonary venous atrial flow reversal. *Circulation* 1991;84 Suppl 2:II–163

8

Transesophageal Echocardiography in Ischemic Heart Disease

Jae K. Oh • Roger L. Click • Patricia A. Pellikka

Echocardiography is an invaluable diagnostic tool in the clinical management of patients with coronary artery disease. Myocardial ischemia is immediately manifested as decreased or absent myocardial systolic thickening detected readily by echocardiography as regional wall motion abnormalities [1,2]. Echocardiography uses multiple tomographic planes to visualize entire left and right ventricular myocardial segmental function. The location and the extent of regional wall motion abnormalities after acute myocardial infarction have been well correlated with other imaging modalities and coronary angiography [3,4]. Semiquantitative wall motion scoring, used to express the extent of regional myocardial function, has been shown to be useful in the identification of high-risk patients after acute myocardial infarction [4,5]. Another important role of echocardiography is the detection of complications of myocardial infarction, such as ventricular septal defect, papillary muscle rupture, true and false aneurysms, left ventricular thrombus, pericardial effusion, and free-wall rupture. Less clearly documented is the role of echocardiography in the visualization of the coronary arteries, but steady progress is being made in this area.

The main limitation of transthoracic echocardiography in patients with ischemic heart disease has been the less than optimal image quality caused by obesity, chronic obstructive lung disease, and distance of the cardiac structures from the precordial surface. Because of the strategic location of the esophagus in relation to the heart, the transesophageal approach provides high-quality images in nearly all patients and is particularly suited for the detection of myocardial ischemia or infarction and postinfarction mechanical complications and for the visualization of the proximal coronary arteries.

REGIONAL WALL MOTION ASSESSMENT: METHODS AND FORMAT

Transesophageal echocardiography (TEE) provides an excellent modality for assessing left ventricular regional wall motion abnormalities. As with transthoracic echocardiography, wall motion is assessed in each of 16 segments recommended by the American Society of Echocardiography [6]. All left ventricular segments can be visualized with a combination of horizontal and longitudinal biplane views (Figs. 8-1, 8-2, and 8-3). The inferoseptal and anterolateral walls are imaged in the transverse four-chamber plane. The anteroseptal and inferolateral segments are seen with anterior angulation from the four-chamber view to the left ventricular outflow view. Transgastric transverse plane imaging displays generally excellent short-axis images of basal and middle portions of the left ventricle and right ventricle and, with lateral probe advancement and angulation, the ventricular apices in 70 to 80% of patients. Longitudinal imaging permits a long-axis, two-chamber image of the inferior and anterior walls.

Fig. 8-1. Horizontal and longitudinal TEE views of the left ventricle from the transgastric position. Horizontal plane: Depending on the position of the transducer and its angulation, short-axis views of the left ventricular basal, middle, and apical levels can be obtained. Longitudinal plane: The long-axis view of the left ventricle is visualized, similar to the transthoracic parasternal long-axis view, and shows the anteroseptal and inferolateral walls. Medial angulation would image the inferior segments and posteromedial papillary muscle. 1. Basal anteroseptum. 2. Basal anterior. 3. Basal anterolateral. 4. Basal inferolateral. 5. Basal inferior (or posterior). 6. Inferobasal septum. 7. Mid-anteroseptum. 8. Mid- anterior. 9. Mid- anterolateral. 10. Mid-inferolateral. 11. Mid- inferior. 12. Mid- inferoseptum. 13. Apical septum. 14. Antero-apex. 15. Lateral apex. 16. Inferoapex. *(P = papillary muscles.)*

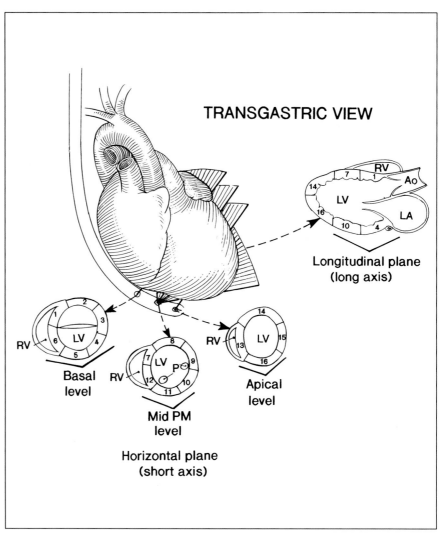

Fig. 8-2. A. Transgastric short-axis view (horizontal plane) of the left ventricle at the middle level. Diastolic frame is shown with the transducer position at the bottom of the sector. The left ventricle is divided into six segments at the basal and middle levels and into four segments at the api-cal level. B. Transgastric longitudinal view of the left ventricle. This view corresponds to the trans-thoracic parasternal long-axis view, showing the anteroseptal *(AS)* and inferolateral walls.

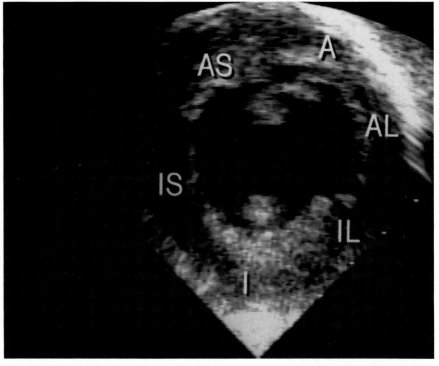

A

Fig. 8-3. Horizontal and longitudinal views of the left ventricle from the midesophagus (30 to 35 cm from incisors) position. Imaging planes analogous to the transthoracic apical two- and four-chamber and left ventricular outflow images are obtained. Horizontal plane: The four-chamber view visualizes the inferior septum and the anterolateral walls. Anterior angulation to the level of the outflow tract and aortic valve visualizes the anteroseptal and inferolateral walls. The true apex may be foreshortened in these views. Longitudinal plane: The left ventricular two-chamber inflow view visualizes the anterior and inferior walls. (See Fig. 8-1 legend for key to numbered segments.)

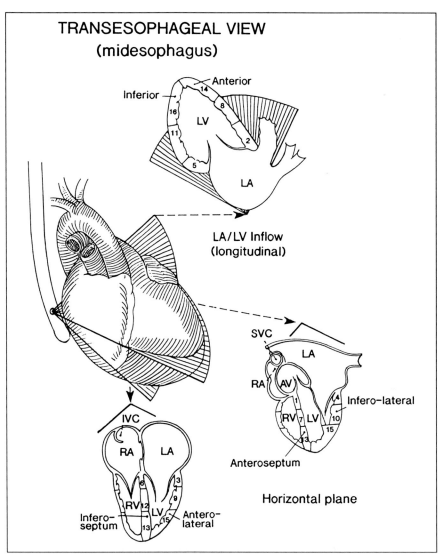

TRANSESOPHAGEAL VIEW
(midesophagus)

LA/LV Inflow
(longitudinal)

Horizontal plane

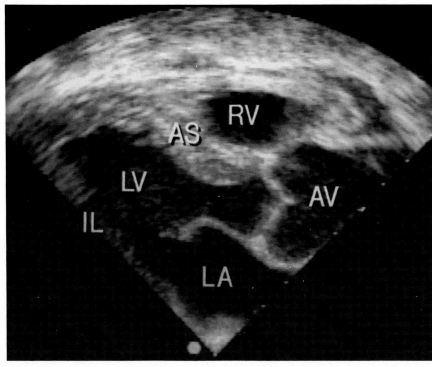

B

Transgastric long-axis imaging delineates the anteroseptum and inferior or inferolateral segments.

The left ventricle is divided into three levels along its long axis: basal, middle, and apical. The basal portion extends from the mitral valve annulus to the tips of the papillary muscles, the midportion extends from the tips to the bases of the papillary muscles, and the apical region constitutes the remainder of the ventricle. At the basal and middle levels, the left ventricle is divided into six segments on the short-axis image, and at the apical level, the ventricle is divided into four segments. The wall motion is graded as normal, hypokinetic, akinetic, dyskinetic, or aneurysmal. For a semiquantitative evaluation of regional wall motion abnormalities, a wall motion score from 1 to 5 (1, normal; 2, hypokinesis; 3, akinesis; 4, dyskinesis; 5, aneurysmal) is assigned to individual segments depending on their contractility. The grading of regional wall motion abnormalities during TEE has been shown to have excellent interobserver and intraobserver variability [7].

Although the short-axis view of the left ventricle at the level of the papillary muscles does not show all segments, it contains segments that are presenting blood flow derived from all three major coronary arteries. Therefore, the transgastric short-axis view at the middle level is conventionally the view of choice for monitoring patients at risk for intraoperative ischemia [7]. The limitation of the monoplane horizontal view with TEE is that the left ventricular apex may not be satisfactorily visualized in as many as 32% of patients [8]. Advancing or retroflexing the TEE probe in the stomach often will enhance visualization of the apical segment. Longitudinal imaging allows a transgastric long-axis view similar to the transthoracic parasternal long-axis view. In some patients, however, the true apex may still be difficult to obtain by TEE.

Transesophageal echocardiography has been extensively used in the perioperative evaluation of patients with known or suspected coronary artery disease [9–12]. Regional wall motion abnormalities detected by two-dimensional TEE during intraoperative monitoring appear to be sensitive indicators of myocardial dysfunction and ischemia. These wall motion abnormalities may be more sensitive than electrocardiographic and hemodynamic measurements, including blood pressure and pulmonary artery wedge pressure monitoring, in predicting perioperative cardiac complications (see Chapter 16).

STRESS TRANSESOPHAGEAL ECHOCARDIOGRAPHY

The accuracy of transthoracic stress echocardiography in the diagnosis and assessment of coronary artery disease is well established [13]. But for patients in whom transthoracic images are difficult to obtain, TEE combined with various forms of stress may permit better endocardial definition and assessment of myocardial contractility. In addition to regional wall motion abnormalities, an increase in left ventricular volume or decrease in ejection fraction is a marker of hemodynamically significant coronary artery disease that may be better detected by TEE [14]. Because neither upright nor supine exercise with TEE monitoring is practical for the patient, a variety of nonphysiologic methods of stress TEE have been described.

The largest experience thus far reported has used atrial-paced TEE [15,16]. A flexible, silicone-coated pacing catheter has been specially designed for attachment to the TEE probe for transesophageal pacing of the left atrium. Pacing is incrementally increased to 85% of the patient's age-predicted maximal heart rate; atropine is administered intravenously as needed for Mobitz I (Wenckebach) atrioventricular nodal heart block that is occasionally observed at higher pacing rates. Segmental left ventricular contraction is monitored by TEE at baseline and during and immediately after maximal transesophageal pacing. This approach has been feasible in 90 to 100% of patients, and preliminary experience suggests a high sensitivity and specificity for detection of coronary artery disease [15,16].

Alternatively, pharmacologic stress TEE with intravenously administered dobutamine [17,18], dipyridamole [19,20], or adenosine may offer a means for diagnosis and evaluation of the functional significance of coronary artery disease. However, this approach is infrequently needed. Thus far, no significant complications have been encountered with incremental infusions of dobutamine (5 to 40 µg/kg/min) during TEE.

DETECTION OF POSTINFARCTION COMPLICATIONS

Life-threatening postinfarction complications include rupture of the ventricular septum, free wall, or papillary muscle and cardiac tamponade. Right ventricular infarction, true left ventricular aneurysm formation, and ischemic mitral regurgitation may also complicate the patient's course during myocardial infarction and lead to potentially high morbidity and mortality. Transthoracic echocardiographic examination has been shown to be capable of detecting these postinfarction complications when echocardiographic images are adequate [21]. Transthoracic echocardiography may be the only test necessary to establish an unequivocal diagnosis of ventricular septal defect or papillary muscle rupture before the patient is taken to the operating room. These complications, although uncommon (2 to 5% of patients with acute myocardial infarction), account for up to 15% of deaths related to myocardial infarction [22]. Studies have shown that the best survival rates can be achieved by surgical intervention immediately after the diagnosis is made [23,24]. However, many of these patients present with pulmonary edema or cardiogenic shock requiring aggressive intervention with mechanical ventilation, hemodynamic monitoring, and intra-aortic balloon counterpulsation. These circumstances can significantly interfere with the transthoracic echocardiographic examination, necessitating an alternative imaging window with TEE [25].

Methods of performing TEE and its clinical impact in hemodynamically unstable and critically ill patients are discussed in Chapter 17. In this chapter, TEE examination of infarct-related mechanical complications is discussed.

Ventricular Septal Defect

Ventricular septal defect occurs in 2% of all acute myocardial infarctions. Although more common with anterior wall myocardial infarction, it also occurs after inferior wall myocardial infarction. The prognosis is poorer in patients with inferoseptal defect because of right ventricular involvement with infarction [26]. The right ventricle is frequently involved with infarction when a ventricular septal defect is present, even with anterior wall myocardial infarction. Usually, right ventricular involvement is small and insignificant with anterior infarctions associated with septal rupture and is generally localized to the anteroapical portion of the right ventricle. Right ventricular infarction is common (30 to 60%) and much more extensive with inferior infarctions complicated by inferior septal rupture. Involvement of the right ventricle usually contributes to significant hemodynamic compromise and is an adverse prognosticator, even after septal defect repair.

The ventricular septum is best seen from the four-chamber and transgastric views during TEE examination. In the four-chamber view, the anteroseptum is seen along with the left ventricular outflow tract, and the transducer must be retroflexed to view the inferoseptum. The four-chamber view may foreshorten the left ventricular apex, and the true apical septum may not be visualized. In the transgastric view, both the anteroseptum and the inferoseptum are visualized at a given tomographic level, so that the transducer has to be advanced and withdrawn to scan the entire length of the left ventricle from the basal to the apical level.

Definite two-dimensional echocardiographic diagnosis of infarct-associated ventricular septal defect is made when discontinuity or disruption of the ventricular septum is detected within a region of myocardial akinesis to dyskinesis (Fig. 8-4). Often, the rupture is contained within a region of localized infarct thinning and expansion. Relatively normal to even hyperdynamic contiguous segmental left ventricular contractility contributes to generation of shear forces responsible for myocardial disruption within the site of rupture. A large defect is quite obvious, but a small, serpiginous ventricular defect may be difficult to detect. Typically, septal ruptures associated with anterior infarctions are relatively well circumscribed and localized to the apical half of the left ventricle. Inferoseptal ruptures most often occur within the basal half of the septum and can be complex, serpiginous, and poorly delineated by two-dimensional imaging. Color-flow imaging supplements two-dimensional echocardiographic imaging in the diagnosis of ventricular septal defect by demonstrating a left-to-right intraventricular shunt through the defect. With the availability of TEE color-flow imaging, transesophageal continuous-wave or pulsed-wave Doppler examinations usually do not provide additional aid in the diagnosis of ventricular septal defect.

From the transgastric format, echocardiographic dropout or discontinuity in the ventricular septum by two-dimensional echocardiography again is diagnostic of ventricular septal defect, even without the help of color-flow imaging (Fig. 8-5). However, demonstration of the shunt from the left ventricle to the right ventricle through the defect by color-flow imaging leaves no doubt in the diagnosis of ventricular septal rupture. On the other hand, color-flow imaging is essential when the defect is small and serpiginous, because two-dimensional echocardiographic imaging alone often does not allow complete confidence in the diagnosis of ventricular septal defect.

Papillary Muscle Dysfunction

Ischemic left ventricular dysfunction, particularly with ventricular dilatation, may precipitate severe mitral regurgitation without actual disruption of the mitral support apparatus. Inferior myocardial infarction with regional dilatation, especially with posteromedial papillary muscle infarction, may cause significant retraction of the mitral support apparatus, disallowing complete systolic coaptation of the mitral leaflets and hence causing incomplete mitral closure and severe regurgitation (Fig. 8-6).

Thus, the mere demonstration of severe mitral regurgitation by Doppler color-flow imaging is not sufficient to diagnose papillary muscle rupture. Papillary muscle rupture is a morphologic mechanical abnormality of the papillary muscle, and it should be demonstrated by two-dimensional echocardiogra-

phy to establish the diagnosis. It is well known that because of its single blood supply, the posteromedial papillary muscle has a much higher (up to 12 times) incidence of rupture than does the anterolateral papillary muscle.

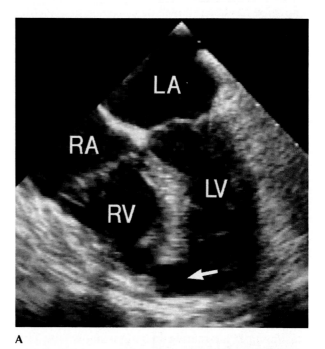

A

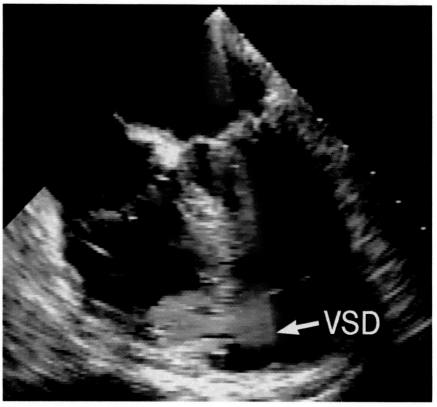

B

Fig. 8-4. Postinfarction ventricular septal rupture *(VSD)*; horizontal four-chamber view. A. The ventricular septal rupture is readily diagnosed in the region of echo dropout *(arrow)*. B. Color-flow imaging shows a shunt from the left ventricle to the right ventricle across this defect.

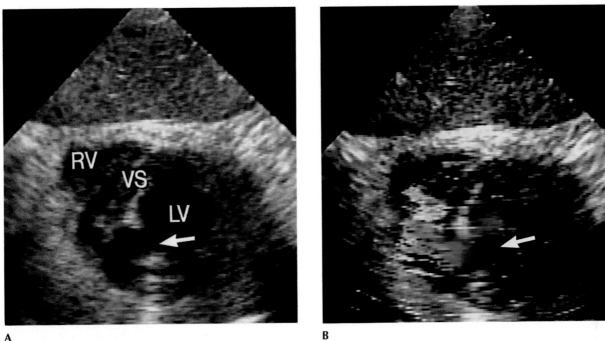

A   **B**

Fig. 8-5.   Postinfarction ventricular septal rupture; transgastric short-axis view.
A. A well-circumscribed anteroseptal postinfarction ventricular septal rupture
(arrow) is visualized at the apical ventricular level, with communication
between the left and right ventricles evident. B. Left-to-right interventricular
shunting *(arrow)* is confirmed by color-flow Doppler mapping.

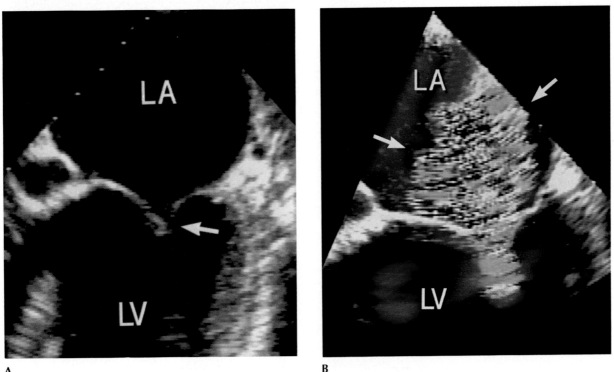

A   **B**

Fig. 8-6.   Mitral regurgitation due to ischemic left ventricular and papillary
muscle dysfunction; focused horizontal four-chamber view. A. The posterior
mitral leaflet is retracted, and mitral valve coaptation in end-systole is
incomplete *(arrow)*. B. Severe central mitral regurgitation *(arrows)*, detected on
color-flow imaging, emanates from the site of incomplete leaflet coaptation.

Usually, the horizontal plane four-chamber view readily demonstrates the ruptured portion of the papillary muscle, which may be either partial (Fig. 8-7) or complete (Fig. 8-8). The unsupported mitral leaflet segment becomes flail. Papillary muscle rupture can also be visualized from the transgastric horizontal short-axis and longitudinal long-axis views; in fact, the rupture is easier to localize from the transgastric window, especially the longitudinal long-axis view, than from the four-chamber horizontal view. Severe mitral regurgitation is expected in patients with papillary muscle rupture, and this can be demonstrated by color-flow imaging. The mitral regurgitant jet is often eccentric, usually in the opposite direction of the flail leaflet segment. Meticulous delineation of the jet in multiple tomographic planes is necessary to determine the severity of the regurgitation.

Once the diagnosis of ventricular septal defect or papillary muscle rupture is established, surgical repair should be performed as soon as possible to optimize the patient's chance of survival. Transesophageal echocardiography is helpful in the operating room to assess the results of ventricular septal defect repair. Since the mitral valve usually is replaced rather than repaired in the setting of papillary muscle rupture, intraoperative TEE is less useful in this situation unless repair is attempted. Intraoperative use of TEE is discussed in detail in Chapter 16.

Right Ventricular Infarct

The right ventricle also is well seen by TEE from the four-chamber and transgastric views. This approach facilitates evaluation of the extent of right ventricular dilatation, regional dysfunction, and abnormal septal displacement by TEE. Because of significant elevation of the right atrial pressure with a large right ventricular infarct, the atrial septum usually is deviated to the left throughout the cardiac cycle unless concomitant left ventricular failure results in high left atrial pressure. The increase in right atrial pressure due to a right ventricular infarct provides a substrate for the opening of a preexisting patent foramen ovale (present in 15 to 30% of the general population), allowing significant right-to-left interatrial shunting resulting in systemic oxygen desaturation and hypoxemia. This abnormality can easily be evaluated by intravenous contrast injection via a peripheral vein into the right atrium (Fig. 8-9).

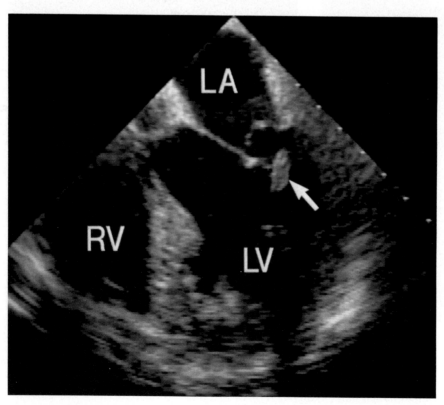

Fig. 8-7. Partial papillary muscle rupture; horizontal four-chamber view. A portion of the posterior papillary muscle head *(arrow)* is partially ruptured, allowing prolapse of the posterior mitral valve leaflet.

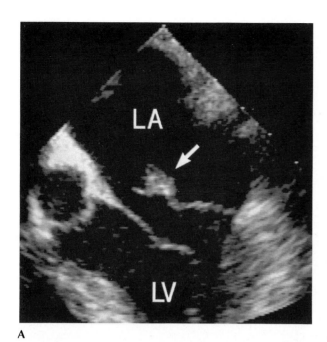

A

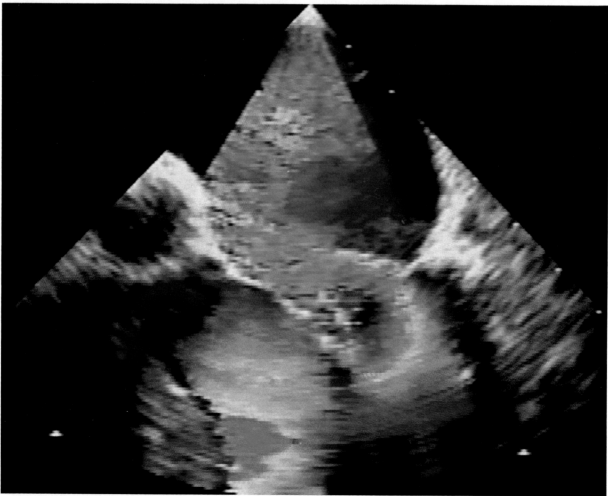

B

Fig. 8-8. Complete papillary muscle rupture; magnified horizontal plane. A. Complete rupture of the posteromedial papillary muscle head *(arrow)* has caused the posterior mitral leaflet to become flail. The triangular mass of the ruptured papillary muscle head *(arrow)* attached to this leaflet is clearly seen within the left atrium. B. An eccentric anteromedial jet of severe mitral regurgitation is demonstrated by color-flow imaging.

Fig. 8-9. Right ventricular infarction; horizontal four-chamber view. A. The right ventricle and the right atrium are markedly dilated. The left ventricle is compressed by septal displacement due to right ventricular pressure overload and dilatation. The atrial septum is bulging far into the left atrium because of increased right atrial pressure. A portion of a hemodynamic monitoring catheter *(arrow)* is seen in the right atrium. B. Indocyanine green injection partially opacifies the right atrium. C. Immediately after the contrast injection, the left-sided chambers are filled with microcavitations because of significant right-to-left interatrial shunting through a patent foramen ovale. Significant systemic oxygen desaturation persisted in this patient despite maximal mechanical ventilatory support.

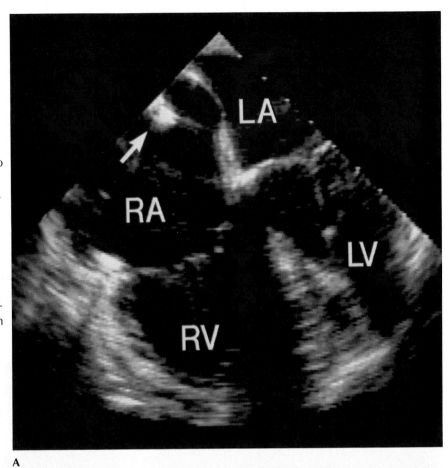

A

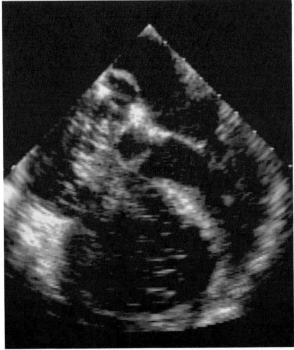

B

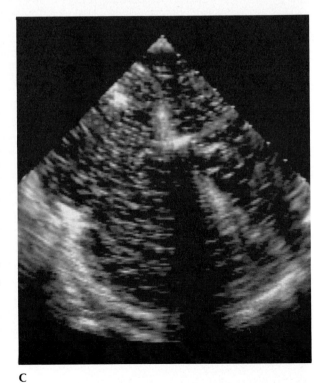

C

Left Ventricular Aneurysms

Both true and false aneurysms may complicate acute myocardial infarction, the latter having a much more ominous prognosis.

True aneurysms typically involve the anteroseptal apical left ventricle and less often the inferobasal portion. A persistent wide-mouthed bulging deformation of the left ventricular cavity contour throughout the cardiac cycle and demonstration of the variably thinned aneurysmal segments by hinge points of adjacent contracting myocardium characterize a true left ventricular aneurysm (Fig. 8-10). Such aneurysms vary greatly in size and often contain laminated thrombus. In patients with large aneurysms and low cardiac output, spontaneous echocardiographic contrast is often evident on TEE (Fig. 8-11).

False left ventricular aneurysms (or pseudoaneurysms) are formed after left ventricular free-wall disruption. The rupture is contained only by adherent pericardium; the risk of further expansion and rupture causing immediate death is high. Left ventricular pseudoaneurysms usually are contiguous with a relatively focal region of infarction, and usually the site of rupture is contained within a region of infarct expansion surrounded by normal to hypercontractile myocardium. The exact site of myocardial disruption is often narrow and produces a small "neck" communicating with the pseudoaneurysm cavity. Such communications may be difficult to visualize not only with transthoracic echocardiography but also with TEE. The pseudoaneurysm cavity itself may be globular or eccentric and may mimic the appearance of a pericardial or pleural effusion. The cavity also usually contains laminated thrombus. Color-

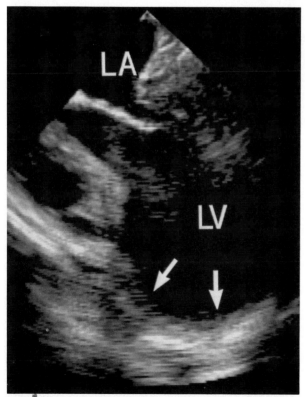

Fig. 8-10.   Left ventricular true aneurysm; horizontal four-chamber view. A large apical aneurysm of the left ventricle is seen with thinned and dyskinetic apical septal walls *(arrows)*. The entire apical aneurysm may not be seen by TEE because of apical foreshortening in this plane, and transgastric imaging should supplement the examination.

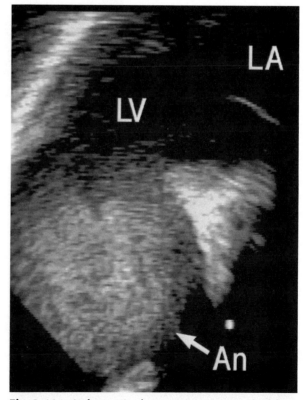

Fig. 8-11.   Left ventricular aneurysm; magnified four-chamber view. A large left ventricular apical aneurysm *(arrow)* is visualized on off-axis imaging. Because of greatly reduced intracavitary blood flow, dense spontaneous echo-contrast opacifies the apical aneurysm.

flow Doppler imaging is often essential to confidently document flow communication between the left ventricular and pseudoaneurysm cavities. A to-and-fro pattern of systolic flow entering the pseu- doaneurysm and diastolic flow reentering the left ventricle firmly establishes the diagnosis of left ventricular rupture with pseudoaneurysm formation (Fig. 8-12).

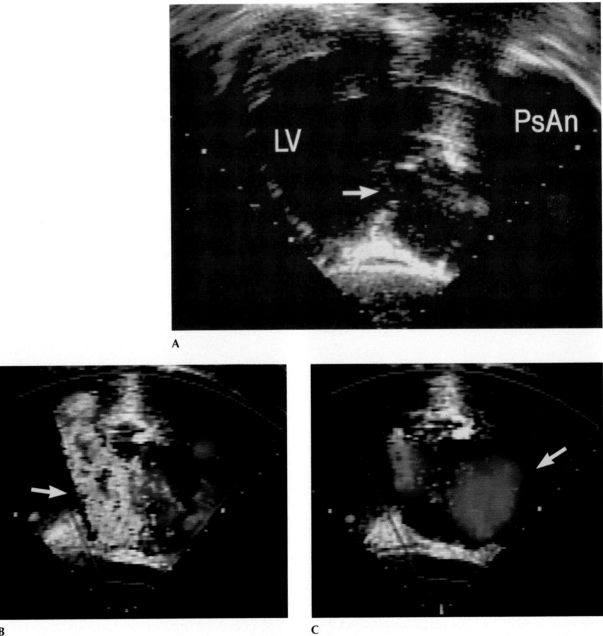

Fig. 8-12. Left ventricular pseudoaneurysm; transgastric horizontal short-axis view, sector apex down. A. Left ventricular free-wall rupture *(arrow)* is present within the middle inferolateral segment, communicating to an adjacent globular pseudoaneurysm. B. Color-flow imaging during systole demonstrates flow from the left ventricle *(arrow)* into the pseudoaneurysm. C. Blood flow exits the pseudoaneurysm *(arrow)* during diastole and reenters the left ventricle through the site of rupture.

CORONARY ARTERY VISUALIZATION

Transthoracic visualization of the coronary arteries was initially described in 1976 by Weyman et al. [27]. Since then, a number of reports have described visualization of the coronary arteries by the transthoracic approach [28–35]. The best success was reported in examining the left main coronary artery, which was visualized in 50 to 75% of patients. The left anterior descending, right, and circumflex arteries were less well visualized. In younger patients, coronary anomalies and aneurysms can be assessed primarily, whereas in older patients, the main goal of coronary artery visualization is determination of the degree of proximal luminal stenosis. Currently, transthoracic echocardiography is not routinely used for visualization and quantification of coronary artery stenoses.

In the past few years, technical advances have improved visualization of the coronary arteries by the transthoracic approach. These include instruments with improved lateral resolution (annular array technology) and digital recording technology [36,37]. During visualization of the coronary arteries, there is constant movement in and out of the imaging plane. When the signal is digitized, only those portions of the cardiac cycle where coronary arteries are best seen can be analyzed in a continuous-loop manner. Even with this technique, the success rate for more detailed visualization of the left anterior descending coronary artery was 70% in one study [37].

Doppler analysis of coronary flow has also been demonstrated and may have potential for quantification of coronary stenosis [38,39]. Even though there have been major advances in the transthoracic evaluation of coronary anatomy and stenosis, significant limitation remains, so that it has not become a reliable or routine part of a transthoracic echocardiographic examination.

Transesophageal Visualization of Coronary Arteries

Coronary arteries can be visualized in both horizontal and longitudinal planes [40–42]. In the horizontal plane, the arteries are visualized in the basal short-axis scan. The coronary arteries lie just above the aortic cusps, and the proximal portions are seen with mild anteflexion of the transducer tip. The course of the left main coronary artery to its bifurcation into the left anterior descending and circumflex arteries can be traced inferior to the left atrial ap-

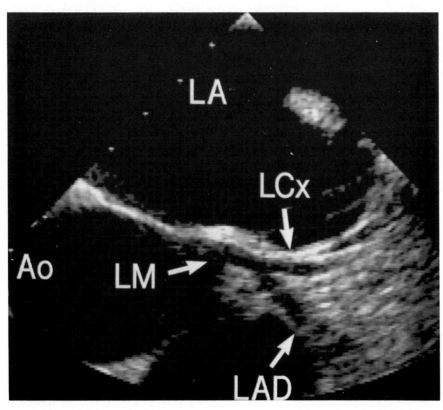

Fig. 8-13. Left coronary arteries; horizontal basal short-axis view. The left main artery *(LM)* and its bifurcation to the left anterior descending *(LAD)* and circumflex *(LCx)* coronary arteries are well visualized.

pendage (Fig. 8-13). Frequently, it is easiest to identify the left atrial appendage first by superior flexion of the endoscope and lateral rotation with slight advancement of the endoscope. Then, slight flexion of the transducer tip inferiorly allows delineation of the course of the left main artery and the bifurcation. Alternatively, from the short-axis view of the aortic valve, slight withdrawal of the transducer reveals the left main coronary artery and bifurcation. The right coronary artery usually arises at a different tomographic level (Fig. 8-14), and the success of right coronary visualization in the horizontal plane is less than that of the proximal left coronary system. From the longitudinal plane, the proximal portions of the coronary arteries are imaged with a short-axis projection of the aortic root with superior and inferior transducer angulation. The left circumflex coronary artery in the left atrial ventricular groove is best imaged by lateral rotation of the transducer in the two-chamber view.

Zwicky et al. [43] described their initial experience with coronary examination by TEE in 50 patients. Using a 5-mHz phased-array transducer with incorporated color-coded Doppler echocardiography, these investigators visualized the right and left coronary arteries in all patients studied. The left main coronary artery could be followed to its bifurcation into the proximal left anterior descending and circumflex arteries, and the proximal 3 cm of the right coronary artery were visualized. Pearce et al. [41] were able to identify the left main coronary artery in 86% of patients, the proximal right coronary artery in 82%, the circumflex artery in 80%, and the left anterior descending coronary artery in 75%. Table 8-1 summarizes studies and success rates in visualization of the coronary arteries by TEE.

It has become clear that the coronary arteries can be visualized more often and in greater detail by the TEE approach than by transthoracic echocardiography. However, quantification of coronary obstruction remains a challenging problem. Pearce et al. [41] found that when the observer believed the vessel could be reliably imaged, TEE was reasonably good at detecting obstructive disease. However, a large number of lesions detected by angiography were missed by TEE or were mistakenly interpreted as

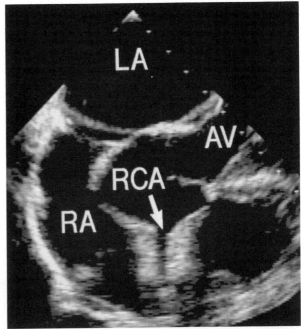

Fig. 8-14. Right coronary artery; horizontal basal short-axis view. At the tomographic level of the aortic valve, the ostium and proximal right coronary artery *(arrow)* are seen anteriorly.

Table 8-1. Visualization of the proximal coronary arteries by transesophageal echocardiography (TEE)

Study	No. of patients	Percent visualized by TEE			
		LM	LAD	LCx	RCA
Memmola et al. [45] (cine loop)	160	70	63	63	—
Ballal et al. [47] (aortic dissection)	18	89	—	—	61
Yamagishi et al. [49]	39	77	77	54	26
Yamagishi et al. [44]	52	90	—	—	—
Pearce et al. [41]	73	86	75	80	82
Zwicky et al. [43]	50	100	—	—	100
Reichert et al. [48]	25	88	52	88	—

Key: LM = left main artery; LAD = left anterior descending artery; LCx = circumflex artery; RCA = right coronary artery.

inadequately visualized vessels. Specifically looking at left main stenosis (Fig. 8-15), Yamagishi et al. [44] studied 20 patients with and 32 patients without left main stenosis documented by angiography. In 70% of the diseased left main arteries that could be seen by TEE, the stenosis was visualized. In 30%, the stenosis could not be seen. Two patients in this series had false-positive images. When a combination of color-flow and pulsed Doppler techniques was used to assess for aliased signals within the left main artery, the sensitivity and specificity for TEE detection of left main coronary stenosis improved [44]. Using cine loop technology with TEE, Memmola et al. [45] evaluated 160 patients before coronary angiography. A stenosis was considered to be present during TEE if hyperrefractile plaques narrowing the coronary lumen were detected. Significant stenosis—that is, narrowing greater than 75%—was detected in 6 of 6 left main, 50 of 63 left anterior descending, and 13 of 24 circumflex artery lesions. False-positive findings were observed in 2 of 105 left main, 5 of 48 left anterior descending, and 14 of 87 circumflex arteries. The sensitivity and specificity, respectively, were 100% and 98% for left main, 79% and 89% for left anterior descending, and 55% and 83% for circumflex coronary artery lesions [45].

In special situations, TEE may be advantageous for assessing coronary artery involvement. Schrem et al. [46] reported four patients with suspicious ostial left main coronary artery stenosis by angiography. Ostial narrowing by plaque and abnormally high flow velocities were seen by TEE. In each case, TEE clarified the ostial abnormality and contributed to subsequent management of the patient. In another use, Ballal et al. [47] described assessment of coronary anatomy in patients with aortic dissection (see Chapter 14). In six type I aortic dissections, TEE diagnosed a flap extending into both the right and the left coronary arteries in three patients and the right coronary artery in two patients. In one patient, the flap was found at surgery to extend down the right coronary artery, which could not be visualized by TEE.

Further advances in TEE assessment of coronary obstruction include use of higher frequency annular array transducers and color-flow Doppler [48] and pulsed Doppler [49] technology. In addition, Iliceto

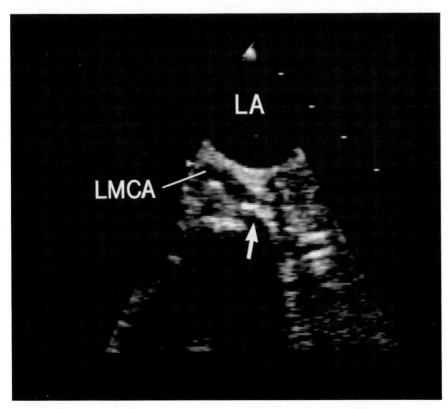

Fig. 8-15. Left main coronary artery stenosis; horizontal basal short-axis view. Severe distal left main coronary artery stenosis *(arrow)* is present immediately proximal to the bifurcation of this vessel.

et al. [50] reported their results in assessing coronary ischemia by use of TEE and pulsed Doppler echocardiography along with intravenous administration of dipyridamole. They concluded that this method has potential in assessing coronary blood flow reserve. These newer technologies may add to the sensitivity and specificity of assessing coronary stenosis.

Transesophageal echocardiography has clearly enhanced the echocardiographic assessment of coronary anatomy. In addition to its potentially use in the evaluation of proximal coronary atherosclerotic disease, TEE may also be helpful in the detection of coronary artery aneurysms (Fig. 8-16) and coronary artery anomalies (Fig. 8-17). The ability to visualize the proximal portion of all three coronary arteries depends greatly on the expertise of the operator. With experience, these arteries can be seen in most patients. Determining the degree and significance of stenosis in a given coronary segment is another significant challenge. As yet, this approach is not

sophisticated enough for routine clinical use to quantify coronary obstructive disease.

SUMMARY

The transesophageal approach has significantly expanded echocardiographic imaging capabilities in patients with ischemic heart disease. In difficult clinical situations involving potentially life-threatening complications of acute myocardial infarction, rapidly obtained and reliable information on cardiac anatomy and function at the bedside is essential. Transesophageal echocardiography overcomes multiple limitations of transthoracic echocardiography and can readily serve this purpose. Furthermore, coronary anatomy can be more frequently visualized by TEE, and with more experience and improved technology, ultrasound detection of significant proximal obstructive coronary lesions is a real possibility in the future.

Fig. 8-16. Coronary artery aneurysm; horizontal basal short-axis view. A large aneurysm *(arrows)* is present within the proximal left circumflex coronary artery *(asterisk)*. The aneurysm contains a large amount of thrombus.

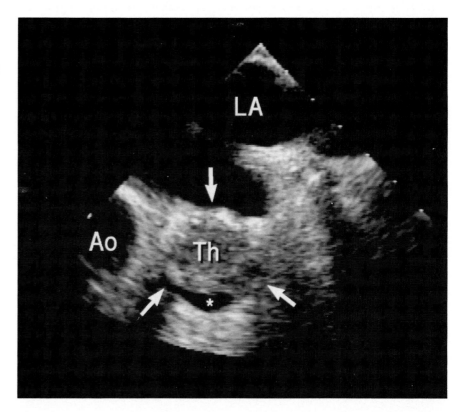

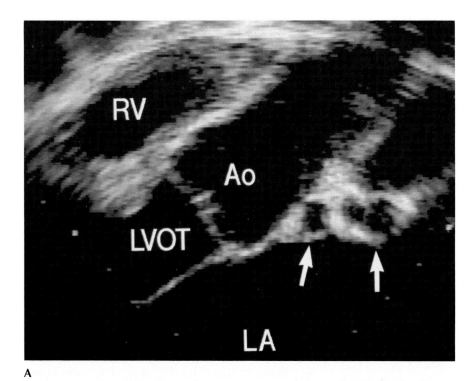

A

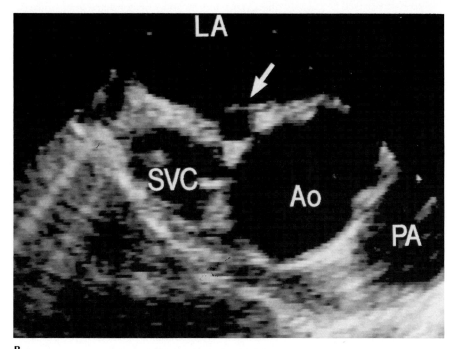

B

Fig. 8-17. Anomalous left coronary artery. A. Longitudinal long-axis view. A large anomalous left coronary artery *(arrows)* is visualized posterior to the ascending aorta. B. Basal short-axis imaging in the horizontal plane. The anomalous coronary artery *(arrow)* courses along the superior vena cava, into which it eventually empties.

REFERENCES

1. Tennant R, Wiggers CJ. The effect of coronary occlusion on myocardial contraction. *Am J Physiol* 1935;112:351–61.

2. Heger JJ, Weyman AE, Wann LS, et al. Cross-sectional echocardiography in acute myocardial infarction: detection and localization of regional left ventricular asynergy. *Circulation* 1979;60:531–8.

3. Van Reet RE, Quinones MA, Poliner LR, et al. Comparison of two-dimensional echocardiography with gated radionuclide ventriculography in the evaluation of global and regional left ventricular function in acute myocardial infarction. *J Am Coll Cardiol* 1984;3:243–52.

4. Shiina A, Tajik AJ, Smith HC, et al. Prognostic significance of regional wall motion abnormality in patients with prior myocardial infarction: a prospective correlative study of two-dimensional echocardiography and angiography. *Mayo Clin Proc* 1986;61:254–62.

5. Nishimura RA, Tajik AJ, Shub C, et al. Role of two-dimensional echocardiography in the prediction of in-hospital complications after acute myocardial infarction. *J Am Coll Cardiol* 1984;4:1080–7.

6. Schiller NB, Shah PM, Crawford M, et al. Recommendations for quantitation of the left ventricle by two-dimensional echocardiography. *J Am Soc Echocardiogr* 1989;2:358–67.

7. Abel MD, Nishimura RA, Callahan MJ, et al. Evaluation of intraoperative transesophageal two-dimensional echocardiography. *Anesthesiology* 1987;66:64–8.

8. Chan KL. Comprehensive assessment of cardiac anatomy in anesthetized patients by transesophageal echocardiography. *Can J Cardiol* 1988;4:397–401.

9. van Daele MERM, Sutherland GR, Mitchell MM, et al. Do changes in pulmonary capillary wedge pressure adequately reflect myocardial ischemia during anesthesia? A correlative preoperative hemodynamic, electrocardiographic, and transesophageal echocardiographic study. *Circulation* 1990;81:865–71.

10. Leung JM, O'Kelly B, Browner WS, et al. Prognostic importance of postbypass regional wall-motion abnormalities in patients undergoing coronary artery bypass graft surgery. *Anesthesiology* 1989;71:16–25.

11. Gewertz BL, Kremser PC, Zarins CK, et al. Transesophageal echocardiographic monitoring of myocardial ischemia during vascular surgery. *J Vasc Surg* 1987;5:607–13.

12. Smith JS, Cahalan MK, Benefiel DJ, et al. Intraoperative detection of myocardial ischemia in high-risk patients: electrocardiography versus two-dimensional transesophageal echocardiography. *Circulation* 1985;72:1015–21.

13. Armstrong WF, O'Donnell J, Dillon JC, et al. Complementary value of two-dimensional exercise echocardiography to routine treadmill exercise testing. *Ann Intern Med* 1986;105:829–35.

14. Berberich SN, Zager JRS, Plotnick GD, Fisher ML. A practical approach to exercise echocardiography: immediate postexercise echocardiography. *J Am Coll Cardiol* 1984;3:284–90.

15. Lambertz H, Kreis A, Trümper H, Hanrath P. Simultaneous transesophageal atrial pacing and transesophageal two-dimensional echocardiography: a new method of stress echocardiography. *J Am Coll Cardiol* 1990;16:1143–53.

16. Zabalgoitia M, Gandhi DK, Abi-Mansour P, et al. Transesophageal stress echocardiography: detection of coronary artery disease in patients with normal resting left ventricular contractility. *Am Heart J* 1991;122:1456–63.

17. Berthe C, Pierard LA, Hiernaux M, et al. Predicting the extent and location of coronary artery disease in acute myocardial infarction by echocardiography during dobutamine infusion. *Am J Cardiol* 1986;58:1167–72.

18. Sawada SG, Segar DS, Brown SE, et al. Dobutamine stress echocardiography for evaluation of coronary disease (abstract). *Circulation* 1989;80 Suppl 2:II–66.

19. Picano E, Lattanzi F, Masini M, et al. Comparison of the high-dose dipyridamole-echocardiography test and exercise two-dimensional echocardiography for diagnosis of coronary artery disease. *Am J Cardiol* 1987;59:539–42.

20. Bolognese L, Sarasso G, Aralda D, et al. High dose dipyridamole echocardiography early after uncomplicated acute myocardial infarction: correlation with exercise testing and coronary angiography. *J Am Coll Cardiol* 1989;14:357–63.

21. Mintz GS, Victor MF, Kotler MN, et al. Two-dimensional echocardiographic identification of surgically correctable complications of acute myocardial infarction. *Circulation* 1981;64:91–6.

22. Vlodaver Z, Edwards JE. Rupture of ventricular septum or papillary muscle complicating myocardial infarction. *Circulation* 1977;55:815–22.

23. Montoya A, McKeever L, Scanlon P, et al. Early repair of ventricular septal rupture after infarction. *Am J Cardiol* 1980;45:345–8.

24. Nishimura RA, Schaff HV, Gersh BJ, et al. Early repair of mechanical complications after acute myocardial infarction. *JAMA* 1986;256:47–50.

25. Oh JK, Seward JB, Khandheria BK, et al. Transesophageal echocardiography in critically ill patients. *Am J Cardiol* 1990;66:1492–5.

26. Moore CA, Nygaard TW, Kaiser DL, et al. Postinfarction ventricular septal rupture: the importance of location of infarction and right ventricular function in determining survival. *Circulation* 1986; 74:45–55.

27. Weyman AE, Feigenbaum H, Dillon JC, et al. Noninvasive visualization of the left main coronary artery by cross-sectional echocardiography. *Circulation* 1976;54:169–74.

28. Chandraratna PAN, Aronow WS, Murdock K, Milholland H. Left main coronary arterial patency assessed with cross-sectional echocardiography. *Am J Cardiol* 1980;46:91–4.

29. Chen CC, Morganroth J, Ogawa S, Mardelli TJ. Detecting left main coronary artery disease by apical, cross-sectional echocardiography. *Circulation* 1980;62:288–93.

30. Rink LD, Feigenbaum H, Godley RW, et al. Echocardiographic detection of left main coronary artery obstruction. *Circulation* 1982;65:719–24.

31. Rogers EW, Feigenbaum H, Weyman AE, et al. Possible detection of atherosclerotic coronary calcification by two-dimensional echocardiography. *Circulation* 1980;62:1046–53.

32. Ogawa S, Chen CC, Hubbard FE, et al. A new approach to visualize the left main coronary artery using apical cross-sectional echocardiography. *Am J Cardiol* 1980;45:301–4.

33. Block PJ, Popp RL. Detecting and excluding significant left main coronary artery narrowing by echocardiography. *Am J Cardiol* 1985;55:937–40.

34. Vered Z, Katz M, Rath S, et al. Two-dimensional echocardiographic analysis of proximal left main coronary artery in humans. *Am Heart J* 1986; 112:972–6.

35. Douglas PS, Fiolkoski J, Berko B, Reichek N. Echocardiographic visualization of coronary artery anatomy in the adult. *J Am Coll Cardiol* 1988;11:565–71.

36. Ryan T, Armstrong WF, Feigenbaum H. Prospective evaluation of the left main coronary artery using digital two-dimensional echocardiography. *J Am Coll Cardiol* 1986;7:807–12.

37. Presti CF, Feigenbaum H, Armstrong WF, et al. Digital two-dimensional echocardiographic imaging of the proximal left anterior descending coronary artery. *Am J Cardiol* 1987;60:1254–9.

38. Fusejima K. Noninvasive measurement of coronary artery blood flow using combined two-dimensional and Doppler echocardiography. *J Am Coll Cardiol* 1987;10:1024–31.

39. Gramiak R, Holen J, Moss AJ, et al. Left coronary arterial blood flow: noninvasive detection by Doppler US. *Radiology* 1986;159:657–62.

40. Seward JB, Khandheria BK, Oh JK, et al. Transesophageal echocardiography: technique, anatomic correlations, implementation, and clinical applications. *Mayo Clin Proc* 1988;63:649–80.

41. Pearce FB, Sheikh KH, deBruijn NP, Kisslo J. Imaging of the coronary arteries by transesophageal echocardiography. *J Am Soc Echocardiogr* 1989;2:276–83.

42. Seward JB, Khandheria BK, Edwards WB, et al. Biplanar transesophageal echocardiography: anatomic correlations, image orientation, and clinical applications. *Mayo Clin Proc* 1990;65:1193–213.

43. Zwicky P, Daniel WG, Mügge A, Lichtlen PR. Imaging of coronary arteries by color-coded transesophageal Doppler echocardiography. *Am J Cardiol* 1988;62:639–40.

44. Yamagishi M, Miyatake K, Yaser T, Nimura Y. Detection of coronary blood flow associated with left main coronary artery stenosis by transesophageal color Doppler imaging technique (abstract). *J Am Soc Echocardiogr* 1990;3:224.

45. Memmola C, Iliceto S, Sublimi L, et al. Detection of proximal stenosis of left coronary artery by digital cine loop transesophageal 2D echo: feasibility, sensitivity and specificity (abstract). *Circulation* 1990;82 Suppl 3:III–245.

46. Schrem SS, Tunick PA, Slater J, Kronzon I. Transesophageal echocardiography in the diagnosis of ostial left coronary artery stenosis. *J Am Soc Echocardiogr* 1990;3:357–73.

47. Ballal R, Nanda NC, Samdarshi T, et al. Transesophageal echo assessment of coronary artery involvement in aortic dissection (abstract). *Circulation* 1990;82 Suppl 3:III-245.

48. Reichert SLA, Visser CA, Koolen JJ, et al. Transesophageal examination of the left coronary artery with a 7.5 MHz annular array two-dimensional color flow Doppler transducer. *J Am Soc Echocardiogr* 1990;3:118–24.

49. Yamagishi M, Miyatake K, Beppu S, et al. Assessment of coronary blood flow by transesophageal two-dimensional pulsed Doppler echocardiography. *Am J Cardiol* 1988;62:641–4.

50. Iliceto S, Marangelli V, Memmola C, Rizzon P. Transesophageal Doppler echocardiography evaluation of coronary blood flow velocity in baseline conditions and during dipyridamole-induced coronary vasodilation. *Circulation* 1991;83:61–9.

9

Transesophageal Echocardiographic Evaluation of Native Valvular Heart Disease

Lyle J. Olson • *William K. Freeman*
Maurice Enriquez-Sarano • *A. Jamil Tajik*

The modern era of evaluation and management of valvular heart disease began with the development of cardiac catheterization and surgical intervention more than 3 decades ago. Cardiac catheterization remains a necessary method for the detection and assessment of the severity of valvular stenosis and regurgitation in selected cases. The development of accurate noninvasive ultrasonic methods for hemodynamic assessment in the echocardiographic laboratory and concomitant advances in percutaneous coronary revascularization techniques have directed the primary objectives of the invasive cardiac laboratory to the evaluation and intravascular treatment of coronary artery disease. Hence, the primary diagnostic role of cardiac catheterization for the evaluation of valvular heart disease has been challenged, and in increasingly numerous clinical settings superseded by echocardiography [1].

Echocardiographic methods enable early detection, assessment of etiology and hemodynamic severity, and characterization of the natural history of valvular heart disease without the risk or cost of cardiac catheterization. Transesophageal echocardiography (TEE) has extended the clinical usefulness of two-dimensional and Doppler echocardiography in the assessment of valvular heart disease [2–5]. Biplane TEE provides comprehensive morphologic and hemodynamic assessment of the patient with native valvular heart disease through use of the methods of tomographic imaging, Doppler spectral analysis (pulsed-wave and continuous-wave), and color-flow imaging [6].

Although echocardiographic methods for hemodynamic assessment and color-flow imaging have greatly advanced the noninvasive assessment of cardiac structure and function, the transthoracic approach may be limited by factors causing ultrasonic interference and suboptimal images. Such factors include acoustic attenuation from the chest wall, thoracic cage, general body habitus, pulmonary disease, and prosthetic material. These impediments to optimal tomographic and hemodynamic assessment are largely overcome by the transesophageal approach; combined transthoracic echocardiography and TEE generally provides a complete morphologic and hemodynamic assessment of valvular heart disease. Moreover, the proximity of the TEE transducer to the heart allows imaging with far greater resolution than can be obtained by the transthoracic technique, thereby enhancing the diagnostic sensitivity of echocardiographic imaging.

In this chapter we describe the complementary roles of transthoracic echocardiography and biplane TEE, including two-dimensional and spectral and color-flow Doppler methods, for the evaluation of native valvular heart disease in adult patients. The indications for and the role of TEE in patients with native valvular heart disease are reviewed.

187

MITRAL VALVULAR STENOSIS

Mitral valvular stenosis is characterized by reduced orifice dimension with obstruction to left ventricular inflow. Rheumatic disease remains the most common cause despite the declining incidence of rheumatic fever in western nations [7]. Rare causes of mitral valvular stenosis are congenital valvular stenosis and the parachute mitral valve. Rarely, mitral valvular stenosis is caused by systemic lupus erythematosus complicated by the anticardiolipin syndrome, and in such cases, nonbacterial vegetations are frequently observed on the atrial surface of the leaflets [8,9] (see Chapter 11, Figure 11-12). Unusual causes of left ventricular inflow obstruction not caused by mitral valve leaflet disease include tumors, thrombi, extensive mitral annular calcification [10], cor triatriatum (see Chapter 13), and supravalvular rings [11–13].

Complete morphologic and hemodynamic echocardiographic assessment of mitral valvular stenosis is usually possible by the transthoracic approach, provided that acoustic windows are adequate. In patients with mitral valve stenosis, TEE provides incremental diagnostic information for the assessment of degree of associated mitral regurgitation, potential suitability for either percutaneous balloon or surgical valvuloplasty, and presence of left atrial thrombus.

Characteristic findings of rheumatic disease include thickened, nonpliable, and deformed leaflets with fusion of the commissures and subvalvular apparatus; the valvular and subvalvular apparatus are frequently calcified [12,13] (Fig. 9-1). Typically, the leaflets have reduced opening excursion with diastolic doming of the bodies of partially pliable leaflets. The posterior leaflet may be severely tethered and even immobilized in severe rheumatic stenosis.

Congenital stenosis may be valvular or subvalvular. Congenital valvular stenosis is characterized by thickened and fibrotic valve leaflets with fused or absent commissures and fibrotic and shortened chordae and papillary muscles [14]. The mitral apparatus is not typically calcified, in contrast to rheumatic disease. Motion abnormalities of the leaflets are similar to those observed in rheumatic disease. The parachute mitral valve, associated with Shone's syndrome, is characterized by a single large papillary muscle with normal chordae and valve leaflets [15].

Convergence of the chordal insertions into the single large papillary muscle produces subvalvular obstruction. Transesophageal echocardiography is generally not necessary in patients with such congenital mitral disease, because these entities are usually readily delineated by transthoracic imaging in the pediatric age group.

Associated morphologic abnormalities often observed in the patient with chronic obstruction to left ventricular inflow are left atrial and right heart enlargement. Left atrial thrombus is frequently present, especially in patients with chronic atrial fibrillation. However, thrombus in the left atrial appendage usually cannot be demonstrated by transthoracic two-dimensional echocardiography (see Chapter 12). Coexistent mitral regurgitation, also frequently present, may be underestimated by transthoracic examination because of acoustic masking from calcification of the mitral leaflets and annulus (Fig. 9-2). These limitations of transthoracic imaging are readily overcome by the transesophageal approach.

On TEE examination, the valvular, subvalvular, and annular portions of the mitral apparatus are imaged in the transverse (horizontal) four-chamber imaging plane, with the probe in the midesophagus in neutral or slightly anteflexed position [16,17]. By sweeping the transducer anteriorly to posteriorly in this view, the examiner inspects the anterior and posterior mitral valve leaflets for morphologic and motion abnormalities. The subvalvular apparatus should be routinely evaluated for chordal retraction, fusion, and calcification but is often shadowed in the horizontal four-chamber view by the calcified mitral leaflets. Imaging in the transgastric longitudinal long-axis plane yields the best images of the subvalvular support structures, and chordal disease associated with both anterolateral and posteromedial papillary muscles is delineated (Fig. 9-3). In the basal short-axis imaging plane, the left atrial appendage is routinely observed and inspected for thrombus. Uncommonly, the left atrial appendage cannot be completely visualized in this plane; this problem is almost always alleviated with evaluation of the appendage in the longitudinal left ventricular inflow plane.

Imaging in the transverse plane and withdrawal of the TEE probe several centimeters with increased anteflexion of the tip yields a tomographic plane of the base of the heart, with left lateral transducer rotation visualizing the left atrial appendage. The

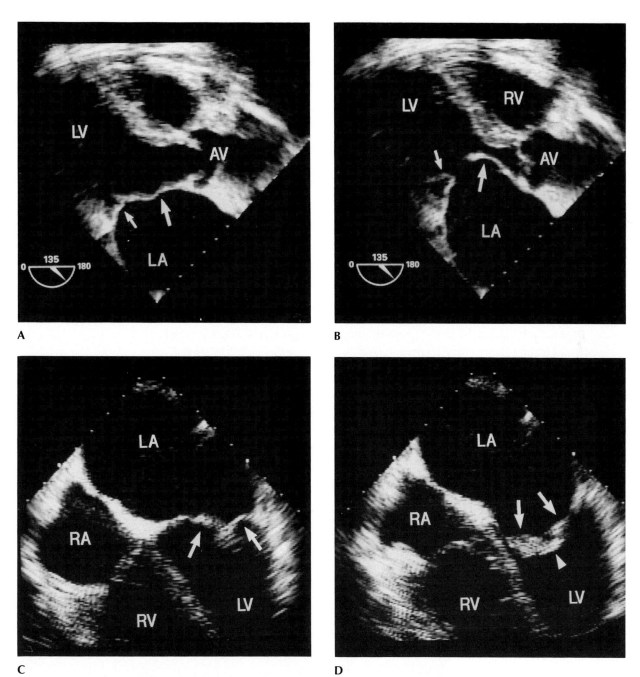

Fig. 9-1. A and B. Mild rheumatic mitral valve stenosis; multiplane imaging at 135 degrees. A. Systolic frame shows intact coaptation of the mildly thickened anterior *(large arrow)* and posterior *(small arrow)* mitral leaflets. B. During diastole there is characteristic diastolic doming of the pliable anterior leaflet *(large arrow)*, with much less diastolic movement of the tethered posterior leaflet *(small arrow)*; a narrowed central inflow orifice is seen between the leaflets. C and D. Severe rheumatic mitral valve stenosis; transverse four-chamber view. C. In systole both leaflets appear considerably thickened *(arrows)*. D. During diastole the severe calcific thickening of the anterior (nearly 1 cm in this view) and, less so, posterior leaflets is evident *(arrows)*; diastolic excursion hinges primarily from the annular insertion of both leaflets. A central diastolic inflow orifice is not even visible *(arrowhead)*.

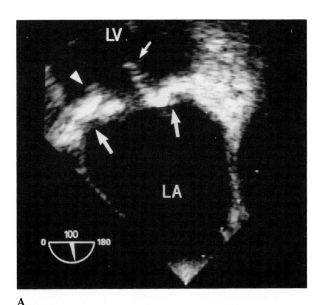
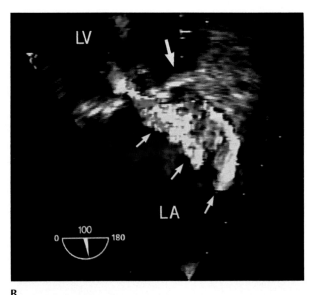

A   B

Fig. 9-2. Mitral annular calcification associated with mild mitral stenosis; longitudinal two-chamber view at 100 degree multiplane imaging. A. Extensive mitral annular calcification *(large arrows)* encompasses the mitral annulus in this view, obscuring visualization of the posterior mitral leaflet *(arrowhead)*. There is mild diastolic doming of the pliable anterior leaflet *(small arrow)*. B. An eccentric anteromedial jet of mitral regurgitation *(small arrows)* is demonstrated on color-flow imaging. A much smaller regurgitant jet was appreciated by transthoracic echocardiography from the apical window because of acoustic shadowing of the left atrium by the extensive mitral annular calcification *(large arrow)*.

Fig. 9-3. Rheumatic mitral valve stenosis; transgastric longitudinal long-axis view. Extensive subvalvular disease is present, with dense thickening and fusion of the chordae *(large arrows)* supporting the posterior leaflet *(small arrow)*. These chordae insert into the posteromedial papillary muscle, which is largely obscured by the subvalvular disease. The anterior mitral valve leaflet *(arrowhead)* is also moderately thickened and coapted poorly with the retracted, tethered posterior leaflet.

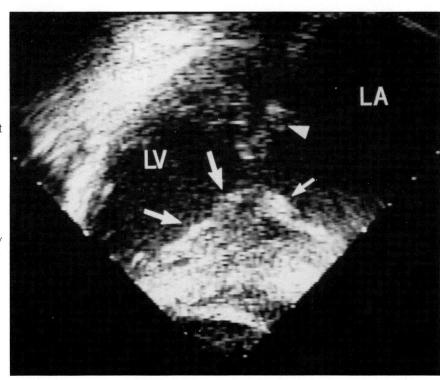

appendage should be tomographically scanned from its most inferior to superior extent to visualize a potentially multilobed apex. Imaging in the longitudinal plane provides additional information on the mitral valve apparatus and body of the left atrium and optimally delineates the left atrial appendage [17]. Left atrial dimension should be routinely measured in both transverse and longitudinal planes, because occasional patients who might otherwise be candidates for balloon valvuloplasty cannot be treated by this technique if the chamber of the left atrium is so large that valvuloplasty catheters are unable to be guided to the mitral orifice.

The body of the left atrium, the atrial septum, and the left atrial appendage should be carefully inspected for thrombus (Fig. 9-4). When observed, thrombus should be characterized as laminated or pedunculated and mobile, as these features may predict thromboembolic potential and provide baseline information for follow-up studies. In the transverse plane, the entire left atrium may be seen by slow withdrawal of the TEE probe during leftward and rightward scanning rotation to visualize the lateral walls. The TEE probe is withdrawn until the right pulmonary artery is seen, assuring visualization of the most superior aspects of the left atrium. Such maneuvers are necessary to allow confident exclusion of laminated eccentric left atrial thrombus. Similarly, in the longitudinal imaging plane, scanning from the orifices of the left to right pulmonary veins (to encompass the extreme lateral aspects of the left atrium) should be performed to detect thrombus (see Chapter 12). A small, laminated thrombus, which may be observed adherent to the dome of the left atrium or atrial septum, is easily overlooked if not specifically sought. However, the most likely site of thrombus is the left atrial appendage [18]. If the left atrial appendage is vertical in orientation, as it often is, imaging in the longitudinal plane with anteflexion of the probe tip better demonstrates the entire appendage.

It is not uncommon to observe spontaneous contrast in the body of the left atrium or the left atrial appendage on TEE examination (Fig. 9-4). This phenomenon is characterized by a smoke-like swirling appearance and may be difficult to discriminate from thrombus if there is "sludging" within the appendage. This abnormality is most likely related to low-velocity blood flow with consequent formation of rouleaux by red blood cells [19,20]. This phenomenon suggests increased risk for thromboembolic events and is attributed to underlying anatomic and

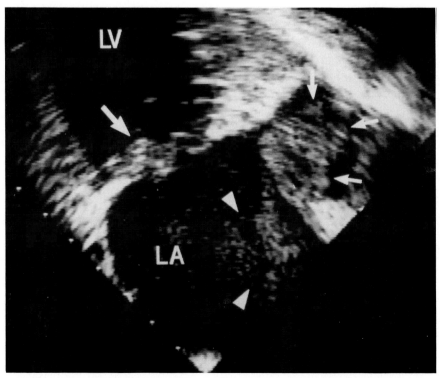

Fig. 9-4. Left atrial thrombus complicating mitral stenosis; longitudinal two-chamber view. A large thrombus *(small arrows)* nearly fills a severely dilated left atrial appendage. Dense, swirling spontaneous echocontrast within the left atrium *(arrowheads)* was present on real-time examination and was associated with atrial fibrillation in a patient with moderately severe mitral stenosis *(large arrow).*

hemodynamic abnormalities (such as left atrial enlargement and mitral stenosis) often coupled with atrial fibrillation, responsible for the low blood flow state.

The atrial septum is routinely evaluated for structural integrity and interatrial shunting. The demonstration of a patent foramen ovale with interatrial shunting may be expected in a significant proportion (20% to 30%) of patients in all age groups. The detection of a patent foramen ovale is helpful in the assessment of potential candidates for balloon valvuloplasty (see below). The atrial septum is best evaluated in the longitudinal plane, because this is the optimal plane of imaging during Doppler color-flow mapping and intravenous contrast echocardiography for the detection of interatrial shunting [17] (see Chapter 13).

Transgastric TEE evaluation of mitral valve stenosis yields useful information about the mitral orifice dimension and the structure of the subvalvular apparatus. After entering the stomach, the tip of the endoscope is anteflexed to optimize contact between the wall of the stomach and the transducer and, thereby, to enhance image quality. Imaging in the longitudinal plane demonstrates the subvalvular apparatus, mitral leaflets, annulus, and posterior and anteroseptal walls of the left ventricle (see Fig. 9-3). Leftward and rightward rotation of the TEE endoscope enables inspection of the entire mitral apparatus. The entire mitral valve apparatus can be scanned by moving the tip of the endoscope from an anteflexed position to a neutral position (i.e., by retroflexion), so that the left ventricular cavity is swept in a superior to inferior arc. Examination in the transverse plane with anteflexion and gradual withdrawal of the TEE probe toward the basal plane enables short-axis visualization of the mitral orifice in some patients. However, because of oblique imaging angles often encountered at this level, a true short-axis view usually cannot be obtained precisely at the tips of the mitral leaflets corresponding to the minimal mitral orifice. Hence, the degree of mitral stenosis generally cannot be reliably estimated by planimetry of the visualized orifice.

Hemodynamic Assessment

Hemodynamic assessment of mitral stenosis by Doppler echocardiography has been well described [21]. Accurate estimates of gradient and orifice dimensions are almost always obtained by the trans-

thoracic approach. For patients in whom evaluation of the hemodynamic severity of mitral stenosis is assessed by TEE, the principles of the Doppler hemodynamic method are identical to those used for transthoracic examination.

Continuous-wave Doppler echocardiography is used to assess mitral inflow because velocity aliasing occurs with pulsed-wave Doppler if the transmitral gradient is increased. Analysis of the mitral valve inflow velocity profile by continuous-wave Doppler echocardiography provides direct hemodynamic assessment of the severity of obstruction to mitral inflow. The optimal Doppler signal is obtained by placing the continuous-wave interrogating beam directly into the inflow jet, parallel to the direction of flow (Fig. 9-5). Examination may be aided by simultaneous color-flow imaging (Fig. 9-6). Either the transverse or the longitudinal plane may provide an ideal display of mitral inflow for hemodynamic evaluation.

The diastolic pressure gradient from left atrium to left ventricle is obtained from the mitral inflow velocity profile by application of the modified Bernoulli equation [21], in which the maximal pressure gradient (ΔP) is estimated by $\Delta P \cong 4V^2$, with V equal to the maximal inflow velocity. The instantaneous pressure gradient between the left atrium and the left ventricle can be estimated at any point in diastole. As has been the convention by invasive techniques, hemodynamic severity is assessed by estimation of the peak, mean, and end-diastolic gradients. The mean mitral inflow gradient is the most clinically useful Doppler-derived pressure measurement obtained by TEE.

Mitral valve area can be estimated by two different Doppler echocardiographic methods: estimation of the pressure half-time and measurement of valve area by the continuity equation. The pressure half-time method, originally described by invasive means [22], has been adapted for the estimation of mitral valve area by Doppler echocardiography. The rate of decline of the diastolic pressure gradient may be described by the pressure half-time, which is the time required for the initial gradient to decline by 50%. Estimation of mitral valve area is based on the observation that as the degree of stenosis becomes more severe, the diastolic gradient is maintained for a longer period and the pressure half-time is prolonged. On continuous-wave Doppler echocardiographic examination, this effect is manifested as a reduced rate of decline and prolongation of the early diastolic inflow signal.

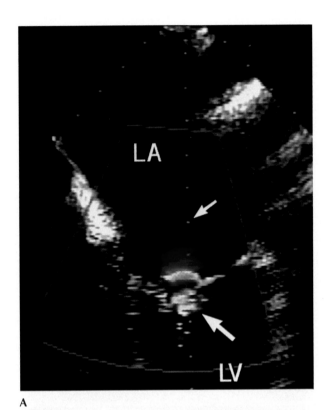

A

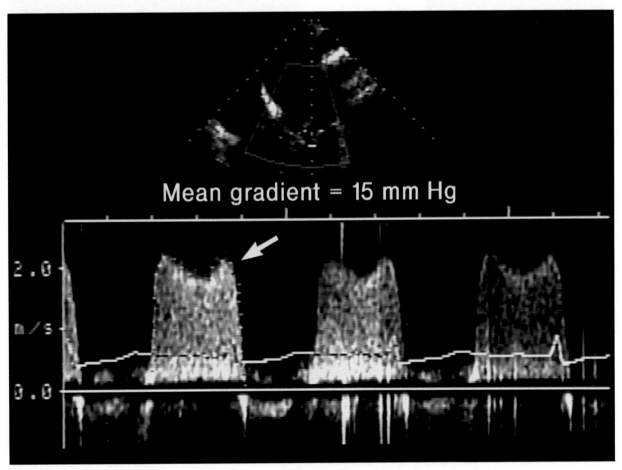

B

Fig. 9-5. Continuous-wave Doppler evaluation of mitral stenosis (same patient as that in Figures 9-1 C and 9-1 D); transverse four-chamber view. A. The dotted cursor line *(small arrow)* is aligned to be colinear with the long axis of mitral inflow *(large arrow)*. B. Continuous-wave Doppler interrogation revealed a mean mitral inflow gradient of 15 mm Hg *(arrow)*, diastolic pressure half-time of 300 msec, and mitral valve area of 0.7 cm²; all findings confirmed severe mitral stenosis.

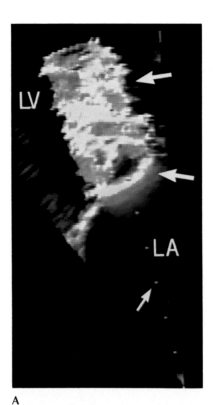

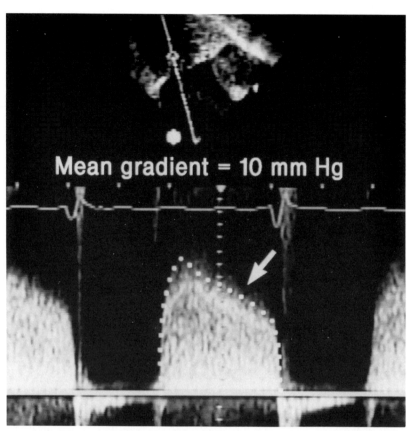

A   B

Fig. 9-6. Continuous-wave Doppler echocardiography in mitral stenosis (same patient as that in Figure 9-4); longitudinal two-chamber view. A. Color Doppler imaging readily identifies the turbulent high velocity jet of stenotic mitral inflow *(large arrows)*, facilitating nearly coaxial alignment of the Doppler cursor (dotted line, *small arrow*). B. Continuous-wave Doppler analysis detects a mean mitral inflow gradient of 10 mm Hg *(arrow)*.

According to the principles of Bernoulli hemodynamics, the relationship between pressure drop and velocity is quadratic. Hence, the pressure half-time is obtained from the Doppler velocity profile by dividing peak velocity by the square root of two and then measuring the time interval from peak velocity to the time of peak velocity divided by the square root of two. Hatle et al. [23] derived an empiric constant that relates pressure half-time to mitral valve area (MVA):

MVA = 220/pressure half-time

In normal persons, the pressure half-time is approximately 50 to 70 msec, whereas it is 110 to over 300 msec in patients with progressively severe mitral stenosis. Mitral valve area determined by the pressure half-time method correlates extremely well with mitral valve area determined by the Gorlin formula in patients undergoing cardiac catheterization for assessment of mitral stenosis without other associated left-sided valvular heart disease (in particular, aortic regurgitation), left ventricular hypertrophy, or significant left ventricular systolic or diastolic dysfunction [23].

Although estimation of mitral valve area by the Doppler half-time method has been widely employed, it cannot be applied to all patients with mitral stenosis. In patients with a prolonged PR interval, increased velocity from atrial contraction earlier in diastole makes it impossible to separate the mitral inflow E and A waves and hence to measure pressure half-time. Similar problems are encountered in patients with sinus tachycardia, atrial flutter, and atrial tachycardia. In patients with atrial fibrillation, pressure half-time should be estimated from an average of at least five inflow signals. Use of the Doppler pressure half-time is also precluded after recent mitral valvuloplasty [24] and if moderate-to-severe aortic regurgitation is coexistent [25,26]. In these two situations, estimates of mitral valve area by the half-time method may differ significantly from estimates based on the Gorlin formula. Significant aortic regurgitation is associated with a rapidly rising left ventricular diastolic pressure, which may decrease the transmitral pressure gradient and thereby abbreviate the pressure half-time and cause overestimation of valve area. Similar abbreviation in the pressure half-time is observed in left ventricular dysfunction associated with increased diastolic filling pressures.

In the absence of significant regurgitant lesions, the limitations of the pressure half-time method for estimation of mitral valve area are overcome by use of the continuity equation. The continuity equation may be applied to mitral stenosis to yield valve area estimates that correlate well with Gorlin formula estimates despite coexistent left ventricular dysfunction or hypertrophy [26]. The method assumes that inflow volume crossing the mitral annulus in one cardiac cycle is equal to left ventricular stroke volume. Hence, mitral valve area (MVA) can be determined as the stroke volume (SV) divided by the time velocity integral of mitral inflow (TVIm):

$$MVA = SV/TVIm$$

Because stroke volume is the product of the cross-sectional area of the aortic or pulmonary annulus and the time velocity integral of aortic (TVIa) or pulmonary (TVIp) flow velocity at the annulus level, MVA = aortic (or pulmonary) annular cross-sectional area $\times$ TVIa (or TVIp)/TVIm. The left ventricular outflow tract can be reliably evaluated by pulsed-wave (or continuous-wave) Doppler echocardiography only in the transgastric long-axis view because of prohibitive angles of incidence of the interrogating beam in other views. If this view is inadequate, the pulmonary valvular flow should be used in the continuity equation; this is best assessed from high basal short-axis imaging in the transverse plane. If mitral regurgitation is significant, this method underestimates mitral valve area. Flow measurements must be made at the level of the pulmonary valve, not the left ventricular outflow tract, if significant aortic regurgitation is present.

Coexistent hemodynamic abnormalities frequently observed in patients with mitral stenosis include tricuspid regurgitation, pulmonary arterial hypertension, and mitral regurgitation. Every patient with mitral stenosis should be systematically evaluated for these associated problems by transthoracic echocardiography. In patients with mitral valvular stenosis who undergo TEE, additional clinically useful information may be obtained for these coexistent hemodynamic abnormalities. Tricuspid regurgitation can be assessed in the transverse or longitudinal planes by color-flow imaging and continuous-wave Doppler echocardiography (Fig. 9-7). Pulmonary artery systolic pressure is estimated by measurement of the peak tricuspid regurgitant jet velocity (V_{TR}) by continuous-wave Doppler echocardiography and application of the modified Bernoulli equation ($\Delta P \cong 4V_{TR}^2$) which yield the pressure gradient (ΔP) between right ventricle and right atrium [27]. Estimated right atrial pressure derived from a regression equation is added to the right ventricular-right atrial gradient to yield peak right ventricular systolic pressure, which is equivalent to pulmonary artery systolic pressure if there is no obstruction to right ventricular outflow. If the continuous-wave Doppler tricuspid regurgitation signal is difficult to obtain or is incomplete, it can be significantly enhanced with intravenous injection of agitated saline (Fig. 9-8).

Extensive calcification of the mitral valve apparatus, especially the annulus, may make transthoracic assessment of associated mitral regurgitation suboptimal because of acoustic masking. This problem is entirely avoided by the transesophageal approach, because the imaging probe is located posterior to the left atrium and thus allows the interrogating Doppler ultrasound to traverse the atrium unimpeded by the calcified valve apparatus. Hence, color-flow imaging for the detection and semiquantitation of mitral regurgitation should be routinely performed in patients with mitral valve stenosis undergoing TEE.

Color-flow examination is performed in both the transverse and the longitudinal imaging planes to avoid underestimation of the severity of regurgitant jets, which may have an eccentric course through the body of the left atrium [17,28–32]. Leftward and rightward rotation of the TEE transducer endoscope, as well as anteflexion and retroflexion and withdrawal and insertion of the endoscope tip, should be routinely performed for complete visualization of the left atrium to fully delineate the spatial extent of mitral regurgitation and thereby avoid underestimation of regurgitant severity. Semiquantitative evaluation of mitral regurgitation is discussed under "Mitral Regurgitation" in this chapter.

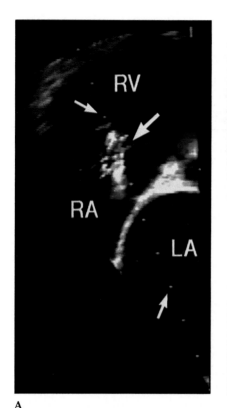
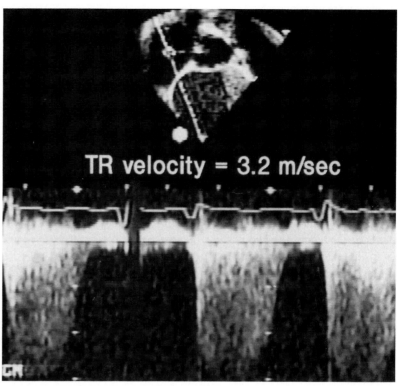

A   **B**

Fig. 9-7.   Continuous-wave Doppler assessment of tricuspid regurgitation velocity; longitudinal short-axis view. A. A narrow jet of mild tricuspid regurgitation *(large arrow)* is identified by color Doppler mapping; the Doppler cursor (dotted line, *small arrows*) is placed within the jet's central portion. B. An average tricuspid regurgitation *(TR)* velocity of 3.2 m/sec is obtained by continuous-wave Doppler evaluation, yielding an estimated right ventricular systolic pressure of 55 mm Hg if the right atrial pressure derived from a regression equation is assumed to be 14 mm Hg. Because of the minor degree of tricuspid regurgitation, a reliable velocity was not obtainable by transthoracic Doppler echocardiography in this patient.

Indications for and Role of TEE

Comprehensive transthoracic two-dimensional echocardiography and Doppler echocardiography are the preferred methods for detection and assessment of the severity of mitral stenosis. Transthoracic two-dimensional echocardiography and Doppler echocardiography completely characterize the morphologic and hemodynamic abnormalities in most patients.

Transesophageal echocardiography is indicated for patients with suspected mitral regurgitation that may be underestimated by the transthoracic technique because of technically limited windows or acoustic shadowing of the left atrium. Transesophageal echocardiography is also indicated for patients in whom balloon valvuloplasty is contemplated to rule out left atrial thrombus before transseptal catheterization and to further stratify candidacy for valvuloplasty. Atrial thrombus is not an indefinite contraindication to balloon valvuloplasty. However, it necessitates vigorous anticoagulant therapy and subsequent documentation of resolution of thrombus on follow-up TEE before balloon valvuloplasty. Similarly, grade I or II mitral regurgitation is not an absolute contraindication to mitral balloon valvuloplasty. However, grade III or IV mitral regurgitation is considered a contraindication to balloon valvuloplasty. In patients with mitral valve stenosis who have undergone previous commissurotomy, the mitral regurgitant jet may be eccentric and must be carefully investigated to avoid underestimation of severity.

Two-dimensional echocardiographic criteria have

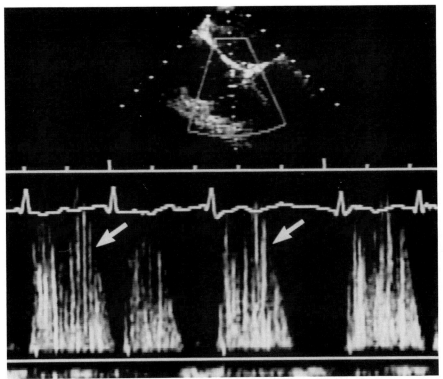

Fig. 9-8. Continuous-wave Doppler evaluation of tricuspid regurgitation; transverse four-chamber view. A. The dotted cursor line is aligned with a small posteromedial jet of tricuspid regurgitation *(sector insert)*; however, the continuous-wave Doppler signals *(arrows)* are fragmented and incomplete for analysis. B. After peripheral intravenous injection of agitated saline, the tricuspid regurgitant signal has been significantly enhanced, producing well-defined spectral envelopes *(arrows)* with variable peak velocities, ranging from 3 to 4 m/sec, in the presence of atrial fibrillation.

A

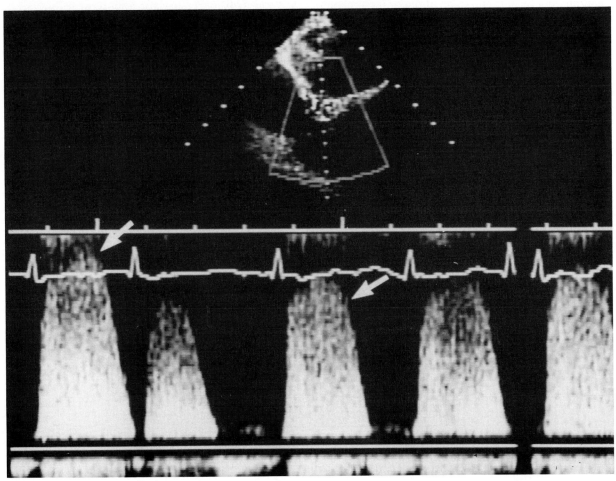

B

been used to identify and stratify patients who may be candidates for mitral valvuloplasty. A scoring system based on transthoracic two-dimensional imaging has been devised for this purpose [33,34] (Table 9-1). The system scores (grades 1 through 4) each of four morphologic characteristics: valve mobility, valve thickness, valve calcification, and subvalvular thickness. Patients with a score of 8 or less have a greater than 90% chance of an initially satisfactory result. Depending on clinical circumstance, patients with mitral scores in the range of 8 to 10 may be treated by balloon mitral valvuloplasty with less predictable success. Diffuse calcification of the mitral apparatus is considered a predictor of poor outcome for valvuloplasty. However, calcification of a single commissure does not necessarily preclude an excellent result with valvuloplasty, because opening of a single commissure may be sufficient to produce a satisfactory hemodynamic result. The mitral scoring system does not reliably predict postdilatation mitral regurgitation [33,34].

Transesophageal echocardiographic scoring of the morphologic features of mitral valve stenosis has generally not been found to be of major incremental value for the prediction of the success of balloon valvuloplasty. However, the marked incremental diagnostic yield for the detection of left atrial thrombus has led investigators to suggest that TEE should be routinely performed in all patients considered candidates for mitral valvuloplasty [35,36].

Transesophageal echocardiography is not routinely indicated during balloon valvuloplasty. However, TEE has been used to facilitate the performance of transseptal cardiac catheterization and the sizing and placement of the balloon dilators during mitral valvuloplasty [37–40] (Fig. 9-9). The observation of a markedly displaced atrial septum due to left atrial enlargement may predict difficulty in passage of catheters into the body of the left atrium in patients considered candidates for valvuloplasty. Other advantages to simultaneous TEE at the time of balloon mitral valvuloplasty are prompt assessment of morphologic and hemodynamic results of valvuloplasty, especially the detection and quantitation of mitral regurgitation, which thereby obviates left ventriculography.

Transesophageal echocardiography is likewise not routinely necessary for long-term follow-up of

Table 9-1. Echocardiographic score index for mitral stenosis

Mitral Valve Morphology
  Mobility
    Grade 1 Highly mobile valve with restriction of leaflet tips only
    Grade 2 Leaflet middle and base portions have normal mobility
    Grade 3 Valve continues to move forward in diastole, mainly from the base
    Grade 4 No or minimal forward movement of the leaflets in diastole
  Leaflet thickening
    Grade 1 Leaflets slightly increased in thickness (3–4 mm)
    Grade 2 Mid-leaflets normal; marked thickening of margins only (5–8 mm)
    Grade 3 Thickening extending through the entire leaflet (5–8 mm)
    Grade 4 Marked thickening of all leaflet tissue (>8–10 mm)
  Subvalvular thickening
    Grade 1 Minimal thickening just below the mitral leaflets
    Grade 2 Thickening of chordal structures extending up to one-third of the chordal length
    Grade 3 Thickening extending to the distal third of the chords
    Grade 4 Extensive thickening and shortening of all chordal structures, extending down to the
             papillary muscles
  Calcification
    Grade 1 A single area of increased echo brightness
    Grade 2 Scattered areas of brightness confined to the leaflet margins
    Grade 3 Brightness extending into the mid-portion of the leaflets
    Grade 4 Extensive brightness throughout much of the leaflet tissue

To determine the echocardiographic score add the grades from the four categories; the minimum score is 4, and the maximum score is 16.
Modified from Wilkins et al. [33] and Abascal et al. [34].

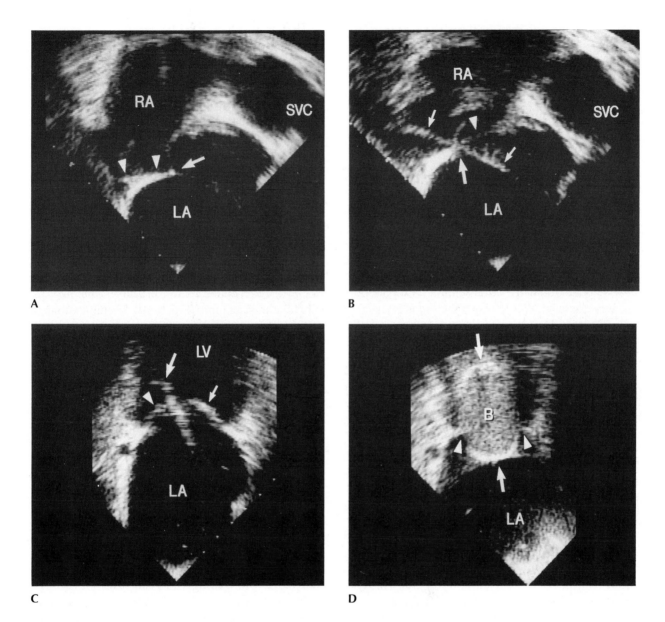

Fig. 9-9. Transesophageal echocardiography during percutaneous balloon mitral valvuloplasty for severe mitral stenosis; longitudinal imaging planes. A. The position of the transseptal needle *(arrowheads)* is confirmed by TEE to be safely within the limbus of the atrial septum. The fossa ovalis membrane is tented *(arrow)* by the needle tip just before entry into the left atrium. B. The transseptal catheter *(small arrows)* is passed across the site of puncture *(large arrow)* of the fossa ovalis membrane *(arrowhead)* along the inferior aspect of the limbus. *C.* The deflated balloon valvuloplasty catheter *(large arrow)* is guided into the stenotic mitral valve orifice; diastolic doming of both the anterior *(small arrow)* and posterior *(arrowhead)* leaflets is evident. D. The valvuloplasty balloon *(B)* is inflated and remains well situated across the mitral valve *(arrowheads)* with its proximal and distal ends within the left atrium and left ventricle, respectively *(arrows).*

balloon mitral valvuloplasty. When complications are suspected after the procedure, however, TEE is the safest and most expeditious method for the detection of the morphologic and hemodynamic abnormalities. Mitral regurgitation associated with balloon dilatation is generally caused by a leaflet tear without opening of a commissure. The tear may involve either the posterior or the anterior leaflet. Less often, mitral regurgitation is due to ruptured chordae tendineae or papillary muscles. The mitral regurgitant jets observed after valvuloplasty may be eccentric, originating at the site of the leaflet tear and taking an oblique direction into the body of the left atrium. Interatrial shunting is typically observed after balloon mitral valvuloplasty and is caused by balloon dilatation of the atrial septum for transseptal catheter passage. The left-to-right shunt is usually transient and, if persistent, is of mild degree and is seldom of clinical significance [41,42].

MITRAL REGURGITATION

Proper coaptation of the mitral valve leaflets depends on the normal function of the leaflets, annulus, chordae tendineae, papillary muscles, and subjacent left ventricular myocardium. Dysfunction of any of these components of the mitral valve apparatus may produce mitral regurgitation. Hence, mitral regurgitation has many causes.

Anatomic assessment of the mitral valve apparatus by TEE provides the basis for diagnostic classification of the cause of mitral regurgitation. The importance of a systematic approach in the sequence in which the various components of the mitral valve apparatus are evaluated cannot be overemphasized [16,17,28]. In this way, potential lesions will not be overlooked. Routine assessment by biplane imaging includes visualization of the leaflets, annulus, and subvalvular apparatus from the transverse and longitudinal planes with the TEE transducer in the mid and distal portion of the esophagus. When examining in the transverse plane, the operator should scan through multiple four-chamber tomographic planes in an anterior-posterior arc by anteflexion and retroflexion of the endoscope tip. Similarly, the heart can be examined in entirety in the longitudinal plane by sweeping in a left-to-right arc by lateral flexion of the transducer. Secondary long-axis and short-axis views in the longitudinal plane (see Chapters 3 and

4) should be routinely obtained in cases of suspected or known mitral valve disease [16,17]. In the imaging of the mitral apparatus by the transesophageal approach, it is important to examine in off-axis planes to optimize detection of morphologic and hemodynamic abnormalities. Systematic evaluation also includes assessment of the valve leaflets, annulus, and subvalvular apparatus from the transgastric longitudinal and horizontal (short-axis) planes. The mitral support structures and left ventricular size, global function, and segmental function are usually best assessed by transgastric biplanar imaging.

Infective endocarditis produces mitral regurgitation by impairing function of the mitral valve apparatus through damage to leaflets, annulus, or subvalvular structures (Fig. 9-10). Complications of endocarditis causing regurgitation include large vegetations preventing leaflet coaptation, leaflet prolapse or flail, leaflet perforation, chordal rupture, and disruption of the annulus. The utility of TEE for the identification of small vegetations, leaflet perforation, perivalvular abscess, and damage to the subvalvular apparatus is well established [43–46] (see Chapter 11).

The demonstration of vegetations less than 3 mm in diameter is generally not possible by transthoracic imaging [47]. Furthermore, because infective endocarditis frequently involves previously diseased valves, it is often impossible to differentiate small sessile valvular vegetations from leaflet thickening, calcification, or myxomatous degeneration. Transesophageal echocardiography has been shown to be highly sensitive and specific for the diagnosis of infective endocarditis and significantly more sensitive than transthoracic echocardiography [43–45]. Furthermore, Shively et al. [44] suggested that the absence of characteristic abnormalities by TEE indicates a very low probability of disease in a patient with intermediate pretest likelihood of endocarditis. In our clinical practice we have found TEE to be instrumental in establishing the diagnosis of endocarditis as well as characterizing morphologic and hemodynamic complications. A complete discussion of TEE in the evaluation of infective endocarditis is found in Chapter 11.

The two-dimensional echocardiographic diagnosis of mitral valve prolapse is usually established by the transthoracic technique and is based on the demonstration of systolic motion of one or both

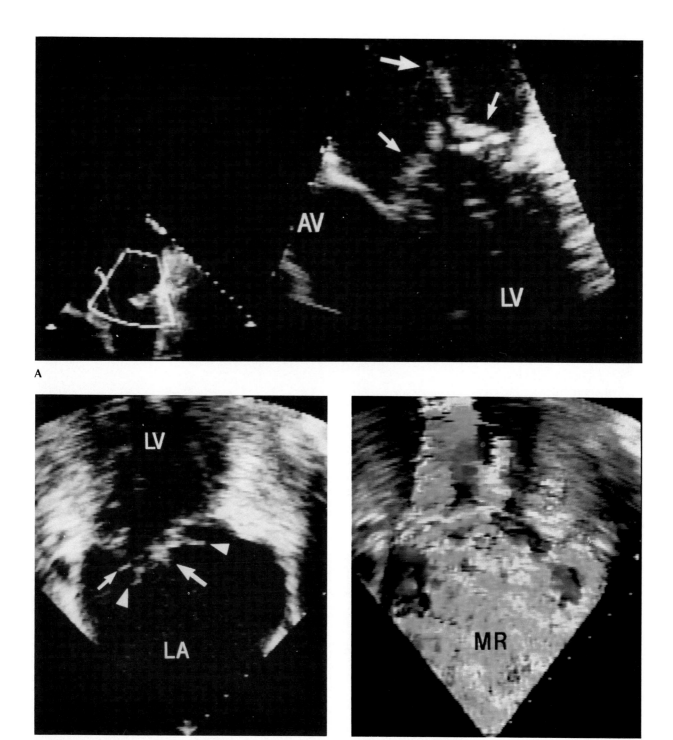

Fig. 9-10. Mitral regurgitation due to prior infective endocarditis. A. Transverse four-chamber magnified view. There is severe prolapse of the mitral leaflets, both of which are encrusted with chronic vegetations *(small arrows)*. A flail segment of the posterior leaflet *(large arrow)* is seen in this view. B. Longitudinal two-chamber view. Flail chordae *(arrowheads)* associated with both the posterior *(small arrow)* and the anterior *(large arrow)* mitral leaflets are demonstrated. C. Torrential mitral regurgitation *(MR)* caused by the flail mitral leaflets nearly fills the entire left atrium in this view.

valve leaflets posterior to the plane of the mitral annulus into the body of the left atrium. However, a great spectrum of morphologic abnormality is observed on echocardiographic imaging, ranging from mild prolapse of a single leaflet scallop to bileaflet disease associated with marked myxomatous changes, chordal rupture, flail leaflet segments, and annular dilatation [48–51]. Transesophageal echo-

Fig. 9-11. Bileaflet mitral valve prolapse; multiplane imaging. A. Imaging at 0 degree rotation of the transducer reveals bileaflet prolapse, which is more prominent in the posterior leaflet *(large arrow)* than in the anterior leaflet *(small arrow)* in this view. B. A narrow central jet of mitral regurgitation *(arrow)* is detected by color Doppler imaging, consistent with grade I/IV (mild) regurgitation in this view. C. Left ventricular inflow view at 70 degrees. Moderate redundancy, thickening, and prolapse of both the anterior *(small arrow)* and the posterior *(large arrow)* leaflets is seen. D. The somewhat broader central mitral regurgitant jet *(arrow)* in this view approaches grade II/IV (moderate) severity. *(asterisk = orifice of left atrial appendage).*

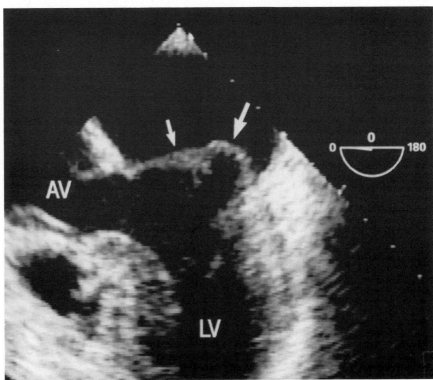

A

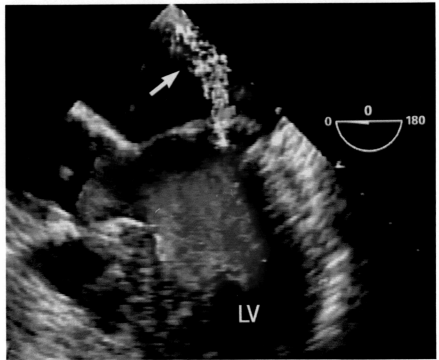

B

cardiographic assessment of the patient with mitral valve prolapse enables more precise characterization of the specific morphologic abnormalities associated with mitral valve prolapse, including identification of ruptured chordae, assessment of annular diameter, elongation of chordae subtending the valvular apparatus and areas of leaflet redundancy, each of which may be surgically repaired [52,53] (Fig. 9-11).

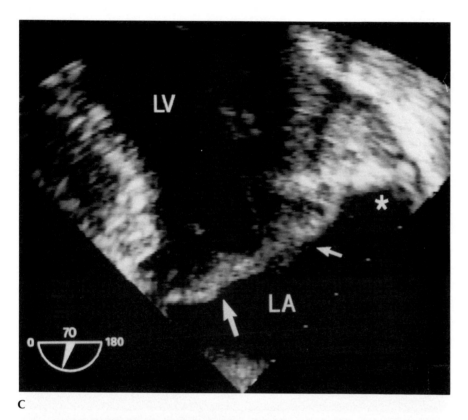

C

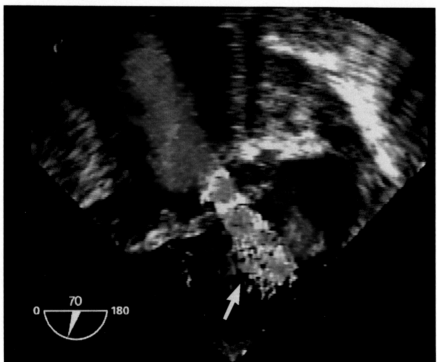

D

Chordal rupture is a well-recognized complication of mitral valve prolapse and may be associated with acute, severe decompensation or chronic progressive regurgitation (Fig. 9-12). Ruptured chordae tendineae are the most common cause of acute severe mitral regurgitation and may be associated with myxomatous degenerative disease, infective endocarditis, rheumatic disease, myocardial infarction, or trauma. A ruptured chorda is recognized echocardiographically as a highly mobile, linear density that appears to move primarily with the leaflet or subvalvular structures, depending on the site of rup-

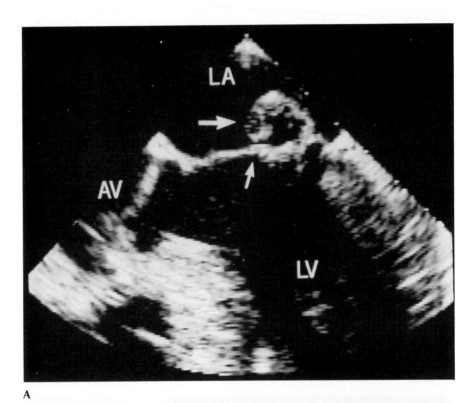

A

Fig. 9-12. Chordal rupture associated with posterior mitral leaflet prolapse. A. Transverse left ventricular outflow view. Marked prolapse of the thickened posterior leaflet *(large arrow)* is evident. The posterior leaflet overrides the anterior leaflet *(small arrow)*; no flail segment could be identified in this view. B. Color Doppler imaging reveals a narrow sheet-like jet of mitral regurgitation *(large arrows)* emanating from the point of override *(arrowhead)* of the posterior leaflet *(small arrow)* and tracking anteromedially. Such eccentric jets may significantly underestimate the severity of mitral regurgitation and should prompt additional imaging in other planes and quantitative Doppler evaluation (see text under "Hemodynamic Assessment"). C. Longitudinal left ventricular outflow view. A ruptured chordae *(small arrow)* attached to a flail portion of the posterior leaflet *(large arrow)* is readily identified. There is no prolapse of the anterior leaflet *(arrowhead)*. D. A broad anteromedial jet of severe mitral regurgitation *(arrows)* is detected by color Doppler mapping. Color Doppler assessment of mitral regurgitation should be done in more than one imaging plane with use of multiple views.

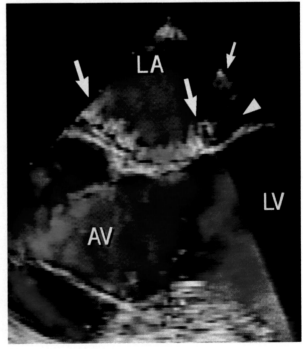

B

ture [54–56]. Ruptured chordae and flail leaflet segments should be carefully looked for in patients with severe mitral regurgitation associated with significant prolapse and especially in patients with acute pulmonary edema (with or without a mitral regurgitant murmur) in whom the cause of left ventricular failure is not otherwise clear. Transesophageal echocardiography will establish the diagnosis if transthoracic echocardiographic findings are indeterminate. The diagnostic yield of TEE for the detection of chordal rupture is much greater than that of transthoracic imaging [54–56]. The TEE examiner should

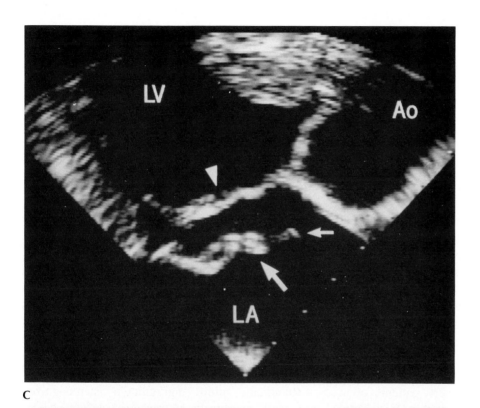

C

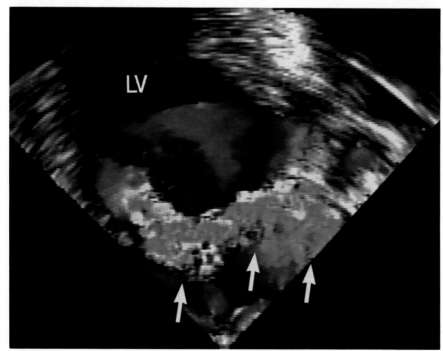

D

be highly suspicious of ruptured chordae in any patient with mitral valve prolapse who has an unsupported leaflet segment. If chordal rupture is chronic, the chordal segments may appear as retracted nodular echodensities attached to an unsupported segment of the valve leaflet (Fig. 9-13).

A flail mitral valve leaflet is associated with acute severe regurgitation due to disruption of either the chordae tendineae or the papillary muscles. The motion of the flail leaflet is usually demonstrated from either the parasternal long-axis or the apical four-chamber view by transthoracic imaging. Transesophageal echocardiography is very useful for high-resolution definition in patients in whom the diagnosis is uncertain; the anatomic abnormality is readily recognized, because the body of the leaflet prolapses into the left atrium [57]. Transesophageal echocardiography is especially useful in patients with acute, severe decompensation, in whom the diagnosis must be obtained rapidly. The safety and utility of TEE in critically ill patients has been well demonstrated [58] (see Chapter 17).

Papillary muscle dysfunction of any cause may produce mitral regurgitation. Abnormalities of the papillary muscles associated with regurgitation and identified by two-dimensional imaging include fibrosis, calcification, dysfunction of the subjacent myocardium, and papillary muscle rupture. Mitral annular calcification is a degenerative disorder and a frequent echocardiographic finding in elderly patients, often in association with mitral regurgitation. It is recognized on transthoracic imaging by dense echoes in the region of the annulus [59]. It may range from mild to severe and typically is most severe at the posterior aspect of the annulus. Rarely, it is associated with mitral inflow obstruction [10]. Calcification of the annulus may impede the transthoracic hemodynamic assessment of the severity of mitral regurgitation because of acoustic shadowing of the left atrium (see Fig. 9-2). Transesophageal echocardiography is useful in this situation because the interrogating beam of ultrasound is posterior to the valve annulus, so that acoustic masking is avoided. Extensive calcification of the walls of the left atrium can complicate advanced rheumatic disease and present a rare cause of acoustic shadowing of the left atrium that could hinder TEE assessment of mitral regurgitation as well as other cardiac structures.

Chronic mitral regurgitation is also caused by congenital anomalies of the mitral valve, including a partial or complete cleft of the anterior or, less commonly, the posterior leaflet. Generally, TEE is not necessary for the morphologic or hemodynamic characterization of this cause of mitral regurgitation in pediatric patients but can be useful in adults. As with transthoracic imaging, the cleft mitral leaflet is visualized only on short-axis imaging of the mitral valve, and good nonoblique transgastric transverse short-axis imaging planes are required for confident diagnosis.

Rheumatic mitral regurgitation is recognized echocardiographically by thickened, deformed leaf-

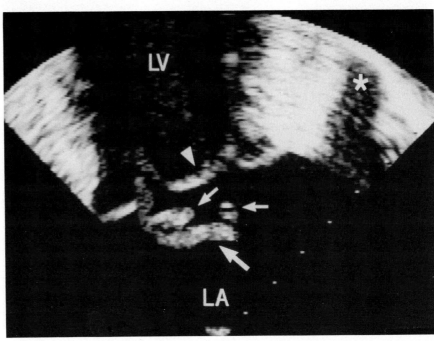

Fig. 9-13. Chronic flail of the posterior mitral valve leaflet; longitudinal two-chamber view. A large flail portion of the posterior leaflet *(large arrow)* and loss of coaptation with the anterior leaflet *(arrowhead)* can be seen. Thickened and retracted ruptured chordae *(small arrows)* are visible along the ventricular aspect of the flail segment; such echodense nodularities may be difficult to differentiate from vegetations. *(asterisk* = left atrial appendage).

lets and subvalvular apparatus with or without associated calcification [60]. Because both leaflets are involved in relatively symmetrical fashion, there is generally a central trajectory of the mitral regurgitant jet within the left atrium (Fig. 9-14). Frequently, there is associated mitral stenosis or aortic valve disease. If rheumatic disease is absent, there is typically little leaflet calcification and no commissural fusion. If dense calcification and associated mitral stenosis are present, TEE may be necessary to characterize the severity of mitral regurgitation because of acoustic masking.

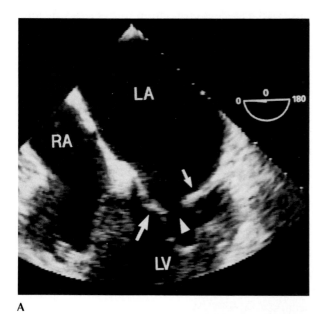

A

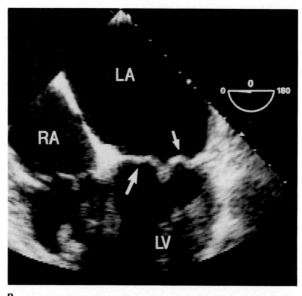

B

Fig. 9-14. Rheumatic mitral stenosis with mitral regurgitation; multiplane imaging at 0 degrees (transverse four-chamber view). A. The tethered posterior leaflet *(small arrow)* and doming anterior leaflet *(large arrow)* restrict the mitral inflow orifice *(arrowhead)* during diastole. B. Coaptation of the equally thickened posterior *(small arrow)* and anterior *(large arrow)* leaflets is intact during systole. C. Color Doppler mapping demonstrates a central jet of mild (grade I/IV) mitral regurgitation *(arrow)* emanating from the point of leaflet coaptation *(arrowhead)*. A central regurgitant jet trajectory characterizes disease processes that involve both leaflets in symmetrical fashion or produce mitral annular dilatation.

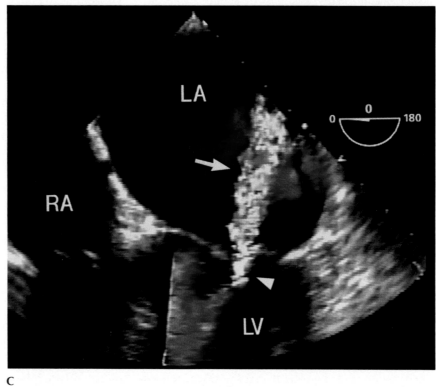

C

Left ventricular enlargement from any cause may be accompanied by mitral annular dilatation, which in the absence of significant asymmetrical mitral leaflet lesions is typically associated with variable degrees of central regurgitation.

Hemodynamic Assessment

Semiquantitative Evaluation

The severity of mitral regurgitation is estimated semiquantitatively by combined color-flow and pulsed-wave Doppler echocardiography. Quantitative methods are also used to assign a semiquantitative grade of regurgitant severity and are particularly useful with eccentric regurgitant jets.

Mitral regurgitant flow signals characteristically have a mosaic appearance because of turbulence and variance associated with high-velocity flow due to the large systolic pressure gradient between left ventricle and atrium. Trivial physiologic mitral regurgitation is commonly detected by TEE and is manifested as a tiny systolic reverse flow signal detected immediately posterior and superior to the mitral valve leaflets [61]. With noneccentric jets, more severe regurgitation is associated with larger areas of turbulent systolic flow within the body of the left atrium. The principles of semiquantitative grading of regurgitant severity on the basis of color-flow imaging are the same as those used in transthoracic imaging [62–64]. It has been shown that TEE more often demonstrates mitral regurgitation than does transthoracic imaging and that Doppler regurgitant jet areas are frequently larger than those demonstrated by transthoracic imaging in comparable scan planes [63]. Biplane TEE yields both longitudinal and transverse (as well as off-axis) views of the regurgitant jet. Transverse imaging provides complementary assessment of the magnitude of regurgitation with the longitudinal plane, but optimal correlation with angiographic assessment is obtained when the maximal spatial extent of the jet is obtained from biplanar imaging [31].

The severity of mitral regurgitation may be expressed as the maximum jet cross-sectional area indexed by left atrial area in the same plane. By transthoracic examination, it has been suggested that a ratio of less than 0.2 corresponds to angiographically mild regurgitation, of 0.2 to 0.4 to moderate regurgitation, and of greater than 0.4 to severe regurgitation [64]. The echocardiographic area method has been demonstrated to correlate extremely well with angiographic grading of mitral regurgitation

when the regurgitant jets are centrally directed. However, this method underestimates regurgitant severity when jets are eccentric and adherent to the walls of the left atrium (directed toward the atrial septum, posteriorly, or toward the lateral wall) because of the Coanda effect [65] (Fig. 9-15).

Studies comparing jet area dimensions assessed by TEE and ventriculography have generally demonstrated excellent correlation for the classification of the semiquantitative severity of mitral regurgitation [66–68]. A variety of measures of jet dimension and specific flow patterns have been used, including absolute jet area, ratio of regurgitant jet area to left atrial area, area of the mosaic aspect of the regurgitant jet only, identification of systolic wraparound flow within the body of the left atrium, and presence of systolic pulmonary venous flow reversal. Castello et al. [67] suggested that the absolute area of the mosaic aspect of the regurgitant jet may be the single best area method for assessment of regurgitant severity by TEE, but further studies are needed to confirm this observation. These investigators found that a maximal mosaic regurgitant jet area of less than 3 cm^2 predicted mild mitral regurgitation with a sensitivity of 96%, a specificity of 100%, and a predictive accuracy of 98%. A maximal regurgitant jet area greater than 6 cm^2 predicted severe mitral regurgitation with a sensitivity of 91%, a specificity of 100%, and a predictive accuracy of 98% [67].

Further refinement of the semiquantitative assessment of mitral regurgitant severity was introduced by Tribouilloy et al. [69] with the measurement of regurgitant jet width at its origin by TEE. When the regurgitant jet diameter exceeded 5.5 mm, this method was found to have a high sensitivity, specificity, and predictive accuracy in comparison with angiography in the classification of patients with severe mitral regurgitation and regurgitant stroke volume of greater than 60 ml [69]. This relation was not significantly affected by the driving pressure or the eccentricity of the regurgitant jets. The advantages of this method over the jet area technique are its simplicity and its independence from the spatial extent of flow in the body of the left atrium, loading conditions, and left ventricular function. Furthermore, the concept is supported by in vitro investigation and may have a more physiologic basis than the jet area method [70]. Limitations include the potential variability due to technical factors, such as color gain, filter and velocity settings, and imaging depth, that may affect the color jet dimension. This method assumes that the regurgitant orifice has a

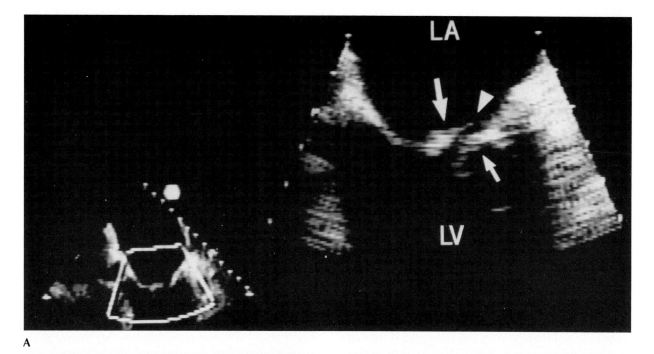

A

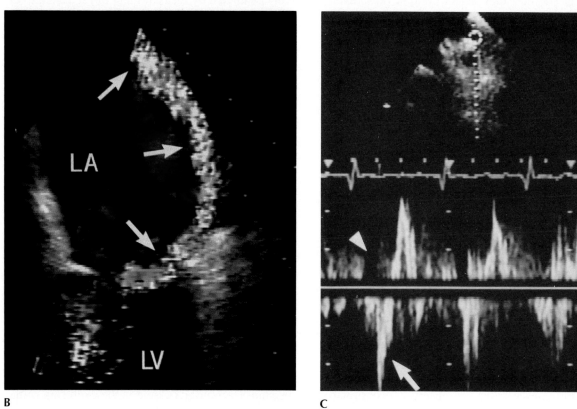

B

C

Fig. 9-15. Eccentric mitral regurgitation; magnified transverse four-chamber views. A. A flail portion of the anterior mitral leaflet *(large arrow)* with a ruptured chordal segment *(arrowhead)* is seen. The posterior leaflet *(small arrow)* is thickened, but without prolapse. B. An eccentric jet of mitral regurgitation *(arrows)*, detected on color-flow mapping, is adherent to the posterolateral left atrial free wall with wraparound to the dome of the left atrium. The size of such eccentric jets significantly underestimates the severity of regurgitation when only ratios of jet to left atrial area are used for assessment. C. Pulsed-wave Doppler analysis of the left upper pulmonary vein. Absence of normal antegrade inflow during systole *(arrowhead)* and aliased systolic flow reversal *(arrow)*, are highly sensitive for severe mitral regurgitation (see text). Such ancillary information is essential for the composite Doppler evaluation of mitral regurgitation.

uniform shape throughout systole, which may not always be the case [70,71].

Pulsed-wave mapping of the body of the left atrium is not routinely performed in the assessment of mitral regurgitation because it is laborious and time-consuming and has been supplanted by color-flow imaging. However, pulsed-wave Doppler assessment of pulmonary vein flow has been demonstrated to be a useful adjunct in the identification of hemodynamically severe mitral regurgitation. Systolic flow reversal in the pulmonary veins indicates severe regurgitation and is the hemodynamic equivalent of angiographic reflux into the pulmonary veins on left ventriculography. It is important to place the pulsed-wave Doppler sample volume well within the pulmonary vein and not at the orifice, as the latter position may detect systolic flow disturbance caused by an eccentric mitral regurgitant jet itself and not reflect true pulmonary venous flow patterns.

Pulmonary venous flow can be readily assessed in virtually all patients by transesophageal pulsed-wave Doppler echocardiography of the right and left upper pulmonary veins [72]. Normal pulmonary venous flow is biphasic, with forward flow in systole and diastole. Alterations of pulmonary venous flow due to significant mitral regurgitation accompanied by increased left atrial pressure include diminished systolic flow and reversal of systolic flow. Correlative studies comparing pulsed-wave interrogation of the pulmonary veins with color-flow assessment by TEE and left ventricular angiography have demonstrated high sensitivity and specificity (compared with ventriculography) for identification of grades III and IV mitral regurgitation; pulmonary venous systolic flow reversal is indicative of grade IV regurgitation, whereas diminished antegrade systolic flow is typical of grade III regurgitation [73–81] (Fig. 9-16).

Discordant flow profiles between right and left upper pulmonary veins are observed occasionally and may be related to various factors, including eccentric mitral regurgitation directed toward certain pulmonary venous orifices, left atrial size, and even left lateral decubitus posture during examination [81]. Hence, it is important to routinely evaluate both right and left pulmonary venous inflow during TEE evaluation of mitral regurgitation.

In our clinical practice of TEE for the assessment of the semiquantitative severity of mitral regurgitation, a grading system comprised of grade I (mild), grade II (moderate), grade III (moderately severe), and grade IV (severe) is used. The final gradation of severity of mitral regurgitation is made after consideration of the hemodynamic data routinely collected during TEE, which at minimum includes delineation of the maximal spatial extent and trajectory of the jet in orthogonal planes and pulsed-wave Doppler assessment of pulmonary venous inflow. If hemodynamic severity of the lesion remains ambiguous after this assessment, quantitative measures of regurgitant volume are performed to aid in establishing the grade of regurgitation. Hence, the final determination of severity of mitral regurgitation is a composite of various methods, and no one technique is solely relied on to the exclusion of others.

Quantitative Evaluation

The severity of mitral regurgitation may be quantitatively evaluated by measurement of regurgitant volume and regurgitant fraction. Combined pulsed-wave Doppler and two-dimensional echocardiography has been used to calculate regurgitant fraction and volume from the difference between mitral and aortic stroke volumes; results have correlated well with those of angiographic and scintigraphic methods [82]. Aortic stroke volume (measured at the subannular left ventricular outflow tract level) is the product of the left ventricular outflow tract time-velocity integral and aortic annular cross-sectional area. Mitral stroke volume (measured at the mitral annular level) is similarly derived as the product of the mitral time-velocity integral and mitral cross-sectional annulus area. Cross-sectional areas for each value are calculated by πr^2; valve orifices are assumed to be circular, with the radius (r) equal to one-half the measured diameter. Regurgitant flow is the difference between mitral flow and aortic flow, and regurgitant fraction is regurgitant flow divided by total mitral inflow [83,84].

The major limitation of the combined Doppler echocardiographic methods for the estimation of regurgitant fraction or volume is the exclusion of patients with other left-sided valvular heart disease, particularly patients with more than mild aortic regurgitation. The most important potential source of error is the estimate of the functional mitral orifice area. When this method is applied with TEE, the major limitation is obtaining adequate pulsed-wave Doppler signals of the left ventricular outflow tract. Because of the angles of incidence of the left ventricular outflow tract with the esophagus, the best view for obtaining pulsed-wave Doppler interrogation of this location is the transgastric long-axis view in the longitudinal plane.

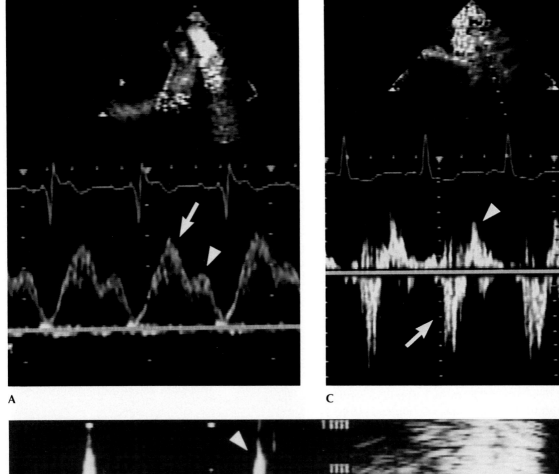

A

C

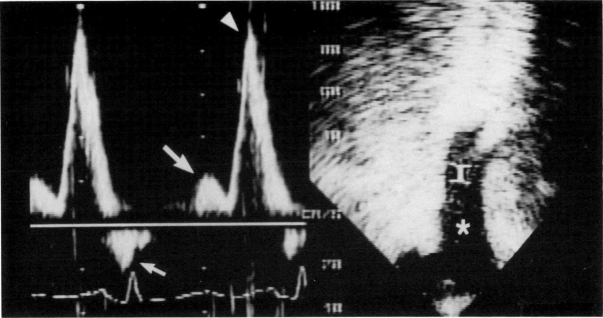

B

Fig. 9-16. Pulsed-wave Doppler analysis of pulmonary venous inflow with various degrees of mitral regurgitation. A. Left upper pulmonary vein, basal short-axis transverse plane. Normal systolic *(arrow)* and lower velocity diastolic *(arrowhead)* antegrade pulmonary venous inflow is observed with mild (grade I/IV) mitral regurgitation. The systolic and diastolic velocities may be equal with moderate mitral regurgitation. B. Longitudinal view; the sample volume is well within the left upper pulmonary vein *(asterisk)*. Significant diminution of systolic filling *(large arrow)* and enhanced diastolic filling *(arrowhead)* are present with increasing left atrial pressures in moderately severe (grade III/IV) mitral regurgitation. Low-velocity end-diastolic flow reversal *(small arrow)* is caused by atrial systole, occurs immediately after the P wave and before the QRS complex on the electrocardiogram, and is a normal finding to a velocity of 0.3 m/sec. C. Left upper pulmonary vein; basal short-axis transverse plane. Turbulent systolic pulmonary venous flow reversal *(arrow)* is observed with severe (grade IV/IV) mitral regurgitation and most likely is generated from a combination of direct reflux of regurgitant blood into the pulmonary vein and significant increase in left atrial pressure during systole causing reversal of the normal left atrial inflow gradient. Increased diastolic pulmonary venous filling *(arrowhead)* is due to the systolic regurgitant flow.

A Doppler color-flow method for the quantitative estimation of regurgitant volume and the severity of valvular regurgitation is based on measurement of volume flow rate proximal to the regurgitant orifice [85–88]. It differs from previously described Doppler color-flow methods in that it does not focus on the spatial extent of the jet distal to the regurgitant orifice but instead identifies a proximal (to the regur-

Fig. 9-17. Quantitative Doppler assessment of mitral regurgitation by the proximal isovelocity surface area (PISA) method. A. Anteriorly directed longitudinal imaging in the plane of left ventricular outflow reveals flail portions of both the posterior *(large arrow)* and, to a lesser degree, the anterior *(small arrow)* mitral leaflets. B. Color Doppler imaging detects an eccentric jet of anteromedial mitral regurgitation *(large arrows)*. The flow entrained into the regurgitant orifice *(small arrows)* is partly visible in this view. C. The proximal isovelocity surface area (PISA) can be significantly enhanced for more accurate measurement by baseline shifting of the aliasing velocity (in this case to 31 cm/sec). The PISA radius is measured from the color-aliased boundary *(large arrow)* to the constriction at the mitral regurgitant orifice. The radius *(r)* in this case is 1.4 cm, and the mitral regurgitant flow is 2π (1.4 cm)^2 (31 cm/sec) = 381 cm^3/sec. D. In a modified longitudinal view, the continuous-wave Doppler signal is aligned with the mitral regurgitant jet; the peak velocity is 600 cm/sec,

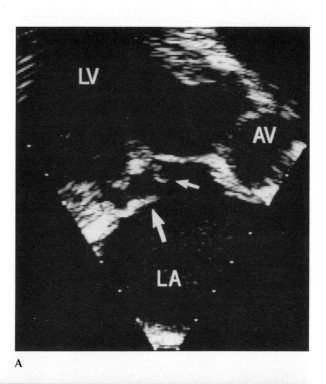

A

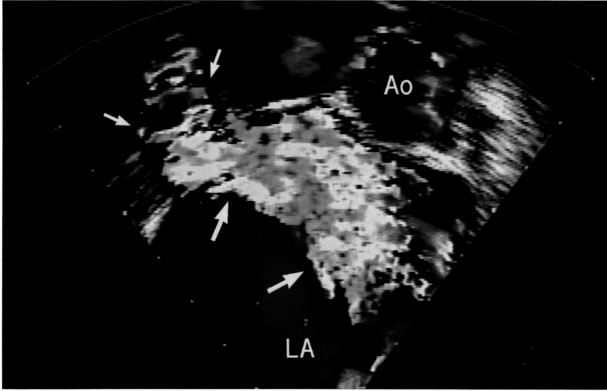

B

gitant orifice) isovelocity surface area (PISA) by depiction of an aliasing interface (Fig. 9-17). Regurgitant volume flow rate (cubic centimeters per second) can be calculated as the proximal isovelocity surface area in square centimeters multiplied by the aliasing velocity (centimeters per second). Assuming that the PISA is a hemispherical shell of accelerating flow proximal to the regurgitant orifice, the

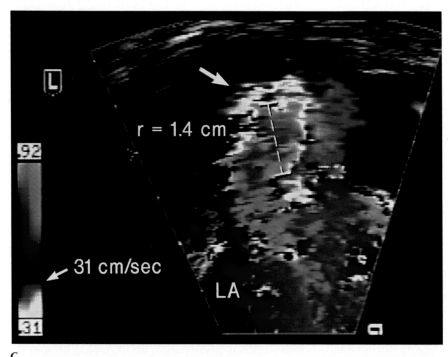

Fig. 9-17 (continued). and the time velocity integral *(TVI)* is 150 cm *(arrow)*. The effective regurgitant orifice (ERO) area is: 381 cm³/sec/600 cm/sec = 0.64 cm². The regurgitant volume per beat can then be calculated: (0.64 cm²) (150 cm) = 95 cm³. All findings are consistent with severe mitral regurgitation.

C

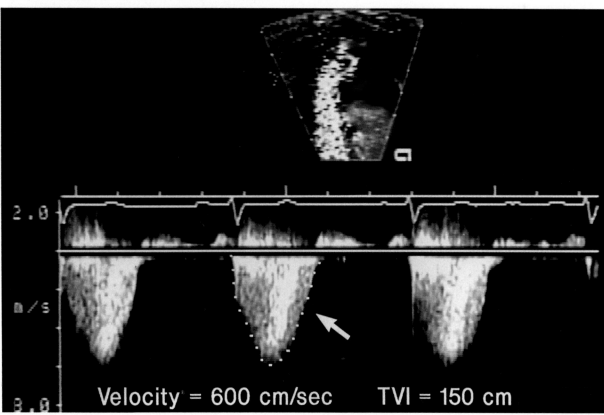

D

mitral regurgitant flow ($Flow_{MR}$) is calculated as

$$Flow_{MR} = 2\pi r^2 \times V_r$$

in which $2\pi r^2$ equals the area of the PISA (square centimeters) having the radius r (centimeters) at the aliasing velocity V_r (centimeters per second) interface. Since flow equals the product of velocity and the area through which it passes,

$$Flow_{MR} = ERO_{MR} \times V_{MR}$$

when ERO_{MR} is the mitral regurgitant effective orifice area (square centimeters) and V_{MR} is the maximal mitral regurgitant velocity (centimeters per second) by color-flow-directed continuous-wave Doppler echocardiography. By rearranging,

$$ERO_{MR} = Flow_{MR}/V_{MR}$$

The mitral regurgitant volume (RV_{MR}) in cubic centimeters may then be calculated by

$$RV_{MR} = ERO_{MR} \times TVI_{MR}$$

in which TVI_{MR} (centimeters) is the time velocity integral of the mitral regurgitant signal obtained by continuous-wave Doppler echocardiography. In severe mitral regurgitation, the ERO_{MR} is usually greater than 0.4 cm² and the RV_{MR} is greater than or equal to 50 cm³.

In principle, the PISA method may be affected by instrumentation factors and the shape of the regurgitant orifice, leading to inaccuracies in the estimate of volumetric flow. However, if a hemispherical model is assumed for the regurgitant orifice, differences in plane or orifice shape do not appear to affect the calculated volume flow rate. Furthermore, changes in instrument factors, including system gain, wall filter settings, frame rate, transmission power, and packet size, do not appear to significantly affect calculations of volume flow rate by the PISA method. Hence, the PISA method may have advantages over previous Doppler color-flow methods in calculating volume flow rate and may be used clinically for estimating regurgitant volume and severity.

The main limitation with the use of any invasive or noninvasive quantitative method based on regurgitant fraction or volume is that no definitive criteria have been defined in large patient populations for the evaluation of disease progression, reproducibility of the methods, or usefulness in clinical decision-making. Cardiac catheterization and angiography have been shown to lack precision; hence, a reference standard is absent [89]. The quantitative methods are generally most useful for the semiquantitative assignment of a grade of regurgitant severity (mild, moderate, or severe) for clinical use.

Continuous-wave Doppler echocardiography enables measurement of the peak mitral regurgitant velocity, which is usually in the range of 5 to 6 m/sec. Application of the modified Bernoulli equation ($\Delta P \cong 4V^2$) enables measurement of the instantaneous pressure difference between left ventricle and left atrium at any point during systole. The instantaneous gradient is not a measure of the severity of mitral regurgitation; the gradient is determined by left ventricular-atrial systolic pressure difference and accurately reflects the pressure gradient throughout systole when compared with catheterization findings [90].

However, the continuous-wave spectral flow profile of mitral regurgitation contains information other than absolute pressure gradient that may eventually prove to have practical clinical utility. The intensity of the regurgitant signal is proportional to volumetric flow and when normalized to mitral inflow enables estimation of regurgitant fraction. The intensity of the mitral regurgitant signal and mitral inflow profile may be measured on-line by investigational computer programs and the regurgitant fraction calculated by the weighted time-velocity integral method [91].

Analysis of the time-velocity profile of mitral regurgitation also enables estimation of the maximal left ventricular dp/dt, a measure of left ventricular contractile reserve, often useful in the setting of severe mitral regurgitation. The time derivative of the left ventricular-left atrial pressure gradient is obtained by differentiating the time course of the ventriculoatrial gradient assessed by continuous-wave Doppler echocardiography (Fig. 9-18). This method has been demonstrated to correlate well with catheter-derived measures and is not substantially affected by orifice size or flow rate [92]; however, dp/dt is load-dependent to a mild degree [93]. The usefulness of these quantitative methods and their role in patient management remain to be clinically validated in prospective clinical studies.

Indications for and Role of TEE in Clinical Decision-Making

The indications for and utility of TEE vary with the clinical setting. In our practice, we recommend TEE

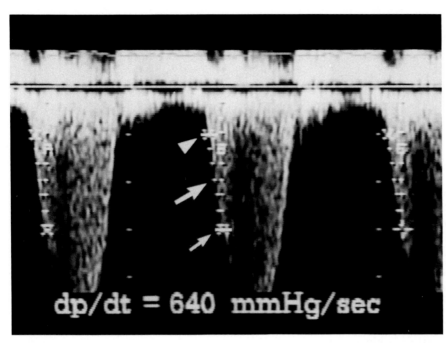

dp/dt = 640 mmHg/sec

Fig. 9-18. Determination of left ventricular dp/dt (pressure/time derivative). A continuous-wave Doppler spectral envelope of mitral regurgitation has been obtained with a well-defined systolic upslope *(large arrow)*. A time of 50 msec elapses between a left ventriculoatrial gradient of 4 mm Hg [4 (1 m/sec)^2] *(arrowhead)* and 36 mm Hg [4 (3 m/sec)^2] *(small arrow)*. The dp/dt is calculated as: 36 − 4 mm Hg/0.05 sec = 640 mm Hg/sec. Decreasing dp/dt values of less than 1000 mm Hg/sec are consistent with increasingly impaired left ventricular contractile function.

in all patients with known or suspected infective endocarditis because of its demonstrated incremental diagnostic yield (compared with that of transthoracic imaging) for both detection of vegetations and demonstration of complications of endocarditis (see Chapter 11). Transesophageal echocardiography may also resolve the differential diagnosis of acute pulmonary edema in the patient who has had myocardial infarction with consequent papillary muscle dysfunction.

Transesophageal echocardiography is of great use in the characterization of valve leaflet structure in patients considered candidates for surgical valvuloplasty or annuloplasty (see Chapter 16). Transesophageal echocardiography aids in the planning of elective surgery for mitral valve repair or in the intraoperative assessment of reparative procedures. Hence, one of the main aims of the TEE examination in the patient with mitral regurgitation is to determine whether valve repair is feasible.

In developed countries, the most common cause of mitral regurgitation requiring surgical intervention is mitral valve prolapse [94]. Generally, mitral valve prolapse is a lesion well-suited to repair, as determined by specific associated morphologic features.

In the examination of the patient with mitral valve prolapse, the TEE operator must assess the extent of prolapse and characterize whether the lesion is focal or diffuse and affects one or both leaflets.

Generally, focal lesions are more easily repaired, whereas the more diffusely diseased valve, characterized by diffuse myxomatous changes of both leaflets, chordal elongation, and annular dilatation, is more difficult to repair [95]. However, elongated chordae can be shortened, annular dilatation can be corrected by ring annuloplasty, and tissue excess (if not diffuse) can be reduced by resection or plication, or both. Hence, the TEE operator must assess all portions of the mitral valve apparatus with potential repair in mind.

A localized flail segment of the posterior leaflet with one or more ruptured chordae and without involvement of the anterior leaflet is the most common subgroup of surgical mitral regurgitation in patients with mitral prolapse [95,96]. Surgical correction requires plication or resection of the flail segment and mitral ring annuloplasty. However, this type of repair may be extremely difficult if there is associated severe annular calcification. The degree of calcification of the mitral annulus should be assessed from both the transverse and the longitudinal planes with the TEE transducer in the midesophageal position. The transgastric view allows complete visualization of the mitral annulus adjacent to the posterior leaflet; anteflexion of the transducer tip and slight withdrawal of the probe in the longitudinal and transverse planes optimize the examination. Annular calcification may be divided into three categories:

1. Localized nodules of calcium of the mitral annulus adjacent to the posterior leaflet; generally not a limitation to valve repair.
2. Diffuse annular calcification of mild to moderate degree; generally not an absolute contraindication to resection or plication of the posterior leaflet.
3. Massive calcification involving the annulus and the base of the leaflets; feasibility of adequate repair poor and even prosthetic replacement difficult.

Flail segments of the anterior leaflet associated with ruptured chordae are more difficult to repair [95,96]. Resection of the flail segment can be corrective, but the degree of resection on the anterior leaflet is much more limited than on the posterior leaflet because of less leaflet tissue and relatively rigid adjacent annulus. For this reason, the incidence of significant residual mitral regurgitation is higher for surgically repaired prolapse or flail of the anterior leaflet [95,96]. Recent technical improvements, including artifical chordae or transposition of chordae from the posterior leaflet to the anterior leaflet, have greatly improved the repairability of these lesions. Depending on the skill of the surgeon, significant anterior leaflet prolapse or flail should not be considered an absolute contraindication to mitral repair.

Perforation of a mitral leaflet due to healed endocarditis (see Chapter 11, Figure 11-14) may also be repaired by excision of organized vegetation and patching of the perforation. Transesophageal echocardiography facilitates the identification of valve perforation before repair. For a more complete discussion on the use of intraoperative TEE during valve repair, see Chapter 16.

AORTIC VALVULAR STENOSIS

The anatomic hallmark of aortic valvular stenosis is a reduced orifice area. The morphologic appearance of the valve depends on the cause of stenosis [97–100]. Senescent aortic stenosis is characterized by a three-cusped valve free of commissural fusion with rigid, calcified nodular excrescences within the valve sinuses that limit opening excursion. The congenitally bicuspid valve is identified by two cusps of unequal size, the larger of which is conjoined and contains a raphe at the site of fusion. Calcification of the raphe, annulus, and valve cusps produces a narrowed ellipsoid orifice. Rheumatic aortic stenosis is characterized by fusion of all three commissural margins, cuspid fibrosis, and calcification [97–100].

In most patients, transthoracic two-dimensional echocardiography reliably demonstrates valve structure and reduced systolic excursion of the cusps, readily differentiating valvular stenosis from left ventricular outflow tract obstruction due to subvalvular or supravalvular disease. Anatomic abnormalities frequently associated with aortic valve stenosis and demonstrated by transthoracic echocardiography include left ventricular hypertrophy, poststenotic dilatation of the aorta, and other associated valvular heart disease. The role of TEE for the assessment of aortic valvular stenosis is limited to patients in whom transthoracic data are suboptimal, the cause of left ventricular outflow obstruction is unclear, or the assessment of associated abnormalities, suspected dissection or coarctation of the thoracic aorta, and coexistent mitral valve disease is necessary.

Transesophageal echocardiography enables examination of the aortic valve in multiple planes [16,17,101]. From the primary longitudinal plane with the tip of the endoscope in the upper to mid esophagus in neutral position (or slightly anteflexed), rightward (clockwise) rotation and left lateral flexion of the endoscope tip image the aortic valve cusps and left ventricular outflow tract in long axis (see Chapter 3, Figures 3-12 and 3-13). This view enables assessment of systolic cusp excursion and inspection of the subvalvular and supravalvular regions in continuum for other causes of left ventricular outflow obstruction. Rightward flexion of the TEE probe tip from this longitudinal view demonstrates the aortic valve cusps in short axis, enabling assessment of cusp number and structure, and allows planimetry of aortic valve systolic orifice dimension. The longitudinal short-axis and transverse basal short-axis imaging planes readily permit morphologic characterization of the bicuspid or even unicuspid aortic valve (Fig. 9-19), allowing demonstration of complete or partial raphe, extent of calcification, and estimation of degree of stenosis. Long-axis imaging reveals characteristic systolic doming of the cusp or cusps. Not uncommonly, imaging in the transverse plane provides only oblique images of the aortic valve in either short or long axis. Such a problem must be recognized and prompt evaluation made in the longitudinal plane for correct morphologic assessment. Transesophageal echocardiography facilitates the identification of valve perforation before repair. For a more complete discussion on the use of intraoperative TEE during valve repair, see Chapter 16.

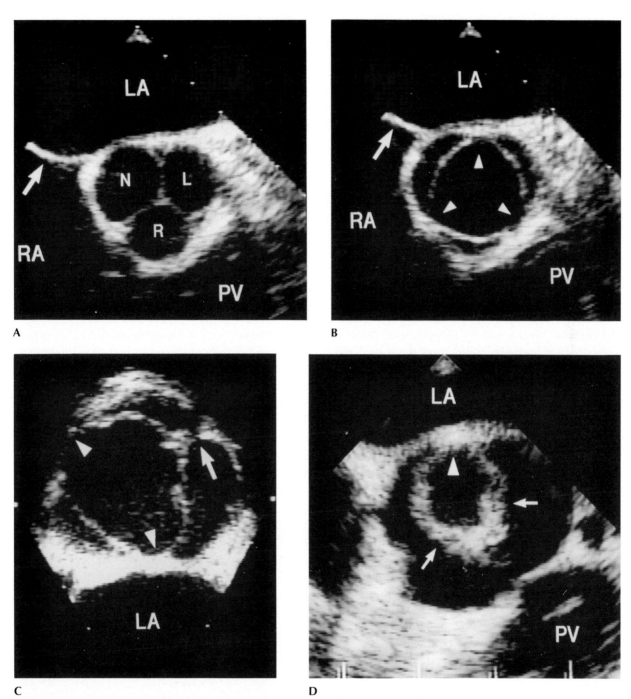

A

B

C

D

Fig. 9-19. Normal aortic valve; basal short-axis view in the transverse plane.
A. The three cusps of the aortic valve are seen during diastole; the noncoronary
cusp *(N)* is always most proximate to the atrial septum *(arrow)* in any imaging
plane, the right coronary cusp *(R)* is most anterior (or farthest from the posterior
TEE transducer at the sector apex), and the left coronary cusp *(L)* is identified
by the left main coronary ostia. B. During systole, three equal commissural
margins *(arrowheads)* are seen along the aortic annulus. C. Bicuspid aortic
valve; longitudinal short-axis magnified view. A partially calcified raphe *(arrow)*
is associated with the larger anterior cusp, and the oval systolic orifice has two
commissural margins *(arrowheads)*. D. Unicuspid aortic valve; transverse basal
short-axis view. The stenotic teardrop-shaped systolic orifice *(arrows)* has only
one commissural margin along the annulus *(arrowhead)*.

yields the best view for TEE two-dimensional guided pulsed- or continuous-wave Doppler evaluation of the aortic valve or outflow tract because of the nearly parallel alignment of these structures to the interrogating ultrasound beam from this window. This imaging plane can generally be obtained easily with multiplanar TEE systems (Fig. 9-20).

Subvalvular disease may cause left ventricular outflow obstruction or coexist with aortic valvular disease. Discrete subvalvular stenosis may be caused by an isolated fibrous membrane just proximal to the aortic valve or by a thicker fibrous ring or collar associated with left ventricular outflow tract narrowing (Fig. 9-21). Severe basal septal hypertrophy associated with severe aortic stenosis also may obstruct the outflow tract. Conventional transthoracic imaging may fail to make the diagnosis, although it should be suspected in the patient with left ventricular outflow obstruction by Doppler evaluation in the absence of impaired excursion of the aortic valve cusps on two-dimensional echocardiographic examination. Transesophageal echocardiographic examination allows clear visualization of the left ventricular outflow tract in the longitudinal plane from both the distal esophagus and the stomach and thereby usually clearly identifies the site and morphologic characteristics of left ventricular outflow tract obstruction [101–103].

Hemodynamic Assessment

The hemodynamic severity of aortic valvular stenosis is best evaluated by comprehensive transthoracic two-dimensional and Doppler echocardiography. The rare patients for whom transthoracic echocardiographic data are unreliable are usually referred for evaluation by cardiac catheterization. For rare patients in whom cardiac catheterization is not advisable, hemodynamic assessment of the severity of aortic stenosis may be accomplished by TEE [104].

Positioning the TEE transducer in the fundus of the stomach in an anteflexed longitudinal orientation provides a long-axis view of the left ventricular outflow tract, allowing continuous-wave interrogation of the aortic valve. In some patients the transvalvular mean gradient may be measurable by continuous-wave Doppler echocardiography (Fig. 9-22). Planimetry of the minimal aortic valve orifice area may be accomplished by short-axis imaging of the aortic valve (Fig. 9-23). Accurate estimation of aortic valve area by planimetry is possible in nearly 90% of patients with aortic stenosis who undergo TEE, and the estimate correlates fairly well with nonsimultaneous measurements of aortic valve area by both transthoracic echocardiography and cardiac catheterization [105].

Pressure gradient estimation by Doppler echocar-

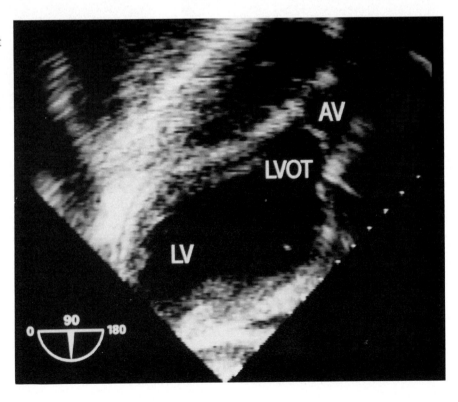

Fig. 9-20. Transgastric longitudinal long-axis view at 90 degrees multiplanar imaging. Anterior angulation can usually develop the left ventricular outflow tract and aortic valve in a projection suitable for pulsed- and continuous-wave Doppler interrogation of these structures.

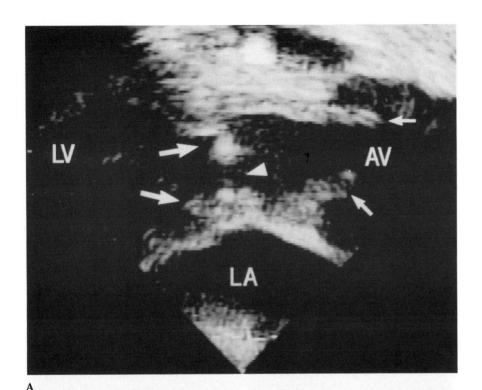

A

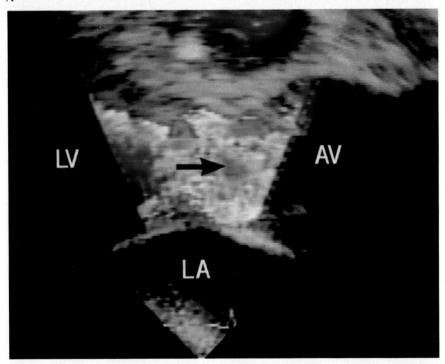

B

Fig. 9-21. Subvalvular left ventricular outflow obstruction; longitudinal left ventricular outflow view. A. Discrete subaortic stenosis is caused by a dense fibrous ring *(large arrows)* that severely constricts *(arrowhead)* the outflow tract at this level. The mildly thickened aortic valve cusps *(small arrows)* cause only minor stenosis at the valvular level. B. Color-flow Doppler imaging is consistent with significant subaortic stenosis; the normal laminar left ventricular outflow (orange-red) becomes highly turbulent (yellow-green mosaic) across the subaortic stenosis *(arrow).*

Fig. 9-22. Continuous-wave Doppler assessment of aortic valve stenosis. A. Transgastric longitudinal long-axis view. The Doppler cursor (fine dotted line, *small arrows*) is aligned with the left ventricular outflow tract and aortic valve *(large arrow)*. B. Continuous-wave Doppler imaging detects a maximal aortic valve velocity of 3.3 m/sec with a mean gradient of 24 mm Hg *(arrow)*, consistent with mild to moderate stenosis in the presence of normal left ventricular function. C. Modified longitudinal long-axis view at the gastroesophageal junction. The aortic valve cusps *(arrows)* are heavily calcified and nearly immobile during real-time examination. D. Continuous-wave Doppler examination reveals a peak aortic valve velocity of 4.7 m/sec, yielding a mean gradient of 56 mm Hg *(arrow)*, consistent with severe aortic stenosis. Note that this signal was obtained by interrogating the eccentric color Doppler jet just above the valve (see *sector insert)*. Not infrequently, the incident angles of interrogation limit Doppler evaluation of the aortic valve from all TEE windows.

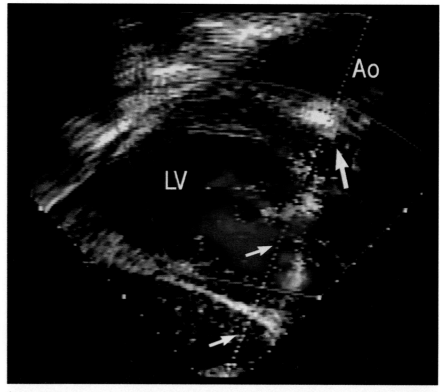

A

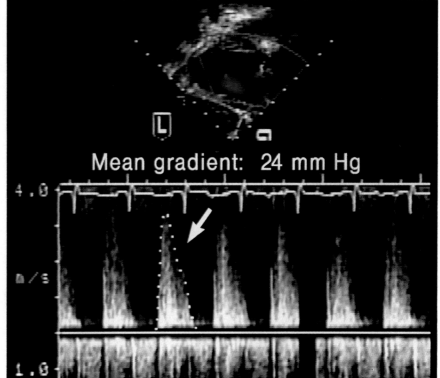

B

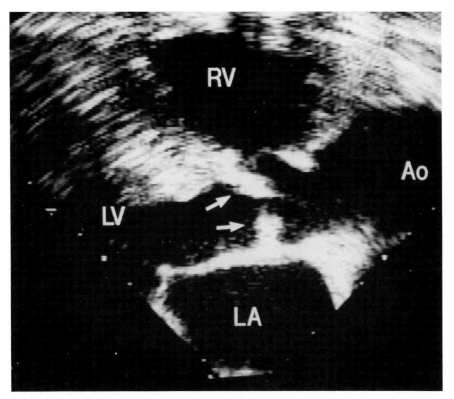

C

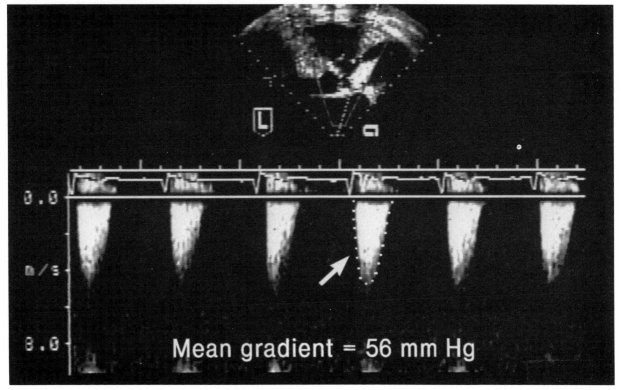

Mean gradient = 56 mm Hg

D

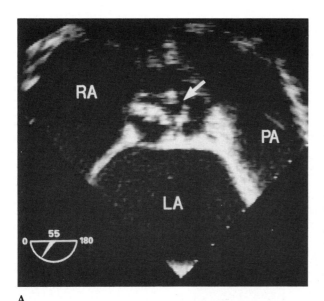
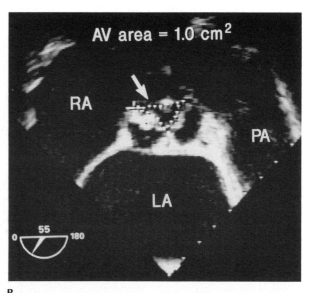

A   B

Fig. 9-23.   Evaluation of aortic stenosis by planimetered aortic valve area; multiplanar longitudinal short-axis imaging at 55 degrees. A. The minimal cross-sectional aortic orifice *(arrow)* is visualized by thorough tomographic short-axis imaging of the valve. The systolic excursion of all three cusps is moderately impaired. B. Planimetry along the inner commissural borders *(arrow)* yields an aortic valve area of 1.0 cm², consistent with moderate stenosis.

diography in aortic valvular stenosis requires measurement of the velocity of blood flow distal to the stenotic valve. This is accomplished by directing the continuous-wave ultrasound beam so that it is within the flow jet and parallel to the velocity vector of transvalvular blood flow. It is often not possible to accomplish this maneuver on TEE because of the orientation of the interrogating ultrasound beam to the orifice of the aortic valve. When a suitable interrogating path is obtained by TEE, analysis of the transvalvular aortic velocity is identical to that performed in the transthoracic examination. Continuous-wave Doppler echocardiography enables estimation of maximal instantaneous and mean transvalvular pressure gradients by application of the modified Bernoulli equation [27]. Only if adequate transgastric windows are available for pulsed- and continuous-wave Doppler evaluation of the left ventricular outflow tract and aortic valve, respectively, can the aortic valve area be assessed by the continuity equation.

Indications for and Role of TEE

Transesophageal echocardiography is not routinely indicated for the evaluation of the patient in whom aortic valvular stenosis has been adequately assessed by transthoracic imaging and hemodynamic evalua-

tion. Its role is limited to the rare patient in whom transthoracic echocardiographic data are inadequate and cardiac catheterization is not possible. Perhaps the greatest uses of TEE in patients with valvular aortic stenosis are for assessment of coexistent mitral valvular or thoracic aortic disease and for the evaluation of suspected infective endocarditis.

However, TEE is useful for resolution of the differential diagnosis of left ventricular outflow obstruction, especially if subaortic obstruction is suspected. Identification of a discrete subaortic membrane or narrowing of the outflow tract as an isolated finding or associated with aortic valvular disease may obviate invasive investigation and aid the cardiac surgeon in devising optimal surgical therapy.

Transesophageal echocardiography is also a useful adjunct for the assessment of the now rare patient considered a candidate for aortic balloon valvuloplasty [106,107]. Transesophageal echocardiographic evaluation allows detailed assessment of cusp function before the procedure and enables direct visualization of the balloon for optimal transannular balloon placement. It also allows immediate assessment of cusp motion after valvuloplasty, eliminates repetitive angiography for assessment of aortic regurgitation, and precludes further dilatation with potentially deleterious larger-sized balloons.

AORTIC REGURGITATION

Aortic regurgitation is classified as either acquired or congenital and is due to disease of the valve or the aortic root or a combination thereof. Regurgitation is subclassified as acute or chronic, each form with characteristic M-mode, two-dimensional, and Doppler echocardiographic findings [108–110]. Two-dimensional echocardiography identifies the anatomic abnormality underlying regurgitation and, hence, forms the basis of diagnostic classification.

Evaluation of the patient with aortic valve regurgitation by TEE requires morphologic assessment of the valve in short-axis and longitudinal planes and complete evaluation of the thoracic aorta. As described for the examination of the patient with aortic valvular stenosis, leftward rotation of the TEE probe in the longitudinal plane from neutral position in the mid esophagus, with slight left or right lateral flexion of the transducer tip, provides a long-axis view of the left ventricular outflow tract that enables assessment of structure and motion of aortic valve cusps and the ascending aorta. This view is also optimal for color-flow imaging assessment of the semiquantitative severity of aortic regurgitation (see below). Rightward lateral flexion of the transducer tip in this plane provides a short-axis view of the valve cusps, enabling assessment of cusp number and structure, and also provides an imaging plane for estimation of the regurgitant orifice area by color-flow Doppler mapping.

In the long-axis view, the caliber and anatomy of the ascending aorta are assessed. Leftward and rightward rotation of the TEE probe effects a tomographic sweep of the lumen of the ascending aorta, optimizing detection of anatomic abnormalities, most notably aneurysm formation or aortic dissection.

Infective endocarditis may cause aortic valve regurgitation due to either vegetations that prevent proper leaflet coaptation or damage to the leaflets by perforation, prolapse, or flail [46]. Combined two-dimensional and color flow imaging are used to characterize the anatomic abnormalities (see Chapter 11, Figure 11-15). Valvular vegetations less than 3 mm in diameter frequently are not identified by transthoracic echocardiography, especially if there is sclerosis, calcification, or myxomatous degeneration of the cusps. Transesophageal echocardiography greatly increases the sensitivity and specificity for the detection of vegetations because of enhanced image resolution made possible by the proximity of the high-frequency transducer to the heart. In combination with color-flow imaging, TEE is useful for localization of the regurgitant jet to the central valvular orifice or perivalvular region. Furthermore, TEE greatly enhances diagnosis of perivalvular abscess and other complications of endocarditis [43] (see Chapter 11).

Enlargement of the aortic root is frequently associated with aortic regurgitation, regardless of cause. Aortic root dilatation may be primary (Fig. 9-24) and cause regurgitation or may be acquired as a consequence of increased flow. Acquired aortic root dilatation causing regurgitation may be accompanied by dilation of the annulus with associated inadequate diastolic valve leaflet coaptation. Other acquired disorders of the aortic root associated with aortic regurgitation are disruption of the aortic apparatus due to aortic dissection and ruptured sinus of Valsalva aneurysm. Dilatation of an aortic sinus associated with a sinus of Valsalva aneurysm may cause prolapse of an aortic cusp and significant aortic regurgitation.

The association of acute valvular aortic regurgitation and dilatation of the aortic root or ascending aorta suggests aortic dissection (Fig. 9-25). The diagnostic sensitivity and specificity of transthoracic echocardiography in the detection of aortic dissection is approximately 80% [111]; the transesophageal approach increases sensitivity and specificity to nearly 99% [111]. Accordingly, TEE has become a diagnostic procedure of choice for the detection of aortic dissection. Retrograde dissection may disrupt the aortic valve apparatus to produce a prolapsing or flail aortic cusp (see Chapter 14). Transesophageal echocardiography should be routinely performed in patients with suspected aortic dissection not clearly demonstrated by transthoracic imaging. Biplane and multiplane imaging probes increase diagnostic sensitivity and specificity by enabling complete visualization of the entire ascending aorta [17].

Rheumatic disease of the aortic valve produces increased leaflet thickening, retraction, and commissural fusion, often causing combined regurgitation and stenosis [112]. Leaflet calcification is prominent if stenosis is present. Characteristic echocardiographic features are increased leaflet thickness, calcification, reduced leaflet excursion, and systolic cusp doming when less than severe stenosis is present. Incomplete diastolic leaflet coaptation may be present, with aortic regurgitation detected at locations of cusp malcoaptation on color Doppler imaging in the short-axis plane.

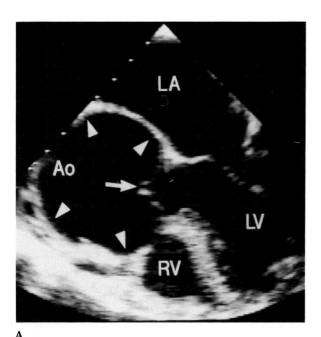
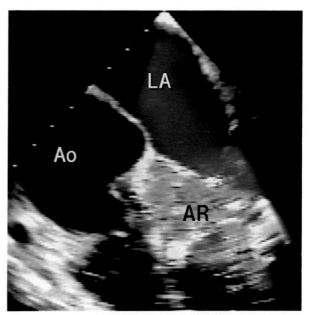

A   **B**

Fig. 9-24. Aortic regurgitation due to aortic dilatation. A. There is severe annuloaortic ectasia *(arrowheads)* with severe dilatation of the aortic root and proximal ascending aorta *(Ao)* to maximal caliber of nearly 6.5 cm. This aneurysmal enlargement has drawn the aortic cusps taut and apart, producing incomplete central diastolic coaptation *(arrow)*. B. Resultant torrential aortic regurgitation fills the entire left ventricular outflow tract on color-flow imaging. This patient had Marfan's syndrome.

Fig. 9-25. Aortic regurgitation complicating aortic dissection; longitudinal long-axis imaging. A. Massive enlargement *(arrowheads)* of the ascending aorta *(Ao)* has been produced by proximal (type A) aortic dissection; a transverse intimal flap *(small arrows)* originates near the sinutubular junction. The aortic cusps have been stretched with loss of diastolic coaptation *(large arrow)*. B. Severe central aortic regurgitation *(large arrow)* fills the left ventricular outflow tract. There is no diastolic prolapse of the intimal flap *(small arrows)*; such prolapse may impinge on or pass through the aortic valve, also causing aortic regurgitation.

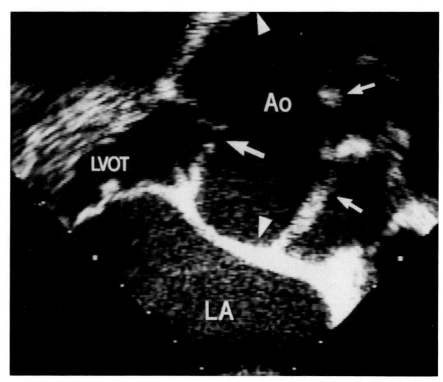

A

Congenital disorders associated with aneurysmal dilatation of the aortic root and secondary aortic regurgitation include Marfan's syndrome and Ehlers-Danlos syndrome [113,114]. In the adult with Marfan's syndrome the aortic root may be massively dilated and the aortic walls thinned. The annulus, sinuses of Valsalva, and aorta are often severely dilated in a "pear-shaped" configuration of annuloaortic ectasia. The aortic cusps are stretched and enlarged yet are often unable to occlude the aortic valve orifice, producing characteristic central aortic regurgitation (see Fig. 9-24).

Hemodynamic Evaluation

In aortic regurgitation, reversal of diastolic flow occurs in the left ventricular outflow tract with the primary velocity vector opposite to normal systolic outflow. Typically, it is holodiastolic and of high velocity, corresponding to the large diastolic pressure gradient between the aorta and the left ventricle. Assessment of the severity of aortic regurgitation by TEE is facilitated by color-flow imaging and is based on the spatial extent of detected regurgitation in the immediate subvalvular left ventricular outflow tract [101].

Ideally, orthogonal imaging planes should be used to characterize the extent of regurgitation, requiring examination by biplane or multiplane TEE. Orthogonal imaging planes are used to characterize the severity of regurgitation in both longitudinal long-axis and short-axis planes. Long-axis examination can be performed with the endoscope tip in neutral position in the mid esophagus and the imaging transducer oriented in the longitudinal array. Rightward rotation from the longitudinal left ventricular inflow view with mild left lateral flexion images the longitudinal long-axis projection of the left ventricular outflow tract, aortic valve, and proximal ascending aorta. Optimal visualization of the aortic valve cusps in the long-axis view frequently requires slight leftward or rightward lateral motion of the transducer tip. Optimal two-dimensional demonstration of the aortic valve cusps in true short axis is obtained by rightward flexion of the transducer tip in the longitudinal plane.

Aortic regurgitant flow appears as a turbulent mosaic signal extending from the aortic valve into the left ventricular outflow tract and left ventricular cavity during diastole. Various measures of the color jet dimension have been described in the estimation of severity, including subvalvular jet width from

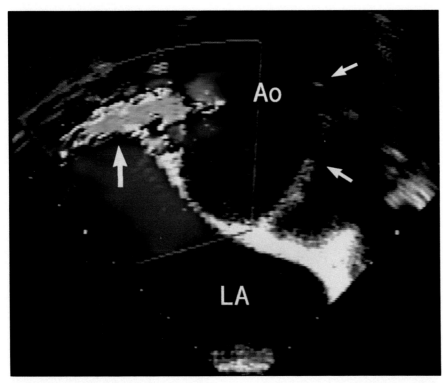

B

the longitudinal plane (Fig. 9-26) and area in the immediate subvalvular short-axis plane. On transthoracic examination, the immediate subvalvular width of the color jet in the long-axis view or the area dimension in the short-axis view have been demonstrated to correlate well with angiographic determination of regurgitant severity [115]. This correlation has been attributed to the relationship of the proximal dimension of the regurgitant orifice to the true regurgitant orifice area. In transthoracic color-flow assessment of aortic valve regurgitation, Perry et al. [115] used a ratio of the minimal subvalvular regurgitant jet width divided by left ventricular outflow tract width in the parasternal long-axis view (analogous to the TEE longitudinal long-axis view of the left ventricular outflow tract). They described four grades of aortic regurgitation by color-flow imaging; using this method, with aortography as the standard for comparison, these investigators correctly classified the severity of regurgitation in more than 90% of patients. Grade I (mild) aortic valve regurgitation corresponded to a ratio of less than 0.25; grade II (moderate), from 0.25 to 0.46; grade III (moderately severe), from 0.47 to 0.64; and grade IV (severe), 0.65 or greater. Semiquantitation of aortic regurgitation by such measurements is appropriate only with centrally directed jets in which the immediate subvalvular jet dimension can be well defined; this is usually not possible with eccentric regurgitant jets.

Instrumentation factors potentially limiting color-flow imaging include variation of the spatial extent of the color jet with transducer frequency, gain settings, and pulse repetition frequency. Physiologic factors not directly related to the severity of regurgitation that may affect the dimensions of the regurgitant jet (particularly length) include the driving diastolic pressure of the aorta, compliance of the left ventricle, duration of diastole, and left ventricular end-diastolic pressure [115,116]. Moreover, color-flow imaging is operator-dependent; small alterations in transducer angulation may substantially influence the dimensions of the regurgitant jet. The dimensions of the regurgitant jet must be maximized in orthogonal planes to avoid underestimation of the severity of the hemodynamic abnormality.

Eccentric aortic regurgitant jets impinging on the walls of the left ventricular outflow tract are difficult to characterize by the color Doppler mapping methods above, and additional quantitative Doppler methods are required to establish severity of regurgitation.

Quantitative methods for the assessment of the severity of aortic regurgitation include analysis of the continuous-wave Doppler profile of regurgita-

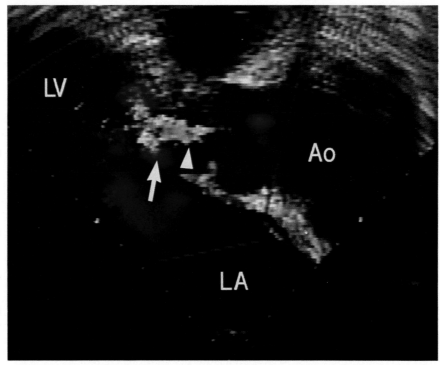

Fig. 9-26. Color Doppler evaluation of aortic regurgitation; longitudinal long-axis view. Measurement of the width of central aortic regurgitant jets on long-axis imaging of the left ventricular outflow tract provides semiquantitation of aortic regurgitation, which correlates well with angiographic methods. The jet should be measured in the immediate subvalvular region *(arrowhead),* as it may broaden considerably *(arrow)* further into the left ventricle. In this patient, the ratio of jet to outflow tract was approximately 0.2, consistent with mild (grade I/IV) aortic regurgitation (see text for details). *(Ao = ascending aorta.)*

tion and measurement of regurgitant fraction and regurgitant volume. Doppler echocardiographic methods for the evaluation of regurgitant orifice area have also been described.

Continuous-wave echocardiography has been used to measure the velocity of aortic regurgitant blood flow throughout diastole, so that the rate of pressure decay between aorta and left ventricle can be estimated. According to the principles of Bernoulli hemodynamics, the pressure gradient across a restricting orifice is proportional to the square of the Doppler velocity. The deceleration slope of the aortic regurgitant signal detected by continuous-wave Doppler imaging reflects the severity of regurgitation in the absence of significant left ventricular dysfunction or rapid peripheral runoff. In mild aortic regurgitation, aortic diastolic pressure decays slowly, left ventricular pressure rises slowly, and a large pressure gradient persists at end-diastole. Accordingly, the Doppler profile of aortic regurgitant velocity also decays slowly through diastole. In severe aortic regurgitation, in contrast, a rapid decrease in pressure gradient between aorta and left ventricle corresponds to a rapid collapse of aortic diastolic pressure and a simultaneous rapid increase in the left ventricular diastolic pressure. This is reflected by a rapidly decreasing aortic regurgitant velocity profile on Doppler assessment.

The rate of pressure decline can be quantified by the pressure half-time method. Accuracy of the Doppler echocardiographic method to derive pressure half-time has been clinically validated by simultaneous Doppler echocardiography and catheterization studies [90]. If other causes of increased left ventricular diastolic filling pressures are absent, pressure half-time measurement by Doppler echocardiography correlates well with the severity of aortic regurgitation assessed by semiquantitative angiography [117,118]. A pressure half-time of less than 300 msec is usually indicative of severe regurgitation, whereas a pressure half-time of greater than 600 msec is consistent with mild aortic regurgitation [118]. Other conditions, such as severe left ventricular systolic or diastolic dysfunction, increase left ventricular end-diastolic pressure and may cause overestimation of the severity of aortic regurgitation by this method because of more rapid decline of the difference in diastolic pressure between aorta and left ventricle [118].

Limitations of the analysis of a continuous-wave Doppler profile of aortic regurgitation by the transesophageal approach may be considerable. As discussed with aortic stenosis, continuous-wave Doppler analysis of the aortic valve depends on adequate transgastric longitudinal long-axis views that minimize the angles of incidence of the interrogating beam to the aortic regurgitant jet (Fig. 9-27).

Quantitative assessment of the severity of aortic regurgitation is also possible by use of combined two-dimensional and Doppler echocardiography for the measurement of either regurgitant fraction or regurgitant volume. Estimation of regurgitant fraction or regurgitant volume requires estimates of total stroke volume and forward stroke volume. The difference between the two measures represents regurgitant stroke volume, and regurgitant fraction is obtained by dividing the regurgitant stroke volume by the total stroke volume [82,83]. The total stroke volume is obtained by two-dimensional echocardiographic measurement of the left ventricular outflow tract area and multiplication of this value by the time velocity integral of left ventricular outflow measured by pulsed-wave Doppler echocardiography. Forward stroke volume is similarily measured by evaluation of a nondiseased mitral or pulmonary valve. In practice, forward stroke volume may be estimated by two-dimensional echocardiographic measurement of the right ventricular outflow tract area and multiplication of the result by the time velocity integral of right ventricular outflow measured by pulsed-wave Doppler echocardiography. Limitations of the echocardiographic determination of regurgitant fraction or regurgitant volume include the ability to obtain adequate left ventricular outflow pulsed-wave Doppler signals, coexistent stenotic or regurgitant disease affecting other valves, and intracardiac or extracardiac shunts. Regurgitant orifice area may be derived by applying the continuity equation to diastolic flow signals associated with aortic regurgitation at the supravalvular and subvalvular levels [119]. This method requires further clinical validation.

Although echocardiographic methods for the estimation of regurgitant fraction and regurgitant volume correlate well with invasive techniques, the quantitative methods are not used routinely in clinical practice because of technical limitations and measurement error associated with the invasive methods that have served as reference standards. Traditionally, quantitative assessment of the severity of regurgitation by invasive techniques has been used to provide a semiquantitative category of regurgitant severity (mild, moderate, severe) rather than true volumetric assessment. The chief limitation of

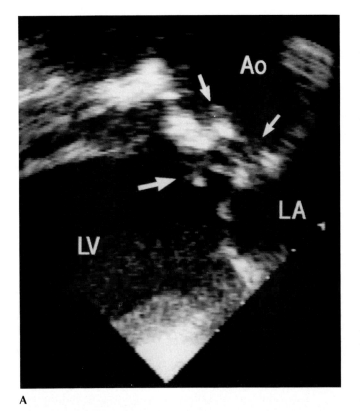

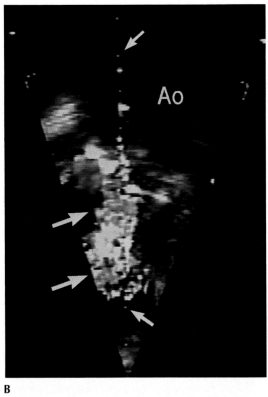

A

B

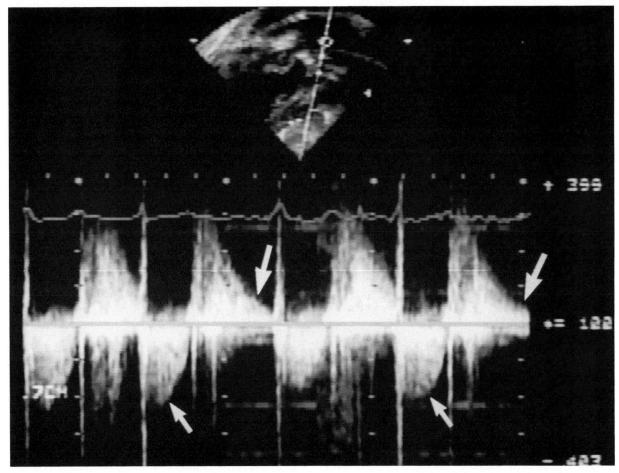

C

Fig. 9-27. ◄ Continuous-wave Doppler assessment of aortic regurgitation; transgastric long-axis view. A. The aortic valve is calcified, with several vegetations on its aortic aspects *(small arrows)*, and a lobulated vegetation prolapses into the left ventricular outflow tract *(large arrow)*. B. Color Doppler imaging demonstrates a broad eccentric jet of aortic regurgitation *(large arrows)*. The Doppler cursor (dotted line, *small arrows*) is aligned coaxially with the regurgitant jet. C. Continuous-wave Doppler study reveals an aortic regurgitant signal with precipitous runoff and an end-diastolic velocity of approximately 1 m/sec *(large arrows)*. The aortic regurgitant diastolic pressure half-time was less than 200 msec, consistent with rapid decay of the diastolic aorta-left ventricular pressure gradient with near end-diastolic pressure equilibration due to very severe aortic regurgitation. Continuous-wave Doppler imaging from this position also reveals insignificant aortic valve functional stenosis, with a systolic velocity of 2.2 m/sec *(small arrows)*. (Ao = ascending aorta.)

the clinical implementation of noninvasive estimates of regurgitant fraction or regurgitant volume has been the lack of a reliable method to establish a precedent for routine use in clinical decision-making.

Indications for and Role of TEE and Clinical Decision-Making

The primary use of TEE in the assessment of aortic regurgitation is to establish the cause of regurgitation. Generally, the semiquantitative severity of aortic valve regurgitation can be established by comprehensive transthoracic Doppler echocardiography. Acoustic shadowing of the left ventricular outflow tract by significant calcification of the mitral apparatus or by a mitral prosthesis presents a major limitation to the evaluation of aortic regurgitation by even multiplane TEE. In some patients, the degree of aortic regurgitation is not appreciated by either physical examination or transthoracic echocardiography. In a higher proportion of patients, these methods may underestimate the severity of established aortic valve regurgitation, which can be more precisely semiquantitated by TEE.

Because of the high-resolution imaging obtained by the TEE technique, particularly of the proximal thoracic aorta, the transesophageal method more reliably defines the cause of aortic valve regurgitation. Transesophageal echocardiography may be useful in the preoperative assessment of the aorta for patients in whom resection or repair of the aortic root is contemplated.

TRICUSPID STENOSIS AND REGURGITATION

The tricuspid valve is larger and more complex than the mitral valve. It consists of three leaflets, an annular ring, and subvalvular components, including chordae tendineae, papillary muscles, and subjacent right ventricular myocardium. It is differentiated from the mitral valve by its trileaflet structure, multiple separate papillary muscles, and annular septal insertion inferior to the mitral annulus [120].

As in mitral stenosis, tricuspid stenosis is characterized by reduced orifice dimension, which impairs right ventricular filling. Obstruction to right ventricular inflow may be due to congenital or acquired disease and may be primarily valvular, subvalvular, or supravalvular in location [6]. Regardless of cause, tricuspid stenosis is frequently associated with tricuspid regurgitation.

Tricuspid valve regurgitation may be due to either intrinsic valvular disease or tricuspid annular enlargement. Functional tricuspid regurgitation is caused by right ventricular volume or pressure overload of any cause with associated dilatation of the right ventricle and the tricuspid annulus. Valvular abnormalities producing tricuspid regurgitation are associated with many diseases because of the anatomic and functional complexity of the valve apparatus.

Rheumatic heart disease is the most common cause of tricuspid stenosis. Stenosis is produced by leaflet fibrosis, commissural fusion, fibrosis, and by increased thickness of the chordae. In tricuspid valve stenosis, unlike in mitral valve stenosis, calcification of the valve apparatus is unusual. Tricuspid regurgitation and rheumatic mitral valvular disease are virtually always also present. Abnormal leaflet motion is characterized by doming at maximal diastolic excursion (Fig. 9-28). Uncommon causes of valvular tricuspid stenosis include carcinoid, methysergide toxicity, and endomyocardial fibrosis [121–124]. Each of these disorders also causes significant tricuspid regurgitation, and, in general, the typical functional abnormality is combined stenosis and regurgitation.

Two-dimensional echocardiographic assessment may not always discriminate among the various causes of combined stenosis and regurgitation, as each is characterized by a thickened valve and shortened and fibrotic supporting structures. In severe cases of carcinoid-induced valvular disease, the tricuspid valve is fixed and immobilized in a semiopen position (Fig. 9-29); such findings would be very

unusual for rheumatic disease but can be seen with methysergide toxicity. Associated morphologic abnormalities generally suggest specific diagnoses; in rheumatic disease, there is virtually always associated mitral valve disease, whereas in carcinoid and methysergide toxicity, combined pulmonic stenosis and regurgitation is frequent. Similarly, endomyocardial fibrosis is associated with thrombotic obliteration of the ventricular apices.

Isolated tricuspid regurgitation generally is associated with degenerative disease with prolapse, endocarditis (uncommonly), and Ebstein's anomaly (rarely). Endocarditis is relatively uncommon but when present may be associated with large vegetations and flail motion of the valvular apparatus (see Chapter 11, Figure 11-7) [125,126]. An unusual cause of tricuspid regurgitation that may be recognized by TEE is traumatic rupture of chordae tendineae or papillary muscles [127] (Fig. 9-30). If the regurgitation is chronic and severe, there is associ-

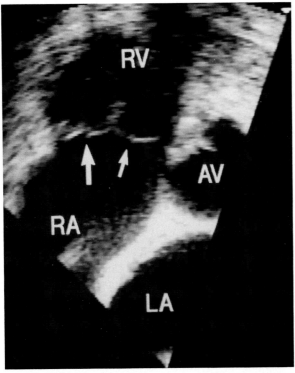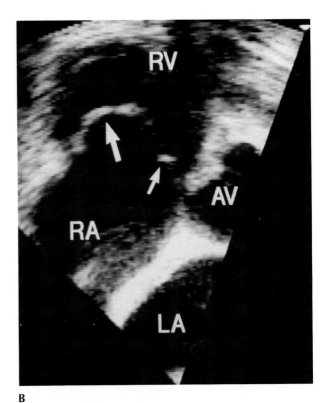

A

B

Fig. 9-28. Rheumatic tricuspid valve stenosis; longitudinal short-axis view. A. During systole, there is normal coaptation of the moderately thickened anterior leaflet *(large arrow)* and mildly thickened septal leaflet *(small arrow)*. B. Prominent doming of the pliable anterior leaflet *(large arrow)* is observed during diastole; the septal leaflet *(small arrow)* is mildly tethered, with decreased diastolic excursion without doming.

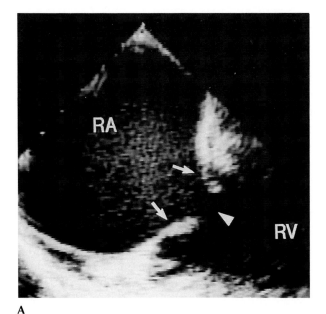
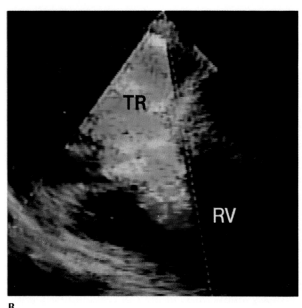

A   B

Fig. 9-29.   Advanced carcinoid tricuspid valve disease; right ventricular inflow view in the transverse plane. A. The septal and anterior tricuspid leaflets *(arrows)* are severely thickened, retracted, and fixed in a semiopen position, resulting in gross deficiency of central systolic coaptation *(arrowhead)*. Depending on the degree of leaflet rigidity and retraction, various degrees of tricuspid stenosis may be present; in contrast to rheumatic tricuspid stenosis, there is no diastolic doming of the leaflets. B. Color-flow Doppler imaging demonstrates severe central tricuspid regurgitation passing through the fixed open tricuspid orifice.

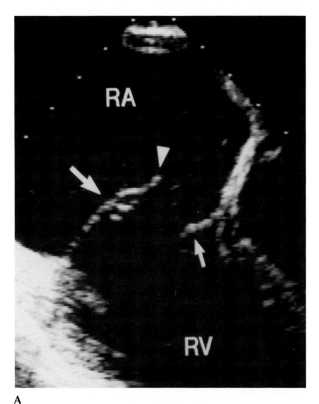
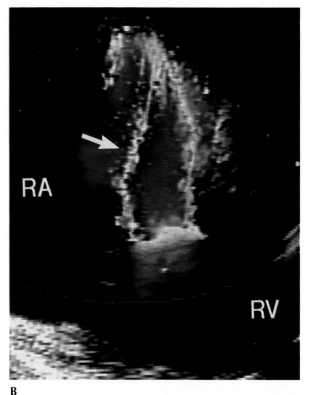

A   B

Fig. 9-30.   Traumatic tricuspid valve disease; right ventricular inflow view in the transverse plane. A. A large flail segment of the anterior tricuspid leaflet *(large arrow)* is present, and a small ruptured chordal segment *(arrowhead)* is visible. There is complete lack of coaptation with the septal leaflet *(small arrow)* in this view. This was a chronic lesion caused by trauma incurred during a motor vehicle accident several years before recognition by echocardiography. The right ventricle and right atrium are severely enlarged because of volume overload. B. Free posteromedial tricuspid regurgitation is shown on color Doppler imaging. Because of the large regurgitant orifice, there is nonturbulent, laminar tricuspid regurgitant flow *(arrow)* between the right ventricle and the atrium during systole; a large region of central aliasing (deep blue) is seen within the regurgitant jet.

ated right atrial and ventricular enlargement. In Ebstein's anomaly, the congenital abnormality of the tricuspid valve is characterized by ventricular displacement of deformed and variably tethered tricuspid leaflets (see Chapter 13).

As in the assessment of other valvular disease, examination is best performed from multiple imaging planes. The tricuspid valve is generally best observed in the transverse plane from the distal esophagus with the endoscope tip in neutral position. In this imaging plane, the septal and anterior leaflets are visualized; the posterior leaflet is seen with transducer tip retroflexion imaging at the level of the coronary sinus. Most of the right ventricular cavity is usually observed, although the subvalvular apparatus may not be seen well. From the longitudinal plane, rightward rotation from the left ventricular two-chamber view yields the foreshortened right ventricular cavity, and further rightward rotation demonstrates the tricuspid apparatus and right ventricular outflow tract, including the pulmonic valve (see Chapter 3, Figure 3-12). This tomographic plane of examination yields an appearance similar to that obtained by standard transthoracic imaging in the parasternal short-axis view at the base of the heart. This view generally yields more optimal orientation for Doppler interrogation of the tricuspid valve, because both antegrade and retrograde flows through the valve orifice are often oriented nearly parallel to the interrogating Doppler beam.

The tricuspid valve may also be imaged from the longitudinal and short-axis planes with the endoscope tip in the stomach. In this view, modified (off-axis) short-axis and long-axis views of the tricuspid valve can be obtained. These views are useful for characterization of the extent of valvular and, particularly, subvalvular disease (Fig. 9-31).

Hemodynamic Evaluation of Tricuspid Valvular Disease

On transesophageal examination, optimal transtricuspid flow signals are generally obtained from a modified longitudinal short-axis view by rightward rotation of the TEE probe. Other views, including the transverse four-chamber view from the distal esophagus and views from the stomach, are generally not as useful because of increased angles of incidence of the Doppler beam and tricuspid valve.

Normal tricuspid valve inflow is qualitatively similar to mitral inflow but of lesser velocities due to a larger valve orifice area. Tricuspid stenosis creates

increased velocity associated with an increased gradient from right atrium to right ventricle throughout diastole (Fig. 9-32). Pressure gradients are reliably estimated by continuous-wave Doppler findings similar to those observed in mitral stenosis.

If systematically sought, tricuspid regurgitation is detected in more than 90% of normal individuals and is attributed to normal physiologic (subclinical) tricuspid regurgitation. These regurgitant jets are easily differentiated from pathologic regurgitation and recognized as physiologic because they are very localized in extent and correspond to a tiny volume of regurgitant flow. Tricuspid regurgitation assessed by color-flow imaging has a mosaic appearance similar to that of mitral regurgitation. The regurgitant flow signal originates at the valve annulus and extends into the body of the right atrium. The trajectory of the tricuspid regurgitant jet in the right atrium is usually directed centrally because of symmetrical annular dilatation or posteromedially because of relative override of the predominant anterior leaflet.

Validation of the accuracy of color-flow imaging for the assessment of the severity of tricuspid regurgitation is not possible because there is no reliable reference standard. If the right heart chambers are of normal dimension, the likelihood of significant tricuspid regurgitation is low unless it is acute. Conversely, patients with severe tricuspid regurgitation that is chronic typically have enlarged right heart chambers consistent with volume overload, with a broad jet of regurgitation occupying most of the right atrium. With free tricuspid regurgitation, there is often mid-to-late systolic pressure equilibration between the right atrium and the right ventricle. In this case, the regurgitant signal has much less turbulence on color-flow Doppler imaging and may even be laminar (see Fig. 9-30).

Hemodynamic Assessment of Right Ventricular Systolic Pressure by Doppler Echocardiography

Continuous-wave Doppler echocardiographic characterization of tricuspid regurgitation enables noninvasive quantitative estimation of right ventricular systolic pressure and pulmonary artery pressure in patients without right ventricular outflow obstruction [128].

The velocity of the tricuspid regurgitant jet is related to the systolic right ventricular-right atrial pressure gradient by the principles of Bernoulli hydrodynamics [27,128]. The systolic maximum in-

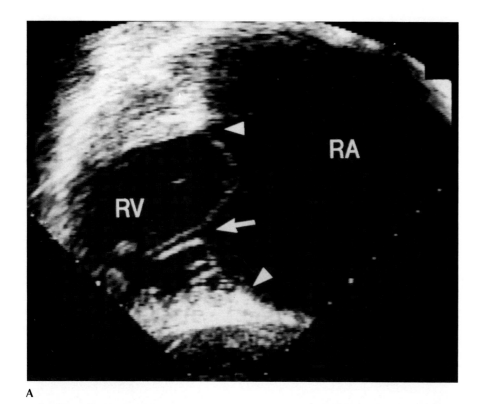

A

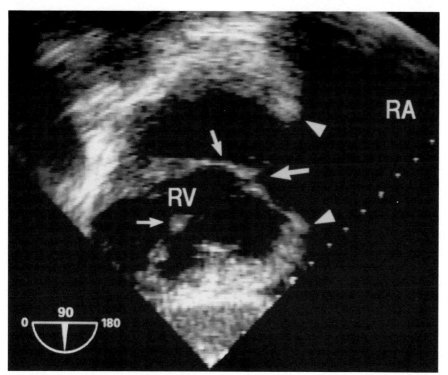

B

Fig. 9-31. Tricuspid valve evaluation; transgastric longitudinal long-axis view. A. Severe tricuspid annular dilatation *(arrowheads)* to a dimension of nearly 5.5 cm in this view results in incomplete central systolic coaptation *(arrow)* of the leaflets. The right ventricle is severely enlarged and the right atrium is giant (>80 mm) because of chronic severe tricuspid regurgitation and volume overload. B. Multiplanar imaging at 90 degrees. Thickened chordae with fusion *(small arrows)* are noted in this patient with rheumatic tricuspid valve disease. The tricuspid annulus is moderately dilated *(arrowheads)*, and loss of central leaflet coaptation *(large arrow)* due to leaflet retraction causes severe tricuspid regurgitation.

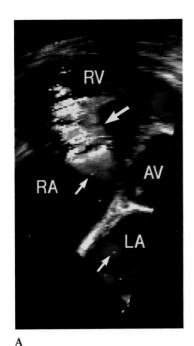
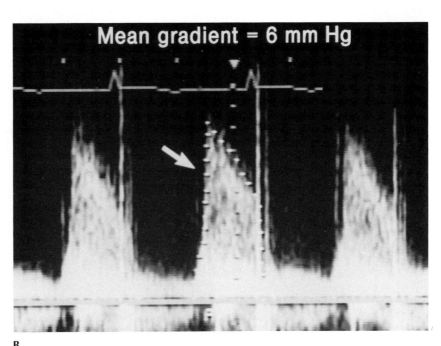

A   B

Fig. 9–32.   Evaluation of rheumatic tricuspid valve stenosis by continuous-wave Doppler imaging; longitudinal short-axis view (same patient as that in Figure 9-28). A. The Doppler cursor (dotted line, *small arrows*) is aligned with the turbulent tricuspid inflow *(large arrow)* detected on color Doppler imaging. B. Continuous-wave Doppler study reveals an early diastolic inflow velocity of 1.6 m/sec with a mean gradient of 6 mm Hg *(arrow)* consistent with mild to moderate tricuspid stenosis.

stantaneous right ventricular-right atrial pressure gradient is estimated by application of the modified Bernoulli equation and velocity data obtained by continuous-wave Doppler echocardiography and added to a regression-equation-derived estimate of right atrial pressure [128] (see Figs. 9-7 and 9-8). The right ventricular systolic pressure (RVSP) is hence obtained by the equation

$$RVSP = 4(V_{TR})^2 + RAP$$

in which V_{TR} is the maximal tricuspid regurgitant velocity and RAP is the estimated right atrial pressure.

Role of TEE

Transesophageal echocardiography is seldom indicated as the primary diagnostic modality in the assessment of isolated tricuspid valvular disease because in the vast majority of patients with significant tricuspid valve disease, a complete morphologic and hemodynamic assessment can be obtained by the transthoracic technique. Transesophageal echocardiography can be very useful in patients with

inadequate transthoracic acoustic windows and also can exclude associated abnormalities, such as an intracardiac shunt, and determine right ventricular systolic pressures.

PULMONARY VALVE STENOSIS AND REGURGITATION

Acquired pulmonic valve disease is extremely uncommon in adult patients. Most often, pulmonary valve stenosis or significant pulmonary valve regurgitation is associated with congenital heart disease recognized in childhood. However, an increasing adult population with treated congenital heart disease may come under the care of the adult cardiologist.

Congenital pulmonic valve stenosis (Fig. 9-33) may occur in isolation or be associated with other congenital cardiac abnormalities [129]. Acquired disease in the pulmonic valve in adult patients is usually associated with combined stenosis and regurgitation due to either rheumatic disease or carcinoid [130]. Rheumatic disease should be suspected

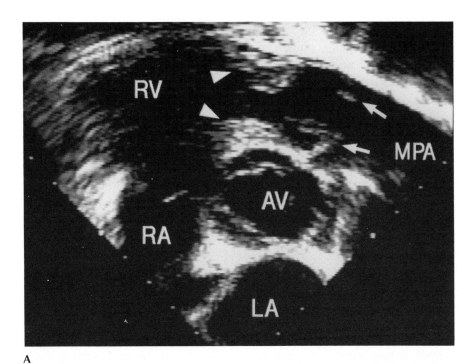

A

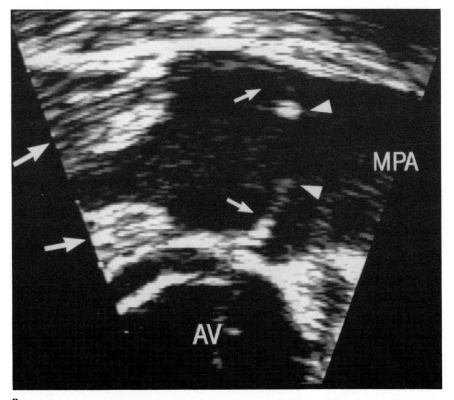

B

Fig. 9-33.   Congenital pulmonary valvular stenosis; longitudinal short-axis view. A. Prominent systolic doming of the pliable and mildly thickened pulmonary valve cusps *(arrows)* is present. Note the distal infundibular muscular stenosis *(arrowheads)* just proximal to the pulmonary valve. B. Magnified view of the pulmonary valve. The characteristic systolic doming of the cusps *(small arrows)* and the stenotic valvular orifice *(arrowheads)* are well visualized. The distal infundibular stenosis *(large arrows)* also contributes to right ventricular outflow obstruction.

in the patient in whom typical left-sided valvular abnormalities are consistent with rheumatic valvular disease. In contrast, carcinoid heart disease is typically isolated to the right side of the heart (unless a right-to-left intracardiac shunt exists), with pulmonary valve involvement (Fig. 9-34) almost always occurring only if obvious carcinoid tricuspid valvular disease (see Fig. 9-29) is present [121,122].

Pulmonic valvular regurgitation is most often functional and due to underlying pulmonary hypertension of any cause. Endocarditis of the pulmonic valve is rare but may be best detected by TEE [131]. The pulmonary valve is best visualized in the longitudinal short-axis plane, a view similar to the parasternal basal short-axis image on transthoracic echocardiography. In this view, pulmonic outflow is nearly perpendicular to the trajectory of interrogating ultrasound, so that steerable pulsed- or continuous-wave Doppler study of the pulmonary valve is impossible. Pulmonary valve stenosis is suspected

on the basis of two-dimensional imaging if systolic doming and reduced excursion of the cusps are observed (see Fig. 9-33). Morphologic abnormalities associated with pulmonic valve regurgitation include vegetations in endocarditis or valve leaflets fixed in a semiopen position with annular contraction in advanced carcinoid pulmonic disease (Fig. 9-34). Abnormalities of the right heart associated with lesions of the pulmonic valve include chamber enlargement that depends on the duration and severity of the hemodynamic abnormality. Concentric right ventricular hypertrophy is anticipated with long-standing severe pulmonic stenosis.

Hemodynamic Evaluation

Pulmonary valve stenosis causes alteration in blood flow velocity qualitatively similar to that observed in other valvular stenoses and can be evaluated from the transthoracic Doppler approach. However, quan-

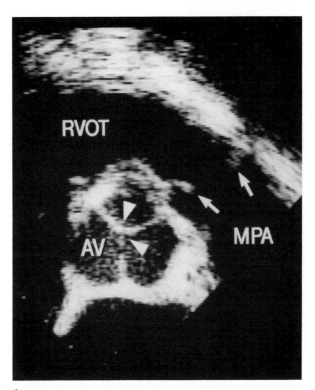
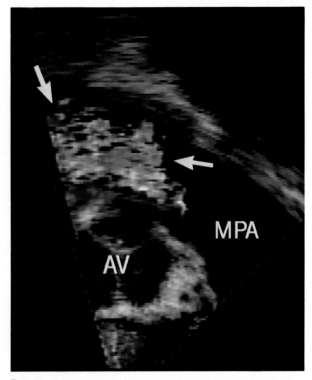

A   **B**

Fig. 9-34. Advanced carcinoid pulmonary valvular disease; longitudinal short-axis view. A. The pulmonary valve cusps *(arrows)* are moderately thickened with marked retraction; minimal mobility of the cusps was detected on real-time examination. This is a diastolic frame with the aortic valve cusps closed *(arrowheads)*. B. Resultant severe pulmonary regurgitation *(arrows)* fills the entire right ventricular outflow tract during diastole.

titative assessment of the peak transpulmonic gradient by TEE is not possible because of orthogonal orientation of the Doppler interrogating beam to the pulmonary outflow tract from all esophageal and transgastric positions.

Color-flow imaging may detect pulmonic regurgitation, and because the interrogating ultrasound beam is typically orthogonal to flow, pulmonic regurgitation can be estimated semiquantitatively in a manner analogous to that for aortic valve regurgitation. At present, however, there are no well-established criteria for the estimation of severity of regurgitation by this approach.

Physiologic pulmonary valve regurgitation may be detected in most normal patients by the transesophageal technique. As in physiologic tricuspid regurgitation, this is without clinical significance and easily discriminated from pathologic regurgitation.

Role of TEE

Transesophageal echocardiography has a limited role in the assessment of pulmonic valve disease. Typically, pulmonic valve disease is best characterized by the transthoracic technique; hence, TEE is seldom indicated for the primary assessment of pulmonic valve disease. However, in occasional patients whose pulmonary valve cannot be adequately visualized by the transthoracic technique, TEE may prove useful in establishing the cause of pulmonary valve disease. Spectral Doppler hemodynamic assessment of the pulmonary valve by TEE is very limited.

SUMMARY

Echocardiography has become the preferred diagnostic modality for the evaluation of patients with valvular heart disease. The clinical application and utility of echocardiography have been greatly broadened by the development of TEE, which has significantly increased diagnostic precision and facilitated clinical decision-making for patients with valvular heart disease. To date, the greatest benefit of TEE has been in mitral valve disease, and this technique has enabled wider application of repair procedures for surgical mitral regurgitant disease and optimal selection of patients for percutaneous balloon mitral valvuloplasty. Because of its safety, superior image

resolution, and the predictable and uniformly excellent image quality, the technique is also an important adjunct in the resolution of difficult diagnostic problems that are unresolved by conventional transthoracic imaging.

Technologic advances, including multiplane probes, miniaturization of the endoscope, and software development, will promote further clinical application.

Although there are limitations to the technique, interpretative errors are avoided by a thorough understanding of methodology, cardiovascular pathoanatomy, and meticulous examination. Combined transthoracic and transesophageal two-dimensional and Doppler echocardiography with color-flow imaging provides a comprehensive and accurate noninvasive assessment of the cause and severity of valvular heart disease.

REFERENCES

1. American College of Cardiology/American Heart Association Task Force on Assessment of Diagnostic and Therapeutic Cardiovascular Procedures. ACC/AHA guidelines for the clinical application of echocardiography. *Circulation* 1990;82: 2323–45.

2. Matsuzaki M, Toma Y, Kusukawa R. Clinical applications of transesophageal echocardiography. *Circulation* 1990;82:709–22.

3. Fisher EA, Stahl JA, Budd JH, Goldman ME. Transesophageal echocardiography: procedures and clinical application. *J Am Coll Cardiol* 1991;18:1333–48.

4. Khandheria BK, Seward JB, Tajik AJ. Transesophageal echocardiography. In Braunwald E, ed. *Heart Disease: a Textbook of Cardiovascular Medicine,* 3rd ed. Philadelphia: Saunders, 1991;Update 12:273–94.

5. Fisher EA, Goldman ME. Transesophageal echocardiography: a new view of the heart. *Ann Intern Med* 1990;113:91–3.

6. Silver MD, ed. *Cardiovascular Pathology,* Vol 1. New York: Churchill Livingstone, 1983:551–74.

7. Annegers JF, Pillman NL, Weidman WH, Kurland LT. Rheumatic fever in Rochester, Minnesota, 1935–1978. *Mayo Clin Proc* 1982;57:753.

8. Nihoyannopoulos P, Gomez PM, Joshi J, et al. Cardiac abnormalities in systemic lupus erythematosus: association with raised anticardiolipin antibodies. *Circulation* 1990;82:369–75.

9. Barbut D, Borer JS, Wallerson D, et al. Anticardiolipin antibody and stroke: possible relation of valvular heart disease and embolic events. *Cardiology* 1991;79:99–109.

10. Hammer WJ, Roberts WC, deLeon AC Jr. "Mitral stenosis" secondary to combined "massive" mitral annular calcific deposits and small, hypertrophied left ventricles: hemodynamic documentation in four patients. *Am J Med* 1978;64:371–6.

11. Weyman AE. *Cross-Sectional Echocardiography.* Philadelphia: Lea & Febiger, 1982:150–7.

12. Pomerance A. Chronic rheumatic and other inflammatory valve disease. In Pomerance A, Davies MJ, eds. *The Pathology of the Heart.* Oxford: Blackwell, 1975:307–26.

13. Roberts WC. Morphologic features of the normal and abnormal mitral valve. *Am J Cardiol* 1983; 51:1005–28.

14. Ruckman RN, Van Praagh R. Anatomic types of congenital mitral stenosis: report of 49 autopsy cases with consideration of diagnosis and surgical implications. *Am J Cardiol* 1978;42:592–601.

15. Snider AR, Roge CL, Schiller NB, Silverman NH. Congenital left ventricular inflow obstruction evaluated by two-dimensional echocardiography. *Circulation* 1980;61:848–55.

16. Seward JB, Khandheria BK, Oh JK, et al. Transesophageal echocardiography: technique, anatomic correlations, implementation, and clinical applications. *Mayo Clin Proc* 1988;63:649–80.

17. Seward JB, Khandheria BK, Edwards WD, et al. Biplanar transesophageal echocardiography: anatomic correlations, image orientation, and clinical applications. *Mayo Clin Proc* 1990;65:1193–213.

18. Matsumura M, Shah P, Kyo S, Omoto R. Advantages of transesophageal echo for correct diagnosis on small left atrial thrombi in mitral stenosis (abstract). *Circulation* 1989;80 Suppl 2:II–678.

19. Chen Y-T, Kan M-N, Chen J-S, et al. Contributing factors to formation of left atrial spontaneous echo contrast in mitral valvular disease. *J Ultrasound Med* 1990;9:151–5.

20. Daniel WG, Nellessen U, Schröder E, et al. Left atrial spontaneous echo contrast in mitral valve disease: an indicator for an increased thromboembolic risk. *J Am Coll Cardiol* 1988;11:1204–11.

21. Olson LJ, Tajik AJ. Echocardiographic evaluation of valvular heart disease. In Marcus ML, Schelbert HR, Skorton DJ, Wolf GL, eds. *Cardiac Imaging: a Companion to Braunwald's Heart Disease.* Philadelphia: Saunders, 1991:430–3.

22. Libanoff AJ, Rodbard S. Atrioventricular pressure half-time: measure of mitral valve orifice area. *Circulation* 1968;38:144–50.

23. Hatle L, Angelsen B, Tromsdal A. Noninvasive assessment of atrioventricular pressure half-time by Doppler ultrasound. *Circulation* 1979;60: 1096–104.

24. Reid CL, McKay CR, Chandraratna PAN, et al. Mechanisms of increase in mitral valve area and influence of anatomic features in double-balloon, catheter balloon valvuloplasty in adults with rheumatic mitral stenosis: a Doppler and two-dimensional echocardiographic study. *Circulation* 1987; 76:628–36.

25. Moro E, Nicolosi GL, Zanuttini D, et al. Influence of aortic regurgitation on the assessment of the pressure half-time and derived mitral-valve area in patients with mitral stenosis. *Eur Heart J* 1988;9:1010–7.

26. Nakatani S, Masuyama T, Kodama K, et al. Value and limitations of Doppler echocardiography in the quantification of stenotic mitral valve area: comparison of the pressure half-time and the continuity equation methods. *Circulation* 1988;77: 78–85.

27. Currie PJ, Hagler DJ, Seward JB, et al. Instantaneous pressure gradient: a simultaneous Doppler and dual catheter correlative study. *J Am Coll Cardiol* 1986;7:800–6.

28. Seward JB, Khandheria BK, Oh JK, et al. Critical appraisal of transesophageal echocardiography: limitations, pitfalls, and complications. *J Am Soc Echocardiogr* 1992;5:288–305.

29. Matsumura M, Kyo S, Shah P, et al. A new look at mitral valve pathology with bi-plane color Doppler transesophageal probe (abstract). *Circulation* 1989;80 Suppl 2:II-579.

30. Rokowski RJ, Niles NW, Nugent WC, et al. Transesophageal color Doppler evaluation of mitral regurgitation: comparison with left ventriculography (abstract). *Circulation* 1989;80 Suppl 2:II–169.

31. Yoshida K, Yoshikawa J, Yamaura Y, et al. Assessment of mitral regurgitation by biplane transesophageal color Doppler flow mapping. *Circulation* 1990;82:1121–6.

32. Stümper O, Fraser AG, Ho SY, et al. Transesophageal echocardiography in the longitudinal axis: correlation between anatomy and images and its clinical implications. *Br Heart J* 1990;64:282–8.

33. Wilkins GT, Weyman AE, Abascal VM, et al. Percutaneous balloon dilatation of the mitral valve: an analysis of echocardiographic variables related to outcome and the mechanism of dilatation. *Br Heart J* 1988;60:299–308.

34. Abascal VM, Wilkins GT, Choong CY, et al. Mitral regurgitation after percutaneous balloon mitral valvuloplasty in adults: evaluation by pulsed Doppler echocardiography. *J Am Coll Cardiol* 1988;11: 257–63.

35. Manning WJ, Reis GJ, Douglas PS. Use of transesophageal echocardiography to detect left atrial thrombi before percutaneous balloon dilatation of the mitral valve: a prospective study. *Br Heart J* 1992;67:170–3.

36. Kronzon I, Tunick PA, Glassman E, et al. Transesophageal echocardiography to detect atrial clots in candidates for percutaneous transseptal mitral balloon valvuloplasty. *J Am Coll Cardiol* 1990;16:1320–2.

37. Kronzon I, Tunick PA, Schwinger ME, et al. Transesophageal echocardiography during percutaneous mitral valvuloplasty. *J Am Soc Echocardiogr* 1989;2:380–5.

38. Jaarsma W, Visser CA, Suttorp MJ, et al. Transesophageal echocardiography during percutaneous balloon mitral valvuloplasty. *J Am Soc Echocardiogr* 1990;3:384–91.

39. Cormier B, Vahanian A, Michel P-L, et al. The contribution of transesophageal echocardiography in the ultrasound assessment of percutaneous mitral valvuloplasty (abstract). *J Am Coll Cardiol* 1989;13:51A.

40. Casale PN, Whitlow P, Currie PJ, Stewart WJ. Transesophageal echocardiography in percutaneous balloon valvuloplasty for mitral stenosis. *Cleve Clin J Med* 1989;56:597–600.

41. Kronzon I, Tunick PA, Goldfarb A, et al. Echocardiographic and hemodynamic characteristics of atrial septal defects created by percutaneous valvuloplasty. *J Am Soc Echocardiogr* 1990;3:64–71.

42. Yoshida K, Yoshikawa J, Akasaka T, et al. Assessment of left-to-right atrial shunting after percutaneous mitral valvuloplasty by transesophageal color Doppler flow-mapping. *Circulation* 1989;80:1521–6.

43. Daniel WG, Mügge A, Martin RP, et al. Improvement in the diagnosis of abscesses associated with endocarditis by transesophageal echocardiography. *N Engl J Med* 1991;324:795–800.

44. Shively BK, Gurule FT, Roldan CA, et al. Diagnostic value of transesophageal compared with transthoracic echocardiography in infective endocarditis. *J Am Coll Cardiol* 1991;18:391–7.

45. Klodas E, Edwards WD, Khandheria BK. Use of transesophageal echocardiography for improving detection of valvular vegetations in subacute bacterial endocarditis. *J Am Soc Echocardiogr* 1989;2:386–9.

46. Ballal RS, Mahan EF III, Nanda NC, Sanyal R. Aortic and mitral valve perforation: diagnosis by transesophageal echocardiography and Doppler color flow imaging. *Am Heart J* 1991;121:214–7.

47. Martin RP, Meltzer RS, Chia BL, et al. Clinical utility of two dimensional echocardiography in infective endocarditis. *Am J Cardiol* 1980;46:379–85.

48. Devereux RB, Kramer-Fox R, Shear MK, et al. Diagnosis and classification of severity of mitral valve prolapse: methodologic, biologic, and prognostic considerations. *Am Heart J* 1987;113:1265–80.

49. Nishimura RA, McGoon MD, Shub C, et al. Echocardiographically documented mitral valve prolapse: long-term follow-up of 237 patients. *N Engl J Med* 1985;313:1305–9.

50. Marks AR, Choong CY, Sanfilippo AJ, et al. Identification of high-risk and low-risk subgroups of patients with mitral-valve prolapse. *N Engl J Med* 1989;320:1031–6.

51. Pini R, Greppi B, Kramer-Fox R, et al. Mitral valve dimensions and motion and familial transmission of mitral valve prolapse with and without mitral leaflet billowing. *J Am Coll Cardiol* 1988;12:1423–31.

52. Joh Y, Yoshikawa J, Yoshida K, et al. Transesophageal echocardiographic findings of mitral valve prolapse. *J Cardiol* 1989;19 Suppl 21:85–95.

53. Gueret P, Lacroix P, Bensaid J. Assessment of mitral valve prolapse by transesophageal echocardiography (abstract). *J Am Coll Cardiol* 1990;15:94A.

54. Turabian M, Chan K-L. Rupture of mitral chordae tendineae resulting from blunt chest trauma: diagnosis by transesophageal echocardiography. *Can J Cardiol* 1990;6:180–2.

55. Hozumi T, Yoshikawa J, Yoshida K, et al. Direct visualization of ruptured chordae tendineae by transesophageal two-dimensional echocardiography. *J Am Coll Cardiol* 1990;16:1315–9.

56. Schlüter M, Kremer P, Hanrath P. Transesophageal 2–D echocardiographic feature of flail mitral leaflet due to ruptured chordae tendineae. *Am Heart J* 1984;108:609–10.

57. Himelman RB, Kusumoto F, Oken K, et al. The flail mitral valve: echocardiographic findings by precordial and transesophageal imaging and Doppler color flow imaging. *J Am Coll Cardiol* 1991;17:272–9.

58. Oh JK, Seward JB, Khandheria BK, et al. Transesophageal echocardiography in critically ill patients. *Am J Cardiol* 1990;66:1492–5.

59. Nestico PF, Depace NL, Morganroth J, et al. Mitral annular calcification: clinical, pathophysiology, and echocardiographic review. *Am Heart J* 1984;107:989–96.

60. Byram MT, Roberts WC. Frequency and extent of calcific deposits in purely regurgitant mitral valves: analysis of 108 operatively excised valves. *Am J Cardiol* 1983;52:1059–61.

61. Akamatsu S, Uematsu H, Yamamoto M, et al. Evaluation of physiological mitral regurgitant flow with transesophageal Doppler echocardiography (abstract). *Jpn Circ J* 1989;53:663.

62. Spain MG, Smith MD, Grayburn PA, et al. Quantitative assessment of mitral regurgitation by Doppler color flow imaging: angiographic and hemodynamic correlations. *J Am Coll Cardiol* 1989;13:585–90.

63. Smith MD, Harrison MR, Pinton R, et al. Regurgitant jet size by transesophageal compared with transthoracic Doppler color flow imaging. *Circulation* 1991;83:79–86.

64. Helmcke F, Nanda NC, Hsiung MC, et al. Color Doppler assessment of mitral regurgitation with orthogonal planes. *Circulation* 1987;75:175–83.

65. Sahn DJ. Instrumentation and physical factors related to visualization of stenotic and regurgitant jets by Doppler color flow mapping. *J Am Coll Cardiol* 1988;12:1354–65.

66. Castello R, Lenzen P, Aguirre F, Labovitz A. Variability in the quantitation of mitral regurgitation by Doppler color flow mapping: comparison of transthoracic and transesophageal studies. *J Am Coll Cardiol* 1992;20:433–8.

67. Castello R, Lenzen P, Aguirre F, Labovitz AJ. Quantitation of mitral regurgitation by transesophageal echocardiography with Doppler color-flow mapping: correlation with cardiac catheterization. *J Am Coll Cardiol* 1992;19:1516–21.

68. Sadoshima J-I, Koyanagi S, Sugimachi M, et al. Evaluation of the severity of mitral regurgitation by transesophageal Doppler flow echocardiography. *Am Heart J* 1992;123:1245–51.

69. Tribouilloy C, Shen WF, Quéré J-P, et al. Assessment of severity of mitral regurgitation by measuring regurgitant width at its origin with transesophageal Doppler color flow imaging. *Circulation* 1992;85:1248–53.

70. Taylor AL, Eichhorn EJ, Brickner ME, et al. Aortic valve morphology: an important in vitro determinant of proximal jet width by Doppler color flow mapping. *J Am Coll Cardiol* 1990;16:405–12.

71. Baumgartner H, Schima H, Kühn P. Value and limitations of proximal jet dimensions for the quantitation of valvular regurgitation: an in vitro study using Doppler flow imaging. *J Am Soc Echocardiogr* 1991;4:57–66.

72. Klein AL, Tajik AJ. Doppler assessment of pulmonary venous flow in healthy subjects and in patients with heart disease. *J Am Soc Echocardiogr* 1991;4:379–92.

73. Klein AL, Obarski TP, Calafiore PC, et al. Reversal of systolic flow in pulmonary veins by transesoph-

ageal Doppler echocardiography predicts severity of mitral regurgitation (abstract). *J Am Coll Cardiol* 1990;15:74A.

74. Klein AL, Stewart WJ, Litowitz H, et al. Pulmonary venous flow assessment of mitral regurgitation: a simultaneous left atrial pressure and transesophageal echo Doppler study (abstract). *Circulation* 1990;82 Suppl 3:III–552.

75. Pearson AC, Castello R, Wallace PM, Labovitz AJ. Effect of mitral regurgitation on pulmonary venous velocities derived by trans-esophageal echocardiography (abstract). *Circulation* 1989;80 Suppl 2:II–571.

76. Kreis A, Lambertz H, Gerish N, Hanrath P. Value of the transesophageal echocardiographic pulmonary venous flow in classification of mitral insufficiency (abstract). *Circulation* 1989;80 Suppl 2:II–577.

77. Bartzokis TC, Lee RJ, Grogin HR, Schnittger I. Assessment of pulmonary venous flow by transesophageal echocardiography (abstract). *Circulation* 1989;80 Suppl 2:II–613.

78. Castello R, Pearson AC, Lenzen P, Labovitz AJ. Effect of mitral regurgitation on pulmonary venous velocities derived from transesophageal echocardiography color-guided pulsed Doppler imaging. *J Am Coll Cardiol* 1991;17:1499–506.

79. Dennig K, Henneke KH, Dacian S, Rudolph W. Estimation of the severity of mitral regurgitation by parameters derived from the velocity profile of pulmonary venous flow using transesophageal Doppler technique (abstract). *J Am Coll Cardiol* 1990;15:91A.

80. Jain S, Moos S, Awad M, et al. Assessment of mitral regurgitation severity using pulmonary venous flow by transesophageal color Doppler (abstract). *Circulation* 1989;80 Suppl 2:II–571.

81. Klein AL, Obarski TP, Stewart WJ, et al. Transesophageal Doppler echocardiography of pulmonary venous flow: a new marker of mitral regurgitation severity. *J Am Coll Cardiol* 1991;18:518–26.

82. Rokey R, Sterling LL, Zoghbi WA, et al. Determination of regurgitant fraction in isolated mitral or aortic regurgitation by pulsed Doppler two-dimensional echocardiography. *J Am Coll Cardiol* 1986;7:1273–8.

83. Enriquez-Sarano M, Bailey KR, Seward JB, et al. Quantitative Doppler assessment of valvular regurgitation. *Circulation* 1993;87:841–8.

84. Enriquez-Sarano M, Tajik AJ, Bailey KR, Seward JB. Color flow imaging compared with quantitative Doppler assessment of severity of mitral regurgitation: influence of eccentricity of jet and

mechanism of regurgitation. *J Am Coll Cardiol* 1993;21:1211–9.

85. Recusani F, Bargiggia GS, Yoganathan AP, et al. A new method for quantification of regurgitant flow rate using color Doppler flow imaging of the flow convergence region proximal to a discrete orifice: an in vitro study. *Circulation* 1991;83: 594–604.

86. Utsonomiya T, Ogawa T, Tang HA, et al. Doppler color flow mapping of the proximal isovelocity surface area: a new method for measuring volume flow rate across a narrowed orifice. *J Am Soc Echocardiogr* 1991;4:338–48.

87. Chen C, Koschyk D, Brockhoff C, et al. Noninvasive estimation of regurgitant flow rate and volume in patients with mitral regurgitation by Doppler color mapping of accelerating flow field. *J Am Coll Cardiol* 1993;21:374–83.

88. Giesler M, Grossmann G, Schmidt A, et al. Color Doppler echocardiographic determination of mitral regurgitant flow from the proximal velocity profile of the flow convergence region. *Am J Cardiol* 1993;71:217–24.

89. Lopez JF, Hanson S, Orchard RC, Tan L. Quantification of mitral valvular incompetence. *Cathet Cardiovasc Diagn* 1985;11:139–52.

90. Nishimura RA, Tajik AJ. Determination of left-sided pressure gradients by utilizing Doppler aortic and mitral regurgitant signals: validation by simultaneous dual catheter and Doppler studies. *J Am Coll Cardiol* 1988;11:317–21.

91. Jenni R, Ritter M, Eberli F, et al. Quantification of mitral regurgitation with amplitude-weighted mean velocity from continuous wave Doppler spectra. *Circulation* 1989;79:1294–9.

92. Chung N, Nishimura RA, Holmes DR Jr, Tajik AJ. Measurement of left ventricular dp/dt by simultaneous Doppler echocardiography and cardiac catheterization. *J Am Soc Echocardiogr* 1992;5: 147–52.

93. Chen C, Rodriguez L, Guerrero JL, et al. Noninvasive estimation of the instantaneous first derivative of left ventricular pressure using continuous-wave Doppler echocardiography. *Circulation* 1991;83: 2101–10.

94. Olson LJ, Subramanian R, Ackermann DM, et al. Surgical pathology of the mitral valve: a study of 712 cases spanning 21 years. *Mayo Clin Proc* 1987;62:22–34.

95. Carpentier A, Chauvand S, Fabiani JN, et al. Reconstructive surgery of mitral valve incompetence: ten-year appraisal. *J Thorac Cardiovasc Surg* 1980;79:338–48.

96. Freeman WK, Schaff HV, Khandheria BK, et al. Intraoperative evaluation of mitral valve regurgitation and repair by transesophageal echocardiography: incidence and significance of systolic anterior motion. *J Am Coll Cardiol* 1992;20:599–609.

97. Davies MJ. Pathology of cardiac valves. London: Butterworths, 1980:18–35.

98. Pomerance A. Pathogenesis of aortic stenosis and its relation to age. *Br Heart J* 1972;34:569–74.

99. Passik CS, Ackermann DM, Pluth JR, Edwards WD. Temporal changes in the causes of aortic stenosis: a surgical pathologic study of 646 cases. *Mayo Clin Proc* 1987;62:119–23.

100. Subramanian R, Olson LJ, Edwards WD. Surgical pathology of pure aortic stenosis: a study of 374 cases. *Mayo Clin Proc* 1984;59:683–90.

101. Dittrich HC, McCann HA, Walsh TP, et al. Transesophageal echocardiography in the evaluation of prosthetic and native aortic valves. *Am J Cardiol* 1990;66:758–61.

102. Schwinger ME, Kronzon I. Improved evaluation of left ventricular outflow tract obstruction by transesophageal echocardiography. *J Am Soc Echocardiogr* 1989;2:191–4.

103. Mügge A, Daniel WG, Wolpers HG, et al. Improved visualization of discrete subvalvular aortic stenosis by transesophageal color-coded Doppler echocardiography. *Am Heart J* 1989;117:474–5.

104. Hofmann T, Kasper W, Meinertz T, et al. Determination of aortic valve orifice area in aortic valve stenosis by two-dimensional transesophageal echocardiography. *Am J Cardiol* 1987;59:330–5.

105. Chandrasekaran K, Foley R, Weintraub A, et al. Evidence that transesophageal echocardiography can reliably and directly measure the aortic valve area in patients with aortic stenosis—a new application that is independent of LV function and does not require Doppler data (abstract). *J Am Coll Cardiol* 1991;17:20A.

106. Derumeaux G, Cribier A, Koning R, Letac B. Transesophageal echocardiographic assessment of valve morphological changes during the procedure of balloon aortic valvuloplasty (abstract). *Circulation* 1989;80 Suppl 2:II–72.

107. Cyran SE, Kimball TR, Schwartz DC, et al. Evaluation of balloon aortic valvuloplasty with transesophageal echocardiography. *Am Heart J* 1988;115:460–2.

108. Edwards JE. Pathologic aspects of cardiac valvular insufficiencies. *Arch Surg* 1958;77:634–49.

109. Edwards JE. Pathology of acquired valvular disease of the heart. *Semin Roentgenol* 1979;14: 96–115.

110. Roberts WC. Left ventricular outflow tract obstruction and aortic regurgitation. *Monogr Pathol* 1974;15:110–75.

111. Erbel R, Engberding R, Daniel W, et al. Echocardiography in diagnosis of aortic dissection. *Lancet* 1989;1:457–60.

112. Olson LJ, Subramanian R, Edwards WD. Surgical pathology of pure aortic insufficiency: a study of 225 cases. *Mayo Clin Proc* 1984;59:835–41.

113. Pyeritz RE, McKusick VA. The Marfan syndrome: diagnosis and management. *N Engl J Med* 1979;300:772–7.

114. Leier CV, Call TD, Fulkerson PK, Wooley CF. The spectrum of cardiac defects in the Ehlers-Danlos syndrome, types I and III. *Ann Intern Med* 1980;92:171–8.

115. Perry GJ, Helmcke F, Nanda NC, et al. Evaluation of aortic insufficiency by Doppler color flow mapping. *J Am Coll Cardiol* 1987;9:952–9.

116. Welch GH Jr, Braunwald E, Sarnott SJ. Hemodynamic effects of quantitatively varied experimental aortic regurgitation. *Circ Res* 1957;5:546–51.

117. Grayburn PA, Handshoe R, Smith MD, et al. Quantitative assessment of the hemodynamic consequences of aortic regurgitation by means of continuous wave Doppler recordings. *J Am Coll Cardiol* 1987;10:135–41.

118. Labovitz AJ, Ferrara RP, Kern MJ, et al. Quantitative evaluation of aortic insufficiency by continuous wave Doppler echocardiography. *J Am Coll Cardiol* 1986;8:1341–7.

119. Yeung AC, Plappert T, St. John Sutton MG. Calculation of aortic regurgitation orifice area by Doppler echocardiography: a new application of the continuity equation (abstract). *Circulation* 1988;78 Suppl 2:II–39.

120. Silver MD, Lam JHC, Ranganathan N, Wigle ED. Morphology of the human tricuspid valve. *Circulation* 1971;43:333–48.

121. Pellikka PA, Tajik AJ, Khandheria BK, et al. Carcinoid heart disease: clinical and echocardiographic spectrum in 74 patients. *Circulation* 1993;87: 1188–96.

122. Lundin L, Landelius J, Andrén B, öberg K. Transesophageal echocardiography improves the diagnostic value of cardiac ultrasound in patients with carcinoid heart disease. *Br Heart J* 1990;64:190–4.

123. Hauck AJ, Freeman DP, Ackermann DM, et al. Surgical pathology of the tricuspid valve: a study of 363 cases spanning 25 years. *Mayo Clin Proc* 1988;63:851.

124. Weyman AE, Rankin R, King H. Loeffler's endocarditis presenting as mitral and tricuspid stenosis. *Am J Cardiol* 1977;40:438–44.

125. Banks T, Fletcher R, Ali N. Infective endocarditis in heroin addicts. *Am J Med* 1973;55:444–51.

126. McKinsey DS, Ratts TE, Bisno AL. Underlying cardiac lesions in adults with infective endocarditis: the changing spectrum. *Am J Med* 1987;82: 681–8.

127. Johnston SR, Freeman WK, Schaff HV, Tajik AJ. Severe tricuspid regurgitation after mitral valve repair: diagnosis by intraoperative transesophageal echocardiography. *J Am Soc Echocardiogr* 1990;3: 416–9.

128. Currie PJ, Seward JB, Chan K-L, et al. Continuous wave Doppler determination of right ventricular pressure: a simultaneous Doppler-catheterization study in 127 patients. *J Am Coll Cardiol* 1985;6: 750–6.

129. Gikonyo BM, Lucas RV, Edwards JE. Anatomic features of congenital pulmonary valvar stenosis. *Pediatr Cardiol* 1987;8:109–16.

130. Altrichter PM, Olson LJ, Edwards WD, et al. Surgical pathology of the pulmonary valve: a study of 116 cases spanning 15 years. *Mayo Clin Proc* 1989;64:1352–60.

131. Shapiro SM, Young E, Ginzton LE, Bayer AS. Pulmonic valve endocarditis as an underdiagnosed disease: role of transesophageal echocardiography. *J Am Soc Echocardiogr* 1992;5:48–51.

10

Echocardiographic Assessment of Prosthetic Heart Valves

Fletcher A. Miller, Jr. • *Bijoy K. Khandheria* • *A. Jamil Tajik*

Accurate evaluation of prosthetic heart valves requires the ability to investigate a variety of different types of prostheses, each of which can be implanted in any of the four positions. In addition, each type of prosthesis is manufactured in several different sizes, and each size has unique hemodynamic characteristics. The complexity of the evaluation is further increased by the number of different pathologic processes that can beset prosthetic valves (Tables 10-1 and 10-2). In the past decade, echocardiography

has developed into a versatile clinical tool that is ideally suited to meeting the challenge of prosthetic valve assessment.

Transesophageal echocardiography (TEE) is critical in the characterization of structural abnormalities

Table 10-1. Pathologic conditions affecting biologic heart valve prostheses

Stenosis
  Degenerative
  Thrombosis (rare)
Regurgitation
  Perivalvular
  Transvalvular (degenerative)
    Simple thickening or calcification
    Leaflet perforation
    Leaflet tear or dehiscence
Endocarditis
  Vegetations
  Valve ring abscess
  Fistula
Hemolysis (usually seen with periprosthetic leak)
Noninfectious valve bed abnormalities
  Pseudoaneurysm
  Hematoma
  Fistula

Table 10-2. Pathologic conditions affecting mechanical heart valve prostheses

Stenosis
  Thrombosis
  Pannus ingrowth
Regurgitation
  Perivalvular
  Transvalvular
    Thrombus
    Pannus
    Disk or poppet variance
    Cloth wear
Mechanical failure
  Disk or poppet variance
  Cage variance
  Strut fracture
Endocarditis
  Vegetations
  Valve ring abscess
  Fistula
Hemolysis
Noninfectious valve bed abnormalities
  Pseudoaneurysm
  Hematoma
  Fistula

of prosthetic heart valves and often critical to the assessment of prosthetic mitral and tricuspid regurgitation. However, the evaluation of prosthetic valvular stenosis and prosthetic aortic regurgitation is largely the domain of transthoracic echocardiography, including spectral Doppler and color-flow imaging. By using an approach that *integrates* all of these modalities, the echocardiographer can thoroughly investigate prosthetic heart valves, thereby obviating cardiac catheterization in the vast majority of cases. The integrated approach to prosthetic heart valves is presented in this chapter.

OVERVIEW

The assessment of prosthetic heart valves should begin with two-dimensional imaging [1–7]. During this portion of the examination, the sewing ring should always be scanned in an attempt to identify dehiscence. Next, the moving parts should be imaged. If the prosthesis is constructed of biologic material, the leaflets should be inspected for thickening, calcification, restriction to opening, and abnormal apposition. In mechanical prostheses, the metal disk or ball creates multiple ultrasound reverberations. Nevertheless, the echocardiographer can assess poppet or disk motion by observing the motion pattern of the reverberations. If a question arises about abnormal occluder motion, M-mode echocardiography can be used to more precisely record the motion pattern [8]. Two-dimensional echocardiography is also used to screen for abnormal mass lesions, such as thrombus or vegetations, associated with the prosthesis. In this evaluation, transthoracic echocardiography and TEE are complementary. These two approaches result in reverberations and shadowing on opposite sides of prosthetic valves, so that abnormalities masked by one technique may be uncovered by the other (Fig. 10-1).

Spectral Doppler imaging provides complete assessment of forward-flow hemodynamics. Continuous-wave Doppler imaging is used to measure prosthetic valve gradients, whereas the combination of pulsed and continuous-wave Doppler echocardiography is used for measurement of effective orifice areas. During the transthoracic study, continuous-wave Doppler imaging is also used to screen for prosthetic valvular regurgitation. In general, the intensity of high-velocity continuous-wave signals is proportional to the amount of regurgitation.

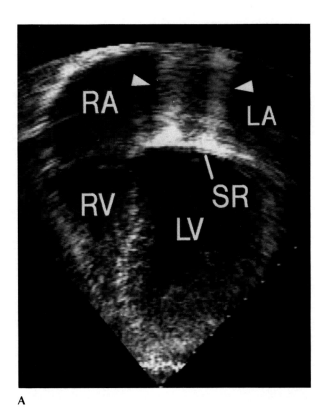

A

Color-flow imaging provides a velocity map of forward flow across the prosthesis. Each type of prosthesis has a characteristic color map (Figs. 10-2 and 10-3). Once the echocardiographer is familiar with normal flow imaging for each of the various types of prostheses, the color-flow examination provides a quick screen for prosthetic valvular stenosis (Fig. 10-4). In addition, color-flow imaging sometimes is necessary to guide placement of the continuous-wave cursor for directed measurement of prosthetic valve gradients.

In most instances, the degree of prosthetic aortic regurgitation can be accurately assessed by color-flow imaging during the transthoracic examination. There is no attenuating prosthetic material between the regurgitant jet and the ultrasound beam with either parasternal or apical transducer positions. For complete assessment of the amount of aortic regurgitation, not only color-flow imaging but also pulsed- and continuous-wave Doppler examinations are necessary. Transesophageal echocardiography provides high-resolution images of the prosthesis itself, allowing the echocardiographer to determine the structural defect causing the regurgitation.

In addition to creating reverberations in the atria, mitral and tricuspid prostheses cause flow masking in the atria. Both of these phenomena limit identifi-

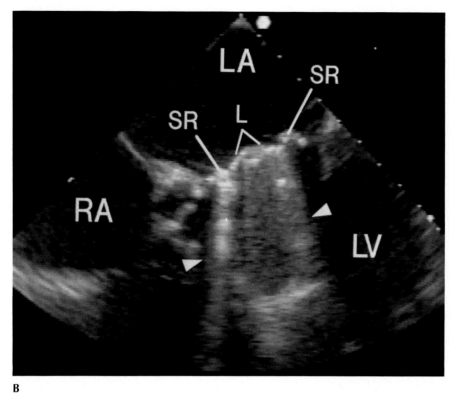

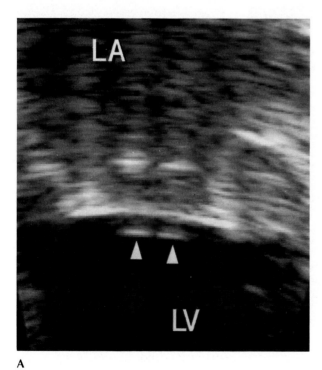

Fig. 10-1.   A. Transthoracic echocardiography. Apex-down four-chamber view of a Medtronic-Hall prosthesis in the mitral position. In this systolic frame, note the reverberations *(arrowheads)* filling the left atrium. B. Transesophageal echocardiography. Horizontal plane, four-chamber view of St. Jude Medical mitral prosthesis. In this systolic frame, the leaflets *(L)* are closed. Reverberations *(arrowheads)* fill the left ventricle. Note that transthoracic echocardiography and TEE are complementary, with transthoracic echocardiography allowing investigation of the ventricular side of mitral prostheses and TEE of the atrial side.

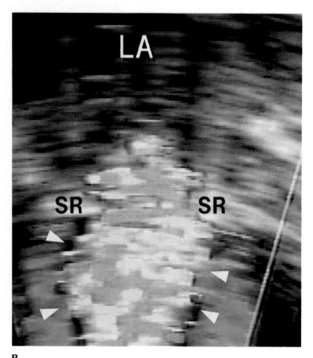

Fig. 10-2.   Transthoracic echocardiographic study with the regional expansion system. A. St. Jude Medical prosthesis is in mitral position, diastolic frame. The two leaflets have opened fully to their parallel positions *(arrowheads)*. Reverberations fill the left atrium. B. Normal diastolic color-flow pattern *(arrowheads)* represents the sum of flow through the two lateral orifices and the larger central orifice.

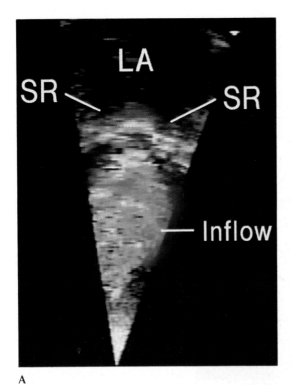

A

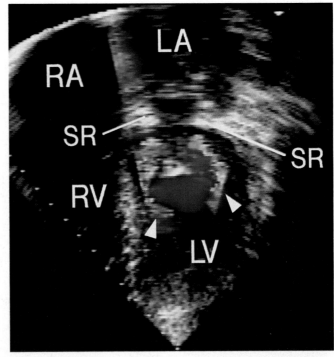

B

Fig. 10-3. Transthoracic echocardiography with apex-down views of normal diastolic flow pattern for various mitral prostheses. A. Heterograft. The normal color-flow pattern *(Inflow)* resembles that of mild native mitral stenosis. Note flow convergence in the left atrium. B. Starr-Edwards prosthesis. The ball is at the apex of the cage. Color jets *(arrowheads)* enter the left ventricle around the poppet. C. Bjork-Shiley prosthesis. The tilting disk is opened into the left ventricle and is surrounded by flow *(arrowheads)* through the major and minor orifices. D. Medtronic-Hall prosthesis. As with the Bjork-Shiley prosthesis, the tilting disk is open and surrounded by diastolic inflow *(arrowheads)*. The yellow portion of the jet indicates that the velocity is slightly higher than that of the Bjork-Shiley prosthesis in C.

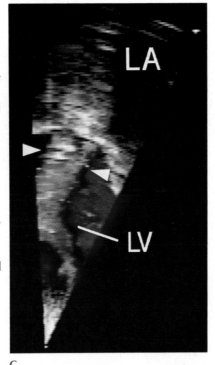

C

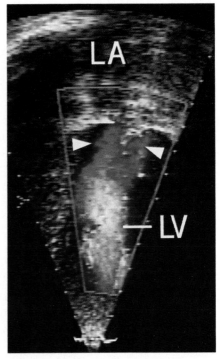

D

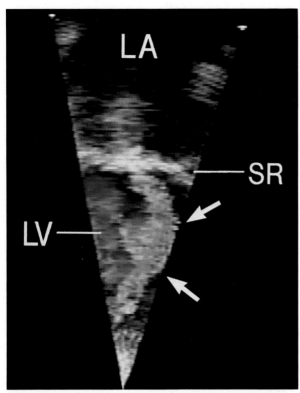

Fig. 10-4. Transthoracic echocardiography, apex-down view. In this Omniscience tilting disk mitral prosthesis, the eccentric, crescent-shaped diastolic jet *(arrows)* in the left ventricle indicates prosthetic stenosis. Note the mosaic appearance of the color jet. Stenosis was confirmed by continuous-wave Doppler analysis. Reduced opening motion for the same prosthesis was demonstrated by TEE (see Fig. 10-32).

cation and semiquantitation of regurgitant lesions by color-flow imaging, particularly for mechanical prostheses. Because the transesophageal transducer can be positioned adjacent to the left atrium, color-flow imaging through this new window has rapidly become the method of choice for assessment of prosthetic mitral and tricuspid regurgitation. As with aortic prostheses, TEE is proving to be a superb technique for identifying structural abnormalities related to mitral and tricuspid prosthetic valves. Thrombus, vegetations, fistulas, ring abscesses, and pseudoaneurysms can usually be clearly imaged from esophageal or gastric transducer positions.

Beyond the information directly related to prosthetic heart valve function, echocardiography supplies important ancillary information about associated lesions of native valves, ventricular size and function, atrial size, and pericardial effusion

among others. Pericardial effusion is of particular importance in instances of hemodynamic compromise in the perioperative period.

We proceed now with a more detailed discussion of echocardiographic assessment of prosthetic valves, beginning with the evaluation of aortic prostheses. We then discuss the evaluation of mitral and tricuspid prostheses. Finally, we describe and illustrate the various structural lesions that can be seen with each of the different types of prostheses.

AORTIC PROSTHESES

Forward Flow Hemodynamics and Obstructive Lesions

Two-dimensional imaging of aortic prostheses is often difficult by transthoracic echocardiography. The increased resolution of transesophageal imaging, however, usually allows analysis of structural detail. For bioprosthetic aortic valves, TEE provides visualization of stents and cusps [9–11]. Cusp thickness and motion can be clearly delineated (Figs. 10-5 and 10-6). Although reverberations from metallic parts are still a problem, TEE usually allows definition of opening and closing motions of mechanical aortic prostheses [12,13]. In fact, the moving parts of disk or bileaflet prostheses are usually seen well enough to allow assessment of the opening angle (Fig. 10-7).

Although imaging of aortic prostheses by TEE is superior to that imaged by transthoracic echocardiography, measuring forward flow hemodynamics with the transesophageal transducer usually is not feasible. It is quite difficult to align a steerable TEE continuous-wave cursor parallel to flow through aortic prostheses. Occasionally, alignment can be accomplished from a long-axis transgastric approach in which the left ventricular outflow tract is viewed (see Chapter 4). Even though this overcomes the angulation problem, Doppler signals are often attenuated because the prosthesis is in the far field. Fortunately, complete hemodynamic assessment of prosthetic aortic valves can almost always be obtained from transthoracic echocardiography [14–20].

Hemodynamic assessment of aortic prostheses should include measurement of peak velocity, mean gradient, and effective orifice area. The mean gradient is determined by continuous-wave Doppler ex-

Fig. 10-5. Transesophageal echocardiography, longitudinal plane short-axis view of normal tissue prosthesis in aortic position. A. Diastolic frame. The three stents *(S)* appear as rounded densities within the aortic root. The three cusps *(arrowheads)* are closed, forming an inverted Y. B. Systolic frame. The three cusps *(arrowheads)* have opened widely.

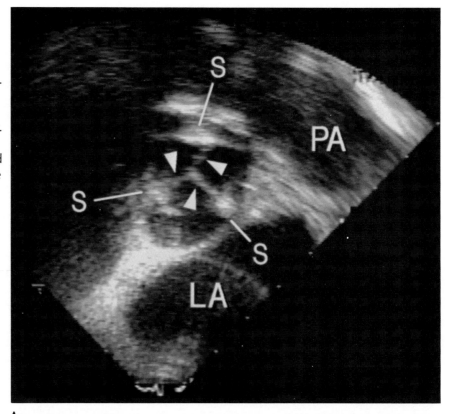

A

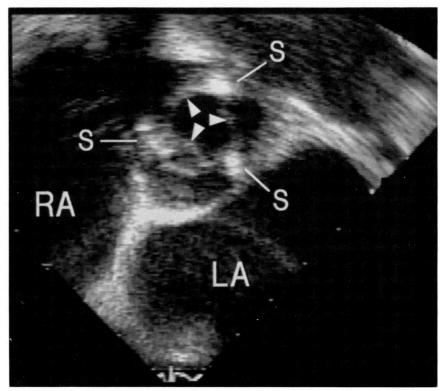

B

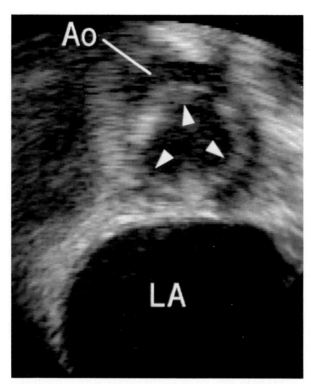

Fig. 10-6. Transesophageal echocardiography, longitudinal plane short-axis view of another normal tissue aortic prosthesis. Expanded view shows normal systolic opening of the cusps *(arrowheads)*, which are also normal in thickness.

amination with use of the simplified Bernoulli equation [21–23]. As with native aortic stenosis, the mean gradient across aortic prostheses is most effectively obtained with a nonimaging transducer (Fig. 10-8). The prosthesis must be interrogated from a number of different transthoracic transducer locations, including apical, right parasternal (with the patient in the right lateral decubitus position), left parasternal, right supraclavicular, suprasternal, and subcostal. In each position, the transducer is manipulated until the velocity spectrum is optimized. Data from all positions are then compared, and the maximal spectrum is selected for calculation of the mean gradient. For patients in regular sinus rhythm, we average the gradients from three to five beats to obtain the mean gradient, which we report to the clinician. For patients in atrial fibrillation, five to ten beats should be averaged.

Table 10-3 lists the transducer positions from which we obtained the optimal and maximal spectral Doppler signals in the analysis of 646 clinically

normal aortic prostheses [24]. Although the apical position had the highest yield, right parasternal and suprasternal positions provided the maximal velocity spectrum in a signficant percentage of patients (Fig. 10-9).

When a prosthesis is first studied just after implantation, all of the transthoracic transducer positions should be used for interrogation. Once the optimal position is identified, it should be recorded in the echocardiographic report. This single position can then be used for measuring the mean gradient and effective orifice area during subsequent echocardiographic evaluations.

By using multiple transducer positions, we can effectively minimize the angle theta in the Doppler equation. In so doing, we obtain gradient information that correlates closely with measurements made during invasive catheterization. This correlation was validated by a Mayo Clinic study. Burstow et al. [25] performed continuous-wave Doppler examination of prosthetic valves, and the velocity spectra were recorded simultaneously with pressures from invasive catheterization. The study group consisted of 36 patients with 42 prostheses, 20 of which were mitral, 20 were aortic, 1 was tricuspid, and 1 was pulmonic. There were 32 mechanical prostheses and 10 bioprostheses. The mechanical valves consisted of 15 Starr-Edwards, 7 Bjork-Shiley, 4 Braunwald-Cutter (mitral), 2 Medtronic-Hall, 2 St. Jude Medical, 1 Sorin, and 1 Smeloff Cutter.

Figure 10-10, an example of a recording from this study, illustrates simultaneous Doppler and pressure tracings from a Starr-Edwards aortic prosthesis. Figure 10-11 graphically displays the correlation between mean gradients obtained by simultaneous catheterization and Doppler study for the 20 aortic prostheses. The correlation is excellent, with a standard error of the estimate of only 3 mm Hg. Valida-

Table 10-3. Transthoracic transducer positions for optimal spectral Doppler signals in echocardiographic assessment of 646 normal aortic prostheses

Position	No.	%
Apical	570	88.2
Right parasternal	50	7.7
Suprasternal	22	3.4
Left parasternal	2	0.3
Subcostal	2	0.3

Fig. 10-7. Transesophageal echocardiography, longitudinal plane long-axis image of a Medtronic-Hall aortic prosthesis. A. In this diastolic frame, the tilting disk is closed and not readily apparent. The sinuses of Valsalva *(S)* are ectatic. B. In systole, the tilting disk *(d)* is fully opened. The opening angle is clearly evident despite the disk reverberations *(arrowheads)* within the aorta.

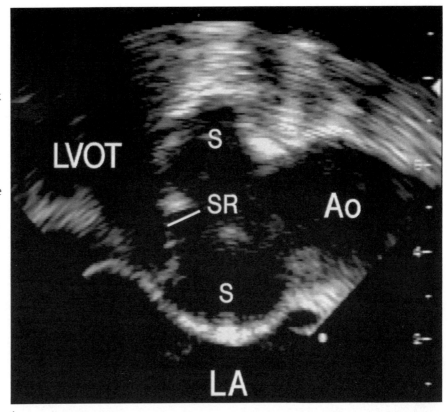

A

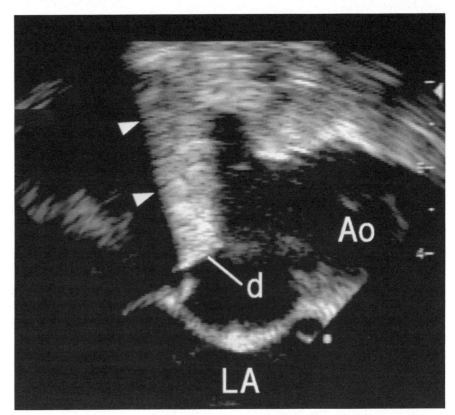

B

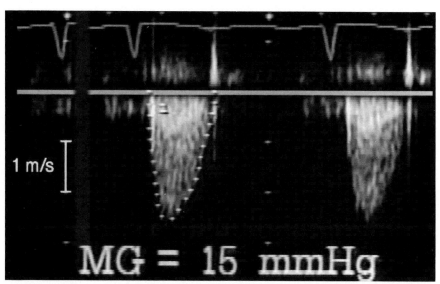

Fig. 10-8. Transthoracic continuous-wave Doppler spectrum from a normal tissue aortic prosthesis. In the apical position for nonimaging transducer, the velocity spectrum is recorded between the opening and the closing clicks. The velocity spectrum has been traced *(small dots)* and the instrument software has used the simplified Bernoulli equation to calculate the mean gradient of 15 mm Hg.

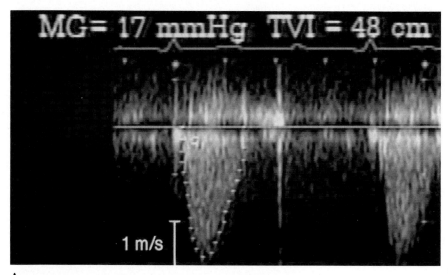

A

Fig. 10-9. Transthoracic continuous-wave Doppler examination of a normal Medtronic Intact aortic prosthesis. A. With the nonimaging transducer at the apex, a mean gradient of 17 mm Hg was obtained with a time velocity integral *(TVI)* of 48 cm. B. The patient was placed in the right lateral decubitus position. With the transducer in a right parasternal position, the true MG of 22 mm Hg and the true TVI of 58 cm were obtained. This illustrates the necessity of using multiple transthoracic transducer positions to obtain the largest velocity spectrum.

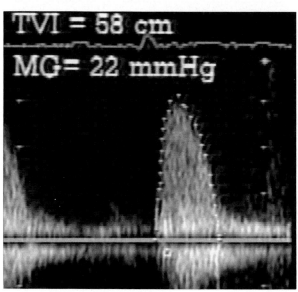

B

tion of Doppler echocardiography for measuring prosthetic valve gradients has also been reported by other investigators [26,27].

Doppler echocardiography has therefore provided us with the first noninvasive means for determining prosthetic valve gradients. This technique can be applied to the study of normal prosthetic valves, thereby allowing comparisons between different types and sizes of prostheses. In 1988, Reisner and Meltzer [28] reviewed the world literature for Doppler evaluation of prosthetic heart valves in patients who were clinically normal. This review included data for more than 1000 prostheses, of which 494 were aortic. Other authors have subsequently de-

Fig. 10-10. Simultaneous Doppler and pressure recordings from a Starr-Edwards aortic prosthesis. Two catheters were used for the invasive hemodynamic assessment, so that left ventricular and aortic pressures were recorded simultaneously. Note that the mean gradient obtained by catheterization (40 mm Hg) closely correlates with that determined by Doppler study when the simplified Bernoulli equation is used (42 mm Hg). (Courtesy of Dr. Darryl Burstow.)

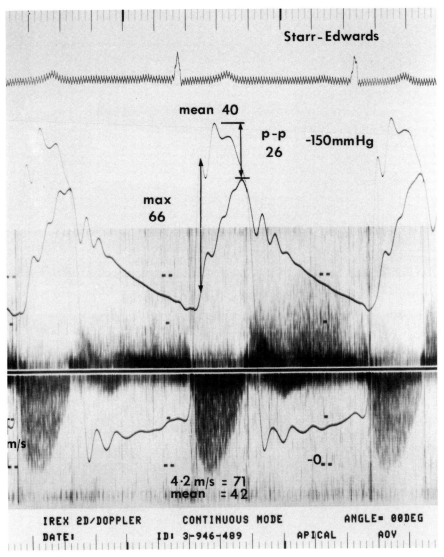

Fig. 10-11. Correlation between mean gradients obtained by Doppler echocardiography and mean gradients obtained by invasive catheterization for 20 aortic prostheses. The *r* value is 0.94, and the standard error of the estimate *(SEE)* is only 3 mm Hg. (From Burstow et al. [25]. By permission of the American Heart Association.)

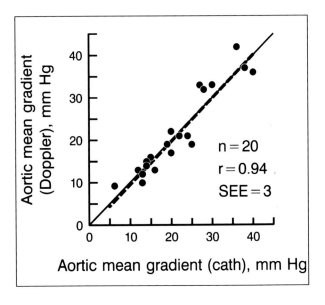

fined normal Doppler gradients for several different prostheses [29–36]. The data from our Mayo Clinic series of 646 clinically and echocardiographically normal aortic prostheses are listed in Table 10-4. These data indicate that normal Starr-Edwards aortic prostheses have a significantly higher mean gradient than heterograft, Bjork-Shiley, and St. Jude Medical valves and that homograft aortic valves are the least obstructive.

When a prosthetic valve is evaluated, identifying its size is always important. Figure 10-12 illustrates the Doppler-derived mean gradients for seven different sizes of St. Jude Medical aortic prostheses [37]. With increasing size, there is a tendency toward decreasing mean gradient. However, within each size is a fairly large range of gradients. In all series

thus far published for clinically normal prosthetic valves, there are a few outliers with seemingly excessive gradients. In our series (Table 10-4), such outliers include Starr-Edwards and heterograft aortic prostheses with mean gradients as high as 48 mm Hg, and Bjork-Shiley and St. Jude Medical prostheses with mean gradients as high as 38 and 39 mm Hg, respectively. Because these persons were all clinically normal at the time of Doppler examination, they have not undergone surgical replacement of their prostheses. It is important to understand that a decision to replace a prosthetic valve should never be made on the basis of gradient data alone. Some normally functioning prostheses yield high gradients because of "patient-prosthesis mismatch" [38]. Our practice is to perform 6-month follow-up evaluations

Table 10-4. Mayo Clinic normal ranges for Doppler measurements of aortic prostheses

Valve type	No.	Peak velocity, m/sec*	Mean gradient, mm Hg*	Effective orifice area, cm²†
Heterograft	212	2.4 ± 0.5/4.5	13.3 ± 6.1/48	1.9 ± 0.7/0.87
Ball-cage	154	3.2 ± 0.6/4.8	22.7 ± 8.3/48	1.5 ± 0.5/0.87
Bjork-Shiley	139	2.5 ± 0.6/4.2	13.8 ± 7.0/38	1.9 ± 0.8/0.75
St. Jude Medical	73	2.6 ± 0.6/3.9	15.1 ± 7.3/39	1.7 ± 0.7/0.81
Medtronic-Hall	24	2.6 ± 0.4/4.0	15.1 ± 5.2/34	1.6 ± 0.6/0.79
Homograft	33	1.9 ± 0.4/3.0	7.8 ± 2.7/16	2.1 ± 0.5/1.40

*Mean ± SD/highest value.
†Mean ± SD/lowest value.
Modified from Miller et al. [24].

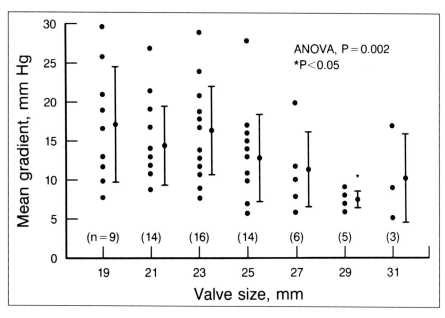

Fig. 10-12. Doppler mean gradients for seven different sizes of normal St. Jude Medical aortic prostheses. Note that the mean value for mean gradient tends to decrease with increasing size. However, there is a large range of gradients within each size, so that there is considerable overlap in gradients among different sizes. (Mean gradient varies with valve size; by analysis of variance, p = .002; * = p < .05.) (From Chafizadeh and Zoghbi [37]. By permission of the American Heart Association.)

of clinically normal individuals known to have high prosthetic valve gradients. This problem is avoided in patients who have more recently undergone prosthetic valve implantation, because we now always obtain a baseline study during the immediate postoperative period. This study defines "normal function" for the individual prosthesis and serves as a baseline for future comparison [39,40].

Calculation of the effective orifice area (EOA) of the prosthetic valve also helps clarify the significance of seemingly excessive mean gradients. As with native aortic valves, the degree of obstruction presented by a prosthetic heart valve can be over-represented or underrepresented by the mean gradient, depending on flow across the valve. For an individual prosthetic valve, the mean gradient can

be relatively large if the patient is in a high-output state (such as postoperative anemia) and much smaller if the patient is in a low-output state [41]. As with native aortic stenosis, we incorporate flow into our assessment of prosthetic valve obstruction by measuring the EOA.

Because of its success in assessing valvular aortic stenosis [42–45] (see Chapter 9), the continuity equation method is being applied to determine prosthetic valve EOAs [37,46–48]. The steps involved in arriving at an EOA are illustrated in Figure 10-13, and the most common pitfalls in determining this area are listed in Table 10-5.

The first step in determining the aortic prosthetic valve area is measurement of the diameter of the systolic left ventricular outflow tract (LVOT) from

Table 10-5. Pitfalls in the determination of effective orifice area (EOA) for an aortic prosthesis

Measurement	Pitfall	Consequence	Solutions
Left ventricular outflow tract (LVOT) diameter	Measuring inside sewing ring	Underestimation of EOA	Identify sewing ring by scanning Measure anteriorly at junction of sewing ring and septum Measure posteriorly at junction of sewing ring and anterior mitral leaflet If in doubt, use sewing ring diameter to approximate LVOT diameter
LVOT velocity	Angle theta error	Underestimation of EOA	Orient apical long-axis image so that pulsed-wave cursor is parallel to LVOT (cursor should be vertical on screen)
LVOT velocity	Measuring too close to sewing ring (region of flow convergence)	Overestimation of EOA	Move pulsed-wave sample volume into ring, and then back off into LVOT until a laminar, nonaliased signal is obtained Use color-flow imaging to identify region of flow convergence Convert LVOT time velocity integral to cardiac output to ensure that a reasonable value is being used for EOA calculation
Prosthesis velocity	Angle theta error	Underestimation of EOA	Use multiple transducer positions At each position, manipulate transducer to optimize Doppler spectrum

the parasternal long-axis view. Geometry is assumed to be circular, and the LVOT diameter is squared and multiplied by the constant 0.785 to arrive at the LVOT area (Fig. 10-13 A). Next, apical long-axis imaging is used to position the pulsed-wave Doppler sample volume in the LVOT. The time velocity integral (TVI) of the resultant velocity spectrum is measured. This represents the stroke distance, and multiplying it by the LVOT area yields the stroke volume. This is the numerator for the EOA formula. The denominator is the TVI of the maximal velocity spectrum for the prosthesis, determined from continuous-wave Doppler interrogation. This is the same velocity spectrum that was used previously to determine the mean gradient. Current instruments measure the TVI and the mean gradient at the same

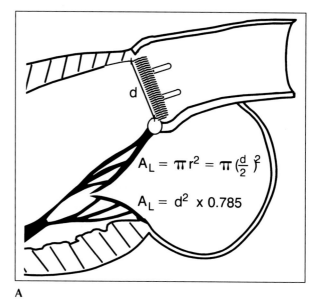

A

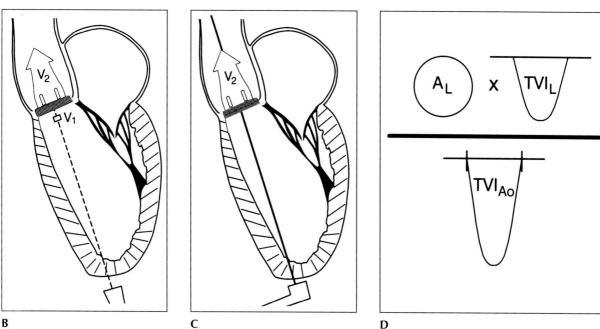

B

C

D

Fig. 10-13. Doppler determination of prosthetic aortic valve effective orifice area by the continuity equation. A. The left ventricular outflow tract diameter is measured from the parasternal long-axis image in systole. The measurement is made in the outflow tract, just below the prosthetic valve sewing ring. The area of the outflow tract (A_L) is calculated by squaring the diameter (d) and multiplying by a constant, 0.785, or $\pi/4$. B. The left ventricular outflow tract velocity is measured by pulsed-wave Doppler echocardiography with the sample volume (V_1) placed in the left ventricular outflow tract below the prosthetic valve sewing ring. From the spectral velocity display, the time velocity integral is measured. C. The prosthetic valve velocity (V_2) is determined by continuous-wave Doppler echocardiography. In this example, an apical transducer position is being used. As described in the text, multiple windows must be sampled to determine that the true maximal velocity is obtained. From the velocity spectrum, the aortic prosthesis time velocity integral is measured. D. Schema of the continuity equation, rearranged to calculate the effective prosthetic aortic valve area, or EOA. The numerator consists of the left ventricular outflow tract area multiplied by the left ventricular outflow tract time velocity integral (TVI_L) (which is the stroke volume). The denominator is the time velocity integral of the prosthesis (TVI_{Ao}).

time (that is, when the maximal velocity spectrum is traced by the examiner). The full EOA formula is

EOA = 0.785 × (LVOT diameter)^2
    × (LVOT TVI) ÷ (aortic prosthesis TVI)

Care must be taken to measure the LVOT diameter rather than the internal diameter of the sewing ring. For this to be accomplished, the sewing ring must be identified before measurement. With the proper parasternal long-axis view, the ultrasound beam slices the sewing ring down the middle, so that it is viewed in cross section (like slicing a lifesaver down the middle and looking directly at the sliced ends). The LVOT diameter should be measured from the junction of the anterior portion of the sewing ring with the ventricular septum to the junction of the posterior portion of the sewing ring with the base of the anterior mitral leaflet (Fig. 10-14).

Rothbart et al. [46] used this method of measuring the LVOT diameter to determine the EOA of 22 aortic bioprostheses by the continuity equation. They compared these Doppler-derived values to those obtained by catheterization and achieved an *r* value of 0.93, as illustrated in Figure 10-15. Kapur et al. [27] compared Doppler EOAs by the simplified continuity equation with those from catheterization for 21 aortic prostheses. They found a somewhat better correlation (*r* = 0.87) for the 10 bioprostheses than for the 11 mechanical prostheses (*r* = 0.76).

At times, the diameter of the LVOT is difficult to measure, particularly if the patient has both mitral and aortic prostheses. In these instances, the LVOT diameter can be approximated from the diameter of the external sewing ring (which, for most prostheses, is identical to the size of the prosthesis). When Rothbart et al. [46] used this sewing ring approximation instead of a measured LVOT diameter, the correlation of Doppler-derived EOA with that determined by catheterization had a *P* value of 0.0001, but the *r* value was reduced to 0.78. Chafizadeh and Zoghbi [37] determined the EOA of 67 St. Jude Medical aortic prostheses shortly after implantation. When they measured the LVOT diameter, the EOAs for the prostheses were 1.63 ± 0.70 cm^2. When they used the sewing ring approximation, the EOAs were 1.87 ± 0.83 cm^2. The findings are likely to be similar for other types of aortic prostheses.

Our preference is to measure the LVOT diameter whenever feasible. The LVOT diameter averages 2.0 cm. Intraobserver and interobserver variations

in measurement of the LVOT diameter for native aortic stenosis have been shown to be 5% and 7%, respectively [44]. For prosthetic aortic valves, the intraobserver and interobserver variations have been determined to average 4% and 7% [37]. Therefore, when a patient is studied on several different occasions, we use the same diameter that was determined at the baseline study unless the new measurement varies by more than 1 mm. Not infrequently, the landmarks for the LVOT measurement are obscured. If the echocardiographer supervising the study is concerned about the accuracy of the LVOT diameter measurement at the time of the baseline study, we use the sewing ring approximation. This same approximation is then used for all subsequent studies for this patient. For Starr-Edwards prostheses, the sewing ring diameter is not always readily apparent from the valve size. Table 10-6 lists the conversions from valve size to sewing ring diameter for both aortic and mitral Starr-Edwards prostheses.

When the LVOT velocity is measured by pulsed-wave Doppler echocardiography, it is important to orient the apical long-axis image in such a way that the Doppler cursor runs vertically down the center of the screen, directly into the LVOT. This orientation prevents underestimation of the true velocity due to angulation. As with native aortic stenosis, it is important to avoid measuring the outflow tract velocity too close to the prosthesis. Because of a zone of central acceleration (flow convergence) just below the prosthesis (Fig. 10-16), the TVI determined in this position does not represent the spatial mean TVI. The sample volume should be moved toward the prosthesis until aliasing occurs. It should then be moved back slightly until a stable, nonaliased velocity is obtained. This position is usually about 1 cm proximal to the sewing ring. It is always worthwhile to verify that the velocity used for the EOA calculation is not too large because of inaccurate sample volume positioning. Color-flow imaging should be used during the pulsed-wave Doppler examination to select a sample volume position that is just below the region of flow convergence. This velocity spectrum represents the spatial mean velocity, and its TVI can be used to determine an accurate EOA. In addition, the TVI measured from the pulsed-wave Doppler examination multiplied by the LVOT diameter is the stroke volume. This value should be multiplied by heart rate to determine cardiac output [49]. If a supraphysiologic value for cardiac output is obtained, one can be certain that

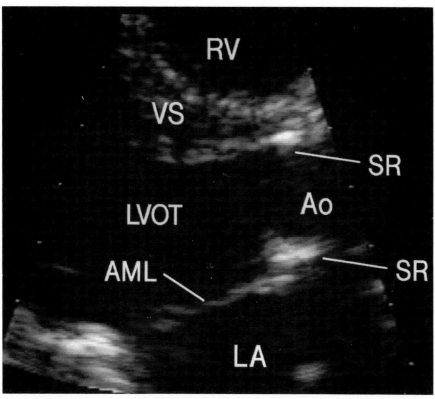

A

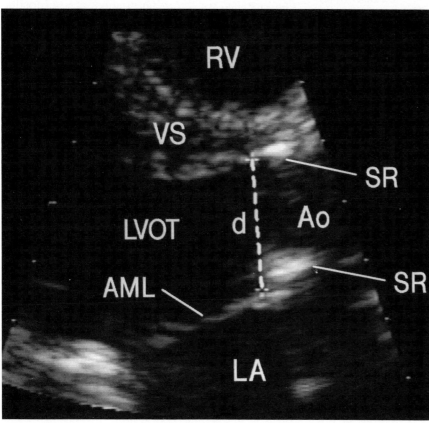

B

Fig. 10-14.   Surface echocardiography, expanded parasternal long-axis view of normal aortic tissue prosthesis. A. The sewing ring has been identified. Note that the ring, particularly the posterior portion, bulges into the aorta. B. The left ventricular outflow tract diameter *(d)* has been measured *(dashed line)*. Note that the anterior cursor has been placed at the junction of the sewing ring and the ventricular septum and the posterior cursor at the junction of the sewing ring and the anterior mitral leaflet. The left ventricular outflow tract diameter will be used for calculation of the effective orifice area of the prosthesis by the continuity equation.

Fig. 10-15. Correlation between Doppler-derived effective orifice area by the continuity equation and catheterization-derived effective orifice area by the Gorlin equation for 22 aortic bioprostheses with various degrees of obstruction. A very reasonable correlation exists both for valves that are unusually obstructed and for normal aortic prostheses. (From Rothbart et al. [46]. Reprinted with permission from the American College of Cardiology. Journal of the American College of Cardiology, 1990, 15:817–824.)

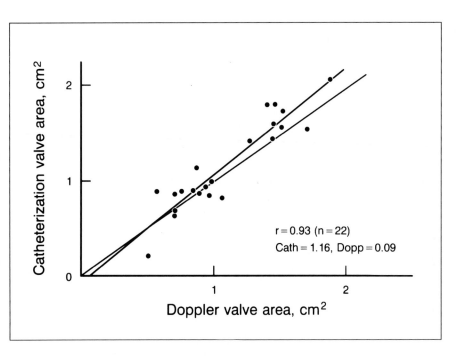

r = 0.93 (n = 22)
Cath = 1.16, Dopp = 0.09

Table 10-6. Conversion from valve size to sewing ring diameter* in Starr-Edwards prostheses

Old code	New code	Diameter (mm)
	Aortic	
6A	16A	16
7A	18A	18
8A	21A	21
9A	22A	22
10A	24A	24
11A	26A	26
12A	27A	27
13A	29A	29
14A	31A	31
	Mitral	
00M	20M	20
0M	22M	22
1M	26M	26
2M	28M	28
3M	30M	30
4M	32M	32
5M	34M	34

*Outer diameter; mounting diameter.

an incorrect sample volume position was used, and the resultant EOA will be falsely large.

The maximal prosthetic valve TVI used in the denominator of the EOA calculation is obtained by the same technique described previously for ob-

taining the mean gradient. Multiple transducer positions must be used at the time of the initial examination. The same maximal velocity spectrum that is traced for the mean gradient is used for the prosthetic TVI in the continuity equation (see Fig. 10-9).

For aortic stenosis, a simplified version of the continuity equation has been shown to be accurate enough for clinical purposes [42–45]. This simplified version uses the ratio of the velocity in the LVOT to the velocity across the aortic valve rather than the ratio of TVIs. Dumesnil et al. [47] validated this simplified version of the continuity equation for aortic bioprostheses, and Chafizadeh and Zoghbi [37] demonstrated its accuracy for St. Jude Medical aortic prostheses. However, this simplification requires an extra assumption in the derivation of a very complex hemodynamic value. Because most instruments now allow easy measurement of TVIs, we prefer the full form of the continuity equation (using the TVI ratio) when calculating prosthetic valve EOAs.

By measuring the mean gradients and EOAs of aortic prostheses, the echocardiographer can fully characterize forward-flow hemodynamics for the clinician. It is most important that these measurements be made within the first few weeks after the valve is implanted. This timing provides a benchmark for the individual prosthesis that serves as a basis for future comparison.

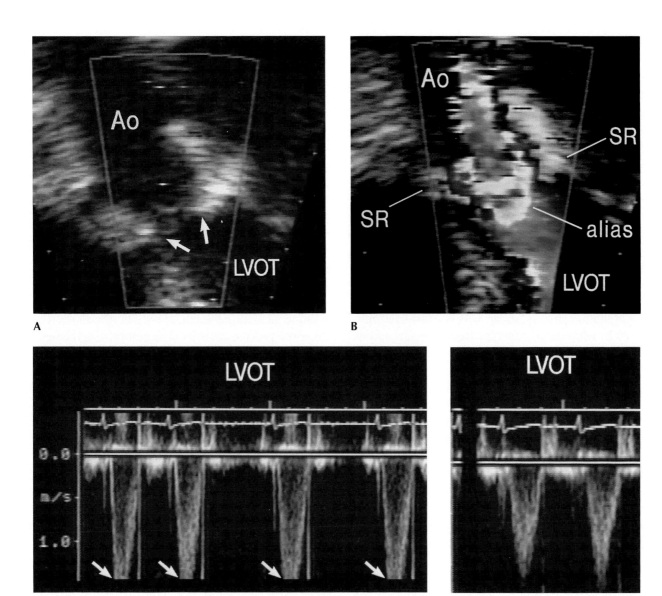

Fig. 10-16. Transthoracic echocardiography, expanded apex-down long-axis view of normal aortic bioprosthesis. A. The prosthesis sewing ring *(arrows)* separates the left ventricular outflow tract from the aorta. B. With color-flow imaging, one sees the expected, slightly turbulent jet in the aorta. Flow convergence creates color aliasing in the left ventricular outflow tract just below the prosthesis. Note that at the level of flow convergence, the velocity profile is not uniform across the diameter of the outflow tract. The velocity becomes uniform (blue) across the diameter just below the zone of color aliasing. C. In this pulsed-wave Doppler spectrum from the left ventricular outflow tract, a sample volume is positioned within the central zone of color aliasing. The left ventricular outflow tract velocity exceeds the Nyquist limit and aliases *(arrows)*. Measuring the time velocity integral of these velocity spectra would result in an erroneously large effective orifice area for the prosthesis. D. The sample volume has been moved to a position below the region of flow convergence (about 1 cm from the sewing ring) in the left ventricular outflow tract. The left ventricular outflow tract velocity is 1.2 mm/sec. This is the correct sample volume position for obtaining this velocity for the effective orifice area calculation. This velocity spectrum would be traced, and the time velocity integral would be used in the numerator of the continuity equation formula.

Regurgitation

Normal prosthetic valve function includes a small amount of regurgitation. As the moving parts of the prosthesis close, blood is displaced back into the receiving chamber. This is referred to as the closing volume of the prosthesis. In addition to the closing volume, tilting disk and bileaflet prostheses normally produce a small amount of transvalvular regurgitation, which is referred to as the leakage volume [50,51]. Therefore, it is not uncommon to detect a small degree of regurgitation during the echocardiographic evaluation of normal prosthetic aortic valves. As with native valves, we score the degree of regurgitation for the clinician on a 0 to 4 scale (Table 10-7). Trivial or mild transvalvular regurgitation (that is, grade 1/4) is considered normal. In addition to semiquantitating regurgitation, we try to differentiate perivalvular from transvalvular regurgitation. All degrees of perivalvular regurgitation are abnormal although not usually clinically significant unless moderate or greater.

Color-flow imaging is the cornerstone for the detection and semiquantitation of prosthetic valve regurgitation. However, to fully characterize the degree of regurgitation, we use an integrated approach that combines color-flow imaging with information from spectral Doppler and two-dimensional imaging. We do not currently calculate and report regurgitant fractions for prosthetic valves in our routine clinical practice.

When evaluating valvular prostheses, one must remember that regurgitant jets are three-dimensional and that color-flow imaging is a tomographic technique. It is therefore necessary to scan the LVOT in as many different planes as possible. In particular, perivalvular jets can have unusual shapes and eccentric trajectories. Interrogation limited to a single imaging plane can result in significant underestimation of severity. The single most important plane for evaluating prosthetic aortic regurgitation is the parasternal short-axis (Fig. 10-17). The dimensions of the jet should be defined just below the prosthetic valve sewing ring. As with native aortic regurgitation, the area of the regurgitant jet should be compared with the area of the LVOT at the same level [52]. In practice, we most often visually estimate the ratio of the jet area to the LVOT area. If the LVOT short-axis view is technically inadequate, the diameter of the jet in long axis should be compared with the LVOT diameter. In the previously mentioned study, Kapur et al. [27] found a high sensitivity (92%) for detection of prosthetic aortic regurgitation by color Doppler echocardiography (compared with catheterization). Furthermore, for 36 aortic prostheses, there was complete agreement with the angiographic grading of regurgitation severity in 25 cases. There was disagreement by one grade in 10 cases and by two grades in only 1 instance.

The grade of prosthetic aortic regurgitation can usually be obtained from surface echocardiography. Comparable imaging planes for prosthetic aortic regurgitation can be achieved during TEE, particularly with biplane or multiplane transducers [9,12,53]. Transesophageal echocardiography is particularly useful for intraoperative studies [54–56]. It provides the added benefit of defining structural abnormalities responsible for regurgitation, such as degeneration of aortic heterograft cusps (Fig. 10-18). Transesophageal echocardiography is also proving to be especially useful in diagnosing dehiscence of aortic prostheses, with resultant severe periprosthetic aortic regurgitation (Fig. 10-19).

As shown in Figures 10-18 and 10-19, jets of aortic regurgitation are most completely defined when biplane (or multiplane) transducers are used. During imaging in the horizontal plane, the transducer should be anteflexed from the four-chamber view to visualize the LVOT (Fig. 10-19 *C* and 10-19 *D*). In the longitudinal plane, medial and lateral flexion of the transducer tip is done to develop both short- and long-axis views of the LVOT (Fig. 10-18, 10-19 *A,* and 10-19 *B*).

The degree of prosthetic aortic regurgitation can also be semiquantitated according to the amount of diastolic flow reversal in the descending thoracic aorta [57]. This can be investigated by transthoracic echocardiography from the suprasternal notch with either color-flow imaging or pulsed-wave Doppler

Table 10-7. Grading prosthetic valve regurgitation

Degree of regurgitation	Grade
Absent	0
Trivial or mild	1/4
Moderate	2/4
Moderately severe*	3/4
Severe*	4/4

*Grades 3/4 and 4/4 are generally considered to be surgical degrees of regurgitation (i.e., sufficient to cause symptoms or ventricular dysfunction).

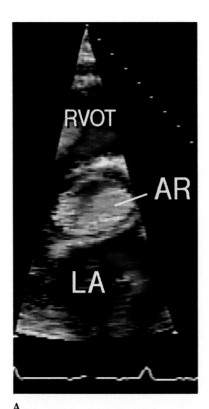 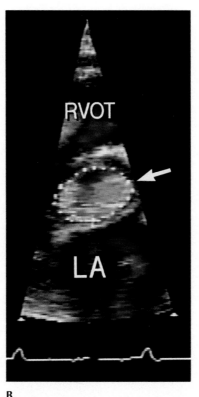 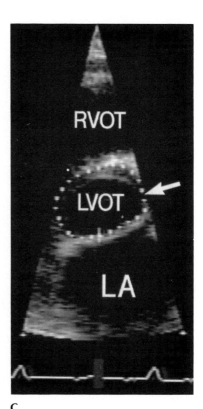

A   B   C

Fig. 10-17. Severe prosthetic aortic regurgitation due to degeneration of Hancock bioprosthesis. A. Transthoracic echocardiography, parasternal short-axis view. Color-flow imaging of aortic regurgitation is performed in the left ventricular outflow tract just below the valve cusps. By visual inspection, the jet fills most of the tract. B. For more precise semiquantitation, the ratio of the aortic regurgitation jet area to the left ventricular outflow tract area can be determined. In this frame, the regurgitant jet has been traced *(arrow, dotted circle).* C. With color-flow signals deleted, the left ventricular outflow tract has been traced *(arrow, dotted circle).* The ratio was 0.7, consistent with severe (grade 4/4) aortic regurgitation.

examination, as discussed in Chapter 9. Significant degrees of regurgitation are associated with reversed flow that persists throughout diastole. It is important to remember to keep the filter settings low when evaluating diastolic flow reversal, since the flow reversal has a relatively low velocity. If evaluation of the aortic arch is technically inadequate, diastolic flow reversal should be evaluated in the abdominal aorta (Fig. 10-20).

Continuous-wave Doppler echocardiography serves as a simple screening tool for prosthetic aortic regurgitation. In addition, the ease with which the velocity spectrum can be fully defined and the intensity of high-velocity continuous-wave signals from aortic regurgitation serve as a clue to severity. Measurement of the pressure half-time of the aortic regurgitant jet is clinically useful [58], but one must

remember that this value is reduced not only by an increased volume of aortic regurgitation but also by elevation of left ventricular diastolic pressure from any cause. The latter increase obviously can occur for reasons independent of regurgitation, such as ischemic heart disease. We have found that the pressure half-time is most useful when prosthetic aortic regurgitation is acute and left ventricular systolic function is normal. This state can occur with infective endocarditis or can arise from degenerative rupture of a bioprosthetic valve cusp. With acute, severe prosthetic regurgitation, the pressure half-time of the regurgitant jet is usually less than 300 msec (Fig. 10-21). Other findings in acute, severe aortic regurgitation are reduction in the mitral valve deceleration time and diastolic mitral regurgitation, both of which can be defined by pulsed-wave Doppler

Fig. 10-18. Transesophageal echocardiographic examination of a degenerated Ionescu-Shiley aortic heterograft prosthesis. A. Longitudinal plane, short-axis view of aortic prosthesis. The three stents *(S)* are well defined. Failure of the cusps in diastole to completely coapt (an inverted Y appearance is lacking) creates two separate regurgitant orifices *(arrows)*. B. Resultant severe aortic regurgitation is clearly demonstrated by short-axis color-flow imaging.

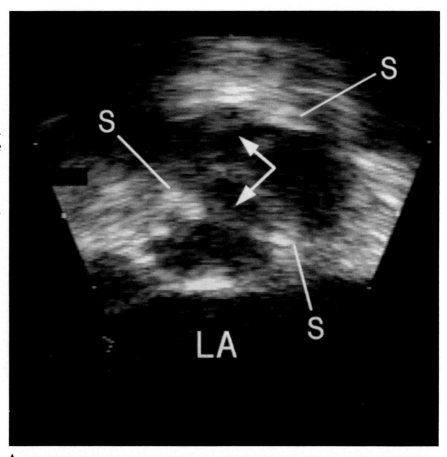

A

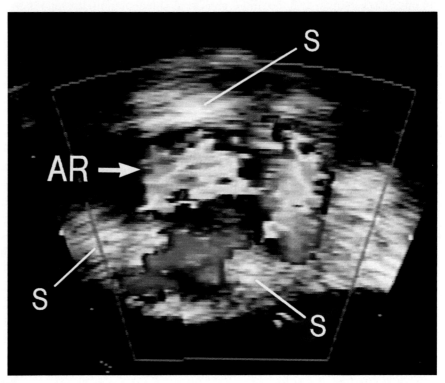

B

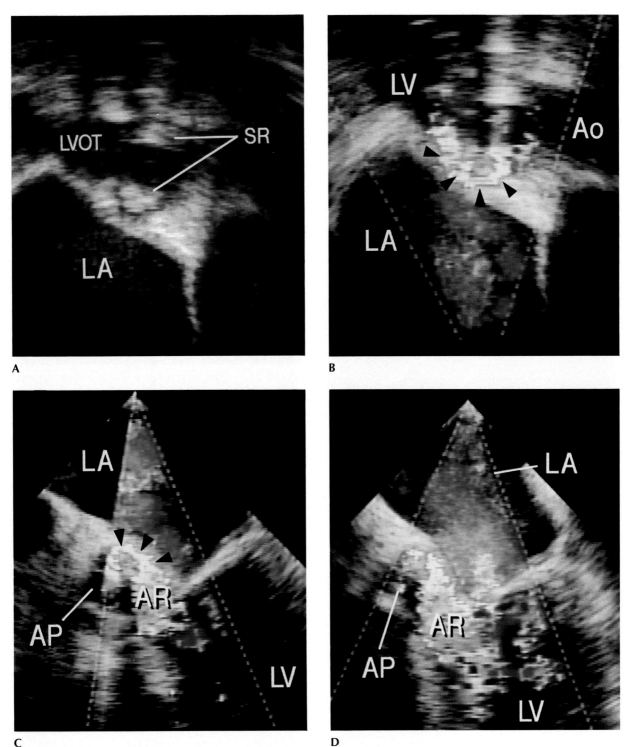

Fig. 10-19. Transesophageal echocardiographic examination demonstrating partial dehiscence of a St. Jude Medical aortic prosthesis. A. Longitudinal plane, long-axis view of the left ventricular outflow tract and the prosthetic valve sewing ring. B. Color-flow imaging demonstrates periprosthetic aortic regurgitation *(arrowheads)* tracking around the dehiscent sewing ring inferiorly. C. Horizontal plane. The periprosthetic aortic regurgitation is again identified with flow around the sewing ring *(arrowheads)* of the aortic prosthesis. D. The transducer has been advanced slightly into the esophagus from its location in C to demonstrate that the aortic regurgitant jet fills the immediate left ventricular outflow tract, consistent with severe regurgitation.

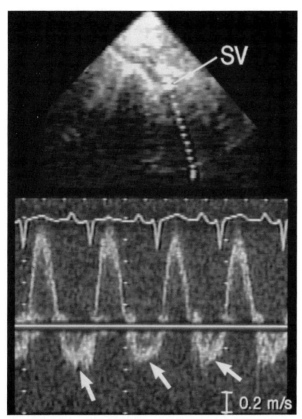

Fig. 10-20. Degeneration of Ionescu-Shiley aortic prosthesis resulting in sudden rupture of one cusp. Transthoracic color-flow imaging was technically difficult, and the descending thoracic aorta could not be adequately evaluated for diastolic flow reversal. Here, the pulsed-wave sample volume *(SV)* has been placed in the abdominal aorta from a subcostal transducer position. The velocity spectrum demonstrates holodiastolic reversal *(arrows)*, confirming the clinical impression of severe prosthetic transvalvular aortic regurgitation.

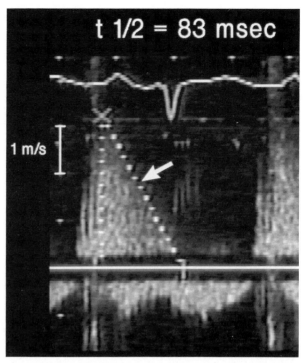

Fig. 10-21. Continuous-wave Doppler interrogation of aortic regurgitant jet from the same patient as in Fig. 10-20; apical transducer position. The pressure half-time has been measured *(arrow)* and is profoundly reduced at 83 msec, consistent with rapid equilibration of aortic and left ventricular diastolic pressures. This finding also confirms that the prosthetic aortic regurgitation is severe, particularly since left ventricular systolic function was normal by two-dimensional imaging.

imaging from either transthoracic or transesophageal studies [59–61]. Diastolic mitral regurgitation can also be seen with color-flow imaging, and the diastolic timing is easily confirmed with color M-mode studies (Fig. 10-22).

Jets of either transvalvular or perivalvular prosthetic aortic regurgitation occur just below the ultrasonic transducer when it is placed in the left parasternal position, and these jets come directly toward the transducer that is placed at the apex. Therefore, transthoracic echocardiography is usually sufficient for characterizing the amount of prosthetic aortic regurgitation by color-flow imaging. In fact, TEE may underestimate the severity of aortic regurgitation by color flow because of acoustic shadowing

in the LVOT created by the prosthetic material (Fig. 10-22 *B*). This is a particular problem if the patient has both aortic and mitral prostheses [62].

Mohr-Kahaly et. al. [63] investigated 136 normal prostheses for regurgitation, comparing transthoracic echocardiography with TEE. Seventy-nine of these prostheses were aortic. Transesophageal echocardiography was more sensitive for detecting prosthetic aortic regurgitation except for Bjork-Shiley prostheses. However, for all types of aortic prostheses, the regurgitant jet area was larger when evaluated by transthoracic echocardiography than it was on the transesophageal examination. This factor must be taken into account when grading the severity of prosthetic aortic regurgitation by TEE color-flow imaging. Color-flow analysis of prosthetic aortic regurgitation by TEE is more frequently used intraoperatively and is also valuable in routine clinical cases when transthoracic imaging is technically inadequate. For both TEE and transthoracic echocardiography, the most complete assessment of aortic regurgitation is obtained when color-flow information is integrated with data from spectral Doppler examination as well as two-dimensional analysis of the malfunctioning prosthesis.

Kapur et al. [27] investigated the accuracy of color-flow imaging by transthoracic echocardiography in determining whether prosthetic regurgitant jets were prosthetic or periprosthetic. The echocardiographic diagnosis was compared with surgical findings for 34 aortic and 45 mitral prostheses. Perivalvular regurgitation was incorrectly diagnosed in only two (4%) of the mitral prostheses and three (9%) of the aortic prostheses. The incorrect diagnoses of perivalvular regurgitation were made when the regurgitant jet originated *at* the stents or suture line or when jets of aortic regurgitation originated at the extreme anterior or posterior margins of the prosthesis. Although such jets are *usually* periprosthetic, these investigators point out that 100% confidence can be achieved only when the origin of the periprosthetic jet is identified *outside* the limits of the prosthesis. This is particularly true for bioprostheses, since tears and perforations of the cusps frequently occur near the point of attachment to the sewing ring. This rule for confidently diagnosing periprosthetic regurgitation certainly applies to both transthoracic echocardiography and TEE.

MITRAL AND TRICUSPID PROSTHESES

Forward Flow Hemodynamics and Obstructive Lesions

For delineation of obstructive characteristics for mitral and tricuspid prostheses, it is important to determine early peak velocity, mean diastolic pressure gradient, pressure half-time, and EOA [31,35,64–72]. The peak velocity, mean gradient, and pressure half-time can almost invariably be obtained with the continuous-wave transducer in transthoracic apical or periapical positions (Fig. 10-23). Measurement of mitral and tricuspid prosthetic EOAs has traditionally been done by the pressure half-time technique [73]. However, there is evidence that in some clinical situations, such as left ventricular dysfunction or significant aortic regurgitation, the continuity equation is more accurate. This is discussed in detail below.

Wilkins et al. [26] studied 11 mitral and 2 tricuspid prostheses, comparing catheterization and Doppler mean gradients. They found an excellent correlation, with an *r* value of 0.96. This close correlation held for both mechanical and porcine prostheses. As previously noted, 20 of the prostheses in the study by Burstow et al. [25] were mitral. Figure 10-24 illustrates simultaneous Doppler and catheterization data from one of these patients. In Figure 10-24 *A*, there is a discrepancy between the mean gradient obtained by Doppler study (3 mm Hg) and the mean gradient obtained by catheterization (9 mm Hg) when pulmonary capillary wedge pressure is used as an estimate of left atrial pressure. The normal pressure half-time of 80 msec is an important clue to the accuracy of Doppler echocardiography as opposed to catheterization in this instance. The tracings in Figure 10-24 *B* are from the same patient after transseptal catheterization to provide a direct measurement of left atrial pressure. With this accurate assessment of left atrial pressure, the diastolic mean gradients measured by Doppler imaging and by catheterization are essentially equal both at rest and when the heart rate is significantly increased with atropine. Figure 10-25 demonstrates the overall correlation between Doppler and catheter mean gradients for the patients with mitral prostheses. When the transseptal technique was used, the *r* value was 0.97 and the standard error of the estimate was only 1.2 mm Hg. Often, when a pulmonary capillary wedge pressure was used as an estimate of left atrial pressure, catheterization significantly overestimated the true mitral mean gradient because of phase delay of the wedge pressure tracing. Fortunately, now that these validation studies have been completed, Doppler echocardiography can replace catheterization in almost every case of suspected mitral or tricuspid prosthesis dysfunction.

In their previously mentioned study, Kapur et al. [27] achieved *r* values of 0.86 and 0.87 for tissue and mechanical mitral prosthesis mean gradients by Doppler echocardiography and catheterization, respectively. As in the Mayo Clinic study, some of the catheterization-derived mean gradients were obtained by wedge pressure instead of direct measurement of left atrial pressure. In this study, mean gradients greater than 14 mm Hg tended to be associated with obstruction at surgery; however, five nonobstructed tissue mitral prostheses had mean gradients in excess of 14 mm Hg. As with aortic prostheses, these outliers represent patient-prosthesis mismatch. All the surgically nonobstructed mitral

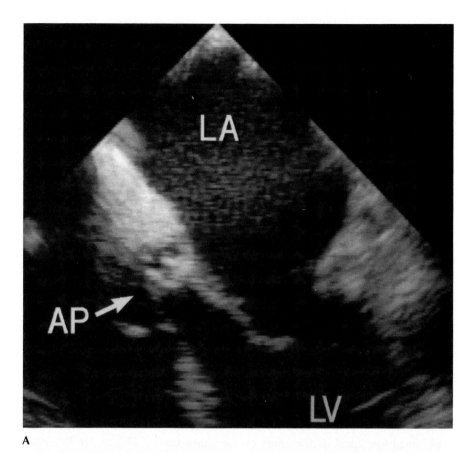

A

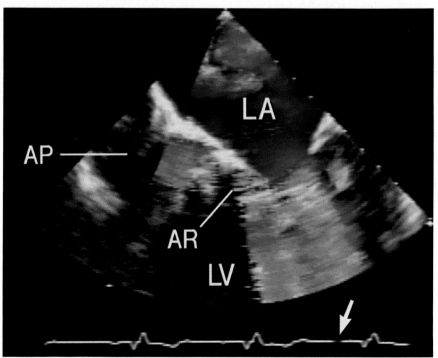

B

Fig. 10-22.   Transesophageal echocardiography in a patient with a degenerated aortic bioprosthesis resulting in severe aortic regurgitation. A. Horizontal plane, left ventricular outflow view. The sewing ring of the aortic prosthesis is identified. B. Color-flow imaging demonstrates mitral inflow. This is an early diastolic frame, as indicated by the sweep on the electrocardiogram *(arrow).* The transvalvular aortic regurgitation is not well appreciated because

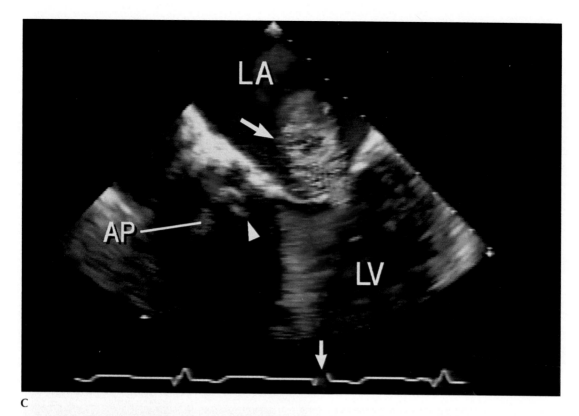

C

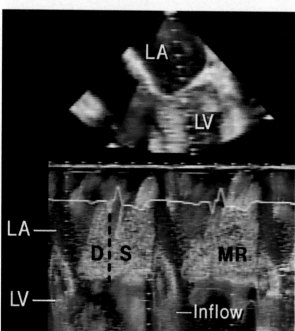

D

of acoustic shadowing by the prosthetic valve sewing ring. C. In this diastolic frame, a flail segment of an aortic cusp *(arrowhead)* is identified. The sweep on the electrocardiogram is on the QRS complex *(arrow)*, indicating an end-diastolic frame. The *arrow* in the left atrium identifies significant diastolic mitral regurgitation, which confirms that the aortic regurgitation is severe and has resulted in marked increase in left ventricular end-diastolic pressure. D. Color M-mode examination. In the upper image, the cursor has been placed across the mitral valve, from left atrium to left ventricle. Below, the color M-mode image provides precise timing for color events. Diastolic flow through the mitral valve into the left ventricle *(Inflow)* is represented in blue. Mitral regurgitation is identified as a turbulent color map in the left atrium. The *dashed line* overlying the left cycle is drawn from the initial portion of the QRS complex on the electrocardiogram. From this it can clearly be seen that a portion of the mitral regurgitation is diastolic *(D)* and a portion systolic *(S)*.

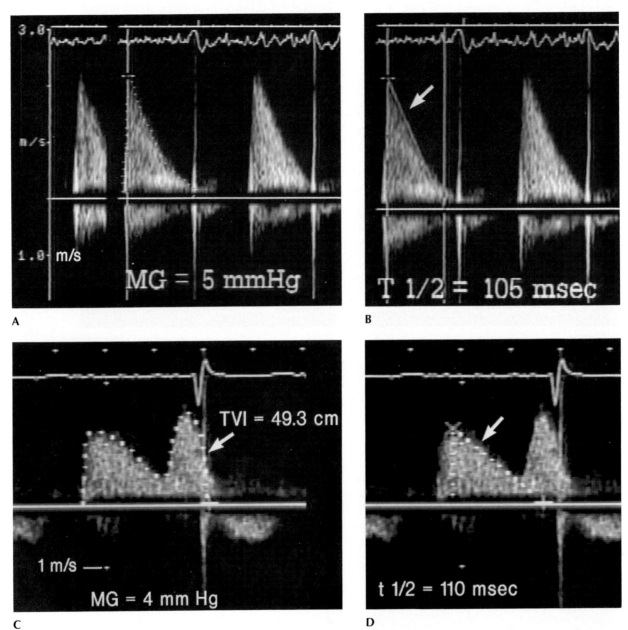

Fig. 10-23. Continuous-wave Doppler analysis of mitral prostheses. A, B. Normal Carpentier-Edwards mitral prosthesis, patient in atrial fibrillation. A. The entire diastolic velocity profile, between the opening and closing clicks, has been traced *(small dots)* and the instrument has calculated the mean gradient as 5 mm Hg. B. The deceleration slope *(arrow)* has been traced. The pressure half-time is normal for this prosthesis at 105 msec. C, D. Normal Starr-Edwards mitral prosthesis, patient in normal sinus rhythm. C. The diastolic velocity profile, including the "a" wave *(arrow)*, has been traced. The time velocity integral is 49.3 cm. From the same tracing, the mean gradient has been calculated as 4 mm Hg. D. The deceleration slope of the early filling profile has been traced *(arrow)*, and the pressure half-time is normal (110 msec) for this prosthesis.

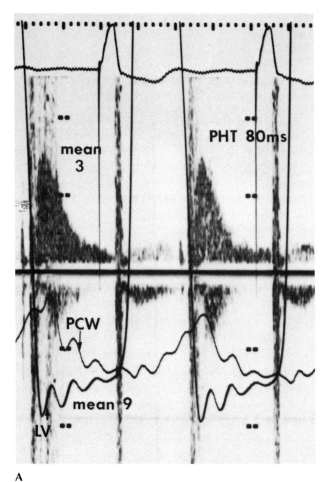

A

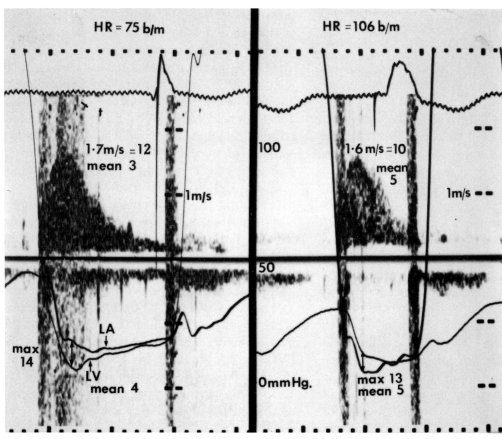

B

Fig. 10-24. Simultaneous Doppler and catheterization tracings for a patient with a normal mitral prosthetic valve. A. The Doppler mean gradient is 3 mm Hg, and the pressure half-time is normal at 80 msec. In this study, the invasive measurement of the mean diastolic gradient was obtained by use of the pulmonary capillary wedge pressure *(PCW)* as an approximation of left atrial pressure. Note that phase delay of the PCW pressure tracing resulted in an excessive mean gradient of 9 mm Hg. B. Doppler and invasive tracings from the same patient. On this occasion, transseptal puncture was performed to provide a direct measurement of left atrial pressure. Now the invasive measurement of mean gradient correlates well with the Doppler-determined gradient, both at a resting heart rate of 75 *(left panel)* and when the heart rate was increased with atropine to 106 *(right panel)*. (Courtesy of Dr. Darryl Burstow.)

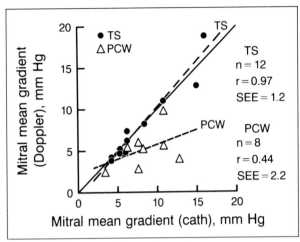

Fig. 10-25. Overall correlation between simultaneous Doppler and catheterization mean gradients for 20 mitral prosthetic valves. When the catheterization laboratory used transseptal *(TS)* puncture for direct measurement of left atrial pressure, the correlation was excellent, with an *r* value of 0.97. The correlation deteriorated significantly when the pulmonary capillary wedge pressure *(PCW)* was used as an approximation of left atrial pressure. This result illustrates the necessity of directly measuring left atrial pressure in those rare instances when invasive assessment of mitral prostheses is necessary. (From Burstow et al. [25]. By permission of the American Heart Association.)

mechanical prostheses had mean gradients of less than 13 mm Hg.

In their review of the world literature related to Doppler evaluation of normal prostheses, Reisner and Meltzer [28] identified 568 mitral prostheses. Our Mayo Clinic study of normal prosthetic valve hemodynamics includes 456 patients with clinically normal mitral valve prostheses [74]. Average values for peak velocity, mean gradient, and pressure half-time from the Mayo Clinic study are given in Table 10-8.

Kapur et al. [27], using the Doppler pressure half-time method, found correlations with *r* values of 0.94 and 0.79 for EOAs of tissue and mechanical mitral prostheses when they were compared with invasively determined EOAs with use of the Gorlin equation. Mitral EOAs of less than 1.1 cm² were associated with obstruction at surgery. These authors also correlated the width of the forward-flow color jet at its origin from the mitral prostheses with Gorlin-derived EOAs (*r* value, 0.81). Jet widths less than or equal to 0.8 cm were usually associated with prosthetic obstruction at surgery.

Dumesnil et al. [75] have raised significant questions about the validity of the pressure half-time method for determining prosthetic EOAs for normal mitral bioprostheses. Using normal mitral Medtronic Intact bioprostheses, they determined the EOA by both pressure half-time and continuity equation methods. The Doppler-derived EOAs were compared with the range of EOAs that could be produced in the in vitro laboratory for the same prostheses. Figure 10-26 illustrates their findings. For each graph, the shaded area represents the range of valve areas that were determined in the in vitro laboratory. It is evident that for many of these prostheses, the pressure half-time method resulted in valve areas that were much larger than those that could be created in the in vitro laboratory—even with very high flow states. However, for the same prostheses, the continuity equation method yielded EOAs that were quite consistent with those determined in vitro.

Our preference is to report the pressure half-time for mitral and tricuspid prostheses as an independent measure of obstruction without converting it to an EOA. The EOA is then measured by the continuity equation method [76]. Determination of mitral (or tricuspid) prosthetic EOAs by the continuity equation is illustrated in Figure 10-27.

The numerator for the EOA calculation is the same used for aortic prostheses (see Fig. 10-13 *D*). The LVOT diameter is measured and used to determine the LVOT area. The area is multiplied by the TVI of flow in the LVOT to yield the stroke volume. The denominator is the TVI of flow across the mitral prosthesis. When the continuous-wave velocity spectrum for the mitral prosthesis is traced to obtain the mean gradient, most instruments now also measure this TVI. It is important to realize that the patient must be free of significant (greater than mild) aortic and mitral regurgitation in order to have continuity of flow from the prosthesis to the outflow tract. Also, since the profiles of the mitral and LVOT velocity spectra are quite different, one no longer has the option of using the LVOT velocity to simplify the numerator. The TVI for the LVOT must be measured. Finally, it is difficult to use this continuity method during TEE, since the alignment of the LVOT with esophageal windows is not favorable for accurate Doppler determination of the LVOT TVI. Transgastric long-axis imaging in the longitudinal plane may provide excellent alignment of the LVOT for Doppler interrogation (see Chapter 3) but is not consistently obtainable.

We recently investigated an alternative method

Table 10-8. Mayo Clinic normal ranges for Doppler measurements of mitral and tricuspid prostheses

Valve type	No.	Peak velocity, m/sec*	Mean gradient, mm Hg*	Pressure half-time, msec*
		Mitral prostheses		
Heterograft	150	1.6 ± 0.3/2.4	4.1 ± 1.5/8	103 ± 26/160
Ball-cage	161	1.8 ± 0.3/2.5	4.9 ± 1.8/10	100 ± 28/183
Bjork-Shiley	79	1.7 ± 0.3/2.5	4.1 ± 1.6/9	91 ± 20/144
St. Jude Medical	66	1.6 ± 0.4/2.5	4.0 ± 1.8/10	80 ± 20/140
		Tricuspid prostheses		
Heterograft	43	1.3 ± 0.2/1.8	3.2 ± 1.1/5.5	145 ± 37/209
Ball-cage	35	1.3 ± 0.2/1.7	3.2 ± 0.8/4.6	140 ± 48/238
Bjork-Shiley	1	1.3	2.2	144
St. Jude Medical	7	1.2 ± 0.3/1.6	2.7 ± 1.1/4.1	108 ± 32/159

*Mean ± SD/highest average value.
Mitral prostheses portion from Lengyel et al. [74]. By permission of the American Heart Association. Tricuspid prostheses portion from Connolly et al. [79]. By permission of the American College of Cardiology.

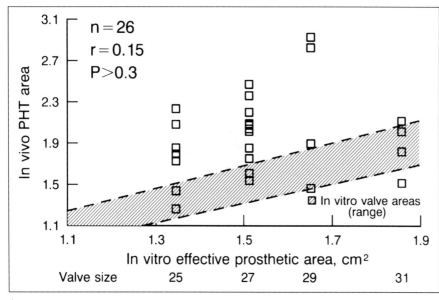

A

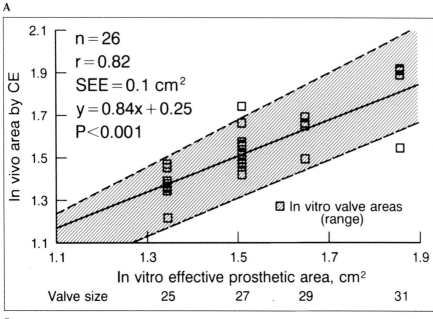

B

Fig. 10-26. Doppler compared with in vitro effective orifice areas for normal Medtronic Intact mitral prosthesis. For each graph, the Doppler-derived values are plotted on the ordinate and the valve size is represented along the abscissa. The shaded area represents the range of valve areas, for each valve size, that was determined in the in vitro laboratory with various simulated cardiac outputs. A. Doppler effective orifice areas were determined by the pressure half-time method. Note that many of the Doppler values fall significantly above the range of values that was determined in the in vitro laboratory, exceeding even those values determined at the highest levels of simulated cardiac output. B. When the Doppler effective orifice area for these same valves was measured by the continuity equation *(CE)*, almost all the values were within the range determined in the in vitro laboratory. (From Dumesnil et al. [75]. By permission of Cahners Publishing Company, a Division of Reed Publishing USA.)

271

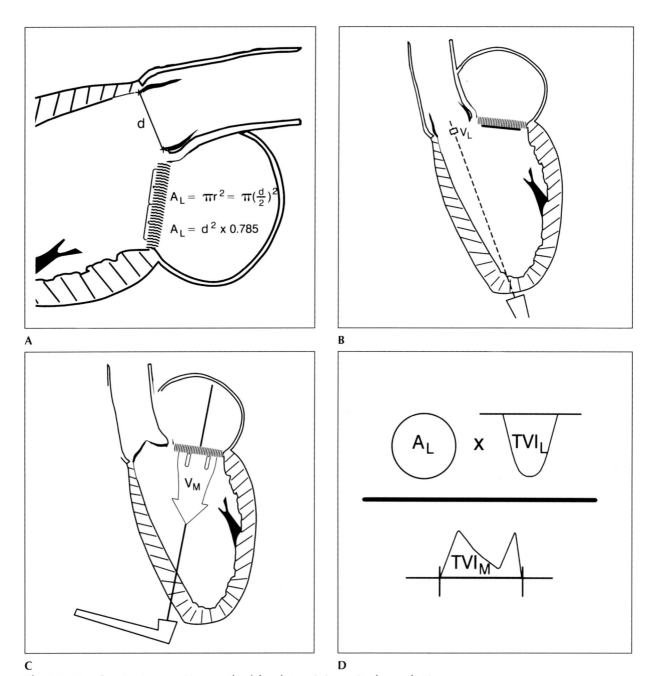

Fig. 10-27. Continuity equation method for determining mitral prosthetic effective orifice area (this method can also be applied to tricuspid prostheses). A. The systolic left ventricular outflow tract diameter *(d)* is measured from a parasternal long-axis view. This diameter is converted to left ventricular outflow tract area *(A_L)* by squaring it and multiplying it by 0.785 (π/4). B. From an apical long-axis view, the velocity in the left ventricular outflow tract *(V_L)* is measured by placing the sample volume at the level of the aortic valve annulus. The time velocity integral is measured from the resultant velocity spectrum. C. From an apical or para-apical transducer position, the mitral prosthesis velocity *(V_M)* is measured by continuous-wave Doppler echocardiography. The resultant time velocity integral is measured from the velocity spectrum. D. Schema of the continuity equation, rearranged to calculate the prosthetic mitral valve area. The numerator is the left ventricular outflow tract area multiplied by the left ventricular outflow tract time velocity integral *(TVI_L)* (which is the stroke volume). The denominator is the time velocity integral of the prosthesis *(TVI_M)*. This method is invalid if the patient has significant aortic or mitral regurgitation.

for using flow continuity to determine the EOA of mitral prostheses [77]. The mitral stroke distance is measured by placement of a pulsed-wave sample volume in the left atrium just above the mitral prosthesis sewing ring and measurement of the TVI of the resultant spectral signal. This TVI is multiplied by the left atrial area at the same level to determine left atrial flow entering the prosthesis. For simplicity, the left atrial area is determined by use of the mitral prosthesis sewing ring diameter (which is squared and then multiplied by 0.785). Because this left atrial flow is continuous with flow through the prosthesis, the mitral EOA can be calculated as

$$\text{Mitral prosthesis EOA} = (\text{sewing ring diameter})^2 \times 0.785 \times (\text{left atrial TVI}) \div (\text{prosthesis TVI})$$

For a small number of cases, we found a very favorable correlation between the mitral prosthesis EOA determined by this method and that derived from the standard continuity method described above. If this correlation holds for a larger number of cases,

this new method will have several advantages: it is quicker than the standard continuity method, it is readily accomplished by TEE, and should be valid even with significant mitral or aortic regurgitation.

Many of the newer TEE transducers have steerable continuous-wave Doppler capability that can be easily used to study mitral prostheses [78]. In particular, TEE-guided continuous-wave Doppler imaging can be used for determining the mean gradient across mitral prostheses (Fig. 10-28). The continuous-wave cursor can be guided across mitral prostheses with use of either horizontal plane four-chamber or longitudinal plane two-chamber views. This approach is supplemented by color-flow mapping to align the cursor directly parallel to mitral inflow. Transesophageal echocardiography should prove particularly useful in the intraoperative evaluation of prosthetic mitral valves.

Occasionally, it is difficult to determine the mean gradient and pressure half-time for tricuspid prostheses by transthoracic echocardiography. In such cases,

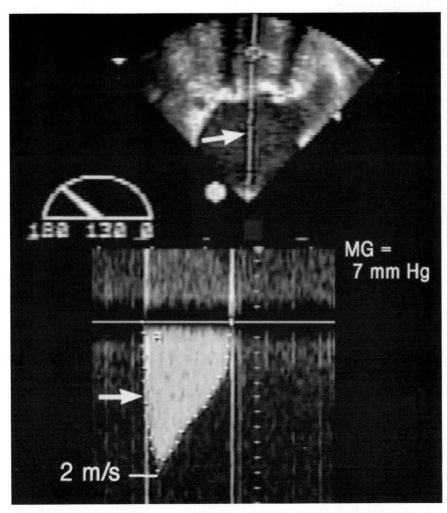

Fig. 10-28. Omniplane TEE-guided continuous-wave Doppler evaluation of a Lillihei-Kaster mitral prosthesis. The small upper image is a longitudinal plane two-chamber view. The continuous-wave cursor *(upper arrow)* has been guided across the mitral prosthesis. The resultant velocity spectrum is recorded below. Since flow through the prosthesis is away from the transesophageal transducer, the diastolic velocity is recorded below the baseline. The profile has been traced *(lower arrow)*, and the resultant mean gradient is 7 mm Hg. See Fig. 10-36 for further discussion.

TEE-guided continuous-wave examination can be done (Fig. 10-29). We have found that it is often easiest to guide the continuous-wave cursor across tricuspid prostheses when a longitudinal-plane short-axis view is used (analogous to the parasternal short-axis view at the base of the heart).

When we determine hemodynamic measurements for mitral prostheses, measuring multiple cycles is particularly important. For patients in sinus rhythm, we average 3 to 5 cycles, and for patients who have atrial fibrillation or other very irregular rhythms, 5 to 10 cycles are used. Measurement of 10 cycles is mandatory for patients with tricuspid prostheses— even when the cardiac rhythm is regular. Table 10-8 also lists Doppler hemodynamic values from the

Mayo Clinic study of 86 clinically normal tricuspid prostheses [79]. Table 10-9 shows the beat-to-beat variation in tricuspid prosthesis hemodynamic values that results from respiratory variation of tricuspid inflow. This variation is most marked for the measurement of pressure half-time.

For all types of prostheses, transthoracic Doppler hemodynamic values can be obtained both at rest and with exercise [80–83]. Measurement is particularly feasible for mitral prostheses because of the ease with which the maximal Doppler spectrum can be obtained from an apical transducer position. The Doppler data can be obtained *during* exercise if a supine or upright bicycle exercise protocol is used. Alternatively, the Doppler data can be obtained immediately after treadmill exercise testing.

By analogy to native valvular lesions, exercise evaluation of prostheses should be considered when the patient has symptoms such as exertional dyspnea but normal resting prosthetic hemodynamic values. Exercise Doppler studies should also be considered for patients who are asymptomatic yet have relatively high gradients across their prostheses. To date, only a small body of data defines normal prosthetic valve hemodynamic values with exercise. Such data are useful not only in the clinical situations mentioned above but also in comparisons of different types of normal prostheses.

Transesophageal echocardiographic imaging of mitral and tricuspid mechanical prostheses complements Doppler hemodynamic measurements by allowing assessment of occluder motion (Fig. 10-30 and 10-31]. This motion may be significantly reduced when the prosthesis is obstructed by thrombus, vegetative material, or pannus [11,84]. In the right panel of Figure 10-32, transesophageal examination shows that an Omniscience mitral prosthesis is obstructed with thrombus. The reduced opening angle for this prosthesis can be compared with the

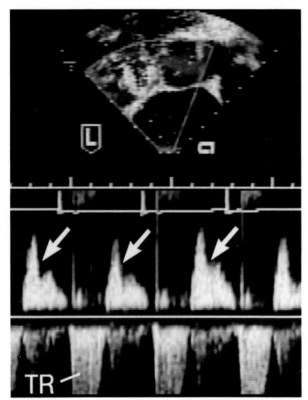

Fig. 10-29. Transesophageal echocardiographic examination of regurgitant Carpentier-Edwards tricuspid valve prosthesis. The small upper image is a longitudinal *(L)* plane, basal short-axis view (for further orientation, see Fig. 10-42). The continuous-wave Doppler cursor has been guided across the tricuspid prosthesis. The resultant Doppler velocity spectrum is shown below and has been inverted so that its appearance is identical to that from a surface study. The diastolic profile *(arrows)* can be traced to obtain mean gradient, time velocity integral, and pressure half-time. Tricuspid regurgitation is recorded below the baseline and is discussed in more detail in Fig. 10-42.

Table 10-9. Maximal beat-to-beat variation for Doppler measurements in 86 normal tricuspid prostheses

Doppler measurement	Maximal beat-to-beat variation (10 beats)
Peak velocity, m/sec	0.5 ± 0.2
Mean gradient, mm Hg	2.3 ± 1.0
Pressure half-time, msec	81.7 ± 37.2

Data from Connolly et al. [79].

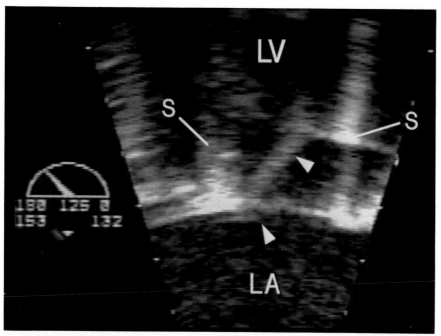

Fig. 10-30. Omniplane TEE image of normal Lillihei-Kaster mitral prosthesis. In this magnified longitudinal two-chamber view, the left ventricle is above and the left atrium below. Two of the stents *(S)* of the prosthesis are imaged. The tilting disk *(arrowheads)* is fully opened. The small image to the left indicates that the crystal array has been rotated to 125 degrees to optimize imaging of the disk. Note that even the small portion of the disk that tilts into the left atrium *(lower arrowhead)* is now evident. From such high-resolution images, the opening angle of the prosthesis can easily be measured.

normal Bjork-Shiley tilting disk prosthesis in the left panel.

For bioprosthetic mitral valves, TEE provides greatly increased resolution for identifying structural and functional abnormalities of the cusps in comparison with that obtained by surface echocardiography [9–11,85]. In Figure 10-33 *A,* a systolic frame from a normal mitral Carpentier-Edwards prosthesis, the two cusps shown are thin, and the point of coaptation is within the stents. Thickening and increased echodensity of the cusps indicate degenerative changes, which often herald progressive prosthetic dysfunction. On occasion, this is stenotic dysfunction, with immobile cusps by TEE two-dimensional imaging. However, degenerative bioprosthetic dysfunction most often is manifested as gradually increasing transvalvular regurgitation. In later stages, degenerated cusps often rupture or perforate. In systole, ruptured cusps flail into the left atrium, as illustrated in Figures 10-33 *B* and 10-33 *C.* This valuable two-dimensional imaging information from transesophageal windows therefore complements the assessment of prosthetic mitral regurgitation by color-flow imaging.

Regurgitation

Regurgitation of mitral and tricuspid prostheses is often very difficult to assess with transthoracic echocardiography. These prostheses lie directly between a transducer that is positioned at the cardiac apex and the regurgitant jet. Therefore, the ultrasound beam is considerably attenuated before it reaches the atria [62]. With mechanical prostheses, detecting prosthetic mitral or tricuspid regurgitation can be very difficult even with color-flow imaging. With bioprostheses, although the regurgitant lesions usually can be detected, the sewing ring and stents create flow-masking within the left atrium, which can lead to significant underestimation of severity.

In many cases, the jet can be better appreciated if color-flow imaging is performed from right and left parasternal positions. Using parasternal long- and short-axis views for mitral prostheses and the right ventricular inflow view for tricuspid prostheses, the examiner can frequently pass the ultrasound beam into the left or right atrium without encountering any prosthetic interference [27]. Continuous-wave Doppler echocardiography can also be used

Fig. 10-31. Transesophageal echocardiographic examination of a normal Starr-Edwards mitral prosthesis; horizontal plane, four-chamber orientation. A. Systolic frame. The ball *(arrow)* is occluding the mitral orifice, which is bounded by the sewing ring. B. Diastolic frame. The ball *(arrow)* has moved to the bottom of the cage, thereby demonstrating full opening motion.

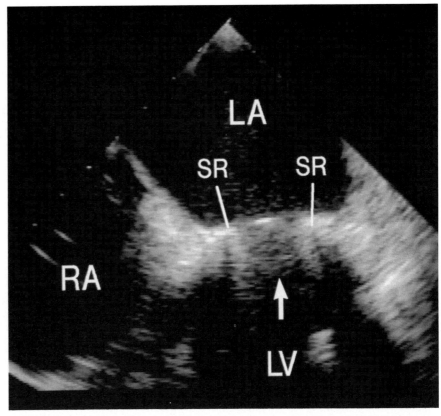

A

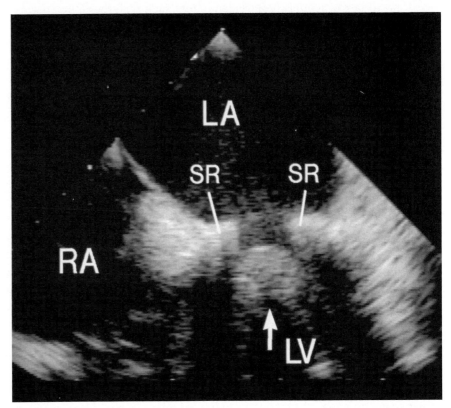

B

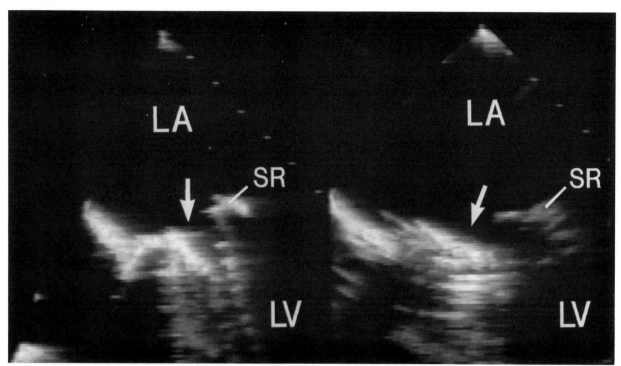

Fig. 10-32. Transesophageal, horizontal plane, four-chamber, side-by-side views. The left panel demonstrates full opening motion of the tilting disk *(arrow)* of a normal Bjork-Shiley mitral prosthesis. The right panel demonstrates reduced opening motion of the tilting disk *(arrow)* of an Omniscience mitral prosthesis. At surgery, this prosthesis was found to be obstructed by thrombus on the ventricular surface. The transthoracic echocardiographic diastolic color-flow image from this prosthesis is shown in Figure 10-4.

to enhance the detection of significant mitral or tricuspid prosthetic regurgitation. Commonly, a very strong signal of regurgitation is obtained by the continuous-wave examination even though color-flow imaging demonstrates no significant regurgitation [86]. In such instances, the examiner can be quite confident that color-flow imaging is underestimating the severity of regurgitation. A further clue to severe mitral or tricuspid regurgitation is an increase in the early diastolic flow velocity or in the diastolic TVI with a normal pressure half-time. The normal half-time indicates that the increase in velocity is due not to obstruction but rather to a large regurgitant volume, which flows back across the prosthesis in diastole. Finally, with color Doppler imaging, flow convergence or flow acceleration adjacent to the prosthesis in the left ventricle can often be appreciated in systole as identifying significant mitral regurgitation—even when color signals in the left atrium are attenuated [87,88].

Kapur et al. [27] compared *detection* of prosthetic mitral regurgitation by color-flow imaging from transthoracic echocardiography with that by contrast

left ventriculography. Despite the difficulties cited above, color Doppler imaging by transthoracic echocardiography had a sensitivity of 89% and specificity of 100% for detecting prosthetic mitral regurgitation. Curiously, there was agreement between echocardiography and angiography in grading the amount of regurgitation for 36 of 40 mitral prostheses. Not surprisingly, echocardiography underestimated the degree of regurgitation for the remaining prostheses—but by only one grade. In our experience, accurately grading the severity of prosthetic mitral regurgitation with transthoracic echocardiography alone has been difficult for a much larger percentage of patients.

Transesophageal echocardiography is ideally suited for detecting and semiquantitating mitral or tricuspid prosthetic regurgitation. The transducer can be positioned directly behind the atria, and regurgitation of prostheses in these two positions can be fully assessed without hindrance [9,89–93]. In a study of 57 mitral prostheses, Mohr-Kahaly et al. [63] found that TEE was far superior to surface echocardiography for the delineation of prosthetic

Fig. 10-33. Transesophageal echocardiography, horizontal plane, four-chamber views of mitral heterograft prostheses. A. Systolic frame, normal mitral bioprosthesis. Two of the three stents *(S)* are identified. Two of the three cusps *(arrowheads)* are seen in the closed position. Note that the cusps are normal in thickness and do not prolapse beyond the sewing ring into the left atrium. B. Another heterograft mitral prosthesis with severe regurgitation due to degenerative changes. A thickened and partially calcified cusp prolapses into the left atrium *(arrow)*. C. Intraoperative study from another degenerated mitral bioprosthesis. Two stents *(S)* are visible in the left ventricle. One of the three valve cusps prolapses into the left atrium and has a sigmoid shape *(arrow)*. In real time, this cusp demonstrated high-frequency vibration during systole. On auscultation, this vibration resulted in a buzzing murmur. This cusp tear was associated with severe mitral regurgitation.

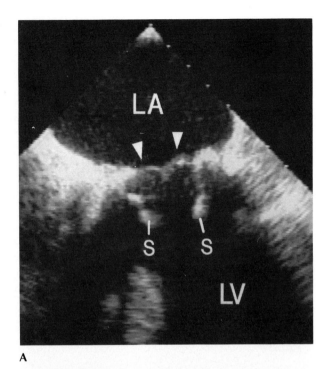

A

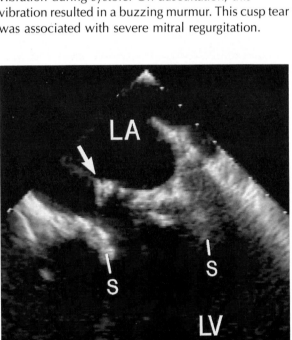

B

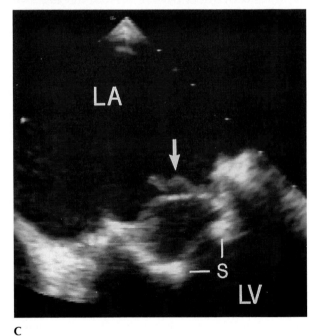

C

mitral regurgitation for both mechanical and tissue prostheses. In addition, for the same valves, the average regurgitant jet area detected by TEE was larger than that detected by transthoracic echocardiography.

Transesophageal color-flow imaging is sensitive enough to detect the normal closing volume of mitral and tricuspid prostheses (Fig. 10-34 and 10-35B). It can also delineate normal transvalvular regurgitation, which is commonly seen with tilting disk and bileaflet prostheses [13,94,95] (Fig. 10-6). The echo-

cardiographer must remember that prosthetic valves often have normal transvalvular regurgitation and that this regurgitation can seem much more prominent on the high-resolution TEE examination than on the familiar transthoracic examination. This impression is particularly true for the Medtronic-Hall prosthesis, because the central hole creates an elongated color jet of normal regurgitation [95].

The foregoing discussion has explained how Doppler echocardiography has been used to establish normal ranges for prosthetic valve forward-flow

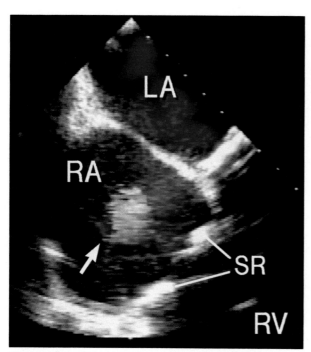

Fig. 10-34. Transesophageal echocardiography, horizontal plane, four-chamber view. Normal Starr-Edwards tricuspid prosthesis. In this systolic frame, the poppet and cage are not visible in the right ventricle. The ball-shaped, low-velocity color map *(arrow)* in the right atrium represents the volume of blood that is displaced as the poppet moves to its closed position against the sewing ring. This color array is therefore referred to as the prosthetic "closing volume."

hemodynamics. Remaining to be defined are the normal ranges for prosthetic regurgitant jet areas for each of the various types and sizes of prosthetic valves. This work is currently under way at several institutions. By comparison with normal regurgitation for each type of prosthetic mitral valve, pathologic regurgitation can usually be distinguished by its location, shape, and more extensive filling of the left atrium. In addition, pathologic prosthetic mitral regurgitation jets tend to be almost entirely mosaic, whereas normal transvalvular jets tend to be uniformly red or blue, consistent with low-velocity, nonturbulent regurgitation (Fig. 10-36).

Ideally, each prosthetic valve will be studied by TEE during implantation. Provided that the patient's hemodynamic milieu at the time of such study is close to physiologic, intraoperative imaging can serve as a baseline for the amount of normal regurgitation. This study can be used for comparison should new symptoms develop that necessitate repeat TEE. Intraoperative TEE also assists the surgeon in identifying *periprosthetic* regurgitation, a significant po-

tential problem with mitral prosthetic replacement, before the sternotomy is closed [54,56].

In contrast to regurgitant lesions affecting native mitral valves, prosthetic mitral regurgitation not uncommonly occurs through two or more separate sites (Figs. 10-35, 10-37, and 10-38). Therefore, imaging of the left atrium should continue even after a single regurgitant lesion has been identified. Because the intent is to reconstruct the volume of a three-dimensional regurgitant jet and because periprosthetic regurgitant jets are frequently eccentric with unusual trajectories, it is critical to scan the atria in as many different planes as possible for complete assessment. In the horizontal plane, flow imaging is performed during anteflexion and retroflexion and while the transducer is tilted laterally and medially. Once a regurgitant jet is identified, it is also important to withdraw the endoscope so that the superior portion of the atrium is inspected. A unique view of the prosthesis can be obtained in the horizontal plane with the transducer at about the esophagogastric junction (Fig. 10-39). In this position, one can often visualize the full circumference of the sewing ring and commonly the site or sites of periprosthetic regurgitation.

Biplane imaging frequently allows more complete visualization of prosthetic mitral regurgitation than does horizontal plane imaging alone. Such a case is illustrated in Figure 10-37, in which the longitudinal plane clearly identifies a larger amount of mitral regurgitation than that seen with the horizontal plane. The longitudinal plane also more clearly delineates a large area of dehiscence of the St. Jude Medical prosthesis. Figure 10-38 illustrates, for a tissue mitral prosthesis, how the combined use of the two planes provides more complete assessment of mitral regurgitation than would isolated use of either plane. It is expected that multiplane probes will provide even more complete flow imaging of prosthetic mitral regurgitation.

By extrapolation from transthoracic echocardiography, the degree of prosthetic mitral regurgitation is determined by transesophageal color-flow imaging according to the percentage of the atrium occupied by the regurgitant jet [27,96]. This assessment is relatively easy and most accurate for centrally directed jets. However, periprosthetic jets often travel along the walls of the atrium, just as jets frequently do in myxomatous mitral valve disease. In such instances, the width of the jet often underrepresents the volume of regurgitation [97]. When scanning the atrium, one should be careful to determine the

Fig. 10-35. Transesophageal echocardiography, horizontal plane views from a patient with a Starr-Edwards mitral prosthesis who was experiencing symptoms of congestive failure and had a murmur of mitral regurgitation. A. Soon after the transducer was introduced into the esophagus, a relatively narrow periprosthetic jet *(arrowheads)* originating around the medial portion of the sewing ring was identified. Note the mosaic appearance. This jet would certainly explain the systolic murmur, but its size seems insufficient to explain the patient's congestive symptoms. B. The transducer has been tilted to visualize the full diameter of the sewing ring. The color signals in the left atrium represent the closing volume of this ball cage prosthesis *(arrowheads)*. C. With further lateral flexion of the tip of the transesophageal probe, a second jet of periprosthetic regurgitation is identified *(arrowheads)*. This is a very large, highly turbulent jet, consistent with severe regurgitation, which certainly explains the patient's symptoms. This case exemplifies the importance of imaging in multiple planes for the complete assessment of regurgitant lesions.

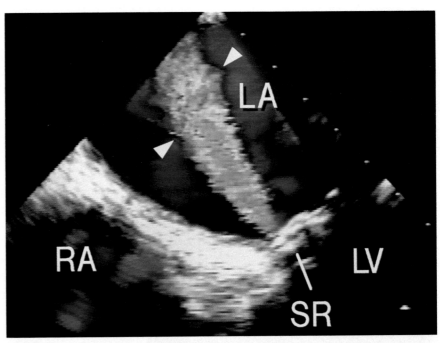

A

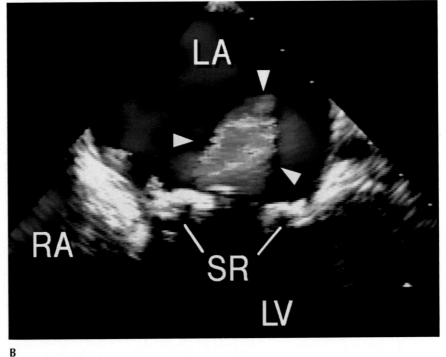

B

entire course of such jets (Fig. 10-40). If they hug the wall, curling entirely around the atrium with a final direction back toward the prosthesis, one can be confident that the regurgitation is severe. Another important marker of severe regurgitation is systolic reflux into the pulmonary veins [98,99]. This is most easily appreciated in the left or right upper pulmonary veins. Regurgitation into the pulmonary veins can be identified by either color-flow imaging or observation of systolic reversal when a pulsed-wave sample volume is placed in the pulmonary vein (Fig. 10-41).

Transesophageal echocardiography also provides increased sensitivity for detecting prosthetic tricuspid regurgitation and increased two-dimensional resolution for identifying the underlying disease. Figure 10-42 illustrates a regurgitant Carpentier-Edwards prosthesis that was implanted in the tricuspid posi-

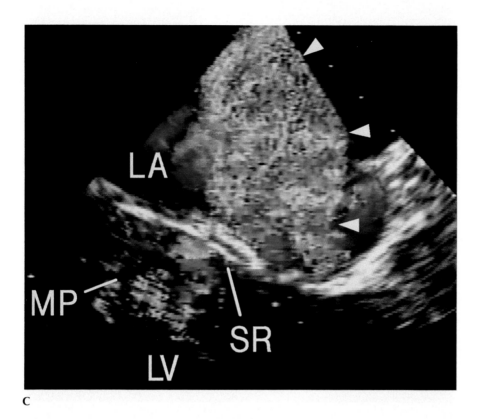

C

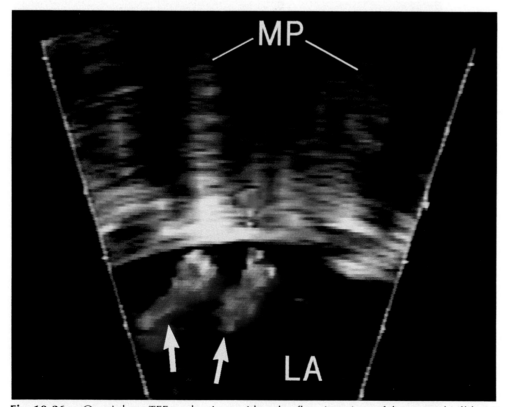

Fig. 10-36.   Omniplane TEE evaluation, with color-flow imaging, of the normal Lillihei-Kaster mitral prosthesis that is also displayed in Figs. 10-28 and 10-30. This tilting disk valve has a normal, small amount of transvalvular regurgitation. Note the two separate jets *(arrows)* in the left atrium. Besides their small size, these jets clearly represent very mild regurgitation, as they are uniformly red (nonturbulent). Very few blood cells are traveling at higher velocities (i.e., above the Nyquist limit); therefore, minimal color aliasing is seen within these jets.

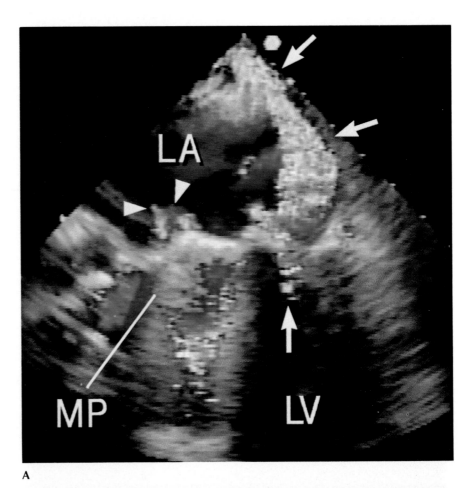

A

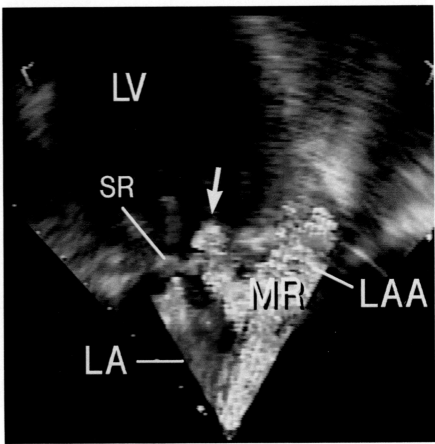

B

282

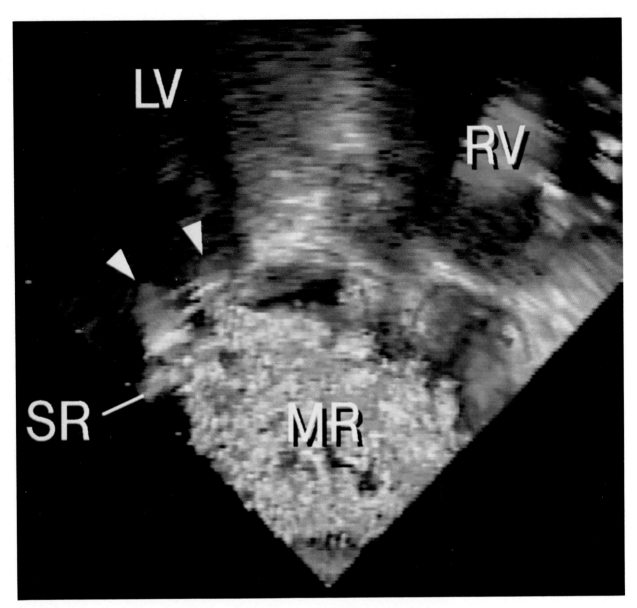

C

Fig. 10-37. Transesophageal examination of a St. Jude Medical mitral prosthesis with severe periprosthetic regurgitation. A. Horizontal plane, four-chamber view. A small periprosthetic regurgitant jet *(arrowheads)* is identified medially. A much larger jet emanates from the lateral portion of the sewing ring and curls along the left atrial wall *(upper arrows)*. The jet in this location is highly turbulent. Note the origin of this jet on the ventricular side of the prosthesis *(lower, vertical arrow)*. B. Longitudinal plane, two-chamber view. Dehiscence is more apparent here as one follows flow *(arrow)* from the left ventricle around the sewing ring and into the left atrium. This particular jet of mitral regurgitation is directed into the left atrial appendage. C. The transducer tip has been tilted slightly medially. Two separate regions of flow convergence *(arrowheads)* are identified in the left ventricle adjacent to the sewing ring. These two periprosthetic jets merge, so that the mosaic color map of mitral regurgitation nearly fills the left atrium in this view. This case illustrates the incremental benefit of adding longitudinal plane imaging to standard horizontal plane views for investigation of prosthetic mitral regurgitation. (Also see Fig. 10-41.)

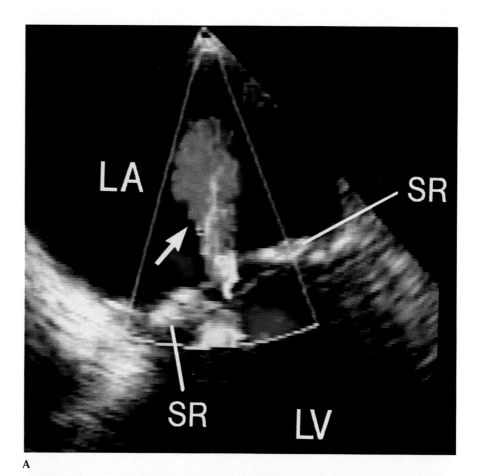

A

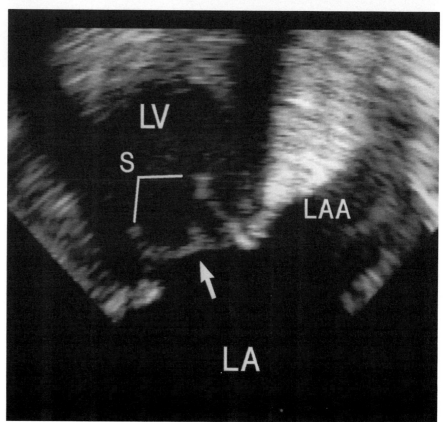

B

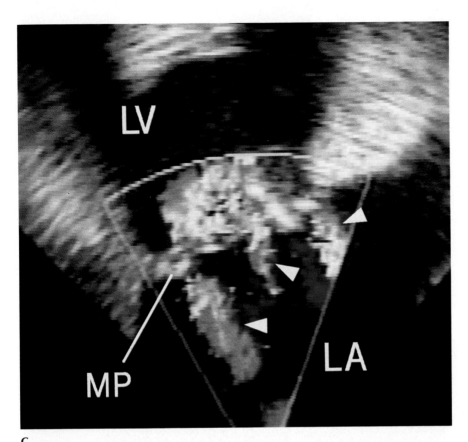

C

Fig. 10-38. Transesophageal echocardiographic examination of a Carpentier-Edwards mitral prosthesis. A. Horizontal plane, four-chamber view. In this systolic frame, the cusps are closed. Mild, central transvalvular regurgitation *(arrow)* suggests mild degenerative dysfunction. B. Longitudinal plane image. Two stents *(S)* are now clearly evident. Cusp closure *(arrow)* appears normal, and the cusps appear normal in thickness and echodensity. C. Color-flow imaging in the longitudinal plane. Three separate jets of mitral regurgitation are identified *(arrowheads)*. The jet on the right is periprosthetic, and the middle and left jets are transvalvular. The latter two jets originate just inside the sewing ring, a common site for perforation of heterograft cusps.

tion because of carcinoid involvement of the native tricuspid valve. At the time of study, this valve had been implanted for 8 years. The stents and cusps appear normal, but significant transvalvular regurgitation was identified by flow imaging. The cause is a pacemaker wire that had been passed through the prosthesis, thereby inhibiting cusp closure (Fig. 10-42 *C*). When prosthetic tricuspid regurgitation is identified by TEE, color-guided continuous-wave examination can be used to record the peak velocity and thus to yield pulmonary artery systolic pressure (Fig. 10-42 *D*).

The addition of TEE with flow imaging and spectral Doppler examination is a tremendous adjunct to surface echocardiography for the assessment of mitral and tricuspid prostheses. In a Mayo Clinic

series, Khandheria et al. [100] analyzed the results of transesophageal examination of 67 mitral prostheses. Thirty-three of these prostheses were found to be abnormal: 12 had perivalvular regurgitation; 11 had severe transvalvular regurgitation; 5 had vegetations or ring abscess; and 5 had thrombus or other obstructing lesions. Twenty-six of the patients underwent surgical repair or replacement. The TEE findings were confirmed at the time of surgery in 24 of the 26 patients (92%). This overall high rate of success in delineating mitral prosthetic abnormalities speaks to the great utility of TEE in this clinical situation.

In two cases from the Khandheria et al. series, the prosthesis was correctly identified as abnormal (by Doppler study) but TEE failed to identify the

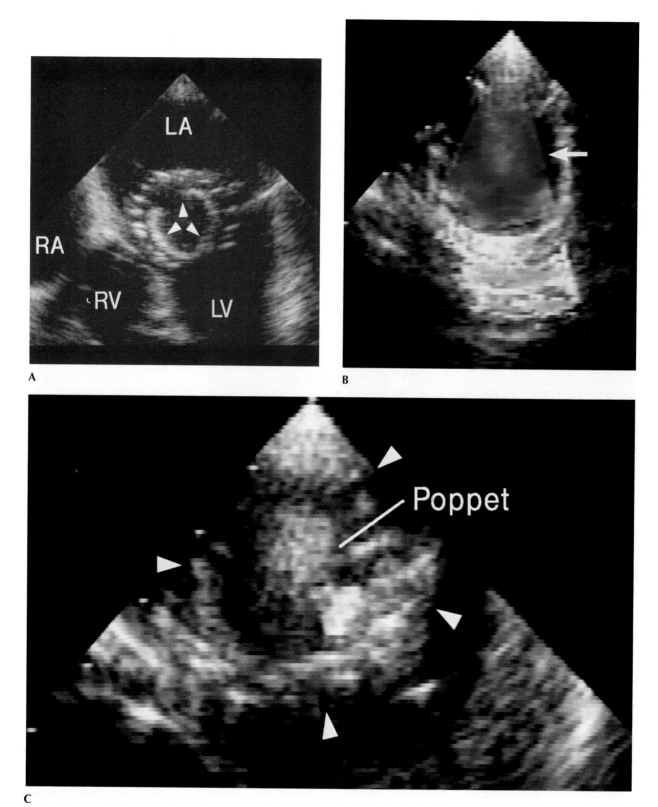

Fig. 10-39. Transesophageal, horizontal plane imaging of Starr-Edwards mitral prostheses. Sewing ring views, with the transducer positioned at the esophagogastric junction. A. The entire circumference of the sewing ring *(arrowheads)* is evident as well as the sewing ring sutures. B. Similar view of a second Starr-Edwards prosthesis, with color-flow imaging. In this diastolic frame, mitral inflow through the sewing ring is represented in blue *(arrow)*. C. In systole, the poppet has closed into the sewing ring *(arrowheads)*. The color signals inside the right lower portion of the sewing ring represent the origin of a small jet of transvalvular mitral regurgitation, which might be due to mild poppet variance or sewing ring cloth wear.

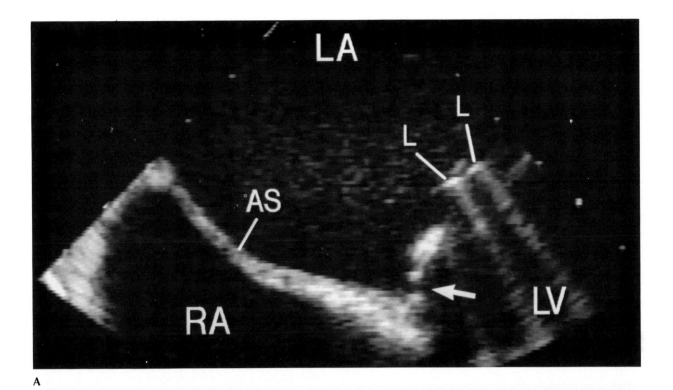

A

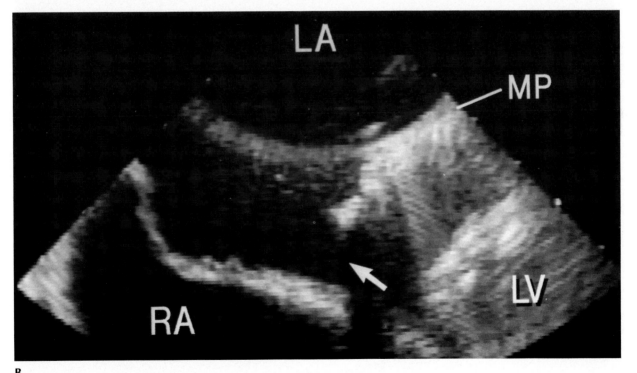

B

Fig. 10-40.   Transesophageal echocardiography, horizontal plane, off-axis four-chamber view of a St. Jude Medical mitral prosthesis. A. In this diastolic frame, the leaflets *(L)* are opened. Separation of the sewing ring from the annulus is evident *(arrow)*. B. In systole, rocking of the prosthesis creates a much larger separation *(arrow)*.

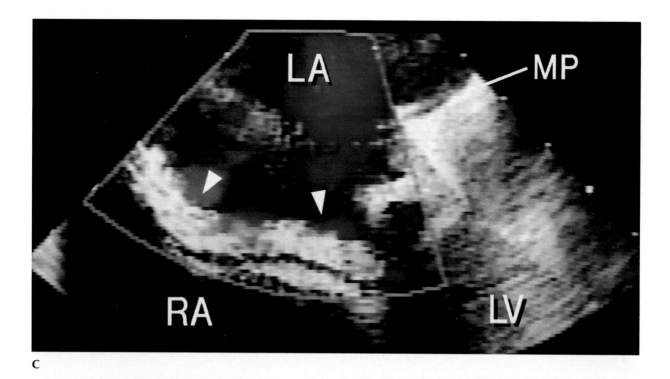

C

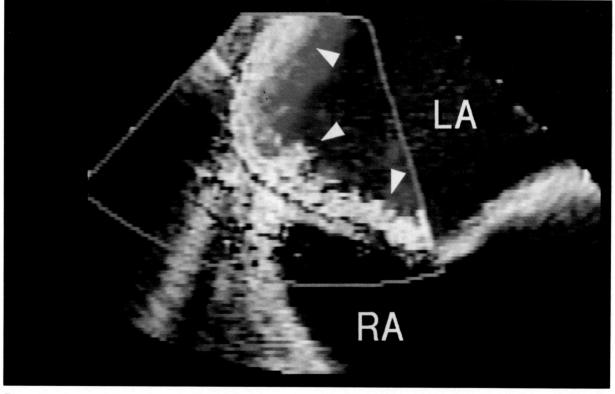

D

Figure 10-40 (continued) C. This large dehiscence results in mitral regurgitation *(arrowheads)* that appears as a narrow jet, hugging the atrial septum. D. The esophageal transducer has been withdrawn to a higher position. The jet of mitral regurgitation *(arrowheads)* curls around the medial left atrium. Note how the jet broadens as it makes the turn from atrial septum to atrial free wall. This is severe periprosthetic regurgitation.

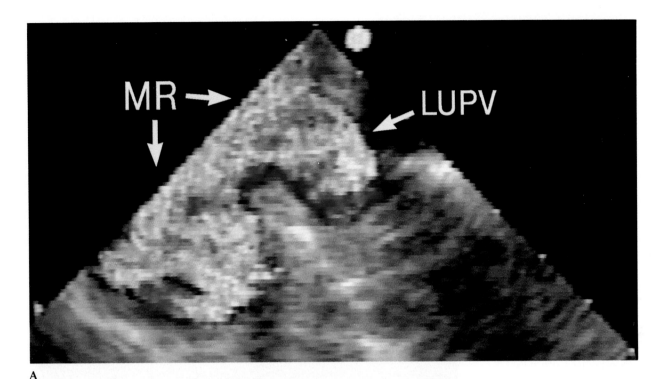

A

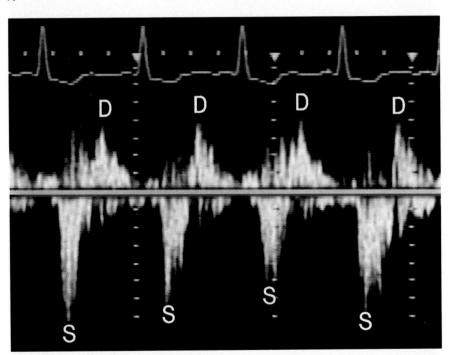

B

Fig. 10-41. Transesophageal echocardiography, systolic reflux into the left upper pulmonary vein. The patient is the same one examined in Fig. 10-37, with perivalvular defects causing severe mitral regurgitation. A. Color-flow imaging demonstrating that the turbulent jet of mitral regurgitation enters the left upper pulmonary vein. B. A pulsed-wave sample volume was placed in the left upper pulmonary vein. Normally, laminar pulmonary venous flow is directed from the pulmonary vein into the left atrium, toward the transesophageal transducer. Therefore, the velocity spectrum is expected to be above the baseline in both systole *(S)* and diastole *(D)*. Here, the severe mitral regurgitation results in complete reversal of systolic flow or flow away from the left atrium.

Fig. 10-42. Transesophageal echocardiography, tricuspid Carpentier-Edwards bioprosthesis. This is the same valve examined in Fig. 10-29. Longitudinal plane, basal short-axis view. The aorta is slightly off-axis. A. Two stents (S) are identified. In this systolic frame, cusp closure (arrowheads) appears normal. B. In diastole, the cusps have opened. A permanent pacemaker wire is directed into the tricuspid orifice (arrow). This pacemaker wire was also evident in the systolic frame, in the right atrium. C. With color-flow imaging, it is evident that the pacemaker wire has resulted in significant tricuspid regurgitation (arrowheads). The regurgitant jet splits in two around the wire. D. In the small upper image, a continuous-wave cursor has been guided through the color-flow image of tricuspid regurgitation. Below, the Doppler velocity spectrum has been inverted to correspond to a normal transthoracic Doppler examination. The diastolic inflow profile of the tricuspid prosthesis is recorded above the baseline (arrows). The tricuspid regurgitation velocity spectrum is recorded below the baseline. The peak velocity of 2 m/sec indicates normal pulmonary artery systolic pressure.

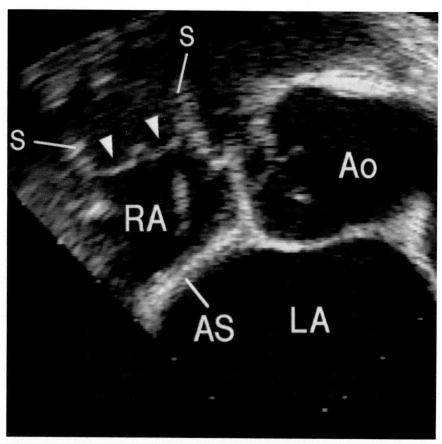

A

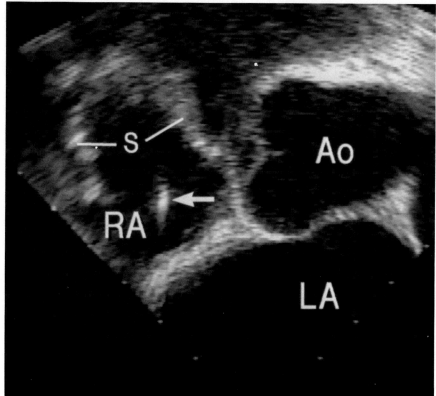

B

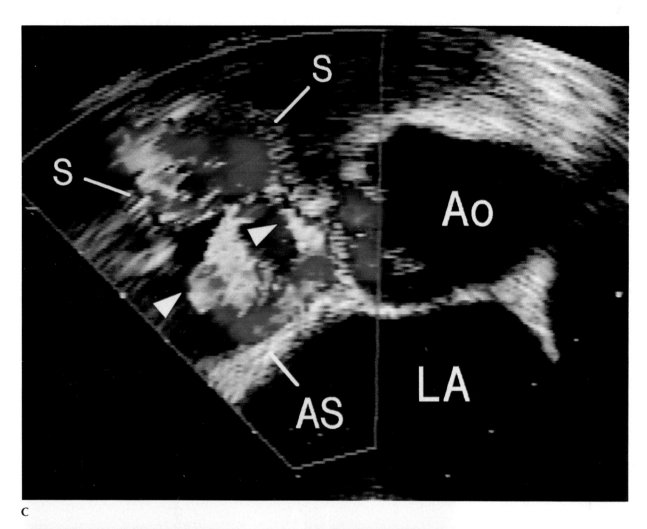

C

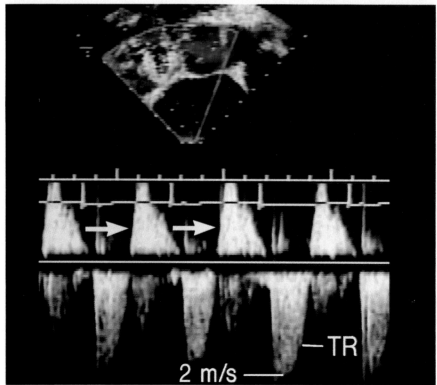

D

specific pathologic process. In both cases, there was a small amount of thrombus at the sewing ring on the ventricular surface of the prosthesis. It is of great importance to realize that this is an expected blind spot for TEE in many views imaging from the left atrium, since reverberations and flow-masking occur on the ventricular side of the prosthesis. This effect not only obscures two-dimensional echocardiographic detail on the ventricular side of the prosthesis but also limits visualization of color events in this location [62] (compare Figure 10-43 with Figure 10-3 *B*). This blind spot can often be overcome by transgastric imaging in the basal left ventricular short-axis or longitudinal long-axis planes. The TEE examination should always be carried out in concert with transthoracic echocardiography to provide complete assessment. With this combination, sensitivity for detection of pathologic processes affecting prosthetic valves should approach 100% [100].

STRUCTURAL LESIONS AND SOURCE OF EMBOLISM

Transesophageal echocardiography provides unique information about structural lesions of prosthetic valves, such as vegetation [101–104]. Even with mechanical prostheses, vegetations can be identified with relative ease (Figs. 10-44 and 10-45). Transesophageal echocardiography has been clearly demonstrated to be superior to surface echocardiography for detection of prosthetic valve vegetations [105,106].

Transesophageal echocardiography has also proven to be a powerful clinical tool for detecting and investigating complications of infective endocarditis, such as valve ring abscess [107]. Abscesses are usually identified as cystic lesions and most commonly result from infection of aortic prostheses or native aortic valves (Figs. 10-46, 10-47, and 10-

Fig. 10-43. Transesophageal echocardiographic examination of the normal Starr-Edwards prosthesis that was depicted in Fig. 10-31. Color-flow imaging demonstrates flow convergence in the left atrium. Note that color signals from left ventricular inflow *(arrowheads)* are incomplete (compare with Fig. 10-3B). The cause is acoustic shadowing by the sewing ring.

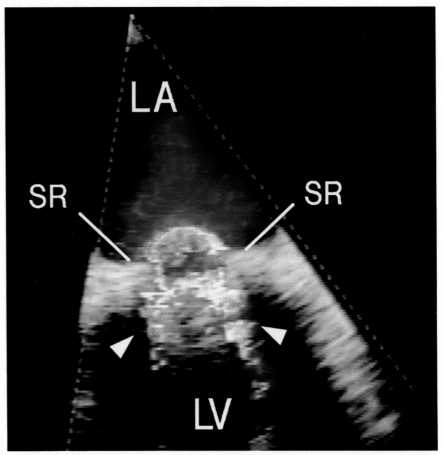

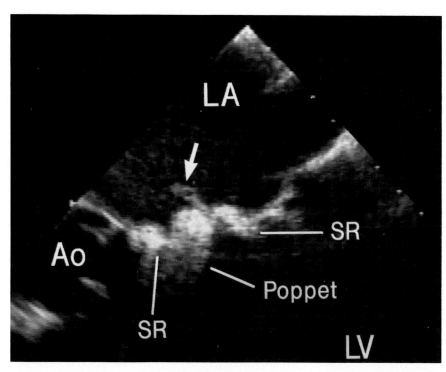

Fig. 10-44. Transesophageal horizontal plane image of Starr-Edwards prosthesis with *Staphylococcus aureus* endocarditis. In this systolic frame, slightly thickened aortic cusps are open in the aorta. The poppet is engaged in the sewing ring. The *arrow* points to a vegetation that originates from the lateral portion of the sewing ring and prolapses into the left atrium.

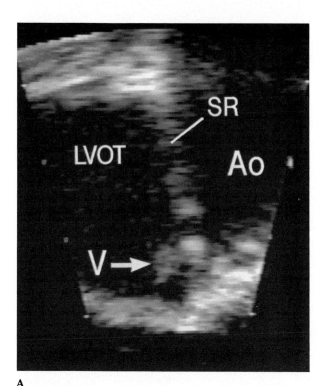

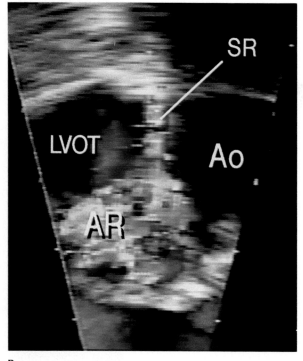

A   B

Fig. 10-45. Transesophageal echocardiography, longitudinal plane, long-axis view, magnified to focus attention on the sewing ring of an aortic Starr-Edwards prosthesis. A. In this diastolic frame, a small vegetation *(V)* is attached to the sewing ring and protrudes into the left ventricular outflow tract. Group G streptococcus grew from blood cultures. B. Color-flow imaging demonstrates moderate prosthetic aortic regurgitation.

Fig. 10-46. Transesophageal echocardiography, longitudinal plane, basal short-axis view at the level of the sewing ring of a Carpentier-Edwards aortic prosthesis. A. *Staphylococcus aureus* endocarditis developed from an infected intravenous line. A large infective mass *(Veg)* surrounds the posterior border of the sewing ring and covers a portion of the orifice. B. Massive left cerebral embolization occurred. Follow-up TEE in the same imaging plane as that in A now shows a multiloculated aortic root abscess *(arrowheads)* adjacent to the prosthetic sewing ring. (*M* = membrane of fossa ovalis.)

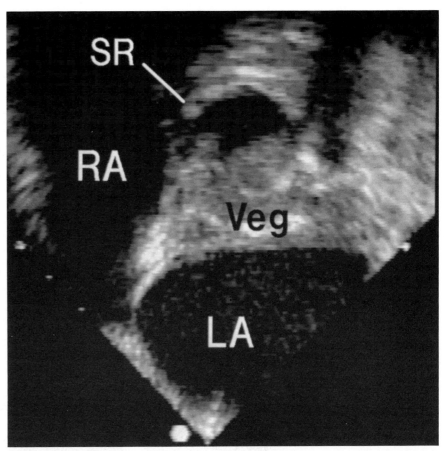

A

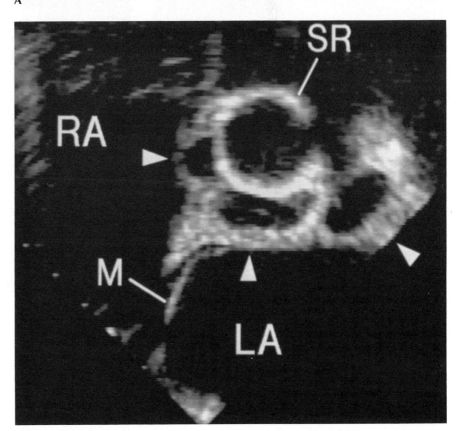

B

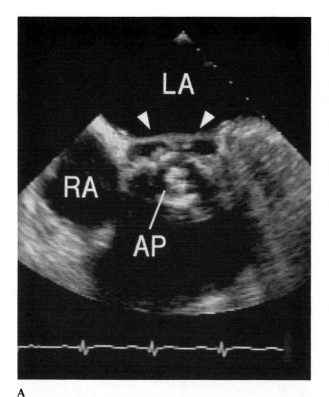
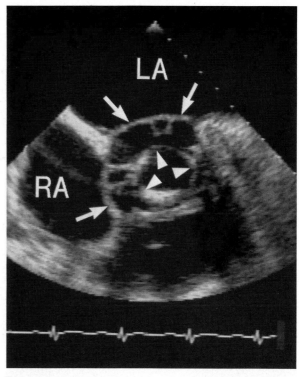

A   **B**

Fig. 10-47.   Transesophageal horizontal plane images of a Carpentier-Edwards aortic prosthesis in a patient with previous streptococcal endocarditis. A. The *arrowheads* point to a nearly circumferential aortic root abscess, which is collapsed in diastole. B. This abscess communicates with the left ventricular cavity. Therefore, in systole the abscess expands *(arrows).* The *arrowheads* point to the prosthesis sewing ring. Along the sewing ring, linear sutures are stretched across the abscess cavity. At 12 o'clock on the sewing ring, there are two sutures that have detached.

48). Less commonly, ring abscesses result from infection of mitral prostheses. Transesophageal echocardiography is useful not only for identifying ring abscesses but also for determining their communications. Figure 10-47 shows systolic expansion and diastolic collapse of an aortic ring abscess that communicates with the left ventricle. Figure 10-48 illustrates the use of color-flow imaging for a similar aortic ring abscess: the abscess fills from the left ventricle during systole and empties into it in diastole.

Several other structural abnormalities of prosthetic valves were very difficult to diagnose before the advent of TEE. These can occur either at implantation or after infective endocarditis. They include pseudoaneurysms of the aorta or left ventricle related to the prosthetic valve sewing ring (Fig. 10-49), fistulas from aorta to right atrium and aorta to left atrium (Figs. 10-50 and 10-51), atrioventricular sep-

tal defects, and aneurysms of the intervalvular fibrosa, which lies at the junction of the aortic annulus and mitral annulus [108,109]. These do not always occur as isolated lesions. In Figure 10-52, a small pseudoaneurysm adjacent to the sewing ring of a St. Jude Medical mitral prosthesis fills in systole from the ventricle but also communicates with the left atrium, so that there is perivalvular regurgitation through the pseudoaneurysm.

Thromboembolic events associated with prosthetic heart valves are frequent. As previously discussed, TEE can be used along with surface echocardiography to delineate prosthetic thrombi or vegetations. Of course, embolic events in patients with prosthetic valves are not always related *directly* to a prosthetic valve lesion. As described in detail in Chapter 15, TEE is also quite useful in identifying associated sources of emboli, including left atrial appendage thrombus and intra-aortic debris.

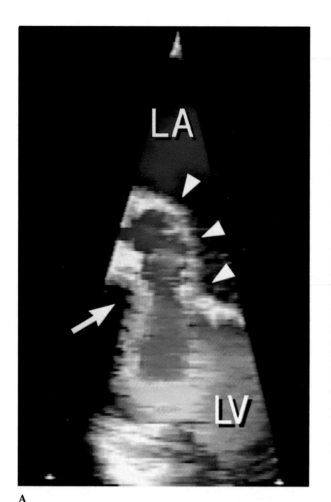 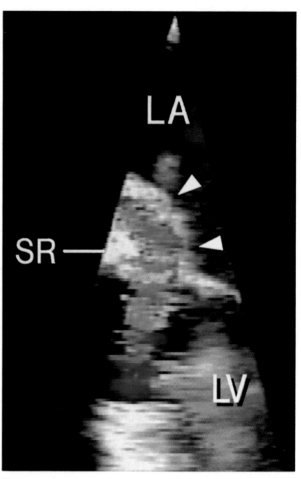

A   **B**

Fig. 10-48. Transesophageal horizontal plane images of a Carpentier-Edwards aortic prosthesis in a patient with *Listeria* endocarditis. The sector has been narrowed to focus attention on the resultant aortic ring abscess. This abscess cavity communicates with the left ventricle. A. In systole, a large amount of flow enters the abscess cavity *(arrow)*. Note the flow convergence in the left ventricular outflow tract, adjacent to the abscess cavity. With this marked inflow, the wall of the abscess has expanded *(arrowheads)*. B. In diastole, the abscess cavity *(arrowheads)* collapses, and color-flow imaging demonstrates regurgitation back into the left ventricle.

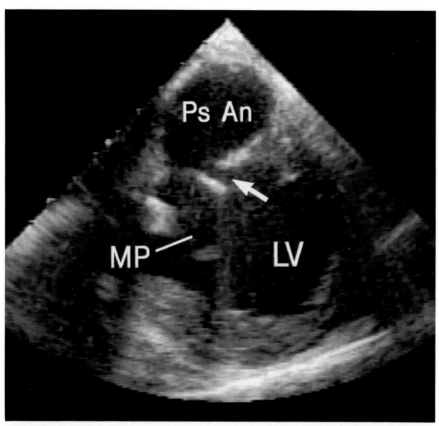

A

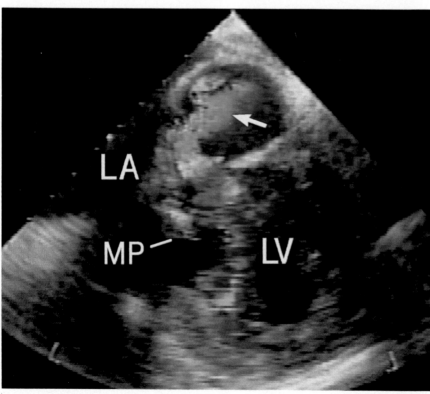

B

Fig. 10-49. Transesophageal horizontal plane view of a Carpentier-Edwards mitral prosthesis from a modified transgastric transducer position. Surgical implantation was complicated by formation of a large pseudoaneurysm adjacent to the prosthesis. A. The *arrow* points to the narrow neck connecting the left ventricle to the pseudoaneurysm B. Color-flow imaging, in systole, demonstrates flow from the left ventricle into the pseudoaneurysm *(arrow).*

Fig. 10-50. Transesophageal horizontal plane view of a Starr-Edwards aortic prosthesis. A. From the usual four-chamber view, the transducer has been pulled higher into the esophagus, providing a view of the proximal ascending aorta, the prosthetic valve sewing ring, and the left ventricular outflow tract *(LV)* as well as the right atrium. B. In systole, blood is ejected from the left ventricle and appears as a color jet in the aorta. There is also a fistula from the aorta to the right atrium, with a left-to-right shunt entering the right atrium *(arrowheads)*. This small fistula probably was created at the time of implantation of the prosthesis; there was no history of endocarditis.

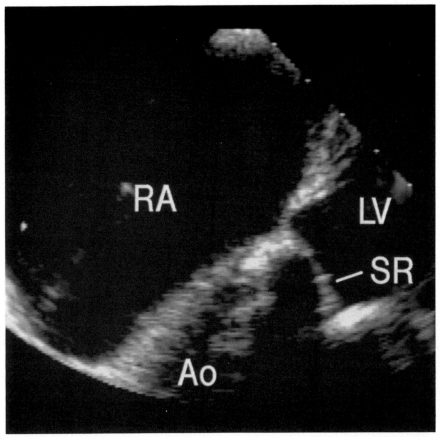

A

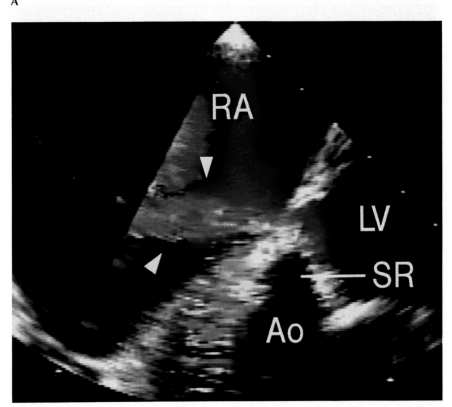

B

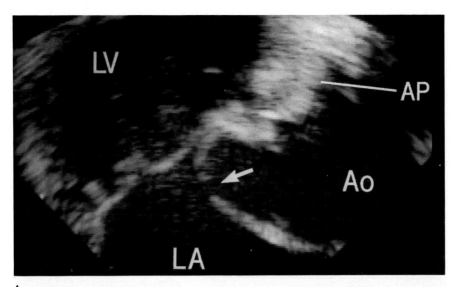

A

Fig. 10-51. Transesophageal longitudinal plane, long-axis view of a St. Jude Medical aortic prosthesis in a patient with *Streptococcus viridans* endocarditis. A. The transducer has been angulated in such a way that prosthetic valve detail is not evident. Attention is focused on a small defect in the wall of the enlarged left coronary sinus of Valsalva *(arrow)*. B. Color-flow imaging confirms communication *(arrowheads)* from aorta to left atrium. This fistula was not apparent with contrast left ventriculography.

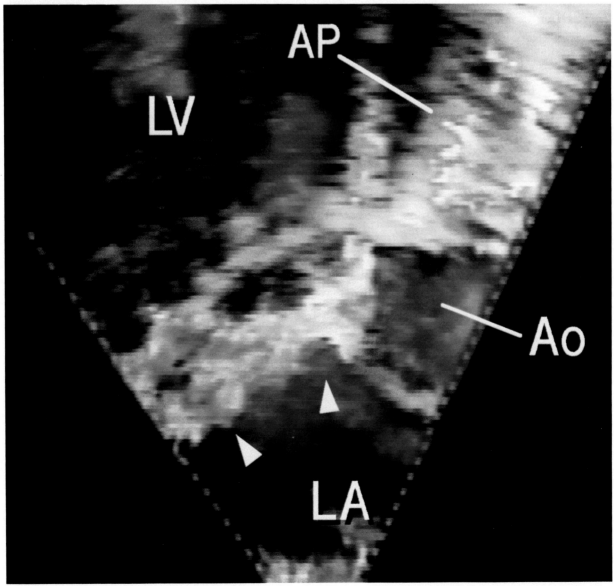

B

Fig. 10-52. Transesophageal horizontal plane, four-chamber view in a patient with a St. Jude Medical mitral prosthesis. A. The small circular cavity (highlighted by *dashed black lines*) lateral to the prosthetic valve sewing ring is a pseudoaneurysm. The *arrow* points to a small separation of the prosthetic valve sewing ring from the annulus. B. In early systole, flow from the left ventricle enters the pseudoaneurysm cavity *(arrowheads)*. C. In this later systolic frame, a moderate jet of periprosthetic mitral regurgitation is identified *(arrows)*. This regurgitant volume travels from left ventricle to left atrium via the pseudoaneurysm. *Arrowheads* identify pseudoaneurysm cavity.

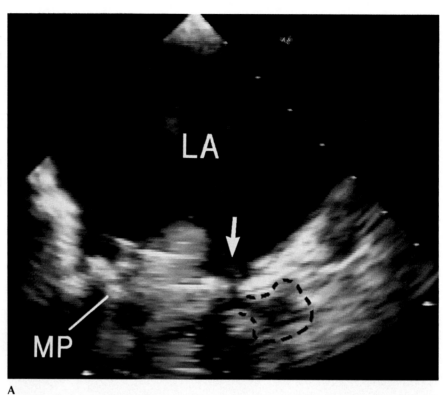

A

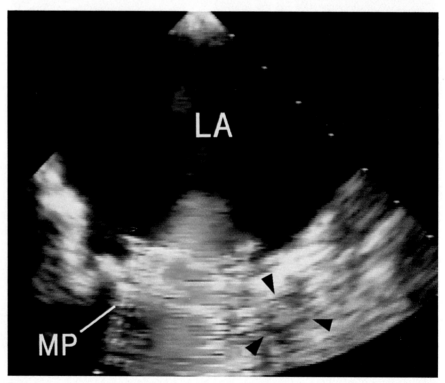

B

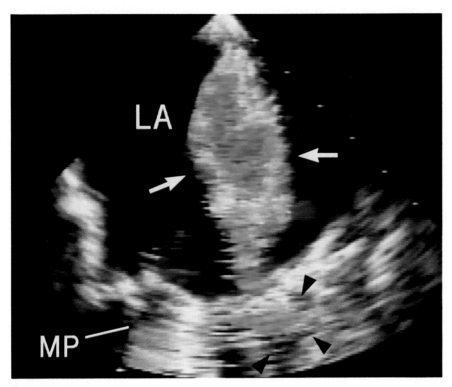

C

SUMMARY

With the addition of transesophageal transducers, echocardiography has become a complete diagnostic modality for patients with prosthetic heart valves. To fully assess prosthetic valves, the echocardiographer must integrate information from two-dimensional, spectral Doppler, and flow-imaging examinations. Transesophageal echocardiography should be performed when one suspects significant prosthetic valve structural abnormalities, including thrombus, vegetations, and bioprosthetic cusp degeneration. Transesophageal echocardiography is particularly useful for assessing prosthetic mitral or tricuspid regurgitation and for evaluating the various perivalvular abnormalities that complicate surgical implantation and infective endocarditis. Furthermore, TEE should be performed whenever the echocardiographer believes that the surface examination provides inadequate answers to clinically important questions. With use of the full complement of currently available cardiac ultrasound modalities, almost all prosthetic valve problems can be defined well enough to allow a recommendation for or against surgical intervention.

Invasive catheterization is still necessary for defining coronary anatomy before prosthetic valve surgery. In addition, invasive procedures are necessary in that small percentage of cases in which both surface and transesophageal examinations fail to provide images of diagnostic quality. Finally, invasive catheterization should be performed if there is significant discordance between the clinical impression and the echocardiographic findings. These cases are clearly in the minority. For prosthetic valve assessment, echocardiography is *not* add-on technology but rather the test of choice. For experimental echocardiographic laboratories, transthoracic echocardiography and TEE have completely supplanted the need for invasive investigation in the vast majority of patients with prosthetic valve dysfunction.

REFERENCES

1. Kotler MN, Segal BL, Parry WR. Echocardiographic and phonocardiographic evaluation of prosthetic heart valves. *Cardiovasc Clin* 1978;9 no. 2:187–207.

2. Alam M, Madrazo AC, Magilligan DJ, Goldstein S. M mode and two dimensional echocardiographic features of porcine valve dysfunction. *Am J Cardiol* 1979;43:502–9.

3. Horowitz MS, Tecklenberg PL, Goodman DJ, et al. Echocardiographic evaluation of the stent mounted aortic bioprosthetic valve in the mitral position: *in vitro* and *in vivo* studies. *Circulation* 1976;54:91–6.

4. Bloch WN Jr, Felner JM, Wickliffe C, et al. Echocardiogram of the porcine aortic bioprosthesis in the mitral position. *Am J Cardiol* 1976;38:293–8.

5. Schapira JN, Martin RP, Fowles RE, et al. Two dimensional echocardiographic assessment of patients with bioprosthetic valves. *Am J Cardiol* 1979;43:510–9.

6. Miller FA, Tajik AJ, Seward JB, et al. Prosthetic valve dysfunction: two-dimensional echocardiographic assessment (abstract). *Circulation* 1981;64 Suppl 4:IV–315.

7. Alam M, Goldstein S, Lakier JB. Echocardiographic changes in the thickness of porcine valves with time. *Chest* 1981;79:663–8.

8. Cunha CLP, Giuliani ER, Callahan JA, Pluth JR. Echophonocardiographic findings in patients with prosthetic heart valve malfunction. *Mayo Clin Proc* 1980;55:231–42.

9. Alam M, Serwin JB, Rosman HS, et al. Transesophageal echocardiographic features of normal and dysfunctioning bioprosthetic valves. *Am Heart J* 1991;121:1149–55.

10. Lanzieri M, Michaelson S, Cohen IS. Transesophageal echocardiography in the diagnosis of mitral bioprosthetic obstruction. *Crit Care Med* 1991;19:979–81.

11. Adamick RD, Gleckel LC, Graver LM. Acute thrombosis of an aortic bioprosthetic valve: transthoracic and transesophageal echocardiographic findings. *Am Heart J* 1991;122:241–2.

12. Alam M, Serwin JB, Rosman HS, et al. Transesophageal color flow Doppler and echocardiographic features of normal and regurgitant St. Jude Medical prostheses in the aortic valve position. *Am J Cardiol* 1990;66:873–5.

13. Alam M, Serwin JB, Rosman HS, et al. Transesophageal color flow Doppler and echocardiographic features of normal and regurgitant St. Jude Medical prostheses in the mitral valve position. *Am J Cardiol* 1990;66:871–3.

14. Sagar KB, Wann LS, Paulsen WH, Romhilt DW. Doppler echocardiographic evaluation of Hancock and Björk-Shiley prosthetic valves. *J Am Coll Cardiol* 1986;7:681–7.

15. Ramirez ML, Wong M. Reproducibility of standalone continuous-wave Doppler recordings of aortic flow velocity across bioprosthetic valves. *Am J Cardiol* 1985;55:1197–9.

16. Cooper DM, Stewart WJ, Schiavone WA, et al. Evaluation of normal prosthetic valve function by Doppler echocardiography. *Am Heart J* 1987;114:576–82.

17. Panidis IP, Ross J, Mintz GS. Normal and abnormal prosthetic valve function as assessed by Doppler echocardiography. *J Am Coll Cardiol* 1986;8:317–26.

18. Weinstein IR, Marbarger JP, Pérez JE. Ultrasonic assessment of the St. Jude prosthetic valve: M-mode, two-dimensional, and Doppler echocardiography. *Circulation* 1983;68:897–905.

19. Williams GA, Labovitz AJ. Doppler hemodynamic evaluation of prosthetic (Starr-Edwards and Björk-Shiley) and bioprosthetic (Hancock and Carpentier-Edwards) cardiac valves. *Am J Cardiol* 1985;56:325–32.

20. Labovitz AJ. Assessment of prosthetic heart valve function by Doppler echocardiography: a decade of experience. *Circulation* 1989;80:707–9.

21. Holen J, Aaslid R, Landmark K, Simonsen S. Determination of pressure gradient in mitral stenosis with a non-invasive ultrasound Doppler technique. *Acta Med Scand* 1976;199:455–60.

22. Hatle L, Brubakk A, Tromsdal A, Angelsen B. Noninvasive assessment of pressure drop in mitral stenosis by Doppler ultrasound. *Br Heart J* 1978;40:131–40.

23. Hatle L, Angelsen BA, Tromsdal A. Non-invasive assessment of aortic stenosis by Doppler ultrasound. *Br Heart J* 1980;43:284–92.

24. Miller FA Jr, Callahan JA, Taylor CL, et al. Normal aortic valve prosthesis hemodynamics: 609 prospective Doppler examinations (abstract). *Circulation* 1989;80 Suppl 2:II–169.

25. Burstow DJ, Nishimura RA, Bailey KR, et al. Continuous wave Doppler echocardiographic measurement of prosthetic valve gradients: a simultaneous Doppler-catheter correlative study. *Circulation* 1989;80:504–14.

26. Wilkins GT, Gillam LD, Kritzer GL, et al. Validation of continuous-wave Doppler echocardiographic measurements of mitral and tricuspid prosthetic valve gradients: a simultaneous Doppler-catheter study. *Circulation* 1986;74:786–95.

27. Kapur KK, Fan P, Nanda NC, et al. Doppler color flow mapping in the evaluation of prosthetic mitral and aortic valve function. *J Am Coll Cardiol* 1989;13:1561–71.

28. Reisner SA, Meltzer RS. Normal values of prosthetic valve Doppler echocardiographic parameters: a review. *J Am Soc Echocardiogr* 1988;1:201–10.

29. Gibbs JL, Wharton GA, Williams GJ. Doppler echocardiographic characteristics of the Carpentier-Edwards xenograft. *Eur Heart J* 1986;7:353–6.

30. Jaffe WM, Coverdale HA, Roche AHG, et al. Doppler echocardiography in the assessment of the homograft aortic valve. *Am J Cardiol* 1989;63:1466–70.

31. Hoffman A, Weiss P, Dubach P, Burckhardt D. Progressive functional deterioration of bioprostheses assessed by Doppler ultrasonography. *Chest* 1990;98:1165–8.

32. Weintraub WS, Clements SD, Dorney ER, et al. Clinical, echocardiographic, continuous wave and color Doppler evaluation of bioprosthetic cardiac valves in place for more than ten years. *Am J Cardiol* 1990;65:935–6.

33. Bojar RM, Diehl JT, Moten M, et al. Clinical and hemodynamic performance of the Ionescu-Shiley valve in the small aortic root: results in 117 patients with 17 and 19 mm valves. *J Thorac Cardiovasc Surg* 1989;98:1087–95.

34. Jaffe WM, Barratt-Boyes BG, Sadri A, et al. Early follow-up of patients with the Medtronic Intact porcine valve: a new cardiac bioprosthesis. *J Thorac Cardiovasc Surg* 1989;98:181–92.

35. Martin GR, Galioto FM Jr, Midgley FM. Doppler echocardiographic evaluation of tilting-disc prosthetic heart valves in children. *Am J Cardiol* 1989;63:964–8.

36. Perin EC, Jin BS, de Castro CM, et al. Doppler echocardiography in 180 normally functioning St. Jude Medical aortic valve prostheses. Early and late postoperative assessments. *Chest* 1991;100:988–90.

37. Chafizadeh ER, Zoghbi WA. Doppler echocardiographic assessment of the St. Jude Medical prosthetic valve in the aortic position using the continuity equation. *Circulation* 1991;83:213–23.

38. Rahimtoola SH. The problem of valve prosthesis-patient mismatch. *Circulation* 1978;58:20–4.

39. Wiseth R, Hegrenaes L, Rossvoll O, et al. Validity of an early postoperative baseline Doppler recording after aortic valve replacement. *Am J Cardiol* 1991;67:869–72.

40. Teoh KH, Ivanov J, Weisel RD, et al. Clinical and Doppler echocardiographic evaluation of bioprosthetic valve failure after 10 years. *Circulation* 1990;82 Suppl 4:IV–110-IV–6.

41. Ren J-F, Chandrasekaran K, Mintz GS, et al. Effect of depressed left ventricular function on hemodynamics of normal St. Jude Medical prosthesis in the aortic valve position. *Am J Cardiol* 1990;65:1004–9.

42. Skjaerpe T, Hegrenaes L, Hatle L. Noninvasive estimation of valve area in patients with aortic stenosis by Doppler ultrasound and two-dimensional echocardiography. *Circulation* 1985;72:810–8.

43. Zoghbi WA, Farmer KL, Soto JG, et al. Accurate noninvasive quantification of stenotic aortic valve area by Doppler echocardiography. *Circulation* 1986;73:452–9.

44. Otto CM, Pearlman AS, Comess KA, et al. Determination of the stenotic aortic valve area in adults using Doppler echocardiography. *J Am Coll Cardiol* 1986;7:509–17.

45. Oh JK, Taliercio CP, Holmes DR Jr, et al. Prediction of the severity of aortic stenosis by Doppler aortic valve area determination: prospective Doppler-catheterization correlation in 100 patients. *J Am Coll Cardiol* 1988;11:1227–34.

46. Rothbart RM, Castriz JL, Harding LV, et al. Determination of aortic valve area by two-dimensional and Doppler echocardiography in patients with normal and stenotic bioprosthetic valves. *J Am Coll Cardiol* 1990;15:817–24.

47. Dumesnil JG, Honos GN, Lemieux M, Beauchemin J. Validation and applications of indexed aortic prosthetic valve areas calculated by Doppler echocardiography. *J Am Coll Cardiol* 1990;16:637–43.

48. Otto CM, Pearlman AS. Doppler echocardiographic evaluation of stenotic bioprosthetic aortic valves (editorial). *J Am Coll Cardiol* 1990;15:825–6.

49. Ihlen H, Mølstad P. Cardiac output measured by Doppler echocardiography in patients with aortic prosthetic valves. *Eur Heart J* 1990;11:399–402.

50. Rashtian MY, Stevenson DM, Allen DT, et al. Flow characteristics of four commonly used mechanical heart valves. *Am J Cardiol* 1986;58:743–52.

51. Yoganathan AP, Chaux A, Gray RJ, et al. Bileaflet, tilting disc and porcine aortic valve substitutes: in vitro hydrodynamic characteristics. *J Am Coll Cardiol* 1984;3:313–20.

52. Perry GJ, Helmcke F, Nanda NC, et al. Evaluation of aortic insufficiency by Doppler color flow mapping. *J Am Coll Cardiol* 1987;9:952–9.

53. Dittrich HC, McCann HA, Walsh TP, et al. Transesophageal echocardiography in the evaluation of

prosthetic and native aortic valves. *Am J Cardiol* 1990;66:758–61.

54. Kyo S, Takamoto S, Matsumura M, et al. Immediate and early postoperative evaluation of results of cardiac surgery by transesophageal two-dimensional Doppler echocardiography. *Circulation* 1987; 76 Suppl 5:V–113-V–21.

55. Bartzokis T, St. Goar F, DiBiase A, et al. Freehand allograft aortic valve replacement and aortic root replacement: utility of intraoperative echocardiography and Doppler color flow mapping. *J Thorac Cardiovasc Surg* 1991;101:545–53.

56. Abbruzzese PA, Meloni L, Cardu G, et al. Intraoperative transesophageal echocardiography and periprosthetic leaks (letter to the editor). *J Thorac Cardiovasc Surg* 1991;101:556–7.

57. Touche T, Prasquier R, Nitenberg A, et al. Assessment and follow-up of patients with aortic regurgitation by an updated Doppler echocardiographic measurement of the regurgitant fraction in the aortic arch. *Circulation* 1985;72:819–24.

58. Teague SM, Heinsimer JA, Anderson JL, et al. Quantification of aortic regurgitation utilizing continuous wave Doppler ultrasound. *J Am Coll Cardiol* 1986;8:592–9.

59. Panidis IP, Ross J, Munley B, et al. Diastolic mitral regurgitation in patients with atrioventricular conduction abnormalities: a common finding by Doppler echocardiography. *J Am Coll Cardiol* 1986; 7:768–74.

60. Rokey R, Murphy DJ Jr, Nielsen AP, et al. Detection of diastolic atrioventricular valvular regurgitation by pulsed Doppler echocardiography and its association with complete heart block. *Am J Cardiol* 1986;57:692–4.

61. Oh JK, Hatle LK, Sinak LJ, et al. Characteristic Doppler echocardiographic pattern of mitral inflow velocity in severe aortic regurgitation. *J Am Coll Cardiol* 1989;14:1712–7.

62. Sprecher DL, Adamick R, Adams D, Kisslo J. In vitro color flow, pulsed and continuous wave Doppler ultrasound masking of flow by prosthetic valves. *J Am Coll Cardiol* 1987;9:1306–10.

63. Mohr-Kahaly S, Kupferwasser I, Erbel R, et al. Regurgitant flow in apparently normal valve prostheses: improved detection and semiquantitative analysis by transesophageal two-dimensional color-coded Doppler echocardiography. *J Am Soc Echocardiogr* 1990;3:187–95.

64. Holen J, Simonsen S, Frøysaker T. An ultrasound Doppler technique for the noninvasive determination of the pressure gradient in the Björk-Shiley mitral valve. *Circulation* 1979;59:436–42.

65. Holen J, Høie J, Semb B. Obstructive characteristics of Björk-Shiley, Hancock, and Lillehei-Kaster prosthetic mitral valves in the immediate postoperative period. *Acta Med Scand* 1978;204:5–10.

66. Holen J, Simonsen S, Frøysaker T. Determination of pressure gradient in the Hancock mitral valve from noninvasive ultrasound Doppler data. *Scand J Clin Lab Invest* 1981;41:177–83.

67. Fawzy ME, Halim M, Ziady G, et al. Hemodynamic evaluation of porcine bioprostheses in the mitral position by Doppler echocardiography. *Am J Cardiol* 1987;59:643–6.

68. Nitter-Hauge S. Doppler echocardiography in the study of patients with mitral disc valve prostheses. *Br Heart J* 1984;51:61–9.

69. Pye M, Weerasana N, Bain WH, et al. Doppler echocardiographic characteristics of normal and dysfunctioning prosthetic valves in the tricuspid and mitral position. *Br Heart J* 1990;63:41–4.

70. Nellessen U, Masuyama T, Appleton CP, et al. Mitral prosthesis malfunction: comparative Doppler echocardiographic studies of mitral prostheses before and after replacement. *Circulation* 1989;79: 330–6.

71. Zoghbi WA, Desir RM, Rosen L, et al. Doppler echocardiography: application to the assessment of successful thrombolysis of prosthetic valve thrombosis. *J Am Soc Echocardiogr* 1989;2: 98–101.

72. Ryan T, Armstrong WF, Dillon JC, Feigenbaum H. Doppler echocardiographic evaluation of patients with porcine mitral valves. *Am Heart J* 1986;111: 237–44.

73. Hatle L, Angelsen B, Tromsdal A. A noninvasive assessment of atrioventricular pressure half-time by Doppler ultrasound. *Circulation* 1979;60: 1096–1104.

74. Lengyel M, Miller FA Jr, Taylor CL, et al. Doppler hemodynamic profiles of 456 clinically and echo-normal mitral valve prostheses (abstract). *Circulation* 1990;82 Suppl 3:III-43.

75. Dumesnil JG, Honos GN, Lemieux M, Beauchemin J. Validation and applications of mitral prosthetic valvular areas calculated by Doppler echocardiography. *Am J Cardiol* 1990;65:1443–8.

76. Nakatani S, Masuyama T, Kodama K, et al. Value and limitations of Doppler echocardiography in the quantification of stenotic mitral valve area: comparison of the pressure half-time and the continuity equation methods. *Circulation* 1988;77: 78–85.

77. Miller FA Jr, Khandheria BK, Freeman WK, et al. Mitral prosthesis effective orifice area by a new

method using continuity of flow between left atrium and prosthesis (abstract). *J Am Coll Cardiol* 1992;19 Suppl A:214A.

78. Gorcsan J III, Kenny WM, Diana P, et al. Transesophageal continuous-wave Doppler to evaluate mitral prosthetic stenosis. *Am Heart J* 1991;121: 911–4.

79. Connolly HM, Miller FA Jr, Taylor CL, et al. Doppler hemodynamic profiles of eighty-six normal tricuspid valve prostheses (abstract). *J Am Coll Cardiol* 1991;17:69A.

80. Tatineni S, Barner HB, Pearson AC, et al. Rest and exercise evaluation of St. Jude Medical and Medtronic Hall prostheses: influence of primary lesion, valvular type, valvular size, and left ventricular function. *Circulation* 1989;80 Suppl 1: I–16-I–23.

81. Jaffe WM, Coverdale HA, Roche AH, et al. Rest and exercise hemodynamics of 20 to 23 mm allograft, Medtronic Intact (porcine), and St. Jude Medical valves in the aortic position. *J Thorac Cardiovasc Surg* 1990;100:167–74.

82. Reisner SA, Lichtenberg GS, Shapiro JR, et al. Exercise Doppler echocardiography in patients with mitral prosthetic valves. *Am Heart J* 1989;118:755–9.

83. van den Brink RBA, Verheul HA, Visser CA, et al. Value of exercise Doppler echocardiography in patients with prosthetic or bioprosthetic cardiac valves. *Am J Cardiol* 1992;69:367–72.

84. Dzavik V, Cohen G, Chan KL. Role of transesophageal echocardiography in the diagnosis and management of prosthetic valve thrombosis. *J Am Coll Cardiol* 1991;18:1829–33.

85. Nellessen U, Schnittger I, Appleton CP, et al. Transesophageal two-dimensional echocardiography and color Doppler flow velocity mapping in the evaluation of cardiac valve prostheses. *Circulation* 1988;78:848–55.

86. Chambers J, Monaghan M, Jackson G. Colour flow Doppler mapping in the assessment of prosthetic valve regurgitation. *Br Heart J* 1989;62:1–8.

87. Appleton CP, Hatle LK, Nellessen U, et al. Flow velocity acceleration in the left ventricle: a useful Doppler echocardiographic sign of hemodynamically significant mitral regurgitation. *J Am Soc Echocardiogr* 1990;3:35–45.

88. Bargiggia GS, Tronconi L, Raisaro A, et al. Color Doppler diagnosis of mechanical prosthetic mitral regurgitation: usefulness of the flow convergence region proximal to the regurgitant orifice. *Am Heart J* 1990;120:1137–42.

89. Nellessen U, Schnittger I, Appleton CP, et al. Transesophageal two-dimensional echocardiography and color Doppler flow velocity mapping in the evaluation of cardiac valve prostheses. *Circulation* 1988;78:848–55.

90. van den Brink RBA, Visser CA, Basart DCG, et al. Comparison of transthoracic and transesophageal color Doppler flow imaging in patients with mechanical prostheses in the mitral valve position. *Am J Cardiol* 1989;63:1471–4.

91. Chen Y-T, Kan M-N, Chen J-S, et al. Detection of prosthetic mitral valve leak: a comparative study using transesophageal echocardiography, transthoracic echocardiography, and auscultation. *J Clin Ultrasound* 1990;18:557–61.

92. Taams MA, Gussenhoven EJ, Cahalan MK, et al. Transesophageal Doppler color flow imaging in the detection of native and Björk-Shiley mitral valve regurgitation. *J Am Coll Cardiol* 1989;13: 95–9.

93. Scott PJ, Ettles DF, Wharton GA, Williams GJ. The value of transesophageal echocardiography in the investigation of acute prosthetic valve dysfunction. *Clin Cardiol* 1990;13:541–4.

94. Lange HW, Olson JD, Pederson WR, et al. Transesophageal color Doppler echocardiography of the normal St. Jude Medical mitral valve prosthesis. *Am Heart J* 1991;122:489–94.

95. Hixson CS, Smith MD, Mattson MD, et al. Comparison of transesophageal color flow Doppler imaging of normal mitral regurgitant jets in St. Jude Medical and Medtronic Hall cardiac prostheses. *J Am Soc Echocardiogr* 1992;5:57–62.

96. Helmcke F, Nanda NC, Hsiung MC, et al. Color Doppler assessment of mitral regurgitation with orthogonal planes. *Circulation* 1987;75:175–83.

97. Vandenberg BF, Dellsperger KC, Chandran KB, Kerber RE. Detection, localization, and quantitation of bioprosthetic mitral valve regurgitation: an in vitro two-dimensional color-Doppler flow-mapping study. *Circulation* 1988;78:529–38.

98. Klein AL, Tajik AJ. Doppler assessment of pulmonary venous flow in healthy subjects and in patients with heart disease. *J Am Soc Echocardiogr* 1991;4:379–92.

99. Klein AL, Obarski TP, Stewart WJ, et al. Transesophageal Doppler echocardiography of pulmonary venous flow: a new marker of mitral regurgitation severity. *J Am Coll Cardiol* 1991; 18:518–26.

100. Khandheria BK, Seward JB, Oh JK, et al. Value and limitations of transesophageal echocardiogra-

phy in assessment of mitral valve prostheses. *Circulation* 1991;83:1956–68.

101. Culver DL, Cacchione J, Stern D, et al. Diagnosis of infective endocarditis on a Starr-Edwards prosthesis by transesophageal echocardiography. *Am Heart J* 1990;119:972–3.

102. Mügge A, Daniel WG, Frank G, Lichtlen PR. Echocardiography in infective endocarditis: reassessment of prognostic implications of vegetation size determined by the transthoracic and the transesophageal approach. *J Am Coll Cardiol* 1989;14:631–8.

103. Van Camp G, Vandenbossche JL. Illustration by transesophageal echocardiography of rapid and important pannus formation during infective endocarditis of a prosthetic valve. *Acta Cardiol* 1991;46:589–92.

104. Sutton MSJ, Lee RT. Diagnosis and medical management of infective endocarditis: transthoracic and transesophageal echocardiography. *J Cardiac Surg* 1990;5:39–43.

105. Taams MA, Gussenhoven EJ, Bos E, et al. En-
hanced morphological diagnosis in infective endocarditis by transoesophageal echocardiography. *Br Heart J* 1990;63:109–13.

106. Pedersen WR, Walker M, Olson JD, et al. Value of transesophageal echocardiography as an adjunct to transthoracic echocardiography in evaluation of native and prosthetic valve endocarditis. *Chest* 1991;100:351–6.

107. Daniel WG, Mügge A, Martin RP, et al. Improvement in the diagnosis of abscesses associated with endocarditis by transesophageal echocardiography. *N Engl J Med* 1991;324:795–800.

108. Bansal RC, Graham BM, Jutzy KR, et al. Left ventricular outflow tract to left atrial communication secondary to rupture of mitral-aortic intervalvular fibrosa in infective endocarditis: diagnosis by transesophageal echocardiography and color flow imaging. *J Am Coll Cardiol* 1990;15:499–504.

109. Meyerowitz CB, Jacobs LE, Kotler MN, et al. Four-year follow-up of a pseudoaneurysm of the mitral-aortic fibrosa. *Am Heart J* 1991;122:589–92.

11

Infective Endocarditis

Evaluation by Transesophageal Echocardiography

Bijoy K. Khandheria • *William K. Freeman* • *Lawrence J. Sinak*

Infective endocarditis is a serious disease that often causes permanent valvular damage, even after effective antimicrobial treatment is instituted. The disease is difficult not only to treat but also to diagnose with certainty. Infective endocarditis is caused by microbial infection of the endocardial lining of the heart. This has been known for over a century, as referenced by Sir William Osler in his Gulstonian Lectures on malignant endocarditis [1]. Vegetations, most often found on the cardiac valves, may extend into support structures and involve the endocardium of the ventricles, atria, or shunt lesions. The definitive diagnosis of endocarditis requires evidence of infection on the basis of histologic examination at surgery or autopsy or bacteriologic study of a vegetation from a peripheral embolization [2].

The characteristic lesion in endocarditis is a vegetation, and no better imaging technique exists for the diagnosis of vegetation than two-dimensional echocardiography. As early as 1973, transthoracic echocardiography was shown to have the capability of detecting valvular vegetations [3]. Since this description, technical advances in cardiac ultrasonography have flourished, and echocardiography now assumes a pivotal role in the evaluation and management of patients with known or suspected endocarditis [4,5]. Comprehensive two-dimensional and Doppler echocardiography not only permits characterization of vegetations but also can provide valuable information about valvular destruction, subsequent hemodynamic sequelae, and complications of endocarditis.

Potential complications resulting from endocarditis, such as valvular destruction, perivalvular extension of infection, and embolization, pose a serious threat to the patient and constitute medical emergencies that mandate rapid diagnosis for effective intervention to minimize otherwise formidable patient morbidity and mortality.

Although echocardiography is the best method for the noninvasive, expeditious diagnosis of infective endocarditis and attendant complications, the transthoracic approach has multiple potential limitations. These limitations occur with inadequate transthoracic acoustic windows, limited sensitivity of detection of small vegetations in diffusely diseased native valves, acoustic shadowing from prosthetic material, and generally unsatisfactory resolution to reliably detect prosthetic valve endocarditis or the details of complicating lesions. Transesophageal echocardiography (TEE), by providing numerous high-resolution biplanar or multiplanar windows to the heart, can overcome most problems limiting the accuracy of transthoracic echocardiography in infective endocarditis.

The role of TEE in the evaluation and management of patients with suspected and proven endocarditis is described in this chapter.

TRANSESOPHAGEAL ECHOCARDIOGRAPHY IN THE PATIENT WITH SUSPECTED ENDOCARDITIS

Diagnostic Accuracy

Multiple reports have appeared in the literature addressing the utility of transthoracic echocardiog-

307

raphy and TEE in the patient with clinically suspected infective endocarditis. Since the development of two-dimensional sector scanning, the sensitivity of transthoracic echocardiography in the detection of native valvular vegetations has been described in numerous reports, some of which are presented in Table 11-1. Vegetations as small as 2 to 5 mm in diameter may be detected in patients with adequate transthoracic images; however, this is possible in only 25% of patients [9]. In general, the overall sensitivity of detection of native valvular vegetations of different sizes in various locations remains approximately 60% to 70% at best [5–11]. Given the multiple problems with acoustic reflectance and shadowing from prosthetic valves, particularly in the mitral position, the sensitivity of transthoracic echocardiography is considerably lower for the diagnosis of prosthetic valvular endocarditis, with sensitivities ranging generally from 20% to 30% [11–13].

All studies of TEE in endocarditis report significantly higher rates of detection of vegetations by TEE than by transthoracic echocardiography; representative studies are summarized in Table 11-2 [9,11,14–19]. Mügge et al. [11] compared transthoracic echocardiography and TEE findings in 105 patients who had clinical signs or histologic evidence of native or prosthetic valvular endocarditis. In a subgroup of 80 patients found to have infected valves at operation or autopsy, the detection rate of "definite" vegetations was 58% by transthoracic echocardiography and 90% by TEE. If the diagnoses of "definite" and "possible" vegetations were combined, the detection rates in this study were 77% by transthoracic echocardiography and 96% by TEE. Despite the clearly increased sensitivity of TEE, these investigators noted that it was not always possible to distinguish between true vegetations and endocarditis-induced valve destruction, such as leaflet rupture or chordal disruption [11]. Nevertheless, even the monoplane TEE technology used in this study was very accurate in the detection of vegetations and a significant improvement over transthoracic echocardiography. In a smaller group of patients, also with confirmation of findings at either autopsy or operation, Erbel et al. [9] reported a

Table 11-1. Sensitivity of transthoracic two-dimensional echocardiography for the detection of vegetations

Authors	Year	No. of patients	Sensitivity (%)
Jaffe et al. [6]	1990	69	78
Stafford et al. [7]	1985	62	73
Stewart et al. [5]	1980	87	54
Mintz et al. [8]	1979	22	41

Data from Stewart et al. [5], Jaffe et al. [6], Stafford et al. [7], Mintz et al. [8].

Table 11-2. Comparison of transthoracic (TTE) and transesophageal (TEE) echocardiography for the detection of vegetations

Authors	Year	No. of patients	Sensitivity (%) TTE	Sensitivity (%) TEE
Daniel et al. [14]	1987	82	40	94
Erbel et al. [9]	1988	51	63	100
Mügge et al. [11]	1989	105	58	90
Taams et al. [15]	1990	33	33	100
Shively et al. [16]	1991	62	44	94
Birmingham et al. [17]	1992	61	30	88

Data from Erbel et al. [9], Mügge et al. [11], Daniel et al. [14], Taams et al. [15], Shively et al. [16], Birmingham et al. [17].

sensitivity of 100% and a specificity of 98% for detection of vegetations by monoplane TEE.

A prospective study comparing the diagnostic values of transthoracic echocardiography and TEE was reported by Shively et al. [16]. Transthoracic echocardiography and monoplane TEE were performed in 62 consecutive patients meeting prespecified clinical criteria for endocarditis. The results demonstrated that TEE provided better visualization of both the mitral and aortic valves than transthoracic imaging. The quality of tricuspid valve visualization was identical by both techniques. Valvular abnormalities were better imaged by monoplane TEE, as was detection of valvular regurgitation. For diagnosis of infective endocarditis, sensitivity was 94% for TEE and 44% for transthoracic echocardiography and specificities were 100% and 98%, respectively. These results were confirmed at operation or necropsy in 88% of patients. Similar data were reported by Birmingham et al. [17], again confirming the important finding of significantly increased sensitivity of TEE over transthoracic echocardiography in the detection of vegetations (Fig. 11-1). Negative results of TEE in patients with clinically suspected endocarditis are also helpful in clinical management. In a retrospective review of 65 such patients with TEE studies negative for endocarditis, 86% were found to have another diagnosis (prompting considerably different therapy) or negative results at follow-up TEE examinations [20]. In the same study, 5% of patients were subsequently found to have endocarditis on follow-up TEE performed because of persistent clinical suspicion of this diagnosis. Re-

sults in this small subgroup suggest an important, yet still incompletely defined, role for serial TEE studies in patients with strongly suspected endocarditis not yet evident during initial TEE early in the course of the illness [20,21]. Repeat TEE within a short follow-up period (from 5 to 7 days) should seriously be considered if the patient's clinical course indicates that infective endocarditis remains in the differential diagnosis.

Diagnostic sensitivity is of paramount importance in evaluation of patients with suspected infective endocarditis because of the serious consequences of missing the diagnosis and thereby delaying therapy of a potentially lethal disease. Transesophageal echocardiography hence should be performed in all patients with clinically suspected endocarditis in whom initial evaluation by transthoracic echocardiography is inconclusive or inadequate to establish or exclude this diagnosis.

The TEE Examination

A generic echocardiographic definition of a vegetation is useful to remember when evaluating a patient with suspected endocarditis, a disease with a widely diverse echocardiographic presentation. In general, the echocardiographic appearance of a vegetation can be described as a discrete, variably mobile mass of echogenic material adherent to a usually abnormal endocardial surface and distinct in character and motion from that surface.

A broad spectrum of vegetation morphologic ap-

Fig. 11-1. Sensitivity and specificity of transthoracic and transesophageal echocardiography in the detection of valvular vegetations in patients with infective endocarditis. A greater than twofold increase in sensitivity with TEE is noted in both studies; the specificities for both modalities are very similar. Left panel data from Shively et al. [16]; right panel data from Birmingham et al. [17].

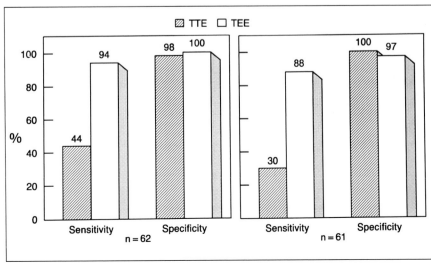

pearances may be seen on TEE, ranging from globular and polypoid to frond-like, shaggy, or even tubular [11,22,23]. Vegetations may appear sessile and nearly immobile, with slight "shimmering" on cardiac motion, or pedunculated and highly mobile, prolapsing in and out of contiguous cardiac chambers throughout the cardiac cycle. Usually vegetations do not change greatly in appearance throughout the course of clinically successful antibiotic therapy, although a minority of vegetations may significantly regress or grow larger [5,24–27]. In a recent preliminary study vegetation size measured by TEE was compared before and after completion of antibiotic therapy. In 184 patients with native valve endocarditis, size did not change significantly in 47% of patients, decreased a mean of 19% to 45% in 39%, and increased a mean of 40% in 14% at the end of antibiotic therapy [27]. Vegetation size and morphol-

ogy have not been found to be consistently correlated with location of endocarditis or a specific causative bacterial organism [11,23,28].

Vegetations associated with infective endocarditis may occur in any location where there is disease or disruption of the endocardium. Because of a variety of degenerative, senescent, rheumatic, congenital, and other causes, there is a marked predilection for the cardiac valves, particularly the left-sided valves, to become involved. The endocardial integrity can also be compromised by trauma caused by high-pressure intracardiac shunt lesions, such as ventricular septal defect, or by basal septal friction lesions due to mitral systolic anterior motion in hypertrophic obstructive cardiomyopathy. Typically, valvular vegetations occur on the regurgitant surfaces, or "upstream" side, of the valve leaflets. Hence, vegetations tend to form on the atrial surfaces of the

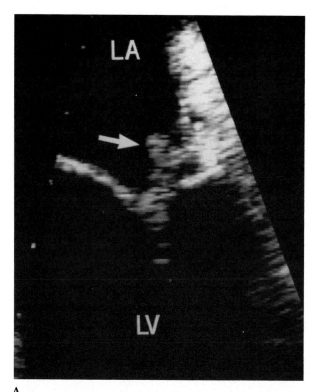

A

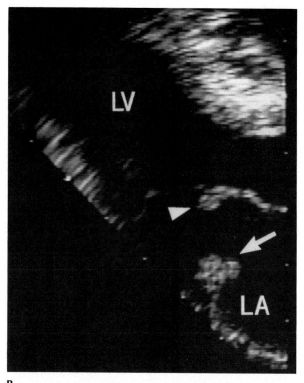

B

Fig. 11-2.   A. Posteriorly directed transverse four-chamber view, narrow sector image of the mitral valve. A polypoid vegetation *(arrow)* is attached to the atrial surface of the posterior mitral leaflet; moderate mobility was present on real-time examination. B. Longitudinal left ventricular inflow view, anterior angulation. Another cluster of vegetations involves both sides of the posterior mitral leaflet *(arrow)*, and a smaller sessile vegetation is attached to the tip of the anterior leaflet *(arrowhead)*.

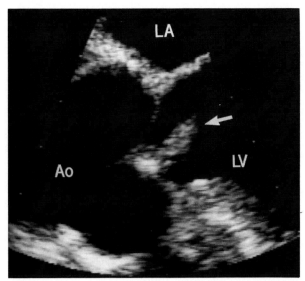

Fig. 11-3. Transverse plane, focused left ventricular outflow tract view of aortic valve. A large vegetation *(arrow)* is attached to the ventricular aspect of the noncoronary cusp. On real-time examination, the vegetation was highly mobile within the left ventricular outflow tract.

mitral valve (Fig. 11-2) and on the ventricular aspects of the aortic valve (Fig. 11-3). The vegetative material occasionally extends to both valvular surfaces and may involve perivalvular and subvalvular support structures in the form of satellite vegetations. Multiplanar imaging [29] and regional expansion capabilities focusing on areas of interest have further enhanced characterization of vegetations by TEE (Fig. 11-4). If mobile and large, the vegetative mass may prolapse across the valve orifice throughout the cardiac cycle (Fig. 11-5). Uncommonly, endocardial lesions caused by a valvular regurgitant jet into the antecedent cardiac chamber may also be a site for vegetative growth [30] (Fig. 11-6).

Right-sided endocarditis is much less common and has been associated with intravenous drug abuse, right heart instrumentation, and immunocompromised patients [31]. Generally, the tricuspid valve is involved, with a broad spectrum of vegetation appearances resembling those of the mitral valve [13,24,32–34]. Tricuspid vegetations are readily rec-

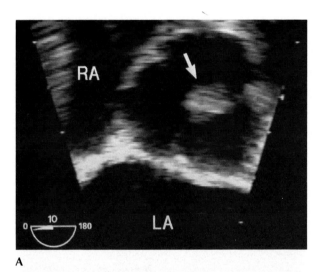

A

Fig. 11-4. Multiplane imaging of an aortic valve vegetation; regional expansion views. A. A true longitudinal short-axis view of the aortic valve is obtained with only 10 degrees rotation of the array in this patient. A vegetation *(arrow)* is seen in the immediate supravalvular region; however, its attachment to the aortic valve is not defined. B. A modified longitudinal long-axis view of the aortic valve is obtained with rotation of the array to 55 degrees. The pedunculated vegetation *(arrow)* was found to attach to the aortic valve by a narrow pedicle *(arrowhead)*. C. In a systolic frame, the vegetation is shown to be attached to the left coronary cusp *(arrow)*, not the right coronary cusp *(arrowhead)*.

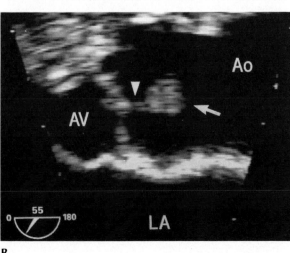

B

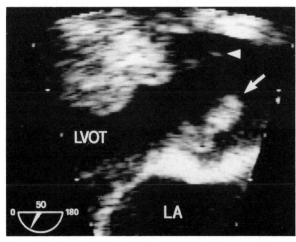

C

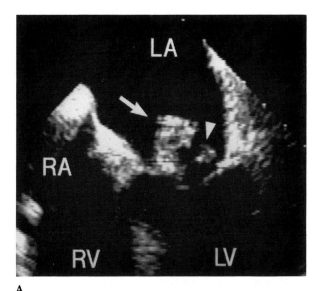
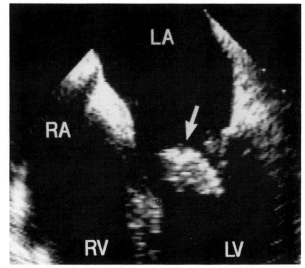

A **B**

Fig. 11-5. A. Transverse four-chamber view during systole. A large cuboid vegetation is attached to the atrial surface of the anterior mitral valve leaflet *(arrow)*. A smaller vegetation is attached to the posterior leaflet *(arrowhead)*. B. With diastole, there is prolapse of the mobile larger vegetation into the left ventricular inflow tract *(arrow)*. Rarely, valvular inflow obstruction is caused by such a lesion. Large prolapsing vegetations of this type have a high incidence of peripheral embolization, especially when located on the mitral valve.

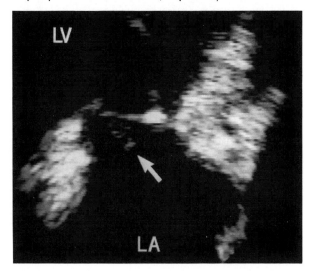
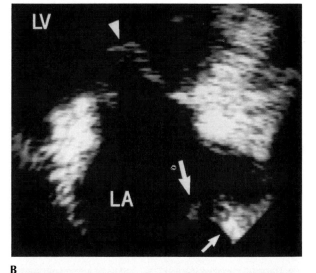

A **B**

Fig. 11-6. A. Modified longitudinal left ventricular inflow view. A veil-like vegetation attached to the mitral valve protrudes into the left atrium during systole *(arrow)*. B. A small endocardial vegetation *(large arrow)* is observed in the vicinity of the limbus of the left upper pulmonary vein entering the left atrium *(small arrow)*. The wispy vegetation is barely visible on the opened anterior mitral leaflet *(arrowhead)*. C. Off-axis anteflexed scanning confirms attachment of this satellite vegetation *(arrow)* to this portion of the left atrium.

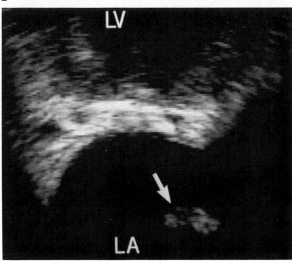

C

ognized in the four-chamber or more posterior right ventricular inflow views with imaging in the transverse plane, and recognition is facilitated by short-axis imaging in the longitudinal plane (Fig. 11-7).

Pulmonary valve endocarditis is particularly rare, most likely because the often limited views of the pulmonary valve on transthoracic echocardiography result in underdetection. Only recently has TEE been recognized to greatly facilitate the diagnosis of pulmonary valvular endocarditis [35]. Only oblique and incomplete views of the pulmonary valve are possible on basal short-axis imaging in the transverse

plane. However, this valve is well visualized along with the entire right ventricular outflow tract in longitudinal short-axis planes. The pulmonary valve should always be examined in this imaging format to exclude pulmonary valve involvement in patients with evidence of tricuspid valve endocarditis.

Patients with chronically indwelling devices, such as infusion catheters or permanent pacemaker leads, within the central systemic venous circulation or right heart chambers are also at risk for endocarditis [36] (Fig. 11-8).

Unquestionably, TEE has been a crucially im-

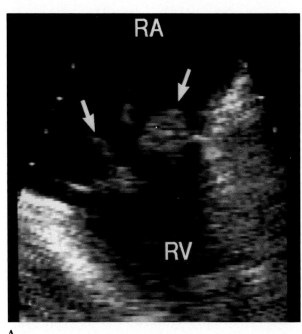

A

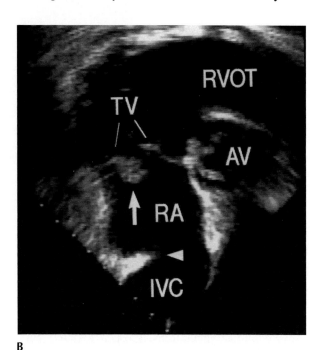

B

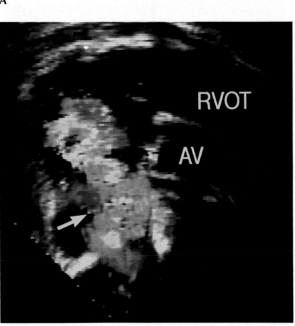

C

Fig. 11-7. A. Transverse plane, right ventricular inflow view obtained at the level of the gastroesophageal junction. Globular vegetations *(arrows)* with mobile filamentous components involve both tricuspid leaflets seen in this view.
B. Longitudinal plane, short-axis view. Prolapse of a large vegetative mass involving the anterior tricuspid leaflet *(arrow)* is best appreciated in this view; the vegetations on the septal tricuspid leaflet are not seen in this plane. The eustachian valve *(arrowhead)* at the orifice of the inferior vena cava may be quite large and mobile and should not be mistaken for a vegetation. C. The gross leaflet malcoaptation causes severe tricuspid regurgitation *(arrow).*

Fig. 11-8. Infective endocarditis complicating permanent pacemaker leads; transverse plane, right ventricular inflow view. Cross sections of both the atrial pacing lead (toward upper left of figure) and the ventricular pacing lead (adjacent to the tricuspid valve) are seen as round hyperrefractile echodensities *(arrowheads)* within the right atrium. Vegetations are attached to both pacing leads and also to the ventricular aspects of the tricuspid valve and annulus *(arrows)*.

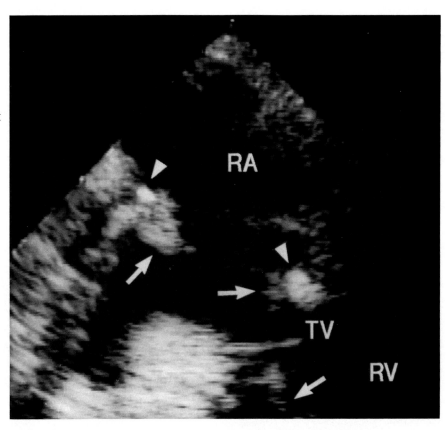

portant advance in the diagnosis of prosthetic valvular endocarditis [11–13,19,37–39]. The formidable problems with acoustic shadowing and artifacts related to transthoracic imaging of prosthetic valves have been largely, but not completely, overcome with biplanar and multiplanar TEE [29,40]. Like native valvular vegetations, those associated with prosthetic valves may vary greatly in appearance on TEE. Vegetations may occur in any location on prosthetic valves, although there is a general tendency for initial infective growth to occur on the sewing ring of mechanical valves (Fig. 11-9). In bioprosthetic valves, diseased or disrupted leaflets more commonly harbor vegetations (Fig. 11-10). All aspects of the prosthesis must be carefully examined for vegetative material. The ventricular aspects of a mitral prosthesis (particularly of the mechanical type) may be very difficult to visualize with standard midesophageal transverse and longitudinal windows, which image the prosthesis from the posterior left atrium (Fig. 11-11). Transgastric long- and short-axis imaging is then essential for complete evaluation. From the transgastric window, the ventricular side of a mitral prosthesis is visualized from a TEE transducer position imaging through the inferobasal left ventricle, avoiding acoustic interference from the prosthetic sewing ring and occluder, which limits

imaging from the esophageal window posterior to the left atrium. The ventricular aspects of aortic prostheses are usually well delineated on longitudinal short- and long-axis imaging. These windows, particularly the long-axis view and transverse left ventricular outflow tract view, may be significantly obscured by a mitral prosthesis, which usually shadows most of the left ventricular outflow tract. Longitudinal short-axis and transgastric longitudinal long-axis views of the subvalvular left ventricular outflow tract usually, but not always, alleviate this problem. Multiplanar long-axis imaging from the transgastric window best facilitates visualization of the subaortic region in this situation [29].

POTENTIAL LIMITATIONS OF TEE IN THE DIAGNOSIS OF INFECTIVE ENDOCARDITIS

Despite the excellent sensitivity of TEE for the high-resolution delineation of vegetations on both native and prosthetic valves, a modicum of caution is necessary in the TEE interpretation of what is or is not a vegetation. The TEE echocardiologist must always keep in mind a differential diagnosis for the finding of a discrete, mobile echodensity, be it attached to a

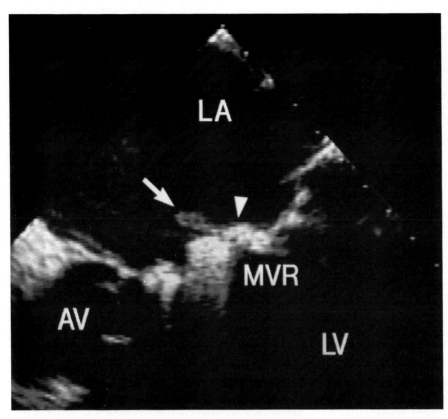

Fig. 11-9. Transverse four-chamber view focused on a mechanical mitral prosthesis *(MVR)*. A pedunculated vegetation *(arrow)* is attached to the lateral sewing ring of the prosthesis *(arrowhead)* and prolapses into the left atrium.

native valve, prosthetic material, or any intracardiac location.

Transesophageal two-dimensional echocardiography usually readily facilitates the differentiation of senescent valvular thickening, nodular sclerosis, and calcification from vegetative lesions, because the former are fixed and variably hyperrefractile and involve the valve in relatively symmetrical fashion. Annular calcification, particularly of the mitral valve, may be quite exuberant but is characteristically highly hyperrefractile and immobile; reverberation artifacts often arise from such calcific deposits and may be mistaken for vegetations.

Degenerative myxomatous disease presents a more difficult problem, especially when it involves the mitral valve. In advanced degenerative disease of the mitral valve, redundancy, thickening, and prolapse of the leaflets usually are marked. When complicated by ruptured chordae and one or more flail leaflet segments, systolic motion and fluttering of disrupted segments may make discernment from vegetations difficult (see Figures 9-11, 9-12, and 9–13). Such cases account for a significant proportion of false-positive and false-negative TEE studies for native valve endocarditis in existing reports [11,16]. Retracted, ruptured chordal segments in the patient with a chronic flail mitral valve often prove difficult to differentially diagnose because such retracted chordae may appear as nodular, pedunculated echodensities attached to the flail leaflet segment.

Patients with a history of endocarditis may have healed vegetations that can be difficult to differentiate from lesions associated with an active infective process. Chronic, healed vegetations are usually involuted, more echodense, and less mobile than active lesions [25,41–43]. Perceived echodensity of vegetations can be gain-dependent, and digital image processing with tissue characterization may allow more confident distinction between active and healed vegetative lesions in the future [43].

Rarely, benign intracardiac tumors mimic the appearance of valvular or endocardial vegetations [44,45]. The most common neoplasm responsible for this potential error in diagnosis is the papillary fibroelastoma (or papilloma), which most often arises from cardiac valves or valvular support structures; myxomas may, but very rarely do, occur on cardiac valves (see Chapter 12).

Sterile native valvular vegetations, which uncommonly cannot be differentiated from typical lesions of bacterial infective endocarditis, are visualized by TEE in multiple conditions causing nonbacterial thrombotic endocarditis [46]. Such illnesses include systemic malignancy ("marantic endocarditis"),

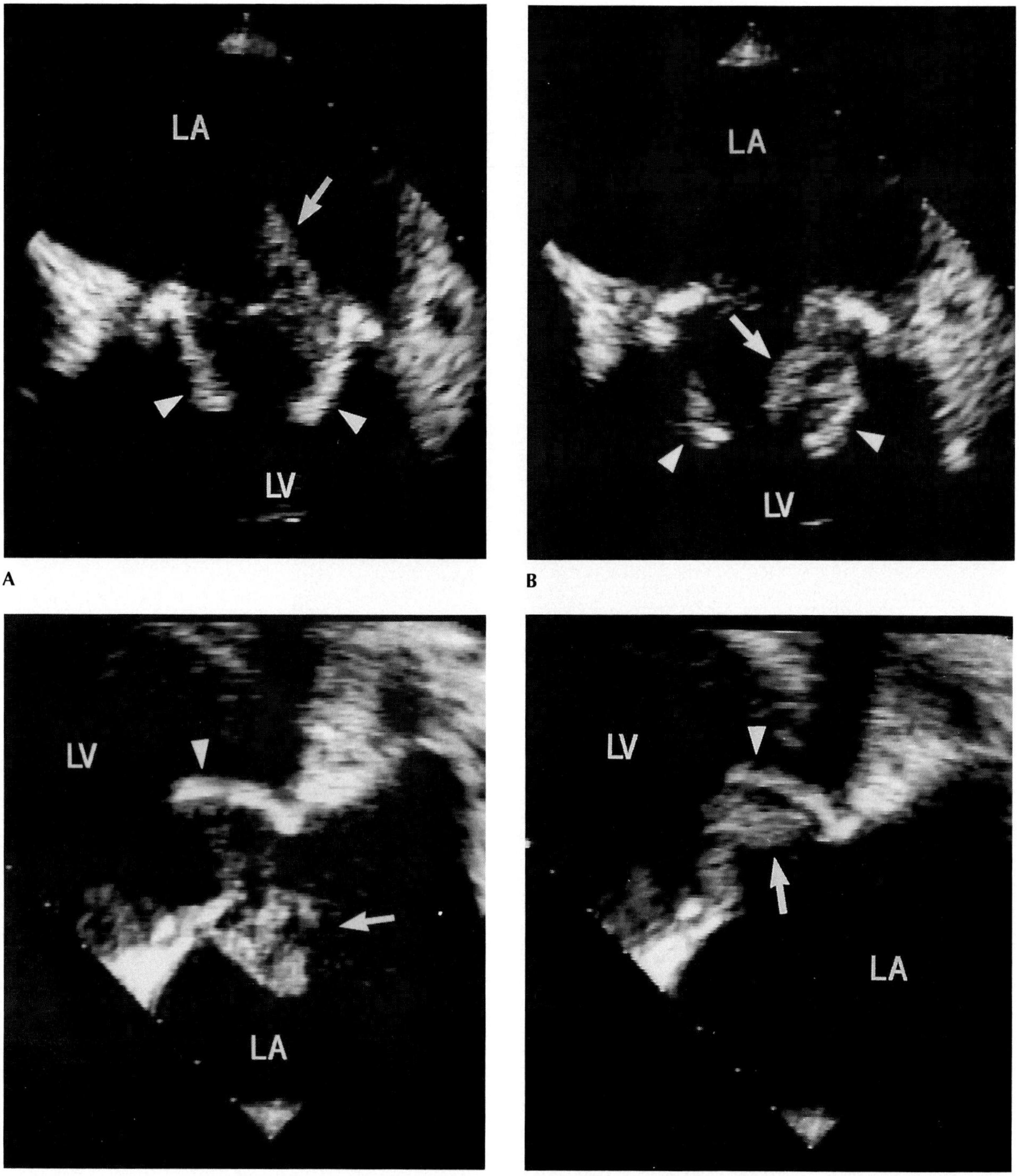

Fig. 11-10.   A. Expanded four-chamber view of mitral prosthetic endocarditis involving a Carpentier-Edwards bioprosthesis. During systole, a shaggy vegetation *(arrow)* attached to a torn prosthetic leaflet prolapses freely into the left atrium. The stents of the bioprosthesis are well visualized *(arrowheads)*. B. During diastole, this large vegetation *(arrow)* falls back into the mitral inflow tract, outlined by the stents *(arrowheads)*. C. Longitudinal images in the same patient. The complex cluster of vegetations on the flail bioprosthetic leaflet *(arrow)* are well seen, as is a medial stent *(arrowhead)* of this prosthesis. D. The significant mobility of this vegetative mass *(arrow)* is appreciated as it descends into the mitral inflow tract at the level of the stent *(arrowhead)*.

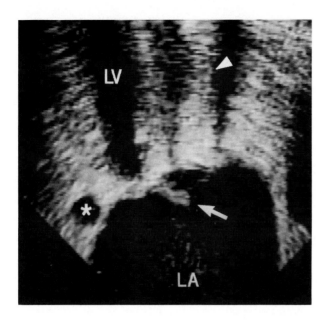

Fig. 11-11. Longitudinal two-chamber mitral inflow view. A pedunculated, mobile vegetation attached to the posterolateral sewing ring of a tilting disc mechanical prosthesis *(arrow)* is readily seen from the transesophageal window posterior to the left atrium. Note that the ventricular aspects of the prosthesis are shadowed in this view *(arrowhead)* and require examination from transgastric windows (which were normal). The sewing ring vegetation was completely obscured by prosthetic shadowing of the left atrium during transthoracic imaging. *(asterisk =* coronary sinus)

uremia, and multiple connective tissue disorders [47]. Usually, vegetations associated with nonbacterial thrombotic endocarditis are small, sessile, and verrucous. Patients with systemic lupus erythematosus who have high anticardiolipin antibody titers associated with the anticardiolipin syndrome are particularly prone to the development of prominent valvular vegetations atypical for usual nonbacterial thrombotic endocarditis lesions [48] (Fig. 11-12).

Valvular prostheses introduce another group of diagnostic considerations. The most common problem, differentiation of prosthetic vegetations from thrombus (see Chapter 10), is most difficult with mechanical prostheses and small lesions detected on TEE. Torn and disrupted sewing ring cloth may have a shaggy appearance and mimic vegetations; the linear appearance of suture material, however, usually allows correct identification (see Fig. 6-10). Mobile, filamentous strands are not uncommonly detected by TEE in association with otherwise structurally and functionally normal prostheses. Such strands, the nature of which is unknown, are observed most commonly with mechanical prostheses and are not associated with endocarditis, thrombosis, or adverse clinical events such as peripheral embolization [49]. Degeneration of bioprosthetic valves is commonly associated with a torn leaflet in the absence of endocarditis. Such torn leaflets are often flail and highly mobile with a vibratory motion, so that differentiation from a vegetation is challenging (Fig. 11-13).

As described in Chapter 6, prominent accumula-

tions of lipomatous tissue within the atrioventricular valvular sulci, atrial septum, and orifices of the systemic and pulmonary veins may occur (see Figures 6-6, 6-7, and 6-8). Such variants of normal anatomy must not be mistaken for vegetative material or perivalvular extension of infection, such as an abscess [50].

Importantly, the findings on TEE must always be integrated with the patient's clinical presentation to optimize the diagnostic capabilities of this technique.

TRANSESOPHAGEAL ECHOCARDIOGRAPHY IN THE PATIENT WITH PROVEN ENDOCARDITIS

Once the diagnosis of infective endocarditis has been established by clinical evaluation and corroborated by microbiologic and echocardiographic data, TEE remains instrumental in further evaluation and management throughout the course of therapy.

An essential role for TEE in this clinical situation is the detection and delineation of potential complications of infective endocarditis, an indication for which TEE unequivocally has been shown to be far superior to transthoracic echocardiography [9,11,21,28,37,39,51–53]. Major structural cardiac complications of endocarditis include progressive destruction of the infected valve or valves and perivalvular extension of infection, which may involve the formation of an abscess, aneurysm, fistula, or, in valvular prostheses, periannular dehiscence. A dreaded complication of endocarditis is peripheral embolization, and TEE has been shown to be helpful in the stratification of patients at risk for such an event [11,28].

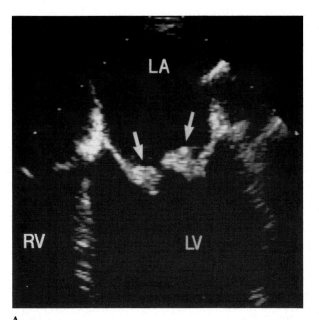

A

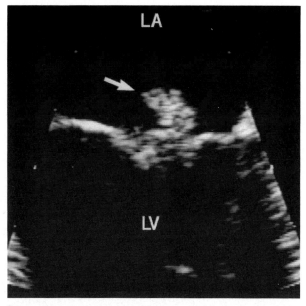

B

Fig. 11-12. Transverse four-chamber views of the mitral valve in a patient with systemic lupus erythematosus and the anticardiolipin syndrome. A. Posteriorly directed view at the crux of the heart. Echodense verrucous and sessile vegetations *(arrows)* extensively involve both leaflets, and the appearance is consistent with, but not diagnostic of, advanced nonbacterial thrombotic endocarditis. B. Anteriorly directed magnified view toward left ventricular outflow tract. A mobile frondlike vegetation *(arrow)* attached to the anterior mitral leaflet is detected. Such an appearance is unusual for nonbacterial thrombotic endocarditis and makes differentiation from infective endocarditis difficult; clinical correlation is essential.

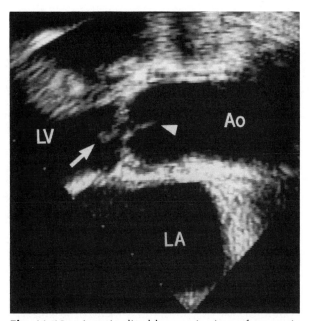

Fig. 11-13. Longitudinal long-axis view of an aortic homograft prosthesis. A large torn leaflet segment *(arrow)* is flail into the left ventricular outflow tract during diastole; the more posterior leaflet in this view is intact and has normal diastolic excursion *(arrowhead)*. The torn prosthetic leaflet had vibratory mobility on real-time examination, and confident differentiation from a vegetation was not possible. No vegetations were found at reoperation. (Ao = ascending aorta)

Valvular Destruction

The degree and time course of progressive native valvular damage due to endocarditis depend largely on the nature of the infecting organism. Preexisting disease and insufficiency of the involved valve and concomitant left ventricular function are also significant contributing factors to the clinical course.

Multiple mechanisms may be responsible for native valvular dysfunction and insufficiency in endocarditis. Progressive, large vegetative growth may engulf and even retract valve leaflets to the extent that adequate systolic or diastolic coaptation is not possible (see Fig. 11-7). Rarely, extensive and large vegetations may cause valvular stenosis [54]. Localized infective erosion through the body of a leaflet leads to perforation (Fig. 11-14), commonly associated with endocarditis. Disruption and flail of an aortic valve cusp may lead to acute severe aortic regurgitation and decompensated left ventricular failure (Fig. 11-15). Disruption of the mitral valvular support apparatus typically occurs at the level of the chordae tendinae and leads to a flail mitral valve leaflet (Fig. 11-16). Rarely, mycotic aneurysms within valve leaflets, a potential precursor to leaflet perforation, can be visualized in extensively infected valves (Fig. 11-17).

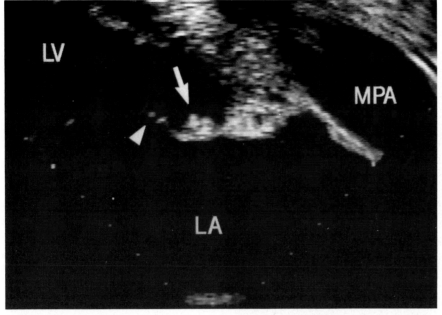

A

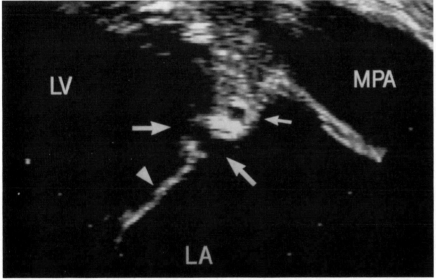

B

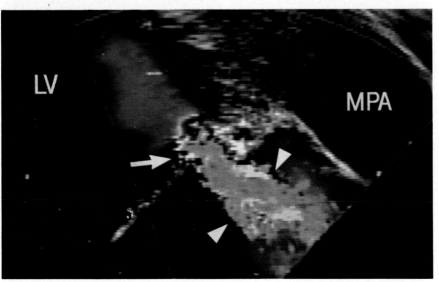

C

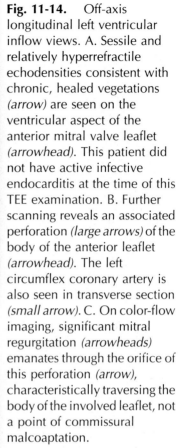

Fig. 11-14. Off-axis longitudinal left ventricular inflow views. A. Sessile and relatively hyperrefractile echodensities consistent with chronic, healed vegetations *(arrow)* are seen on the ventricular aspect of the anterior mitral valve leaflet *(arrowhead)*. This patient did not have active infective endocarditis at the time of this TEE examination. B. Further scanning reveals an associated perforation *(large arrows)* of the body of the anterior leaflet *(arrowhead)*. The left circumflex coronary artery is also seen in transverse section *(small arrow)*. C. On color-flow imaging, significant mitral regurgitation *(arrowheads)* emanates through the orifice of this perforation *(arrow)*, characteristically traversing the body of the involved leaflet, not a point of commissural malcoaptation.

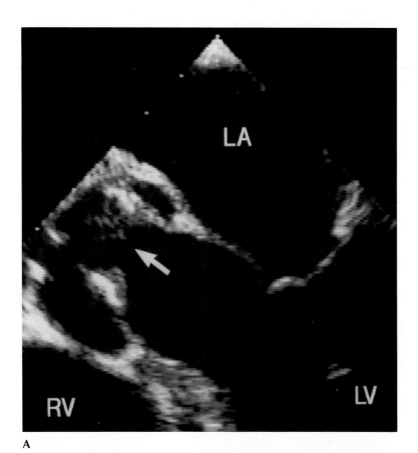

A

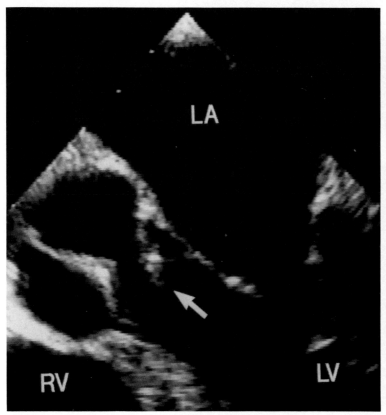

B

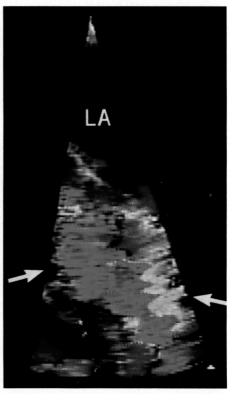

C

Fig. 11-15.   Transverse plane, left ventricular outflow views. A. The aortic valve *(arrow)* is encrusted with minimally mobile vegetations. B. During diastole, an unsupported, flail left coronary cusp *(arrow)* caused by infective destruction of the valve is evident. C. Resultant severe aortic regurgitation is present, with a broad eccentric jet on color Doppler imaging *(arrows)*. This patient had severe acute left ventricular failure.

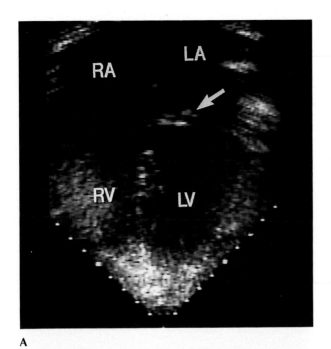

A

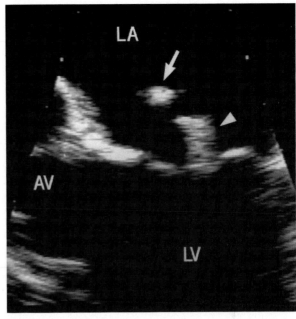

B

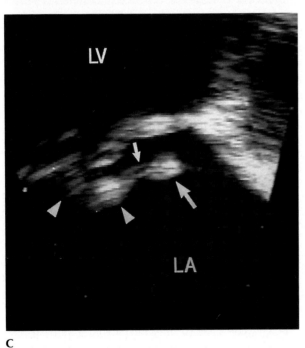

C

Fig. 11-16. Native mitral valve endocarditis associated with a flail posterior leaflet. A. Apex-down transthoracic apical four-chamber view. The posterior mitral leaflet *(arrow)* is abnormal, but the cause is poorly defined. B. Transverse plane, magnified four-chamber TEE view. A thickened tubular mass *(arrowhead)* with a highly mobile echodensity *(arrow)* at its tip protrudes into the left atrium; its exact nature is still unclear in this view. C. Magnified mitral inflow view in the longitudinal plane. The tubular mass is demonstrated to be a flail posterior leaflet segment, grossly thickened with vegetations of varying echodensity *(arrowheads)*. The mobile mass *(large arrow)* at its tip is a vegetation attached to ruptured chordae *(small arrow)*.

Perivalvular Extension of Infection

Extension of infective endocarditis into adjoining perivalvular structures, such as the valve annulus and adjacent myocardium, is a serious complication of this disease and often accounts for clinical failure of antibiotic therapy and need for operative intervention. Simple perivalvular satellite vegetative lesions that remain confined to the endocardial surfaces generally have a far less ominous prognosis than does the formation of an abscess or related complications.

The most common manifestation of significant perivalvular extension of infection complicating endocarditis is the periannular abscess, which may be found in 20% to 30% of patients undergoing surgery or necropsy [55,56]. In a recent study of TEE in

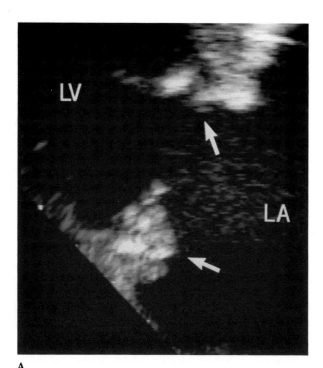
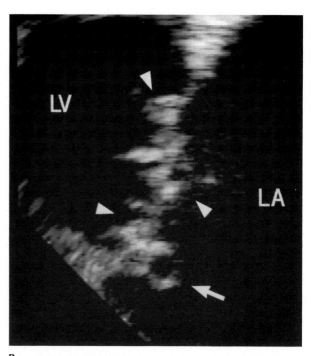

A   B

Fig. 11-17. Valvular mycotic aneurysm complicating infective endocarditis; magnified longitudinal views of the mitral valve. A. Numerous vegetations have deformed both mitral leaflets *(arrows)* shown in diastole. B. During systole, a narrow-necked mycotic aneurysm of the body of the posterior mitral leaflet *(arrow)* is visualized along with multiple vegetations on both sides of the leaflets *(arrowheads)*. This rare valvular complication of endocarditis was confirmed at the time of mitral valve replacement.

the evaluation of anatomically confirmed abscesses, abscess formation complicating endocarditis was found to be localized to the periannular region in nearly 90% of patients, with 75% of all abscesses occurring in the aortic position in either prosthetic or native aortic valve endocarditis [37]. In this study, the overall sensitivity for the detection of abscess was 87% for TEE but only 28% for transthoracic echocardiography; the specificities were 95% and 99%, respectively. Transesophageal echocardiography greatly improved the detection of anatomically proven abscess complicating native or prosthetic valve endocarditis in either the aortic or the mitral position; all ventricular septal abscesses were detected by TEE, with the transthoracic approach visualizing only 22% [37] (Fig. 11-18).

Echocardiographically defined, a perivalvular abscess may appear as either an echodense or an echolucent region within, but distinct from, normal annular or perivalvular tissue in the patient with valvular endocarditis [37,39]. Before diagnosis an abscess should be imaged in several views and tomo-

graphic planes for both confirmation and delineation of its extent. If large enough, an abscess may have a mass effect and displace normal perivalvular tissue planes (Fig. 11-19). Very early in the course of formation an abscess usually has a homogeneous echodense appearance, analogous to an inflammatory mass, or phlegmon. With progressive necrosis and formation of purulent material, such abscesses typically become heterogeneous and echolucent (Fig. 11-20). The lack of echolucency in a perivalvular region suspect for abscess hence by no means excludes this diagnosis. Meticulous scanning of the entire perivalvular region is indicated, because abscesses may occasionally be multicentric (Fig. 11-21).

Abscesses may also disrupt their perivalvular confines, forming communications or fistulae with other cardiac chambers or the intravascular space (Fig. 11-22). Such abscess cavity communications may be visualized directly by two-dimensional examination or be appreciated indirectly by the observation of systolic expansion and diastolic collapse of the

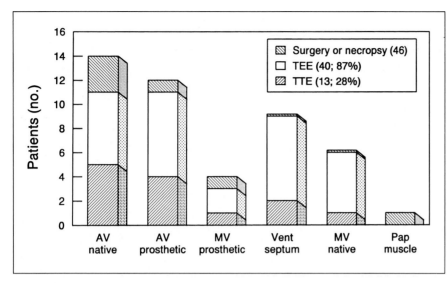

Fig. 11-18. Comparison of the usefulness of transesophageal and transthoracic echocardiography in the detection of anatomically confirmed abscesses complicating infective endocarditis. The major incremental increase in sensitivity of TEE in the diagnosis of abscess in left-sided native or prosthetic valvular endocarditis and ventricular septal abscesses is apparent. (Data from Daniel et al. [37].)

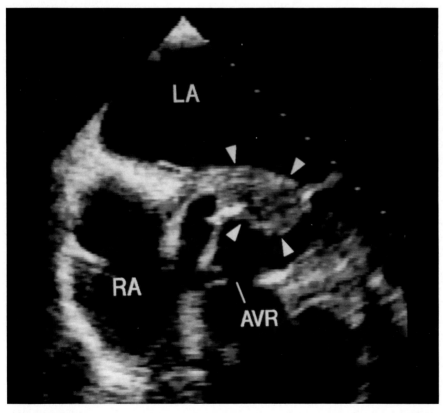

Fig. 11-19. Periannular abscess complicating aortic prosthetic valve endocarditis; modified basal short-axis view in the transverse plane. A large perivalvular abscess (encircled by *arrowheads*) distorts the periannular anatomy adjacent to the aortic valve prosthesis *(AVR)*.

perivalvular cavity throughout the cardiac cycle (Fig. 11-23). Color-flow Doppler imaging confirms the communication with the demonstration of to-and-fro flow in and out of the abscess cavity.

The subaortic complications of native or prosthetic aortic valve endocarditis have been well described by Bansal et al. [51] and Karalis et al. [39]. Abscesses complicating aortic valve endocarditis may extend into the aortic-mitral intervalvular fibrosa, with subsequent formation of a mycotic aneurysm within this region, often with extension both below and above the aortic annulus (Fig. 11-24). Communication between the left ventricular outflow tract and the intervalvular fibrosa aneurysm is best visualized in the longitudinal long-axis view (Fig. 11-25). Such a mycotic aneurysm may rupture into

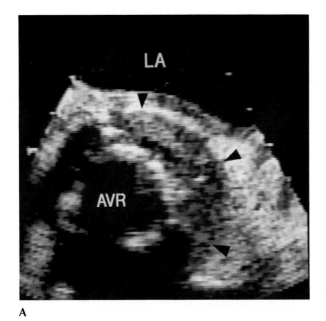

A

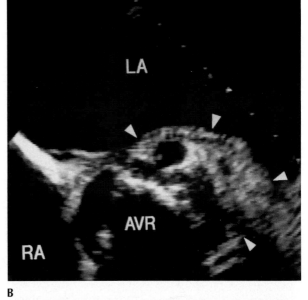

B

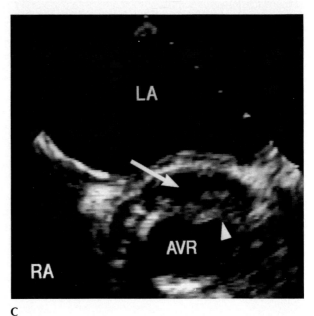

C

Fig. 11-20. Serial TEE examinations of perivalvular abscess complicating aortic prosthetic valve endocarditis; basal short-axis views in the transverse plane. A. Examination early in this patient's course revealed a relatively homogeneous echodense perivalvular extension of infection *(black arrowheads)* bordering the sewing ring of the bioprosthetic aortic valve *(AVR)*, consistent with early abscess formation. B. Follow-up examination in the same patient 2 days later. There is a more heterogeneous appearance to the abscess *(white arrowheads)*, which now contains several regions of echolucency. C. A third TEE examination (4 days after initial diagnosis) before operative intervention. A large echolucent abscess cavity *(arrow)* adjacent to the aortic prosthesis is now present; some debris *(arrowhead)* is contained within this cavity.

the left atrium, forming a shunt from the left ventricular outflow tract into the left atrium (Fig. 11-26). Direct rupture of the aortic-mitral intervalvular fibrosa abscess with fistulous connection into the left atrium can also occur without mycotic aneurysm formation. Subaortic extension of infection can also go directly into the anterior mitral valve leaflet, leading to mycotic aneurysm formation in the body of this leaflet or perforation [39].

Perivalvular abscess formation complicating prosthetic valve endocarditis commonly precipitates significant periprosthetic regurgitation on disruption of the abscess cavity (Fig. 11-27). If extensive, an

abscess may undermine considerable periannular support and cause dehiscence of the involved prosthesis. In prosthetic endocarditis, small regions of periprosthetic annular disruption due to perivalvular extension of infection should always be sought by meticulous scanning of the entire circumference of the prosthetic sewing ring (Fig. 11-28). Not uncommonly, such small periprosthetic defects may not be readily appreciated even by two-dimensional TEE imaging. Color-flow Doppler examination readily facilitates correct identification with the demonstration of a localized periannular regurgitant jet emanating from such a defect (Fig. 11-28).

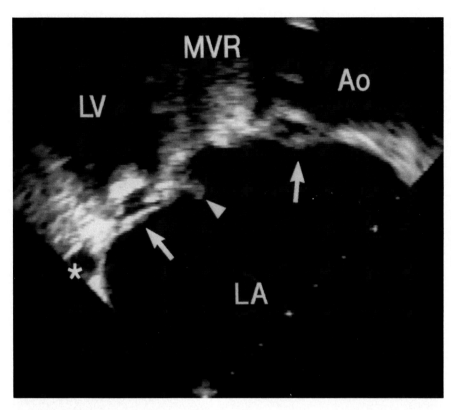

Fig. 11-21. Multicentric perivalvular abscess associated with mitral prosthetic endocarditis; modified longitudinal mitral inflow view. Two echolucent periprosthetic abscess cavities *(arrows)* are seen in this imaging plane. A small vegetation *(arrowhead)* attached to the atrial surface of the mitral prosthesis *(MVR)* is also observed. The coronary sinus *(asterisk)* in the posterior atrioventricular groove must not be mistaken for an abscess. *(Ao* = ascending aorta)

Peripheral Embolization and Other Complications

Transthoracic echocardiographic recognition of valvular vegetations has long been known to be associated with a less favorable outcome than clinically suspected endocarditis without detectable vegetations. Early transthoracic echocardiographic studies have shown that echocardiographically detected vegetations are related to a higher incidence of not only peripheral embolization but also congestive heart failure and need for cardiac surgery [4,5,7,25,57–60] (Table 11-3).

Using detailed two-dimensional transthoracic echocardiographic analysis, Sanfilippo et al. [23] found that vegetation size, extent of valvular involvement, and mobility were multivariate predictors of complications such as embolization, heart failure, need for surgery, and death in left-sided native valvular endocarditis. Vegetations at higher risk for complications were pedunculated or prolapsing, multiple, and involved more than one valve leaflet, especially with perivalvular extension. The cumulative probability of complications increased directly with vegetation size and was estimated to be 50% for vegetations of 11 mm and over 90% for vegetations larger than 16 mm [23].

Mügge et al. [11] employed TEE to examine the prognostic implications of vegetation size. These investigators found that the overall incidence of embolic events was significantly higher with vegetations greater than 10 mm in diameter (47%) than with smaller vegetations (19%). This difference in incidence of embolism was even greater in patients in whom TEE was performed before an embolic event (Fig. 11-29). Eighty-five percent of vegetations larger than 10 mm, but only 48% of smaller vegetations, were mobile. This relation was particularly striking in patients with native mitral valve endocarditis, and statistically nonsignificant trends were present in the native aortic valve and prosthetic valve groups (Fig. 11-30). Embolic episodes were more frequent with mobile (38%) than with sessile (19%) vegetations [11]. Although vegetation size was sensitive in the identification of patients at risk for embolic events, it did not correlate with heart failure or death in this study [11].

By multivariate analysis of 118 patients with left-sided native valve vegetations detected by TEE, Rohmann et al. [28] also found that vegetation size greater than 10 mm and mitral valve location were independent predictors of embolic complications. In their study, the incidence of embolism was 25% with

Fig. 11-22. Perivalvular abscess in bioprosthetic aortic valve endocarditis; longitudinal long-axis imaging plane. A. A large abscess *(arrowheads)* distorts the aortic annulus posterior to the aortic bioprosthesis *(AVR)*. B. Repeat TEE examination in the same patient several days later after an embolic cerebrovascular accident. The abscess *(arrow)* has ruptured into the left ventricular outflow tract, and mobile debris from the disintegrated abscess wall is visible in the outflow tract *(arrowhead)*.

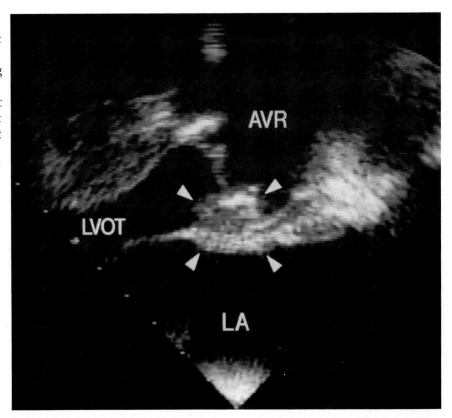

A

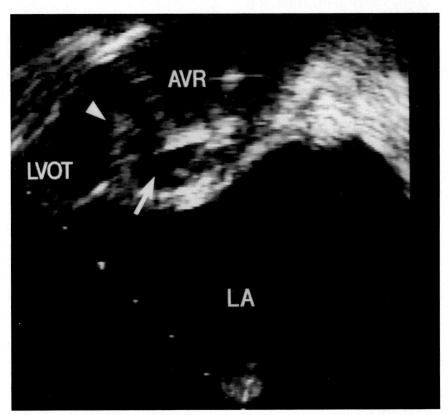

B

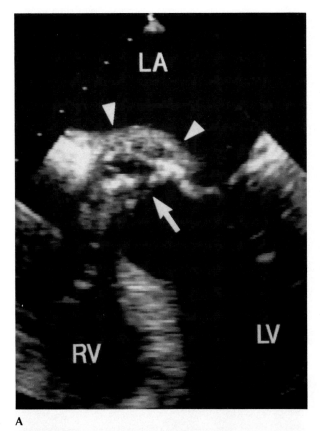

A

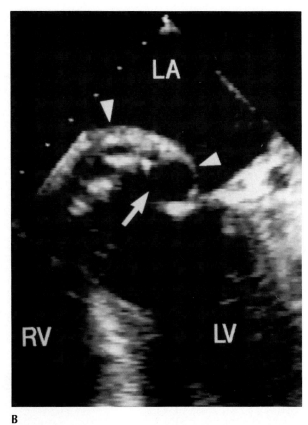

B

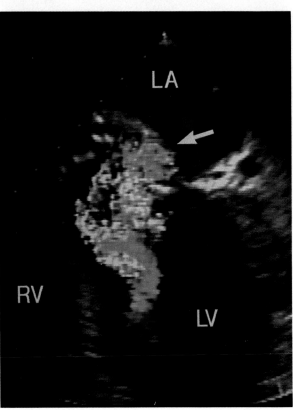

C

Fig. 11-23. Aortic periprosthetic abscess; left ventricular outflow view in the transverse plane. A. A partially collapsed echodense mass *(arrowheads)* is seen adjacent to the obscured aortic prosthesis in end-diastole. A fistulous connection to the left ventricular outflow tract is suggested in this view *(arrow)*. B. With systole, the abscess cavity *(arrowheads)* has expanded and the fistulous connection is well visualized *(arrow)*. C. Color-flow Doppler study demonstrates systolic flow entering the abscess cavity *(arrow)*.

Fig. 11-24. Mycotic aneurysm of the aortic-mitral intervalvular fibrosa; longitudinal long-axis view. As a result of perivalvular extension of infection and abscess formation complicating native aortic valve endocarditis *(arrow)*, a mycotic aneurysm *(A)* has developed within the intervalvular fibrosa, extending both above and below the level of the aortic valve annulus. Such complications involving the intervalvular fibrosa are best delineated by longitudinal long-axis imaging. *(asterisk = right pulmonary artery; Ao = ascending aorta.)*

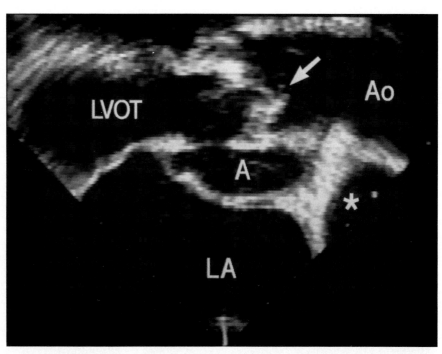

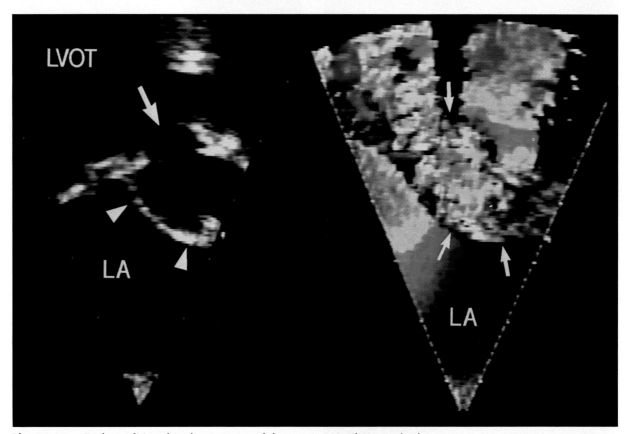

Fig. 11-25. Endocarditis-related aneurysm of the aortic-mitral intervalvular fibrosa; magnified longitudinal long-axis plane. A large mycotic aneurysm *(arrowheads)* within the intervalvular fibrosa bulges into the left atrium, having a wide communication (nearly 1 cm) *(large arrow)* with the left ventricular outflow tract. Color Doppler imaging during systole reveals flow from the left ventricular outflow tract filling this aneurysm *(small arrows)*.

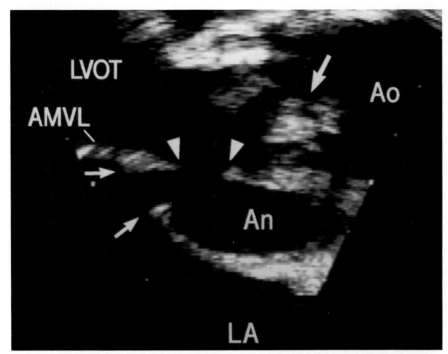

A

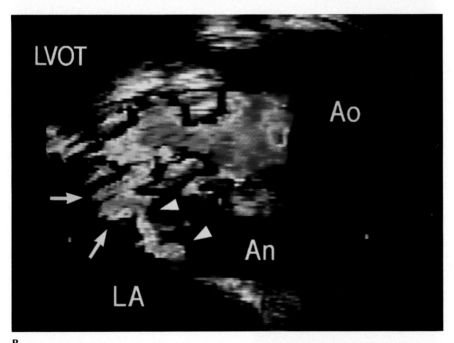

B

Fig. 11-26.   Endocarditis-related aneurysm complicated by an intracardiac shunt; longitudinal long-axis magnified views. A. A large mycotic aneurysm *(An)* is visualized within the aortic-mitral intervalvular fibrosa. The communication from the left ventricular outflow tract into the aneurysm is noted by *arrowheads* just below the aortic valve, which is grossly deformed by vegetations *(large arrow)*. The communication from aneurysm to left atrium is identified by the *small arrows* adjacent to the insertion of the anterior mitral valve leaflet *(AMVL)*. B. Color-flow imaging during systole in the same imaging plane reveals flow entering the mycotic aneurysm *(arrowheads)* from the left ventricular outflow tract and exiting the aneurysm into the left atrium *(small arrows)*, resulting in a shunt from the outflow tract to the left atrium.

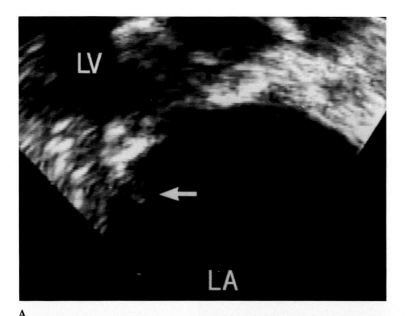

A

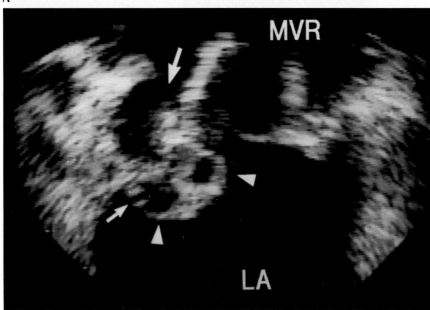

B

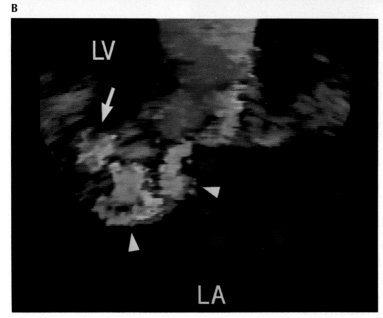

C

Fig. 11-27. Serial TEE studies in a patient with mitral prosthetic endocarditis complicated by periannular abscess formation and periprosthetic dehiscence; longitudinal mitral inflow views. A. The initial TEE study demonstrates a small vegetation *(arrow)* attached to the atrial surface of the posterolateral sewing ring. No periannular abscess was detected. B. Follow-up TEE examination, 14 days later, reveals the formation of a large multiseptated posterolateral periannular abscess *(arrowheads)* bulging into the left atrium. A small defect in the abscess wall is present along its lateral margin *(small arrow)*. A large area of periprosthetic dehiscence *(large arrow)* is present just lateral to the mitral bioprosthesis *(MVR)*. C. Color Doppler imaging reveals diastolic inflow coursing through the serpiginous abscess cavity *(arrowheads)* into the left ventricle *(arrow)*; normal diastolic inflow is also crossing the mitral prosthesis. D. Off-axis longitudinal view in the same patient before reoperation. The posterolateral periprosthetic abscess *(asterisk)* has ruptured into the left atrium *(arrow)*. E. Resultant severe periprosthetic mitral regurgitation *(arrow)* emanates from the region of abscess-induced dehiscence.

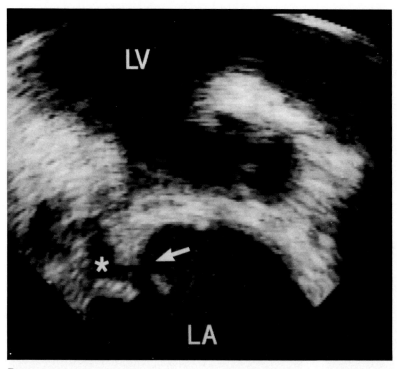

D

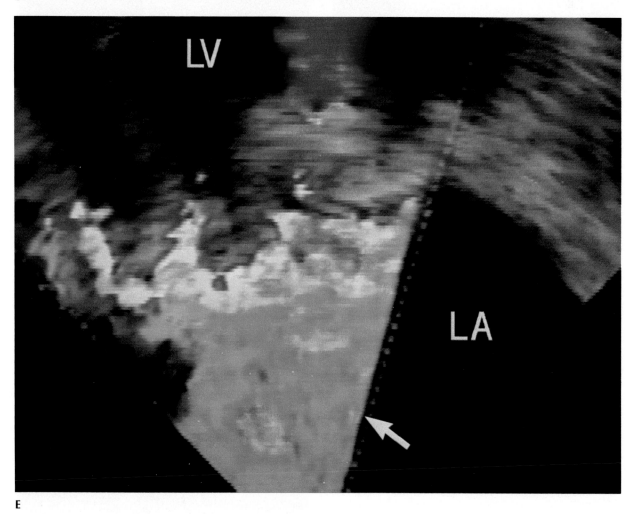

E

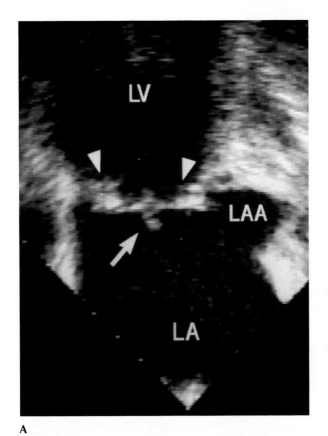

A

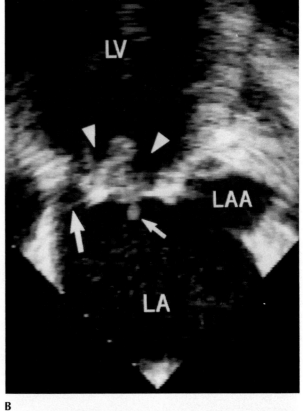

B

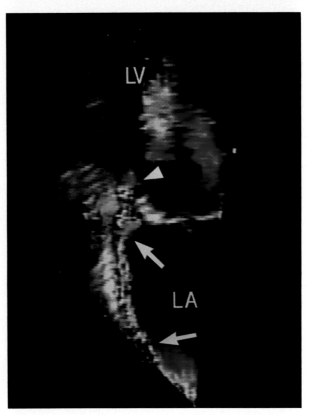

C

Fig. 11-28. Periprosthetic dehiscence complicating mitral periprosthetic endocarditis; longitudinal left ventricular inflow views. A. A small vegetation *(arrow)* is detected on the atrial aspect of the mitral bioprosthesis. No periprosthetic abnormalities are noted adjacent to the prosthetic sewing ring *(arrowheads)* in this imaging plane. B. Further scanning of the circumference of the sewing ring reveals a localized region of periprosthetic disruption *(large arrow)*. The small vegetation *(small arrow)* is seen attached to the bioprosthesis *(arrowheads)*. C. Periprosthetic dehiscence is confirmed by the color Doppler demonstration of periprosthetic mitral regurgitation entrained into this defect *(arrowhead)* and tracking along the posterolateral wall *(arrows)* of the left atrium. *(LAA = left atrial appendage (orifice)).*

Table 11-3. Transthoracic echocardiography and the risk of endocarditis complications

Authors	Year	No. of patients		No. of patients with complications					
		With vegetation	Without vegetation	Embolization		Congestive heart failure		Cardiac surgery	
				Vegetation	No vegetation	Vegetation	No vegetation	Vegetation	No vegetation
Wann et al. [60]	1976	22	43	4	0	22	12	18	0
Stewart et al. [5]	1980	47	40	14	4	15	1	12	2
Hickey et al. [58]	1981	22	14	11	5	18	4	14	3
Lutas et al. [59]	1986	43	34	11	6	23	12	5	7

Data from Stewart et al. [5], Hickey et al. [58], Lutas et al. [59], Wann et al. [60].

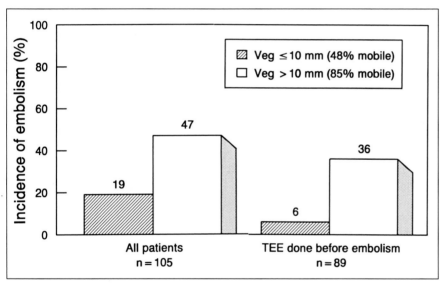

Fig. 11-29. Vegetation size measured by TEE and risk of embolism. Vegetation size of greater than 10 mm was associated with a significantly higher incidence of embolism; the difference in risk compared with that of smaller vegetations is even more noticeable in patients evaluated by TEE before an embolic event. (Data from Mügge et al. [11].)

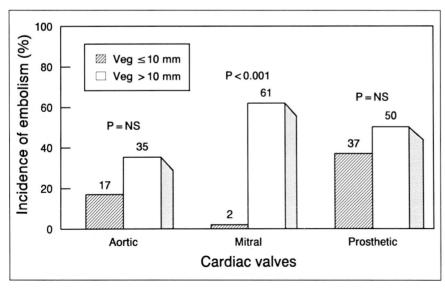

Fig. 11-30. Incidence of embolism related to valvular vegetation location and size. Vegetations greater than 10 mm involving the native mitral valve have the highest risk of embolism. Similar but far less striking trends for aortic and prosthetic vegetations did not reach statistical significance. (Data from Mügge et al. [11].)

mitral vegetations and 10% with those involving the aortic valve. Conversely, abscess formation, need for operative intervention, and mortality were all greater in patients with aortic valve endocarditis. Endocarditis involving both the aortic and the mitral valves was associated with the highest incidences of embolic events (50%), abscess formation (15%), need for surgery (35%), and overall mortality (10%) [28].

A recent preliminary report confirmed the finding that risk of embolic events is greater with larger vegetations measured by either maximal length or planimetered area on TEE [61]. Vegetation mobility, as determined by the maximal angle of displacement of the long axis of the vegetation in relation to the site of attachment, was associated with risk of both embolization and death [61].

Spontaneous echocontrast on TEE in patients with infective endocarditis has been suggested to be a multivariate risk factor for embolization and for operation for valve replacement [62]. Presumably because of a low-flow state and increased spontaneous platelet aggregation (documented by increased aggregability with adenosine diphosphate in this study), spontaneous echocontrast was also associated with prolonged healing of vegetative lesions on serial TEE examinations [62].

CLINICAL USE OF ECHOCARDIOGRAPHY IN INFECTIVE ENDOCARDITIS

Suspected Endocarditis

A frequently asked question is, Should every patient with suspected or known endocarditis have TEE? Although no large, controlled clinical studies have been done to answer this question, we have developed an approach based on our clinical experience and practice. This approach is outlined in Figure 11-31.

Because of its complementary value in making the diagnosis and its ability to define valvular hemodynamics and left ventricular function, a transthoracic echocardiographic examination should be done in all patients with suspected endocarditis. If the images are too poor in quality to allow confident identification or exclusion of a vegetation, TEE should be directly performed.

If the transthoracic images are of good quality and the study shows no evidence of endocarditis,

this examination is probably sufficient for patients with native valves in whom the clinical suspicion of endocarditis is low. However, if clinical suspicion is high or if the patient has a prosthetic valve, it is recommended that TEE be done even though a transthoracic study of good quality yields negative findings. This group of patients benefits the most from the higher sensitivity of infective endocarditis detection offered by TEE.

If the transthoracic images are of good quality and vegetations are identified, the decision to perform TEE depends on clinical variables and the results of transthoracic examination. If there is no evidence of complications (e.g., valve destruction or perivalvular extension of infection), valvular regurgitation has been adequately defined, and the patient is clinically stable, the transthoracic study should serve as an adequate baseline. If there is discordance between clinical and transthoracic echocardiographic impressions, the possibility of complications, inadequate definition of valvular regurgitation, or clinical instability, TEE should be done expeditiously for further evaluation.

A guiding question in deciding whether to perform TEE in infective endocarditis should be, Does the transthoracic echocardiogram provide all the information needed to make decisions in the clinical management of the patient? If not, TEE should be done to obtain the needed additional information.

Proven Endocarditis

Once a patient has been proven to have infective endocarditis, deciding what serial studies to perform and when to perform them depends on the clinical course of the patient and the results of earlier studies.

If the patient is clinically stable, a follow-up study should be done about 1 week after the initial study to assess the effectiveness of antimicrobial therapy. This study should be by the same approach (transthoracic or transesophageal) as that which originally defined the endocarditic lesions.

If the patient is clinically unstable or new physical signs develop (e.g., change in murmur, congestive heart failure, recurrent refractory fever, and embolization), a repeat study is indicated at that time. The type of study to be performed depends on the information needed and the quality of the initial transthoracic images. If worsening valvular regurgitation or possible left ventricular dysfunction is the primary concern, transthoracic study may be adequate. If the concern is progression of vegetative lesions, the

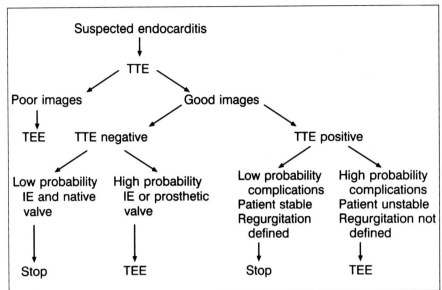

Suspected endocarditis
↓
TTE

Poor images | Good images

TEE | TTE negative | TTE positive

Low probability IE and native valve | High probability IE or prosthetic valve | Low probability complications Patient stable Regurgitation defined | High probability complications Patient unstable Regurgitation not defined

Stop | TEE | Stop | TEE

Fig. 11-31. Algorithm for the use of transthoracic echocardiography and transesophageal echocardiography in the patient with clinically suspected infective endocarditis *(IE)*; see text for details.

serial study should correspond to the original study that defined the vegetations. Transthoracic examination may be appropriate if images are adequate, but TEE should be performed if there are any doubts about the status of vegetations and valvular regurgitation. Once again, all patients with prosthetic valve endocarditis require TEE for adequate evaluation. If the primary concern is of perivalvular extension of infection or other complications, TEE will provide the most accurate information and should be performed in all patients.

SUMMARY

As the resolution of cardiac ultrasonography improves, its diagnostic accuracy in infective endocarditis continues to increase, permitting not only higher sensitivity but also detection of smaller lesions, ideally early in the course of the disease. Data substantiating the benefits of early detection and therapeutic intervention are currently lacking and should be the subject of intensive investigation.

The time has come for a change in the diagnostic criteria for infective endocarditis. Case definition should include diagnostic criteria from transthoracic echocardiography and now TEE, which has greatly enhanced the utility of echocardiography in this disease. With the multiple major advantages of TEE, this imaging technique has become a cornerstone in the evaluation and management of the patient with infective endocarditis.

REFERENCES

1. Osler W. The Gulstonian Lectures on malignant endocarditis. *Br Med J* 1885;1:467–70; 522–6; 577–9.

2. Von Reyn CF, Levy BS, Arbeit RD, et al. Infective endocarditis: an analysis based on strict case definitions. *Ann Intern Med* 1981;94:505–18.

3. Dillon JC, Feigenbaum H, Konecke LL, et al. Echocardiographic manifestations of valvular vegetations. *Am Heart J* 1973;86:698–704.

4. Roy P, Tajik AJ, Giuliani ER, et al. Spectrum of echocardiographic findings in bacterial endocarditis. *Circulation* 1976;53:474–82.

5. Stewart JA, Silimperi D, Harris P, et al. Echocardiographic documentation of vegetative lesions in infective endocarditis: clinical implications. *Circulation* 1980;61:374–80.

6. Jaffe WM, Morgan DE, Pearlman AS, Otto CM. Infective endocarditis, 1983–1988: echocardiographic findings and factors influencing morbidity and mortality. *J Am Coll Cardiol* 1990;15:1227–33.

7. Stafford WJ, Petch J, Radford DJ. Vegetations in infective endocarditis: clinical relevance and diagnosis by cross sectional echocardiography. *Br Heart J* 1985;53:310–3.

8. Mintz GSA, Kotler MN, Segal BL, Parry WR. Comparison of two-dimensional and M-mode echocardiography in the evaluation of patients with infective endocarditis. *Am J Cardiol* 1979;43:738–44.

9. Erbel R, Rohmann S, Drexler M, et al. Improved diagnostic value of echocardiography in patients with infective endocarditis by transoesophageal ap-

proach. A prospective study. *Eur Heart J* 1988;9: 43–53.

10. Gilbert BW, Haney RS, Crawford F, et al. Two-dimensional echocardiographic assessment of vegetative endocarditis. *Circulation* 1977;55:346–53.

11. Mügge A, Daniel WG, Frank G, Lichtlen PR. Echocardiography in infective endocarditis: reassessment of prognostic implications of vegetation size determined by the transthoracic and the transesophageal approach. *J Am Coll Cardiol* 1989;14:631–8.

12. Scanlon JG, Seward JB, Tajik AJ. Valve ring abscess in infective endocarditis: visualization with wide angle two dimensional echocardiography. *Am J Cardiol* 1982;49:1794–800.

13. Daniel WG, Schröder E, Mügge A, Lichtlen PR. Transesophageal echocardiography in infective endocarditis. *Am J Card Imaging* 1988;2:78–85.

14. Daniel WG, Schröder E, Nonnast-Daniel B, Lichtlen PR. Conventional and transoesophageal echocardiography in the diagnosis of infective endocarditis. *Eur Heart J* 1987;8 (Suppl J):287–92.

15. Taams MA, Gussenhoven EJ, Bos E, et al. Enhanced morphological diagnosis in infective endocarditis by transoesophageal echocardiography. *Br Heart J* 1990;63:109–13.

16. Shively BK, Gurule FT, Roldan CA, et al. Diagnostic value of transesophageal compared with transthoracic echocardiography in infective endocarditis. *J Am Coll Cardiol* 1991;18:391–7.

17. Birmingham GD, Rahko PS, Ballantyne F III. Improved detection of infective endocarditis with transesophageal echocardiography. *Am Heart J* 1992;123:774–81.

18. Klodas E, Edwards WD, Khandheria BK. Use of transesophageal echocardiography for improving detection of valvular vegetations in subacute bacterial endocarditis. *J Am Soc Echocardiogr* 1989;2: 386–9.

19. Pedersen WR, Walker M, Olson JD, et al. Value of transesophageal echocardiography as an adjunct to transthoracic echocardiography in evaluation of native and prosthetic valve endocarditis. *Chest* 1991; 100:351–6.

20. Sochowski RA, Chan K-L. Implications of negative results on a monoplane transesophageal echocardiographic study in patients with suspected infective endocarditis. *J Am Coll Cardiol* 1993;21:216–21.

21. Khandheria BK. Suspected bacterial endocarditis: to TEE or not to TEE. *J Am Coll Cardiol* 1993; 21:222–4.

22. Berger M, Gallerstein PE, Benhuri P, et al. Evaluation of aortic valve endocarditis by two-dimensional echocardiography. *Chest* 1981;80:61–7.

23. Sanfilippo AJ, Picard MH, Newell JB, et al. Echocardiographic assessment of patients with infectious endocarditis: prediction of risk for complications. *J Am Coll Cardiol* 1991;18:1191–9.

24. Berger M, Delfin LA, Jelveh M, Goldberg E. Two-dimensional echocardiographic findings in right-sided infective endocarditis. *Circulation* 1980;61: 855–61.

25. Rohmann S, Erbel R, Darius H, et al. Prediction of rapid versus prolonged healing of infective endocarditis by monitoring vegetation size. *J Am Soc Echocardiogr* 1991;4:465–74.

26. Vuille C, Nidorf M, Weyman AE, Picard MH. Natural history of vegetations in successfully treated endocarditis (abstract). *J Am Coll Cardiol* 1993;21: 200A.

27. Rohmann S, Erbel R, Darius H, et al. Influence of antibiotics on vegetation size in infective endocarditis: a comparative study (abstract). *J Am Coll Cardiol* 1993;21:391A.

28. Rohmann S, Erbel R, Görge G, et al. Clinical relevance of vegetation localization by transoesophageal echocardiography in infective endocarditis. *Eur Heart J* 1992;13:446–52.

29. Job FP, Lethen H, Franke S, et al. Benefit of bi- or multiplane versus monoplane TEE for the assessment of endocarditic lesions (abstract). *J Am Coll Cardiol* 1993;21:488A.

30. Schwinger ME, Tunick PA, Freedberg RS, Kronzon I. Vegetations on endocardial surfaces struck by regurgitant jets: diagnosis by transesophageal echocardiography. *Am Heart J* 1990;119:1212–5.

31. Roberts WC, Buchbinder NA. Right-sided valvular infective endocarditis: a clinicopathologic study of twelve necropsy patients. *Am J Med* 1972;53:7–19.

32. Bayer AS, Blomquist IK, Bello E, et al. Tricuspid valve endocarditis due to *Staphylococcus aureus*: correlation of two-dimensional echocardiography with clinical outcome. *Chest* 1988;93:247–53.

33. Ginzton LE, Siegel RJ, Criley JM. Natural history of tricuspid valve endocarditis: a two dimensional echocardiographic study. *Am J Cardiol* 1982;49: 1853–9.

34. Robbins MJ, Frater RWM, Soeiro R, et al. Influence of vegetation size on clinical outcome of right-sided infective endocarditis. *Am J Med* 1986;80:165–71.

35. Shapiro SM, Young E, Ginzton LE, Bayer AS. Pulmonic valve endocarditis as an underdiagnosed disease: role of transesophageal echocardiography. *J Am Soc Echocardiogr* 1992;5:48–51.

36. Cohen GI, Klein AL, Chan K-L, et al. Transesophageal echocardiographic diagnosis of right-sided cardiac masses in patients with central lines. *Am J Cardiol* 1992;70:925–9.

37. Daniel WG, Mügge A, Martin RP, et al. Improvement in the diagnosis of abscesses associated with endocarditis by transesophageal echocardiography. *N Engl J Med* 1991;324:795–800.

38. Alam M, Rosman HS, Sun I. Transesophageal echocardiographic evaluation of St. Jude Medical and bioprosthetic valve endocarditis. *Am Heart J* 1992;123:236–9.

39. Karalis DG, Bansal RC, Hauck AJ, et al. Transesophageal echocardiographic recognition of subaortic complications in aortic valve endocarditis: clinical and surgical implications. *Circulation* 1992; 86:353–62.

40. Roelandt JRTC, Thomson IR, Vletter WB, et al. Multiplane transesophageal echocardiography: latest evolution in an imaging revolution. *J Am Soc Echocardiogr* 1992;5:361–7.

41. Stafford A, Wann LS, Dillon JC, et al. Serial echocardiographic appearance of healing bacterial endocarditis. *Am J Cardiol* 1979;44:754–60.

42. Stratton JR, Werner JA, Pearlman AS, et al. Bacteremia and the heart: serial echocardiographic findings in 80 patients with documented or suspected bacteremia. *Am J Med* 1982;73:851–8.

43. Tak T, Rahimtoola SH, Kumar A, et al. Value of digital image processing of two-dimensional echocardiograms in differentiating active from chronic vegetations of infective endocarditis. *Circulation* 1988;78:116–23.

44. Mügge A, Daniel WG, Haverich A, Lichtlen PR. Diagnosis of noninfective cardiac mass lesions by two-dimensional echocardiography: comparison of the transthoracic and transesophageal approaches. *Circulation* 1991;83:70–8.

45. Reeder GS, Khandheria BK, Seward JB, Tajik AJ. Transesophageal echocardiography and cardiac masses. *Mayo Clin Proc* 1991;66:1101–9.

46. Blanchard DG, Ross RS, Dittrich HC. Nonbacterial thrombotic endocarditis: assessment by transesophageal echocardiography. *Chest* 1992;102:954–6.

47. Lopez JA, Ross RS, Fishbein MC, Siegel RJ. Nonbacterial thrombotic endocarditis: a review. *Am Heart J* 1987;113:773–84.

48. Nihoyannopoulos P, Gomez PM, Joshi J, et al. Cardiac abnormalities in systemic lupus erythematosus: association with raised anticardiolipin antibodies. *Circulation* 1990;82:369–75.

49. Stoddard MF, Dawkins PR, Longaker RA. Mobile strands are frequently attached to the St. Jude Medical mitral valve prosthesis as assessed by two-dimensional transesophageal echocardiography. *Am Heart J* 1992;124:671–4.

50. Seward JB, Khandheria BK, Oh JK, et al. Critical appraisal of transesophageal echocardiography: limitations, pitfalls, and complications. *J Am Soc Echocardiogr* 1992;5:288–305.

51. Bansal RC, Graham BM, Jutzy KR, et al. Left ventricular outflow tract to left atrial communication secondary to rupture of mitral-aortic intervalvular fibrosa in infective endocarditis: diagnosis by transesophageal echocardiography and color flow imaging. *J Am Coll Cardiol* 1990;15:499–504.

52. Nomeir A-M, Downes TR, Cordell AR. Perforation of the anterior mitral leaflet caused by aortic valve endocarditis: diagnosis by two-dimensional, transesophageal echocardiography and color flow Doppler. *J Am Soc Echocardiogr* 1992;5:195–8.

53. Massey WM, Samdarshi TE, Nanda NC, et al. Serial documentation of changes in a mitral valve vegetation progressing to abscess rupture and fistula formation by transesophageal echocardiography. *Am Heart J* 1992;124:241–8.

54. Charney R, Keltz TN, Attai L, et al. Acute valvular obstruction from streptococcal endocarditis. *Am Heart J* 1993;125:544–7.

55. Arnett EN, Roberts WC. Valve ring abscess in active infective endocarditis: frequency, location, and clues to clinical diagnosis from the study of 95 necropsy patients. *Circulation* 1976;54:140–5.

56. Buchbinder NA, Roberts WC. Left-sided valvular active infective endocarditis: a study of forty-five necropsy patients. *Am J Med* 1972;53:20–35.

57. Buda AJ, Zotz RJ, LeMire MS, Bach DS. Prognostic significance of vegetations detected by two-dimensional echocardiography in infective endocarditis. *Am Heart J* 1986;112:1291–6.

58. Hickey AJ, Wolfers J, Wilcken DEL. Reliability and clinical relevance of detection of vegetations by echocardiography in bacterial endocarditis. *Br Heart J* 1981;46:624–8.

59. Lutas EM, Roberts RB, Devereux RB, Prieto LM. Relation between the presence of echocardiographic vegetations and the complication rate in infective endocarditis. *Am Heart J* 1986;112:107–13.

60. Wann LS, Dillon JC, Weyman AE, Feigenbaum H. Echocardiography in bacterial endocarditis. *N Engl J Med* 1976;295:135–9.

61. Meriç M, Castello R, Ofili EO, et al. Transesophageal echocardiography in infective endocarditis: prognostic implications of vegetation size and mobility (abstract). *J Am Coll Cardiol* 1993;21:391A.

62. Rohmann S, Erbel R, Darius H, et al. Spontaneous echo contrast imaging in infective endocarditis: a predictor of complications? *Int J Card Imaging* 1992;8:197–207.

12

Cardiac Neoplasms and Thrombi

Evaluation by Transesophageal Echocardiography

William K. Freeman • Guy S. Reeder

The most commonly encountered intracardiac mass lesions are thrombi and vegetations, which are followed by a variety of uncommon cardiac neoplasms and, rarely, foreign bodies. Extracardiac masses adjacent to the heart include neoplasms of noncardiac origin, congenital cysts, abscesses, and loculated fluid collections with a masslike appearance.

Transthoracic two-dimensional echocardiography has become the initial procedure of choice in the evaluation of the patient with a suspected intracardiac mass lesion [1–3]. However, technically difficult images, loss of far-field resolution, or incomplete delineation of detected lesions commonly warrants further investigation. Having the capability of high-resolution imaging in multiple unique planes [4,5], transesophageal echocardiography (TEE) is ideally suited for the evaluation of cardiac masses and thrombi.

Herein, the utility of TEE in the evaluation of cardiac neoplasms and thrombi is discussed. Vegetations and abscesses are detailed under infective endocarditis (Chapter 11), and the detection of thrombi as potential sources of emboli is reviewed in Chapter 15.

PRIMARY CARDIAC NEOPLASMS

Primary tumors of the heart are rare, with an occurrence of approximately 0.15% in various necropsy series [6,7]. The frequency and distribution of be-

nign and malignant cardiac neoplasms found at postmortem examination [6] are shown in Table 12-1.

A compilation of five recent series [8–12] with a cumulative total of 1529 patients who had cardiac surgery for cardiac tumors showed that the vast majority of operations (94%) were for benign neoplasms. The overwhelming majority of excised

Table 12-1. Primary cardiac neoplasms

Type	%
Benign (n = 319)	
Myxoma	41
Lipoma	14
Papillary fibroelastoma	13
Rhabdomyoma	11
Fibroma	5
Hemangioma	5
Teratoma	4
Mesothelioma of AV node	4
Miscellaneous	3
Malignant (n = 125)	
Angiosarcoma	31
Rhabdomyosarcoma	21
Mesothelioma	15
Fibrosarcoma	11
Other sarcomas	9
Lymphoma	6
Miscellaneous	7

Modified from McAllister and Fenoglio [6].

benign neoplasms were myxomas (90%); the frequency of other benign tumors, such as lipoma, fibroma, angioma, rhabdomyoma, and papillary fibroelastoma, was 1% to 2% [8–12]. In the same combined surgical series, only 6% of all patients were operated on for malignant primary cardiac neoplasms [8–12]. The small operative incidence of primary cardiac malignant lesions was four to five times lower than that reported by postmortem examination [6,7], a reflection of preoperative selection of patients thought to have resectable rather than inoperable neoplasms [10].

Benign Cardiac Neoplasms

Myxomas

Myxomas are the most common primary cardiac tumor, accounting for generally 50% and 90% of all tumors diagnosed at autopsy [6,7] and at operation [8–12], respectively. Among 1214 patients operated on for intracardiac myxoma in four recent surgical series [9–12], most myxomas (86%) were located within the left atrium (Table 12-2). The second most common location for myxoma was the right atrium (7%), and multiple locations occurred in approximately 3% of cases. Rarely, myxomas were located within the chambers of the right and, less often, left ventricles, were attached to valves (most commonly the mitral [10], or even occurred within the pulmonary artery [12]. Similar anatomic localization of intracardiac myxomas has been reported in series of patients studied by transthoracic echocardiography [2,13].

Echocardiographic characterization of intracardiac myxoma has largely been done by investigators using transthoracic echocardiography. Only recently has the usefulness of TEE been described, primarily

Table 12-2. Location of cardiac myxoma in 1214 patients undergoing surgical resection

Location	%
Left atrium	86.5
Right atrium	7.4
Right ventricle	1.9
Left ventricle	0.3
Multiple locations	2.7
Valvular attachment	1.1
Pulmonary artery	0.1

Data from Molina et al. [9], Blondeau [10], Sezai [11], and Guang-ying [12].

in case reports [14–19] or in small series [20–23].

Both left and right atrial myxomas are usually (70% to 80%) attached to the interatrial septum [1,2] (Fig. 12-1) but may uncommonly arise from any location along the atrial free walls, along the valvular annuli, near the orifices of venous inflow, or near the atrial appendages [2] (Fig. 12-2). Very important for the diagnosis of myxoma is the finding of a stalk or pedicle attached to the wall of the involved cardiac chamber. Such a characteristic finding is visualized by transthoracic echocardiography in approximately three-quarters of myxomas; in the remaining cases, the myxoma attachment is not evident by this approach, especially with larger, broader-based tumors [1,2,23]. Definition of the location and type of myoxma attachment is possible in essentially all patients evaluated by biplane TEE [20,23] (Figs. 12-3 and 12-4).

Detailed TEE examination incorporating multiple imaging planes, preferably with biplaner imaging, is warranted to exclude the unlikely (approximately 3%) possibility of multiple intracardiac myxomas. Transesophageal echocardiography is particularly useful in the detection of small, sessile, multicentric myxomas, which are often beyond the resolution of far-field transthoracic imaging (see Fig. 12-3). Multiple myxomas in atypical locations may also suggest the diagnosis of "syndrome myxoma," which is associated with cutaneous lesions, endocrine neoplasms, familial occurrence, and a high rate of postoperative recurrence [24].

Imaging with TEE also enhances tumor characterization and differentiation from intracardiac thrombus. Myxomas are often polypoid, gelatinous in appearance, and deformable throughout the cardiac cycle (Fig. 12-5) or less often are relatively fixed, with a firm, nondeformable contour (Fig. 12-6). Cystic echolucent vacuolations may give the myxoma a "mottled" appearance in contrast to thrombus, vegetations, or other neoplasms. Cystic echolucencies are characteristic but not pathognomonic of myxoma [25] and are detectable in only about 25% of myxomas by transthoracic echocardiography [2]. Such echolucencies may be evident only by TEE examination [26] (Fig. 12-7), although the incidence of this finding in myxomas studied by TEE is currently unknown.

The size and consistency of atrial myxomas may allow various degrees of tumor prolapse (see Fig. 12-5) across the respective atrioventricular valve [27,28], inciting valvular leaflet trauma that is often

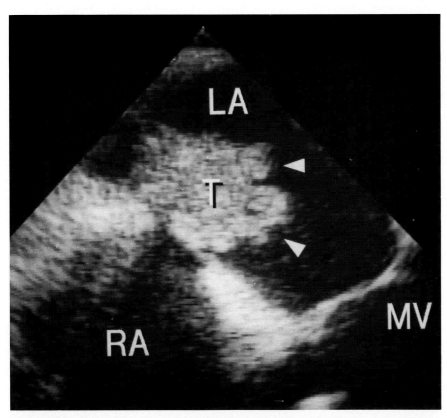

A

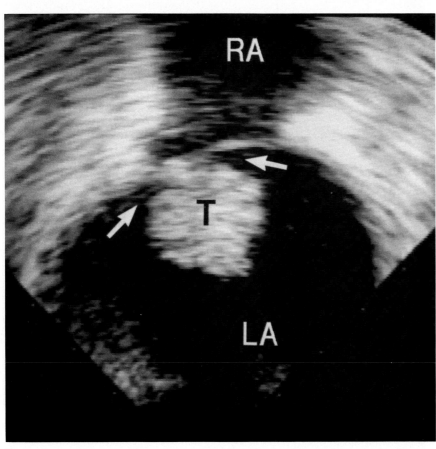

B

Fig. 12-1. A. Expanded TEE imaging of a left atrial tumor *(T)* in the transverse plane. Attachment to the interatrial septum, polypoid appearance *(arrowheads)*, and "gelatinous" mobility on real-time imaging are characteristic of myxoma. B. Another left atrial myxoma; longitudinal TEE plane. A broad-based pedicle attaches the myxoma *(T)* to the margin of the fossa ovalis membrane *(arrows)* of the atrial septum.

Fig. 12-2. Left atrial myxoma; basal transverse TEE plane. There is an atypical site of myxoma *(T)* attachment near the orifice of the left atrial appendage. The prominent limbus *(arrow)* of the orifice of the left upper pulmonary vein is a normal anatomic finding and should not be mistaken for a mass within the left atrium.

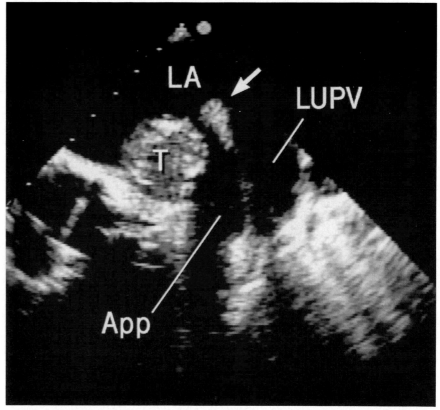

Fig. 12-3. Multicentric right atrial myxomas; modified basal transverse TEE plane. Two of three right atrial myxomas *(T)* are visible in this plane. The larger has a well-defined slender stalk *(arrow)* attaching the tumor to the lateral wall of the right atrium. The smaller myxoma has a broad-based attachment to the posterior atrial septum.

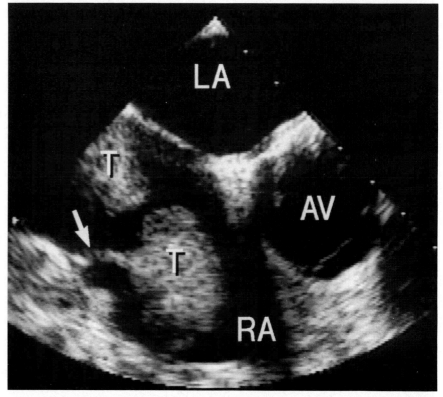

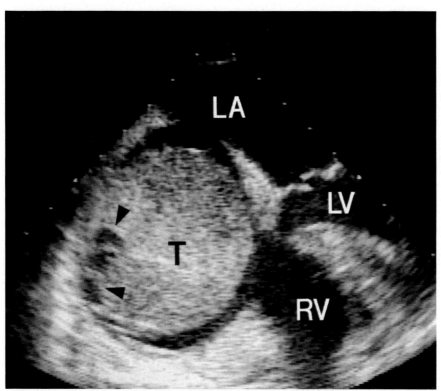

A

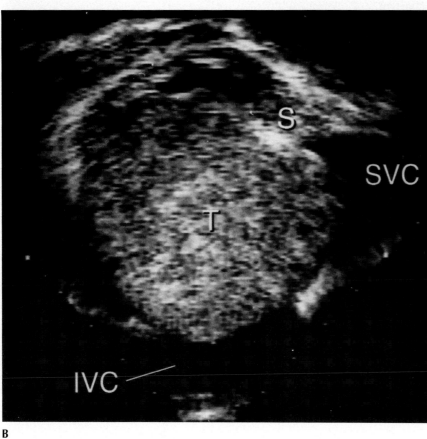

B

Fig. 12-4. Right atrial myxoma. A. Transverse TEE plane. A very large tumor *(T)* nearly fills the entire right atrium. Hypoechoic vacuolations *(arrowheads)* along the lateral margins of the mass are consistent with myxoma. The mass is so large that a site of attachment cannot be seen in this imaging plane. B. Longitudinal TEE plane. In this view the tumor again occupies almost the entire right atrium. A clearly defined stalk *(S)* attachment near the orifice of the superior vena cava confirms the diagnosis of myxoma.

Fig. 12-5.   Right atrial myxoma; transverse TEE plane. A. A large, lobulated myxoma *(T)* occupies the right atrium during systole; the tricuspid valve is closed. B. During diastole, the mobile and deformable myxoma prolapses into the tricuspid inflow tract from the right atrium.

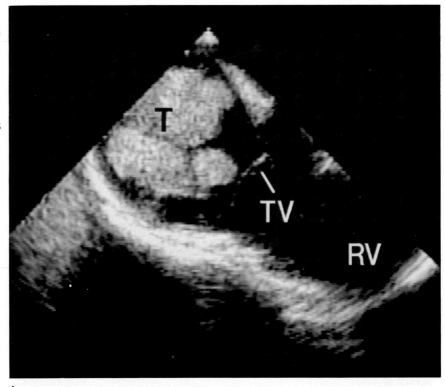

A

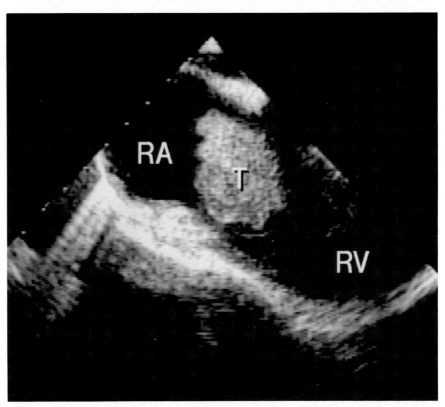

B

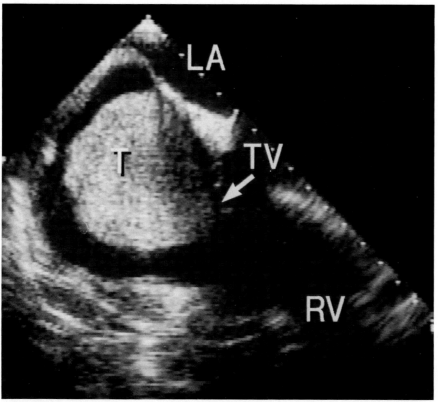

Fig. 12-6. Right atrial myxoma; transverse TEE plane. In contrast to Fig. 12-5, minimal motion of this large nondeformable myxoma *(T)* within the right atrium or toward the tricuspid valve *(arrow)* was noted throughout the cardiac cycle on real-time examination.

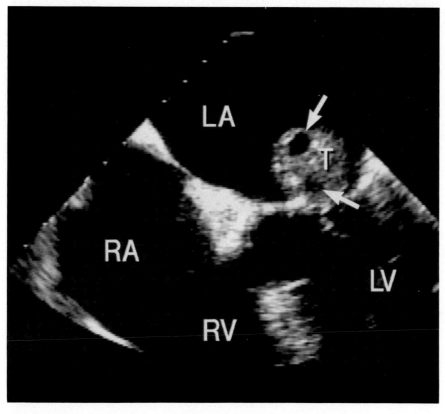

Fig. 12-7. Left atrial myxoma; transverse four-chamber TEE plane. Cystic echolucencies *(arrows)* are clearly seen within this myxoma *(T)*; they were not evident on transthoracic examination. The myxoma appears to be attached to the mitral valve but was found to be attached to the mitral annulus on off-axis imaging.

Fig. 12-8. Right atrial myxoma; transverse TEE plane. A. A large myxoma *(T)* encroaches on the tricuspid valve inflow tract but does not prolapse into the right ventricle. B. Turbulent mosaic tricuspid inflow signals *(arrows)* are evident on color-flow Doppler imaging, consistent with obstruction. C. Mild tricuspid inflow obstruction is documented by continuous-wave Doppler examination. The mean pressure gradient is approximately 4 to 5 mm Hg, varying, as does the flow across the tricuspid valve, throughout the respiratory cycle.

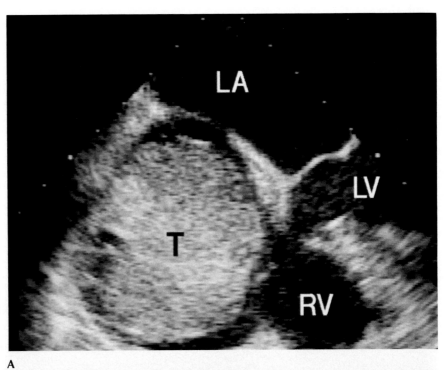

A

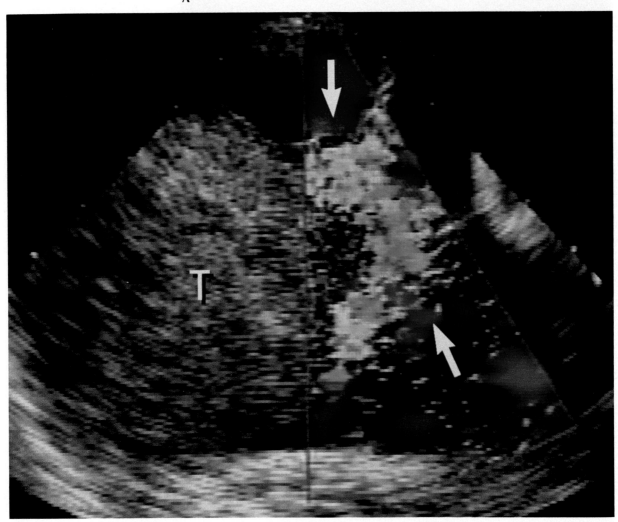

B

trivial but may be extensive, as seen with a large, often calcified "wrecking ball" myxoma [15]. Delineation of associated atrioventricular valvular regurgitation by TEE color Doppler imaging may be difficult, especially with large myxomas, because of the tumor's atrial space occupation and motion artifact. The effects of an atrial myxoma on mitral or tricuspid valve function and competency are best examined by intraoperative TEE [14–16] (see Chapter 16). In this situation the valve leaflets, annulus, and residual regurgitation can be evaluated after myxoma resection to determine whether additional valvular repair is necessary before the operation is complete.

Large myxomas may also cause various degrees of obstruction to atrioventricular valvular inflow. Such obstruction can be demonstrated by turbulent mosaic inflow signals on color Doppler images;

quantitation of the mean inflow gradient is also possible by steerable continuous-wave Doppler interrogation (Fig. 12-8).

Lipoma

Second to the incidence of intracardiac myxoma in pathology series [6] are cardiac lipomas. Lipomas may occur throughout the heart or pericardium but are usually well encapsulated within the myocardium in a subendocardial or subepicardial location [7]. In contrast to myxomas, lipomas are not mobile intracavitary lesions and are without a stalk or pedicle attachment. Most lipomas are relatively small, solitary, asymptomatic, and without clinical significance. These lesions are generally discovered incidentally during echocardiographic examination for other indications. They have a well-demarcated,

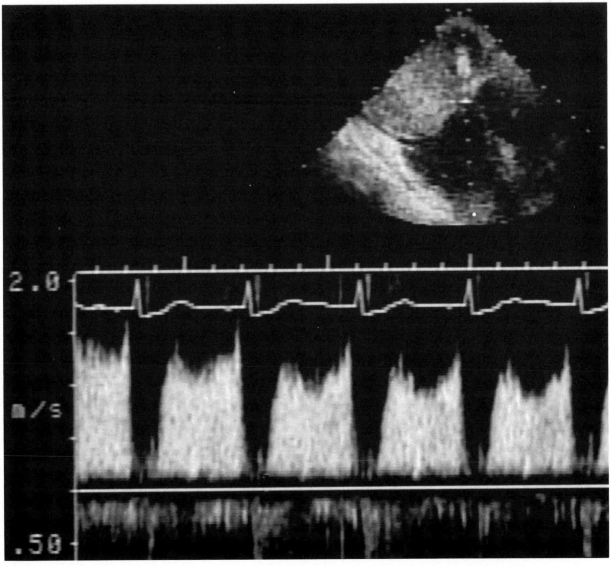

C

firm, echodense, nodular appearance [7]. Occasionally, lipomas become quite large (Fig. 12-9) and mimic the appearance of other cardiac neoplasms. Magnetic resonance imaging may be necessary to define the lipomatous tissue characterization of such lesions [29].

Lipomatous Hypertrophy of the Interatrial Septum

Proliferation of mature adipose tissue within the atrial septum may produce the appearance of a tumor in this location. Much more common than cardiac lipomas, lipomatous atrial septal hypertrophy is not actually a true neoplastic process, because the fatty infiltration is neither homogeneous nor encapsulated; hence, such masses are not classified as true cardiac lipomas [7].

Typically, the fatty infiltration accumulates within the muscular portion of the septum, sparing the fossa ovalis membrane, and gives the atrial septum an echodense, bilobed dumbbell configuration (Fig. 12-10). Such an appearance may not be fully evident with oblique monoplane transverse imaging of the atrial septum; longitudinal biplane imaging enhances delineation for the exclusion of a true intracardiac mass or thrombus. Previously published transthoracic echocardiographic criteria for the diagnosis of lipomatous atrial septal hypertrophy include (1) an echodense bilobed appearance of the atrial septum on images through the region of the fossa ovalis, (2) maximal atrial septal thickness of 15 mm or greater, and (3) the clinical absence of other potential causes of atrial septal infiltration, such as amyloidosis or metastatic malignant disease [30]. Rarely, magnetic resonance imaging is needed to further confirm the lipomatous tissue character of the massively thickened atrial septum so that other diagnostic possibilities can be excluded [31,32].

Lipomatous infiltration also commonly occurs variously in other intracardiac locations, particularly within the limbus of the orifices of the pulmonary veins (most notably, left upper pulmonary vein; see Fig. 12-2), vena cavae, and coronary sinus. Fatty infiltration may also occur within the annular sulcus of the tricuspid and (less so) mitral valves, producing a masslike appearance in these locations (Fig. 12-11). Such findings may suggest an intracardiac mass on transthoracic echocardiography and can be readily delineated by transesophageal imaging. As discussed in Chapter 6, these findings should be recognized as anatomic variants of no clinical significance and not be mistaken for a neoplasm, a thrombus, or an infectious process.

Papillary Fibroelastoma

Papillary fibroelastomas, or papillomas, usually arise from the semilunar or atrioventricular valves and rarely from mural endocardium [7,33]. Although most often a benign echocardiographic finding, papillary fibroelastomas have been associated with a variety of systemic embolic phenomena to the cerebral and coronary circulations [7,33–36].

The high-resolution imaging capabilities of TEE are well suited for the delineation of the characteristic shimmering mobility of the fronds of these pompom-like masses (Figs. 12-12 and 12-13). A short pedicle may be evident [35], and the polypoid mass may prolapse across the valvular orifice. Other neoplasms of this type have a broad base attachment and appear relatively sessile (Fig. 12-14). Although the stalklike attachment of these neoplasms may mimic the appearance of a small myxoma, the characteristic valvular involvement is consistent with papillary fibroelastoma.

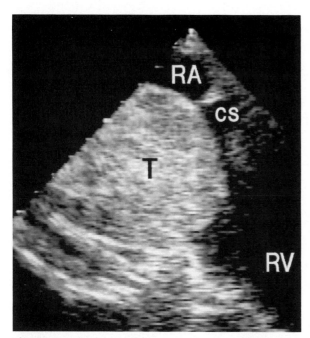

Fig. 12-9. Right atrial lipoma; transverse TEE plane, right ventricular inflow view. A large, immobile, echodense tumor *(T)* arises from the lateral free wall of the right atrium and extends medially to the orifice of the coronary sinus. Magnetic resonance imaging confirmed the lipomatous tissue composition of this neoplasm. Most of the right atrial free wall was resected during surgical excision of this extensive intramural lipoma [29].

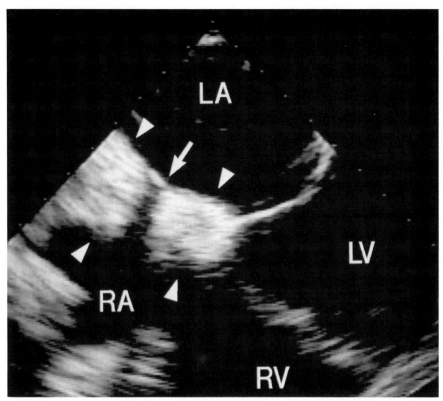

Fig. 12-10. Lipomatous hypertrophy of the atrial septum; transverse TEE plane, four-chamber view. Extensive fatty tissue accumulation within the atrial septum *(arrowheads)* spares the fossa ovalis membrane *(arrow)*, imparting the typical dumbbell appearance of lipomatous atrial septal hypertrophy.

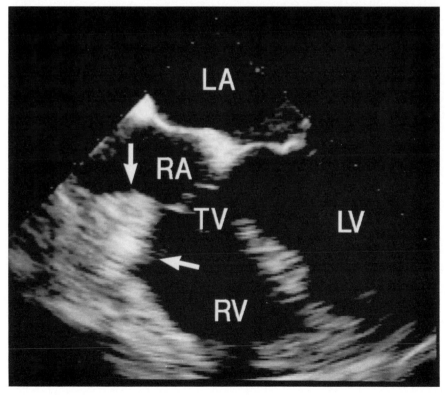

Fig. 12-11. Lipomatous infiltration of the tricuspid annulus; transverse TEE plane. Prominent hyperrefractile fatty infiltration of the tricuspid annulus *(arrows)* is shown in characteristic relationship to the tricuspid valve.

Fig. 12-12. Papillary fibroelastoma of the tricuspid valve; transverse TEE plane. A broad-based mass *(arrow)* is attached to the atrial surface of the septal leaflet of the tricuspid valve. The "shimmering" mobility of its fronds on real-time examination was typical of papillary fibroelastoma.

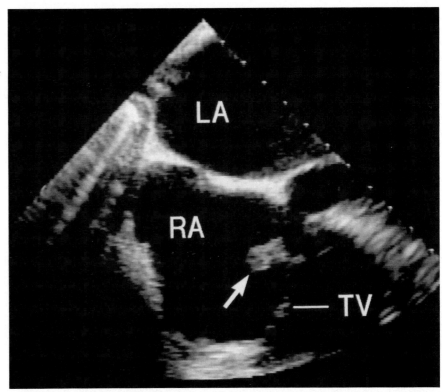

Fig. 12-13. Papillary fibroelastoma of the ventricular septum; longitudinal TEE plane. A pedunculated, fronded papillary fibroelastoma *(arrow)* is attached to the basal ventricular septum. This neoplasm was very mobile within the left ventricular outflow tract during the cardiac cycle. Patch repair *(arrowheads)* of a paramembranous ventricular septal defect had been done long ago; papillary fibroelastoma was confirmed at reoperation.

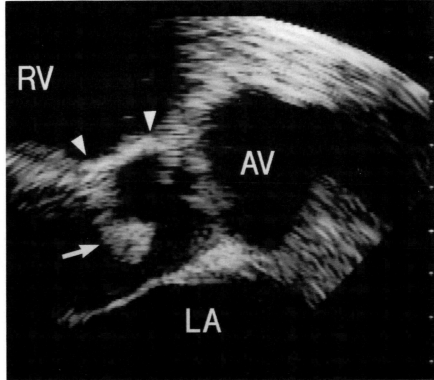

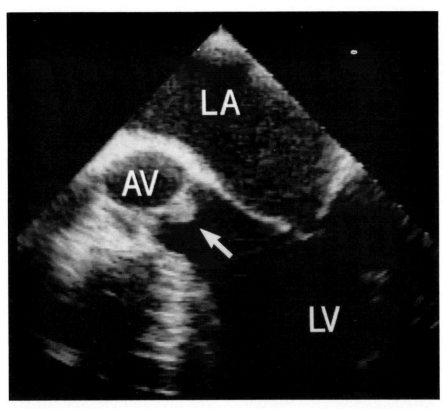

Fig. 12-14. Papillary fibroelastoma of the aortic valve; transverse TEE plane. A small, sessile papillary fibroelastoma *(arrow)* is attached to the ventricular aspects of the aortic valve. Such neoplasms have a predilection for the "upstream" surfaces of the cardiac valves.

Cardiac Rhabdomyoma

Rhabdomyomas are the most frequently encountered benign cardiac neoplasms of the pediatric population [7]. A 35% to 50% incidence of cardiac rhabdomyomas has been reported in patients with tuberous sclerosis evaluated by transthoracic echocardiography [37,38]. Rhabdomyomas have a well-circumscribed, echodense echocardiographic appearance. Most often they are located within the ventricles, generally protruding from the endocardial surfaces of the ventricular septum or apices; rarely, they are located within the atria and have not been reported to involve the cardiac valves [7,37,38]. Multiple tumors are detected in approximately 75% of patients with tuberous sclerosis who have rhabdomyomas [8]. Because intracardiac rhabdomyomas are generally well evaluated through the excellent transthoracic echocardiographic windows available in this young age group, TEE is usually not indicated for further evaluation.

Cardiac Fibroma

Cardiac fibromas, like rhabdomyomas, have a predisposition to occur in children [7]. Fibromas are nearly always solitary and are located within the walls of the ventricular myocardium. Cardiac fibro-

mas occur most frequently within the left ventricular free walls, next most frequently in the interventricular septum and right ventricle, and very rarely in the atria [39].

Transgastric TEE imaging of the left and right ventricles in both the transverse short-axis and the longitudinal long-axis planes should permit full delineation of this neoplasm. Fibromas are generally well demarcated by a homogeneous, hyperrefractile echocardiographic appearance that differentiates the neoplasm from surrounding normal myocardium (Fig. 12-15). Anatomic displacement of normal cardiac structures without neoplastic destruction may also be evident if the fibroma is large.

Malignant Primary Cardiac Neoplasms

Malignant primary neoplasms of the heart are far less common than benign ones. In a large necropsy series reported by McAllister and Fenoglio [6], the overall incidence of malignant primary cardiac neoplasms was 28%, and 72% of cases were sarcomas (Table 12-1). Cumulative surgical experience reported in 1990 involving 1529 patients operated on for cardiac neoplasms revealed that only 6.2% of

Fig. 12-15. Left ventricular fibroma; transverse TEE plane, transgastric window. A well-circumscribed, hyperrefractile intramyocardial fibroma *(T)* is visualized within the inferolateral wall of the left ventricle on short-axis imaging. The liver and diaphragm are near the apex of the inverted sector, and the left ventricular walls are as follows: inferior *(IN)*, inferoseptal *(IS)*, anteroseptal *(AS)*, and anterolateral *(AL)*.

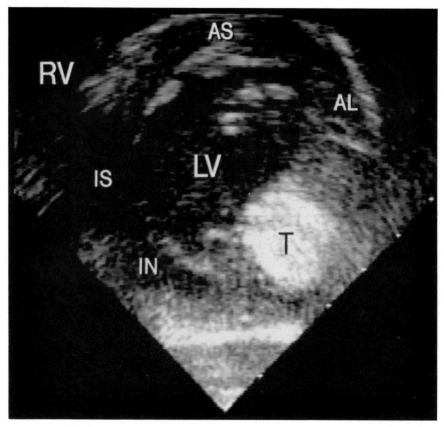

patients had malignant disease, 88% of whom had sarcomas [8–12]. The 4.5-fold lower operative incidence of primary cardiac malignant lesions in this combined series is consistent with the frequent finding of obvious inoperability of such tumors at the time of initial presentation and diagnosis, portending a generally dismal short-term prognosis [8,10,40].

The overwhelming majority of malignant primary cardiac neoplasms are sarcomas, and angiosarcoma is the most common type [6,7,40]. Angiosarcomas have a well-documented predilection to arise from or extend into the right atrium, which is involved in approximately 80% of cases [40]. Angiosarcomas may be polypoid, protruding far into the right atrial cavity, or may infiltrate extensively from or along the epicardial and pericardial surfaces [40]. Transesophageal echocardiography may be more useful than transthoracic echocardiography in the detection of the latter type of neoplasm [41] (Fig. 12-16). Both rhabdomyosarcomas and fibrosarcomas have an equal distribution of occurrence between the right- and left-sided cardiac chambers, often with multicentric myocardial involvement and valvular obstruction [7]. Myxosarcomas usually arise in the

left atrium and frequently infiltrate the mitral valve apparatus, causing either inflow obstruction or regurgitation [10] (Fig. 12-17).

Aside from malignant mesothelioma, which generally arises from the pericardium, lymphoma is the most common nonsarcomatous primary cardiac malignant lesion [6] but remains exceedingly rare [7]. Primary cardiac lymphomas usually appear as a large mass infiltrating the heart (Fig. 12-18) at the time of initial diagnosis [42].

The higher resolution of TEE than of transthoracic echocardiography offers several potential advantages for the differentiation of malignant from benign cardiac disease. Benign intracardiac masses are generally well circumscribed and have a discrete attachment (such as a stalk in most myxomas) to a mural endocardial or valvular surface. Although benign masses may distort cardiac anatomy or obstruct inflow or outflow tracts of the heart (see Fig. 12-8), there is no direct extension or invasion of the mass into surrounding structures. Malignant tumors typically disrupt, infiltrate, and obscure the tissue planes of adjacent cardiac anatomy (see Figs. 12-16, 12-17, and 12-18). Unlike benign neoplasms,

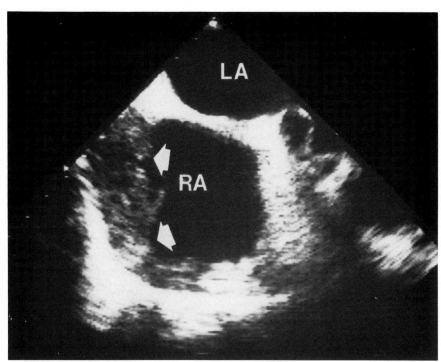

Fig. 12-16. Pericardial angiosarcoma; modified transverse TEE plane. The infiltrating angiosarcoma *(arrows)* has invaded and replaced most of the right atrial free wall in this imaging plane. Because protrusion into the right atrial cavity was only mild, this tumor was not recognized on transthoracic echocardiography. (From Frohwein et al. [41]. By permission of Mosby-Year Book.)

malignant tumors are usually poorly demarcated, immobile, and fixed to adjoining cardiac structures. Direct extension into venous inflow tracts, such as the vena cavae and pulmonary veins, is consistent with a malignant process (Fig. 12-19) and is distinct from the behavior of benign masses, such as myxoma and intracavitary thrombus. An adjacent pericardial effusion is also worrisome for malignant disease.

SECONDARY CARDIAC NEOPLASMS

Essentially all secondary cardiac neoplasms are formed by metastatic spread from a primary malignant tumor of another organ system. The overall incidence of these secondary neoplasms exceeds that of primary cardiac tumors by as much as 40-fold in some series [7,43,44].

Secondary neoplastic invasion of the heart may occur by several mechanisms [6,7,45]. Direct extension is a common mode of spread of neoplasms from organs in close proximity to the heart, most often bronchogenic, esophageal, and breast carcinomas (Figs. 12-20 and 12-21). The same malignant tumors also metastasize to the heart by lymphatic spread (as is typically the case with breast carcinoma). Venous extension into the right heart chambers by way of

the inferior vena cava may occur with genitourinary neoplasms, most notably renal cell carcinoma (Fig. 12-22), and with hepatocellular and adrenal malignant tumors. The superior vena cava may also be an avenue of venous extension for metastatic bronchogenic or thyroid carcinoma. Metastatic invasion of the left side of the heart may occur through spread of neoplasms involving the pulmonary parenchyma into the pulmonary venous system. Hematogenous dissemination is the typical mechanism of metastasis of the two most common malignant diseases of the heart, melanoma and leukemia; lymphoma may spread to the heart by lymphatic and hematogenous routes. Although such malignant diseases frequently infiltrate myocardial tissues without formation of significant space-occupying lesions that are evident on echocardiographic imaging (as in essentially all cases of leukemia), large intracavitary metastatic deposits occasionally are observed (Fig. 12-23).

Whereas transthoracic echocardiography can identify gross metastatic disease involving the heart [45], pericardium [46], or mediastinum [47], TEE is often required for further characterization and differentiation from other diagnostic possibilities. Occasionally, large metastatic lesions invading the heart may not even be detectable by the transthoracic approach [48] (see Fig. 12-21). In patients with a known primary malignant lesion, especially neoplasms with a propensity for metastasis to the heart

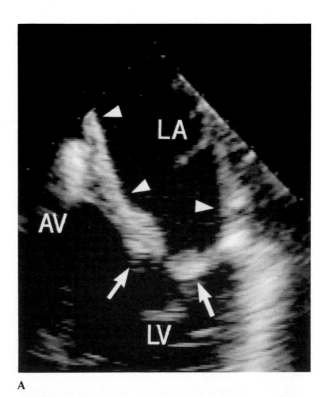

A

Fig. 12-17. Myxosarcoma of the left atrium and mitral valve. A. Transverse TEE plane. Diffuse thickening of the walls of the left atrium *(arrowheads)* and mitral valve leaflets *(arrows)* is due to infiltrating myxosarcoma. Moderate mitral inflow stenosis and regurgitation were precipitated by the gross deformation of the mitral valve. B. Longitudinal TEE plane. Extensive tumor infiltration is evident along the mitral annulus *(arrows)*, with nodular deposition *(arrowhead)* within the left atrial appendage. C. Longitudinal TEE plane. A fungating tumor *(T)* is evident in the more superior aspects of the left atrium, with compression of the left upper pulmonary vein *(PV)*.

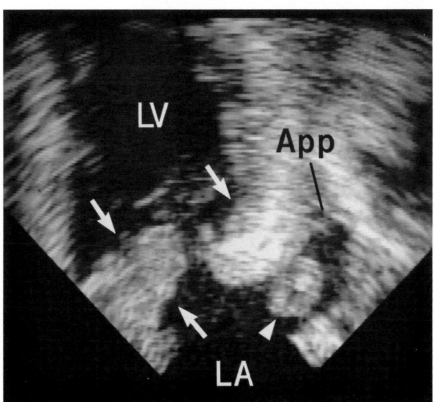

B

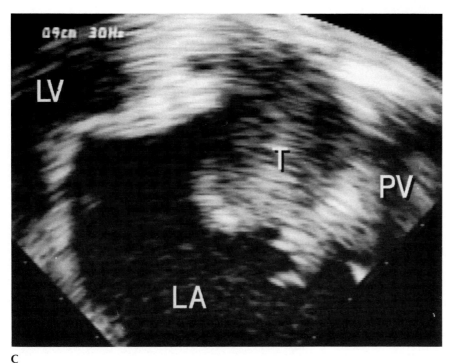

C

and mediastinum (e.g., melanoma, lymphoma, and breast, bronchogenic, and gastroesophageal carcinomas), an intracardiac mass detected by transthoracic echocardiography should strongly suggest metastatic disease until proven otherwise. The details of the location and extent of metastatic invasion are generally much better delineated by TEE than by transthoracic echocardiography. As with primary cardiac malignant disease, secondary neoplastic disease typically disrupts and distorts normal cardiac tissue planes and boundaries, and a heterogeneous echocardiographic appearance differentiates infiltrating neoplasm from surrounding structures (Fig. 12-24). Consistent with a malignant process, metastatic tumor also may encroach upon systemic or pulmonary venous return (Fig. 12-24) or may extrinsically compress the aorta or pulmonary arteries (see Fig. 12-20). Metastatic disease commonly involves the pericardium and is often difficult to directly visualize by transthoracic echocardiography [46]. The improved resolution of TEE should allow better detection of pericardial infiltration and metastatic deposits, especially if highlighted by surrounding pericardial or pleural effusions.

Uncommonly, metastatic disease within the mediastinum distorts or compresses the esophagus, precluding passage of the TEE probe [49]. Examination by TEE is clearly contraindicated if there is any clinically evident esophageal compromise or if the primary malignant lesion is of esophageal origin or involves the gastroesophageal junction (see Chapter 3).

OTHER EXTRACARDIAC MASSES

Benign mass lesions within the mediastinum adjacent to but not directly involving the heart or great vessels can also be visualized and characterized echocardiographically from the transesophageal window.

Pericardial cysts are usually asymptomatic and incidentally discovered on chest radiography. These congenital cysts rarely communicate with the true pericardial space and are most commonly located adjacent to the right atrium near the right cardiophrenic angle [7,50]. Pericardial cysts are found less often in the left cardiophrenic angle in the vicinity of the left atrium and rarely in the anterior or posterior mediastinum [50]. Pericardial cysts generally have an echolucent unilocular cavity that can vary widely in dimension and uncommonly causes significant extrinsic compression of either atrium (Fig. 12-25).

Other congenital cysts of the mediastinum include enterogenous duplication cysts and bronchogenic cysts. Such cysts may have a grossly heterogeneous

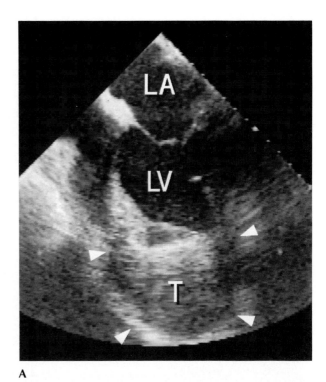

Fig. 12-18. Primary cardiac lymphoma; transverse TEE. A. Four-chamber view. A large tumor *(T)* involves the apical portions of both the right and the left ventricles *(arrowheads)*. B. Transgastric short-axis view. The right ventricular apex has been obliterated by tumor, which has extended far into the cavity of the left ventricle *(white arrow* and *arrowhead)* and into all myocardium at this level *(black arrowheads)* except the inferolateral left ventricle *(LV)*.

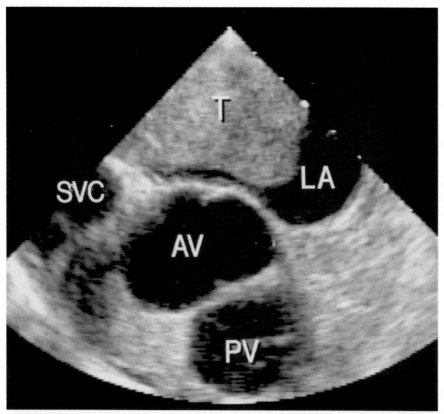

A

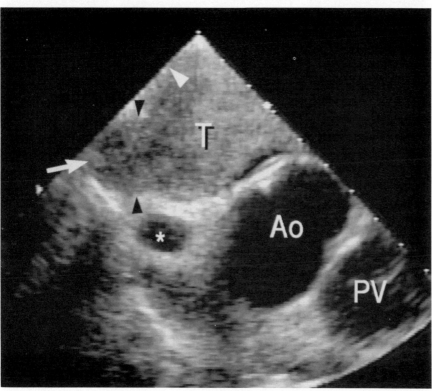

B

Fig. 12-19. Leiomyosarcoma of the left atrium; transverse TEE plane, basal short-axis view. A. A large tumor *(T)* is visualized in the superior aspects of the left atrium. B. The malignant nature of this tumor is evident because it extends *(arrow)* far into the right upper pulmonary vein *(black arrowheads)* adjacent to the superior vena cava *(asterisk)* and obscures the tissue planes of the posterior wall of the left atrium *(white arrowhead)* *(PV = pulmonary valve).*

Fig. 12-20. Metastatic bronchogenic carcinoma involving the right pulmonary artery. A. Transverse TEE, basal short-axis view. Extrinsic constriction *(arrow)* of the proximal right pulmonary artery is caused by direct extension of metastatic tumor *(T)*. B. Turbulent flow across this neoplastic constriction is depicted by color Doppler imaging *(arrow)*, consistent with obstruction. Transthoracic continuous-wave Doppler examination revealed a maximal instantaneous pressure gradient of 45 to 50 mm Hg across this lesion.

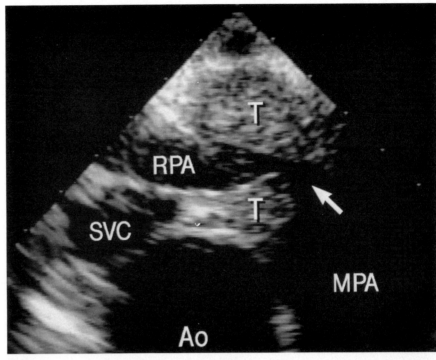

A

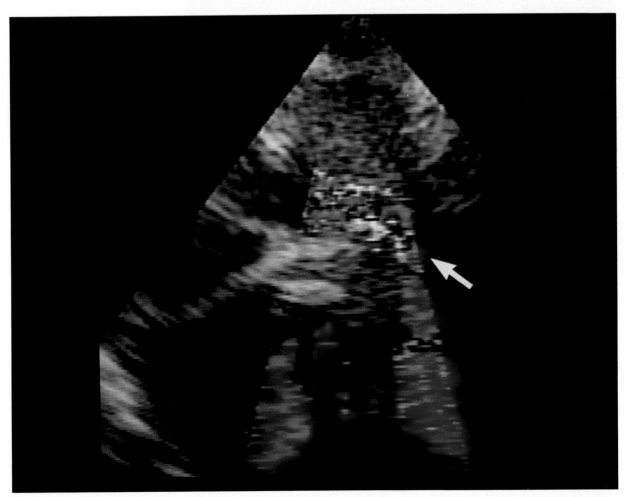

B

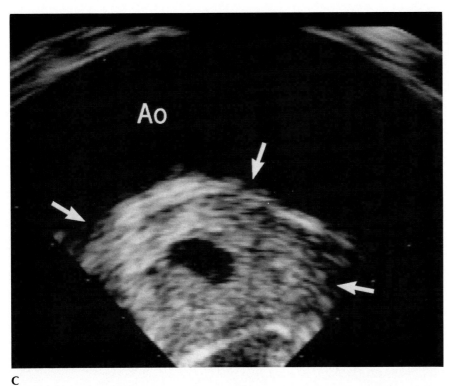

C

Fig. 12-20 (continued). C. Longitudinal TEE plane. Circumferential annular tumor constriction *(arrows)* of the right pulmonary artery is clearly demonstrated.

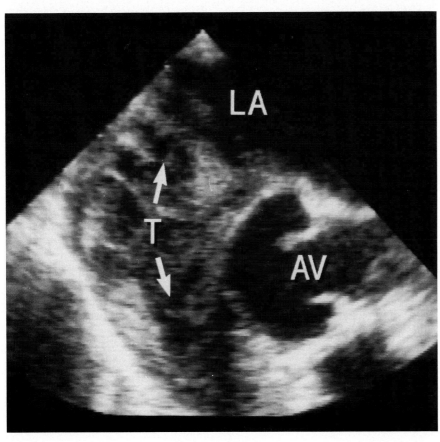

Fig. 12-21. Metastatic adenocarcinoma of the breast; modified transverse TEE plane. A large, grossly heterogeneous metastatic tumor *(T, arrows)* has replaced the superior aspects of the right atrium and right atrial appendage (at the bottom of the sector). This extensive metastatic invasion was not evident on transthoracic echocardiography.

Fig. 12-22. Metastatic renal cell carcinoma. A. Longitudinal TEE plane. A large metastatic tumor *(T)* extends from the inferior vena cava into the right atrium. This tumor was mobile within the right atrium and without direct cardiac infiltration. B. Transgastric off-axis transverse TEE plane. Short-axis imaging of the inferior vena cava reveals tumor metastasizing by direct venous extension. All intracaval metastatic tumor was removed at the time of nephrectomy for renal cell carcinoma.

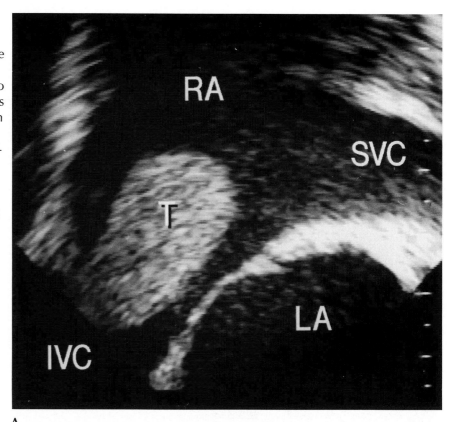

A

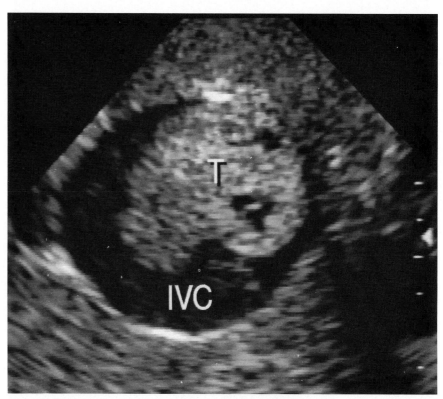

B

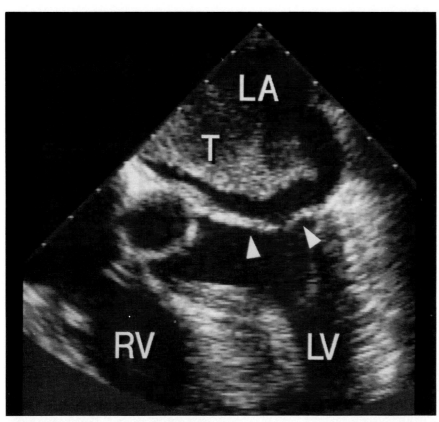

A

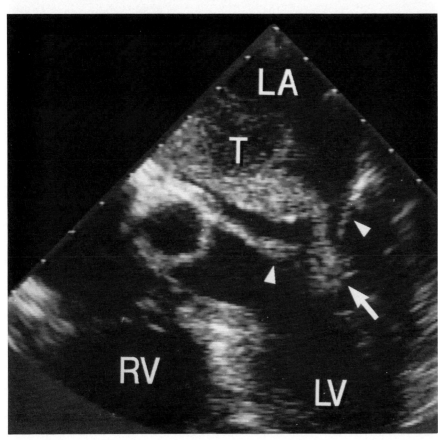

B

Fig. 12-23. Metastatic melanoma to the left atrium; transverse TEE plane. A. A large metastatic tumor *(T)* is visualized within the left atrium. The mitral valve leaflets are closed *(arrowheads)* during systole. B. During diastole, a mobile extension of tumor/thrombus *(arrow)* prolapses across the opened mitral leaflets *(arrowheads)* into the left ventricle.

Fig. 12-24. Metastatic gastric lymphoma to the heart; longitudinal TEE plane. A. Massive metastatic tumor *(T)* infiltration has grossly distorted the region of the atrial septum between the left and right atria. Tumor has also filled most of the right atrium and extended *(arrow)* along the orifice of the superior vena cava. An associated small pericardial effusion *(PE)* is present. B. Color-flow Doppler imaging of the right atrium in a more inferior longitudinal plane reveals turbulent flow interdigitated between metastatic tumor deposits *(T)*. Small intra-atrial pressure

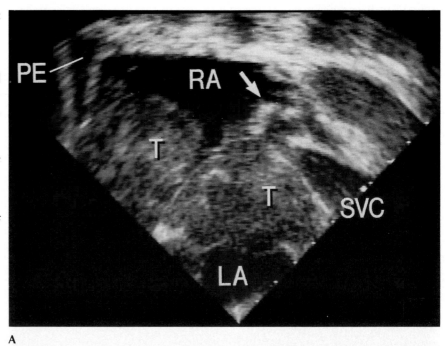

A

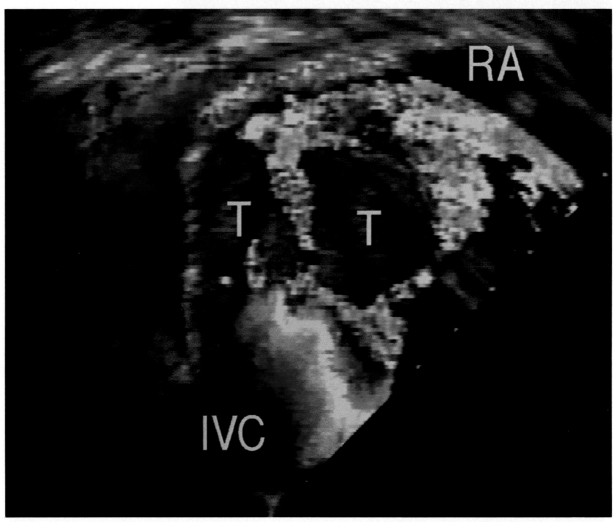

B

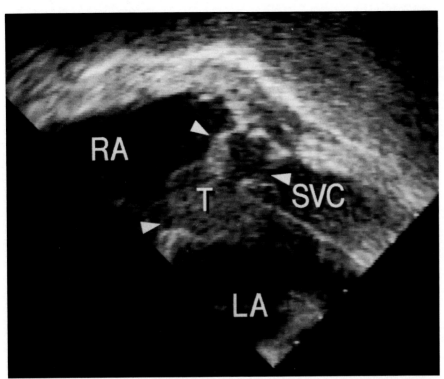

C

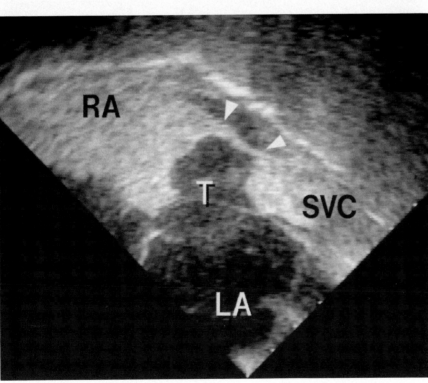

D

Fig. 12-24 continued
gradients were demonstrated by continuous-wave Doppler analysis in the areas of turbulent flow. C. Imaging of the superior right atrium demonstrates subtotal tumor encroachment *(arrowheads)* into the orifice of the superior vena cava. D. The resultant severely narrowed superior vena caval orifice is highlighted *(arrowheads)* by peripheral intravenous injection of contrast agent, which opacifies both the cava and the right atrium.

Fig. 12-24 continued
E. Further evidence of malignant infiltration is seen encompassing the aortic root *(arrows)*. F. Longitudinal short-axis imaging clarifies the extent of malignant invasion *(T, arrows)* at the level of the aortic valve. As above, neoplastic disruption and distortion of normal anatomy and tissue planes are readily evident. The echocardiographically heterogeneous appearance of the metastatic tumor is typical of malignancy.

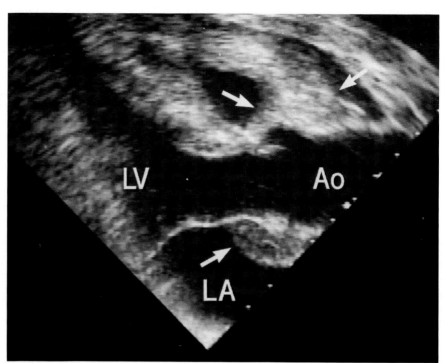

E

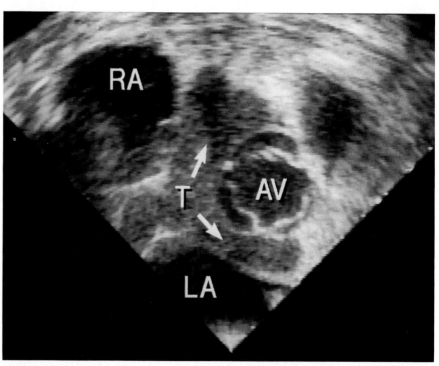

F

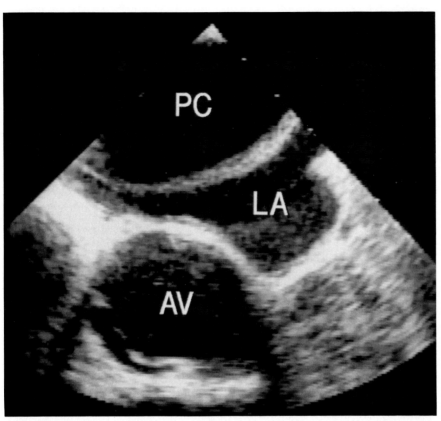

A

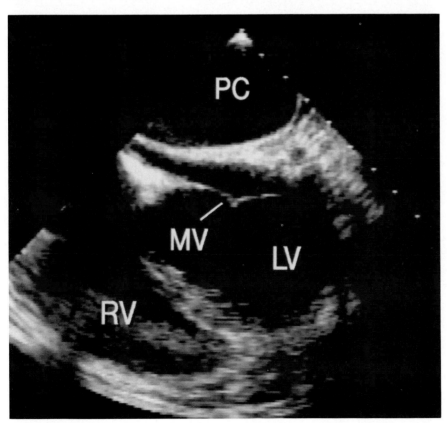

B

Fig. 12-25. Pericardial cyst; transverse TEE plane. A. Basal short-axis view. Severe extrinsic compression by a pericardial cyst *(PC)* nearly obliterates the left atrial cavity. B. Extrinsic compression nearly to the plane of the mitral valve is evident on four-chamber imaging.

echodense appearance on TEE [51] quite likely due to the collection of mucilaginous, inspissated material and other embryonic residua within the cyst (Fig. 12-26). Mobility and "layering out" of the sludgelike material within these cysts may be evident by placing the patient in various positions (e.g., left lateral to supine) during TEE examination [51].

Anterior mediastinal tumors, such as thymoma, lymphoma, and teratoma, and posterior mediastinal tumors, generally of neurogenic origin, may be visualized by TEE. A wide variety of benign mesenchymal neoplasms, such as hemangioma and lymphangioma, are rarely encountered within the mediastinum [52]; when large, they may cause significant extrinsic compromise of the great vessels (Fig. 12-27).

In a recent study of 30 patients with a variety of mediastinal masses, monoplane TEE detected 90% of all masses diagnosed by computed tomography or magnetic resonance imaging of the chest, whereas transthoracic echocardiography detected 73% [53]. Two of the three undetected masses in this study were thymomas located anterior to the distal ascending aorta (and hence shadowed by the inter-posed trachea and bronchi), and the third was a chordoma associated with the high thoracic vertebrae. The composition and contents of the mediastinal masses (e.g., solid neoplasm, fluid-filled cyst) were correctly identified in all masses detected by TEE. The relationship of the mediastinal mass to contiguous structures and associated displacement or invasion were correctly delineated in 89% of patients with masses detectable by TEE, who formed 80% of the entire study population [53].

In our experience [22], only 50% of extracardiac mass lesions delineated by TEE are detectable by transthoracic echocardiography. Even though computed tomography scanning was performed in nearly all patients in this report, TEE was thought to add significant information in 75% of cases and prompted a change in treatment strategy in 33% of patients [22].

Although TEE is useful in the detection and characterization of mediastinal masses in most patients, ultrafast computed tomography and magnetic resonance imaging of the chest are likely to remain the standard means of diagnosis and delineation of such lesions [53–55].

MIMICS OF EXTRACARDIAC MASSES

Other extracardiac findings may mimic the appearance of a mass or cyst. An eccentric false aneurysm of the left ventricle (see Chapter 8, Fig. 8-12) may be mistaken for a pericardiac cyst, as may large descending thoracic aortic aneurysms that impinge on the left atrium. A left pleural effusion may also masquerade as a pericardiac cyst or cavity, and the lower medial portion of a partially collapsed left lung may be mistaken for an extracardiac mass (Fig. 12-28). Commonly the gastric fundus or a diaphragmatic hernia is imaged from the more distal esophageal or transgastric windows. The normal gastric rugae and occasionally evident peristaltic motion readily permit correct recognition (Fig. 12-29).

Vertebral bodies of the spinal column are commonly visualized adjacent to the descending aorta (see Chapter 14, Fig. 14-7), and occasionally entire vertebrae, including the spinal canal and cord, are visible (Fig. 12-30), clarifying this anatomic finding.

Calcification of the pericardium, especially if exu-

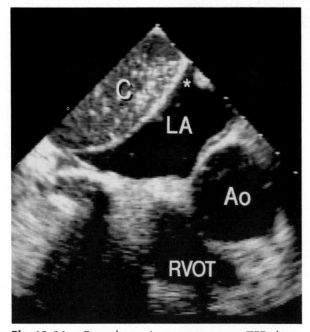

Fig. 12-26. Bronchogenic cyst; transverse TEE plane. A large bronchogenic cyst *(C)* containing mucilaginous material with hyperrefractile spicules extrinsically impinges on the left atrium and compresses the left upper pulmonary vein *(asterisk)*.

berant within a localized region, may have the appearance of an extracardiac mass. In advanced constrictive pericarditis, the pericardium may be severely thickened in a circumferential fashion; the distribution of the hyperrefractile, echodense pericardium should suggest the diagnosis on two-dimensional imaging (Fig. 12-31). Dissociation of intrathoracic and intracardiac pressures can also be demonstrated by pulsed-wave Doppler examination of mitral and pulmonary venous inflow velocities (Fig. 12-31), confirming the hemodynamics of constriction [56].

Copious epicardial fat may mimic an epicardial mass; however, this tissue has a characteristic echolucent texture stippled with granular hyperrefractilities, is sharply demarcated from normal anatomic boundaries of the myocardium, and moves in synchrony with the heart.

INTRACARDIAC THROMBUS

The echocardiographic appearance of intracardiac thrombus is generally readily recognized by the high-resolution capabilities of TEE. Thrombus is usually homogeneous and well demarcated, with variably increased echodensity compared with surrounding myocardial boundaries. Typically, thrombus has a laminated or "layered" appearance of deposition along the involved endocardial surface without a discrete attachment (e.g., the stalk or pedicle of benign tumors) or evidence of tissue invasion and infiltration (e.g., that with malignant neoplasms). Not uncommonly, a thin border of relative echolucency can be identified along the margins of thrombus apposition with the endocardial surface, demarcating myocardium from the thrombus; the same finding confirms absence of myocardial infiltration.

Associated anatomic findings also highly favor the diagnosis of intracardiac thrombus rather than a primary or secondary neoplastic process. Such findings include enlargement of the involved cardiac chamber, usually with significant regional or global ventricular dysfunction, and a low blood flow state, as evidenced by spontaneous echocontrast within the affected cardiac chamber. The additional presence of atrial fibrillation further promotes blood stasis and thrombus formation, particularly within the left atrial appendage.

Left Atrial Thrombus

Thrombus within the left atrium has been associated with atrial fibrillation, significant left atrial enlargement, rheumatic mitral stenosis, and mitral valve prostheses [57–61].

Two earlier studies of transthoracic echocardiography reported sensitivities from 33% [57] to 59% [58] in the detection of left atrial thrombus, usually with a specificity of greater than 90%. Although relatively large thrombi within the body of the atrium are usually evident on technically adequate transthoracic images, major limitations exist in the delineation of left atrial appendage thrombus and even the appendage itself by this approach. Visualization of the left atrial appendage is important, because 22% to 46% of all left atrial thrombi have been shown to be confined to the appendage in echocardiographic studies correlated with findings at the time of mitral valve surgery [58,61]. Despite the use of goal-directed parasternal basal short-axis imaging planes [62], transthoracic visualization of the left atrial appendage with adequate resolution to diagnose or exclude a thrombus is possible in only 3% to, at most, 19% of patients [63–65].

Because of the immediate proximity of the left atrium to the esophagus, TEE allows outstanding high-resolution delineation of the body and appendage of the left atrium [4,5]. Uncommonly, basal short-axis imaging with monoplane systems yields oblique images of the left atrial appendage; more orthogonal scans of the appendage are almost always obtainable on longitudinal imaging. In both TEE imaging planes, the apex of the appendage tapers to a discrete tip, and often comblike pectinate muscular ridges are evident (Fig. 12-32).

If the tip of the left atrial appendage appears truncated or blunted on nonoblique imaging, thrombus should be highly suspect (Fig. 12-33). Stagnated blood flow within the appendage can produce a similar appearance, although sluggish motion of blood, seen as dense, spontaneous echocontrast, is usually present (Fig. 12-34). Often, such conditions of blood stasis produce thrombotic "sludge" within the tip of the appendage. Biplanar examination of the left atrial appendage is preferable, as occasionally laminated thrombus along the lateral appendage walls is not appreciated in the monoplane transverse view alone (see Chapter 15, Fig. 15-5). Large thrombi within the appendage are usually obvious, filling in

Fig. 12-27. Mediastinal lymphangioma. A. Transverse TEE plane, basal short-axis view. A large multiseptated cystic tumor *(T)* anterior to the aorta and right pulmonary artery compresses the superior vena cava into a slitlike channel. B. Longitudinal imaging displays the extrinsic compression, but not invasion, of the superior vena cava by this benign tumor. C. Off-axis longitudinal imaging of the superior vena cava. There is marked extrinsic narrowing of the cava *(arrow)* by the multiseptated tumor. Severe dilatation of the more distal cava dwarfs the left atrium in this view.

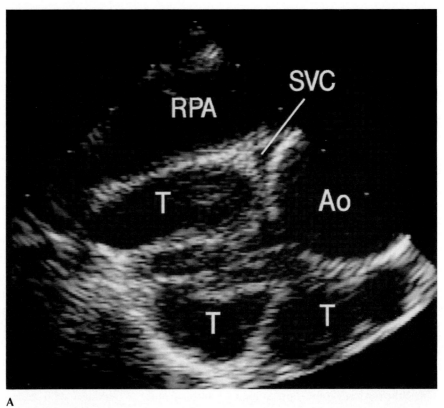

A

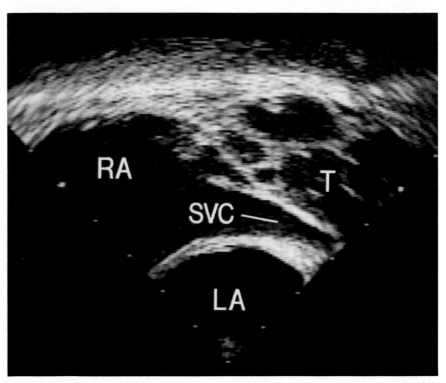

B

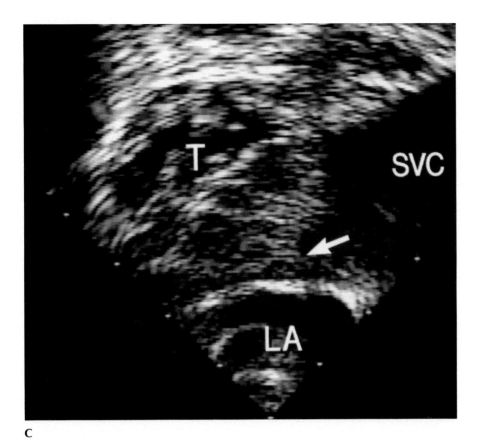

C

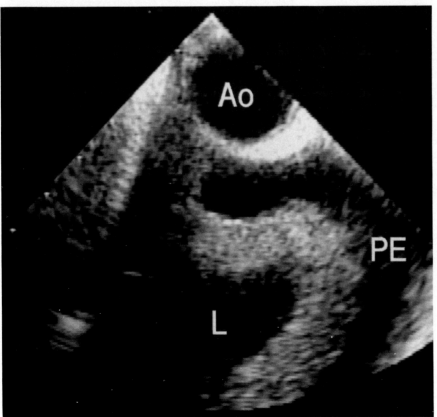

Fig. 12-28. Left pleural effusion; transverse TEE plane. A posteromedial left pleural effusion is visualized adjacent to the descending thoracic aorta. Occasionally such an effusion mimics an extracardiac cyst; the highlighted left lower lung (L) may be mistaken for a mediastinal mass in this situation.

Fig. 12-29. Stomach; transgastric transverse TEE imaging. The stomach *(S)* may be mistaken for a paracardiac cyst or effusion adjacent to the left ventricle. The gastric rugae *(arrowheads)* should readily allow correct identification. In the absence of a diaphragmatic hernia, the diaphragm *(arrow)* is seen to separate the stomach from the heart.

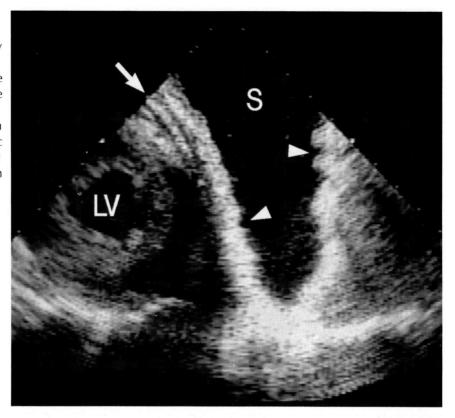

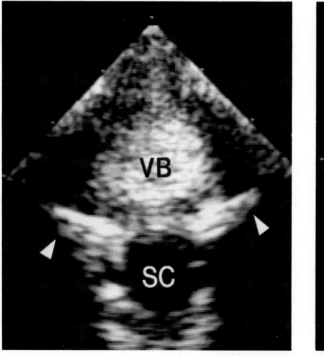
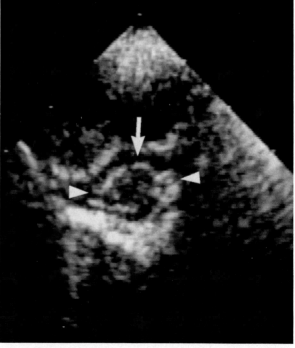

A   B

Fig. 12-30.   Vertebra of the thoracic spinal column. A. Off-axis imaging directly posteriorly may detail the anatomy of the vertebral body *(VB)*, spinous processes *(arrowheads)*, and spinal canal *(SC)*. B. Directed imaging of the spinal canal occasionally reveals the spinal cord *(arrow)* and even spinal roots *(arrowheads)*.

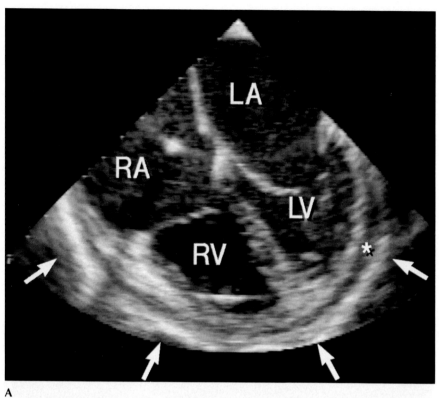

A

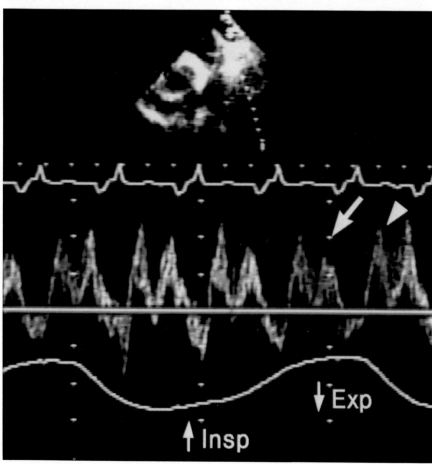

B

Fig. 12-31. Constrictive pericarditis; transverse TEE plane. A. Four-chamber view. Circumferential echodense and hyperrefractile thickening of the pericardium *(arrows)* is causing constriction. A small pericardial effusion *(asterisk)* is adjacent to the left ventricle. B. Pulsed-wave Doppler analysis of the left upper pulmonary vein. Significant diminution of pulmonary venous inflow *(large arrow)* is seen after inspiration, and increased inflow *(arrowhead)* is noted the first beat after expiration. These findings reflect dissociation of intracardiac and intrathoracic pressures, consistent with the hemodynamics of constriction.

Fig. 12-32. Left atrial appendage. A. Transverse TEE plane, expanded basal short-axis view. The appendage of the left atrium is enlarged, and pectinate muscle ridges *(arrowheads)* are evident. Sharp delineation of the pectinate structures and a discrete tip *(asterisk)* of the appendage confirm the absence of thrombus. B. Longitudinal TEE plane, expanded view. Pectinate ridges are evident *(arrowhead)*, as is a discrete apical tip *(asterisk)* within the left atrial appendage.

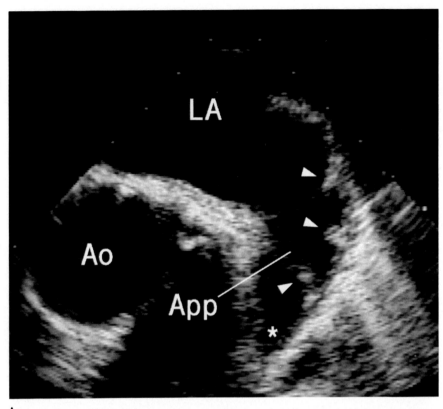

A

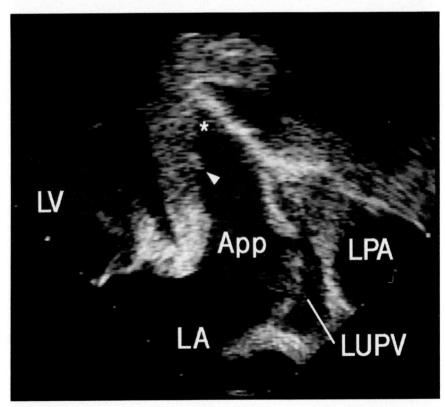

B

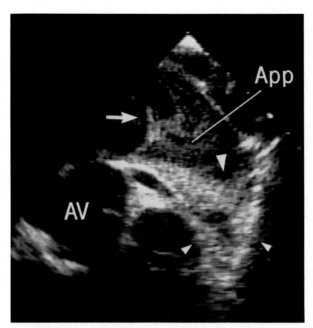

Fig. 12-33. Left atrial appendage thrombosis; transverse TEE plane, expanded basal short-axis view. The left atrial appendage is enlarged and contains dense spontaneous echocontrast *(arrow)*; the tip of the appendage *(small arrowheads)* has been blunted with thrombus deposition *(large arrowhead)*.

the body of the appendage in either a laminated or a protruding fashion (Fig. 12-35).

Large thrombi are readily identified within the body of the left atrium (Fig. 12-36); examination in multiple TEE planes often reveals multicentric thrombus deposition. Not infrequently, some degree of thrombus mobility can be appreciated in protruding left atrial thrombi. Rarely, a free-floating, mobile left atrial "ball thrombus" may be present, and systemic embolization is prevented by mitral inflow stenosis. The lack of any attachment to the left atrial walls strongly supports the diagnosis of thrombus instead of neoplasm.

In a study of 21 patients undergoing mitral valve replacement, TEE was 100% sensitive and specific for the diagnosis of left atrial appendage thrombus, which was verified at surgery; all thrombi were undetected by transthoracic echocardiography [63]. In a series of 2000 consecutive patients undergoing TEE for a wide variety of clinical indications, the incidence of left atrial appendage thrombus was 3.8%; all such thrombi were undetected by transthoracic echocardiography [65]. Of the patients with left atrial appendage thrombus, 69% were in atrial

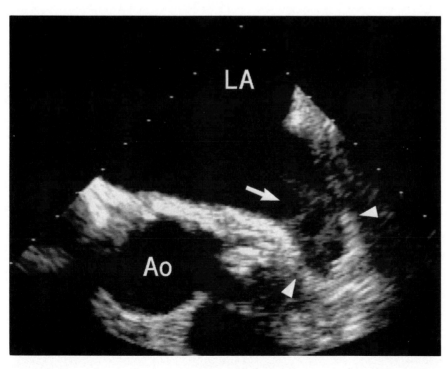

Fig. 12-34. Left atrial appendage spontaneous echocontrast; transverse basal short-axis TEE plane. Dense spontaneous echocontrast *(arrow)* is present within the appendage *(arrowheads)* of the left atrium. Sluggish movement of this echocontrast was noted during real-time examination.

Fig. 12-35. Left atrial appendage thrombus; transverse TEE plane, basal short-axis view. A protruding thrombus *(arrowheads)* fills the appendage of the left atrium. This thrombus was slightly mobile on real-time evaluation.

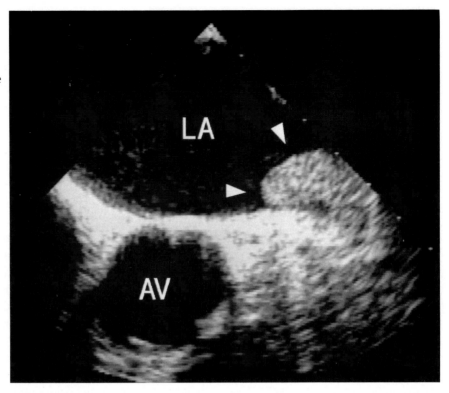

Fig. 12-36. Left atrial thrombus. A. Transverse TEE plane, high basal short-axis view. A large thrombus is present within the dome of the left atrium. Sculpturing of the thrombus *(arrowheads)* by inflow from the left upper pulmonary vein *(asterisk)* is evident.

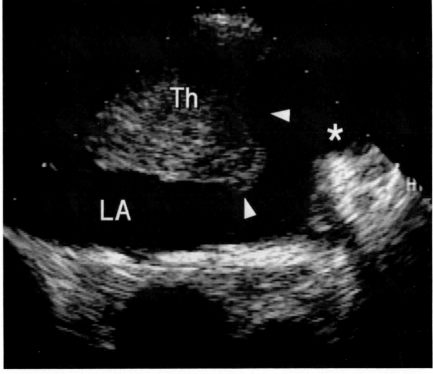

A

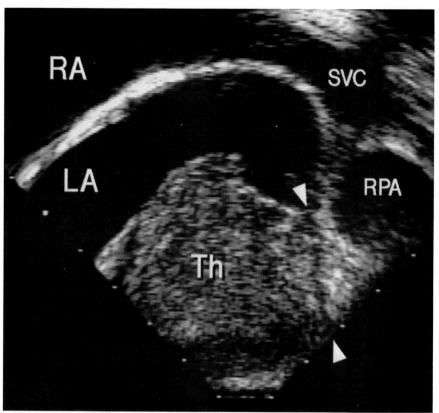

B

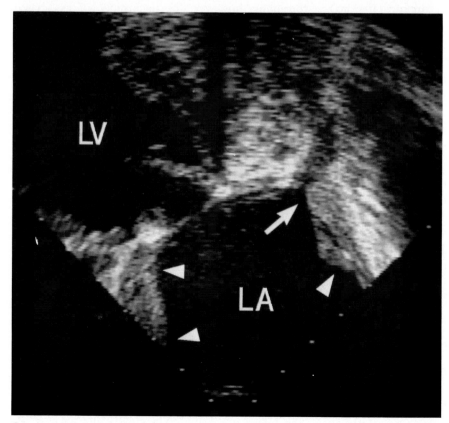

C

Fig. 12-36. continued
B. Longitudinal TEE plane. The large thrombus within the left atrium is well demarcated from adjoining walls of the left atrium *(arrowheads)*, a characteristic of thrombus and not malignancy. C. Further scanning in the longitudinal two-chamber plane reveals additional laminated thrombus *(arrowheads)* encompassing the walls of the left atrium in this view. Thrombus has also encroached on the orifice of the left atrial appendage *(arrow)*.

fibrillation; 49% had mitral stenosis or a mitral prosthesis, and another 21% had ischemic heart disease or another cause of depressed left ventricular function. Curiously, 14 patients (19%) had left atrial appendage thrombus without morphologic or functional cardiac disease, and one-half of these patients (9% of all patients with thrombus) were in normal sinus rhythm at the time of TEE [65]. Mügge et al. [23] also reported the detection rate of thrombus within the body of the left atrium to be 100% by TEE, compared with 69% by transthoracic study; thrombus within the appendage was detected in 100% of patients by TEE and missed in all patients by transthoracic study.

In our experience [22] of 37 patients with left atrial thrombus diagnosed by TEE, 84% had chronic atrial fibrillation, 73% had associated native or prosthetic mitral valve disease, and 62% had spontaneous echocontrast within the left atrium. In only 27% of cases was the diagnosis of left atrial thrombus possible by the transthoracic approach. Transesophageal echocardiography was judged to provide significant additional information in 84% of cases and altered the management in 51% of these patients [22].

Spontaneous echocontrast (or microcavitations) within the body of the left atrium is readily detectable by TEE and rarely is appreciated by transthoracic echocardiography [60]. This finding is associated with stasis of blood flow in patients with atrial fibrillation, a low cardiac output state, or significant left atrial enlargement. In patients with mitral valve disease, left atrial spontaneous echocontrast is quite uncommon (2%) if the left atrial diameter is smaller than 60 mm but is frequently (66%) detected if the diameter is 60 mm or larger [60]. Not only is the incidence of left atrial thrombus significantly increased if spontaneous echocontrast is present [22,60] but this finding is also a probable independent risk factor for systemic embolic events [60,64] (see Chapter 15).

Exuberant mitral annular calcification may be mistaken for a left atrial thrombus, neoplasm, or abscess cavity. The hyperrefractile, echodense appearance localized along the posterolateral aspects of the mitral annulus with acoustic shadowing of portions of the left ventricle is characteristic of mitral annular calcification (Fig. 12-37). Occasionally, extensive mitral annular calcification may have a non-hyperrefractile, homogeneous appearance; a tail-like extension of this "mass" along the posterior mitral annulus prompts the correct diagnosis.

Left Ventricular Thrombus

Provided that adequate acoustic windows are present, transthoracic echocardiography has been shown to have a sensitivity of 92% to 95% and a specificity approaching 90% in the diagnosis of left ventricular thrombus [66,67]. Continued significant improvements in the resolution of transthoracic imaging systems over the decade since the initial anatomically validated studies were published have made transthoracic echocardiography the current standard for the diagnosis of left ventricular thrombus.

Left ventricular thrombi nearly always occur in patients with significant regional or global left ventricular dysfunction. Left ventricular thrombus can complicate 30% to 35% of "transmural" anterior myocardial infarctions and is distinctly unusual in inferior myocardial infarctions [68,69]. Thrombus complicating myocardial infarction hence is located within the apex of the left ventricle in 85% to 98% of cases [70,71], adjacent to the ventricular septum in approximately 10%, and in the inferior free wall in less than 5% [71].

The echocardiographic characteristics of left ventricular thrombus are similar to those of left atrial thrombus; however, the occurrence of associated spontaneous left ventricular echocontrast is probably lower than that observed for left atrial thrombus. Transthoracic studies have demonstrated that thrombus mobility, protrusion into the left ventricular cavity, adjacent left ventricular hyperkinesia, thrombus stranding, and abrupt postectopic thrombus motion are strong predictors of embolic potential [70,71].

Transesophageal echocardiography may offer an advantage over the transthoracic approach for the detection of small, laminated left ventricular thrombi (Fig. 12-38). However, because of far-field location of the left ventricular apex in both the transverse four-chamber and the longitudinal two-chamber views, visualization of relatively small left ventricular thrombi by TEE may be difficult, especially if tangential imaging planes truncate the true apex. This problem is usually overcome by transgastric imaging of the left ventricle in both the transverse short-axis and the longitudinal long-axis planes with careful advancement and retraction of the transducer tip with lateral flexion maneuvers as needed.

Consistent with this experience, TEE monoplane imaging in the four-chamber and transgastric short-axis planes was found to be clearly inferior to transthoracic echocardiography in detection of left ventricular apical thrombi in a small group of patients

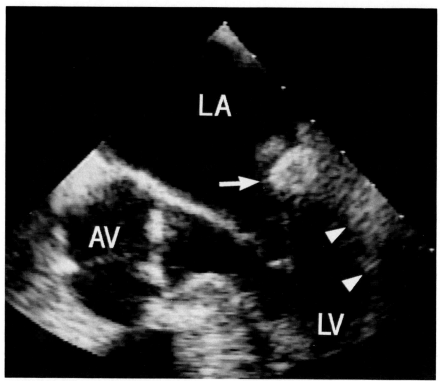

Fig. 12-37. Mitral annular calcification; transverse TEE plane. Extensive mitral annular calcification *(arrow)* protrudes from the lateral annulus. In this location, the immobile, hyperrefractile, echodense appearance with acoustic shadowing *(arrowheads)* of the left ventricle prompts differentiation from thrombus and neoplasm.

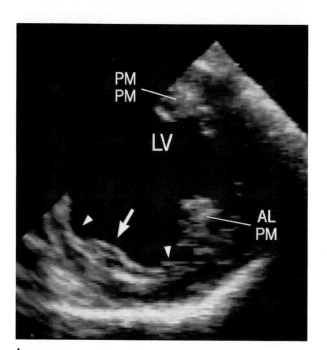

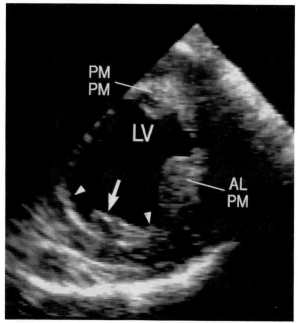

A   B

Fig. 12-38. Left ventricular mural thrombus; transverse TEE plane, transgastric apex-up short-axis view. A. Diastole. A thrombus *(arrow)* is present along the thinned anterior left ventricular wall *(arrowheads)*. The posteromedial papillary muscle *(PMPM)* and anterolateral papillary muscle *(ALPM)* are noted for orientation. Most of the ventricular septum is not seen in this view. B. Systole. The anterior left ventricular wall *(arrowheads)* remains akinetic. Mild mobility of the thrombus *(arrow)* with a change in shape is noted as the remaining left ventricular walls contract.

Fig. 12-39. Advanced dilated cardiomyopathy, right ventricular thrombus. A. Transverse TEE plane, transgastric apex-down view. Echodense thrombus *(arrowheads)* is visualized in the medial inferoapical portion of the right ventricle; the liver *(L)* is adjacent to the inferior walls of the ventricles. B. Longitudinal TEE plane, transgastric long-axis view. The right ventricular apical thrombus *(arrowheads)* is better delineated from the surrounding prominent right ventricular trabeculations and tricuspid valve support apparatus.

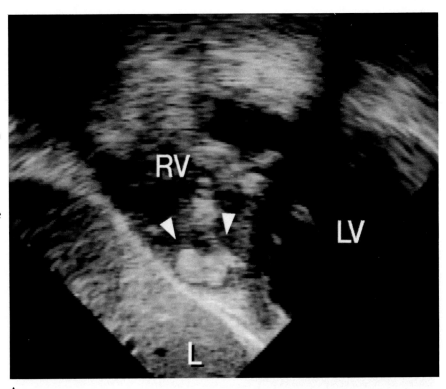

A

recently studied by both methods [23]. In this study, definite identification of left ventricular apical thrombus was possible in only 20% of patients examined by TEE but in all patients imaged transthoracically [23].

The addition of multiplane transgastric imaging, particularly in goal-directed, off-axis planes, is expected to further improve the sensitivity of TEE in the detection of left ventricular apical thrombus.

Right Heart Thrombus

Analogous to left ventricular thrombi, right ventricular thrombus may occur in any situation involving significant right ventricular dysfunction, again with the thrombus most often being apical in location. The more common causes of right ventricular dysfunction associated with thrombus formation are extensive right ventricular infarction, myocardial contusion, advanced dilated cardiomyopathy, and cor pulmonale.

As with left ventricular thrombus, the true sensitivity and specificity of TEE compared with transthoracic echocardiography or other imaging modalities in the detection of right ventricular thrombus remains to be established. Transesophageal echocardiography may be helpful in the delineation of smaller right ventricular apical thrombi (Fig. 12-39), which may be obscured from view by promi-

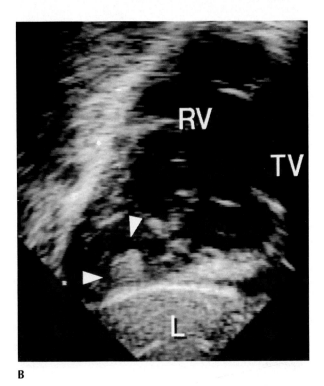

B

nent trabeculations or the moderator band on transthoracic imaging. Transgastric TEE imaging with both the transverse short-axis and the longitudinal long-axis planes optimizes visualization of the apical half of the right ventricle and hence detection of thrombus.

Thrombus originating in the right atrium is rare and is usually associated with chronic indwelling catheters, pacemaker leads, or trauma from instrumentation. Although such a thrombus may be identified from transthoracic windows, TEE offers a

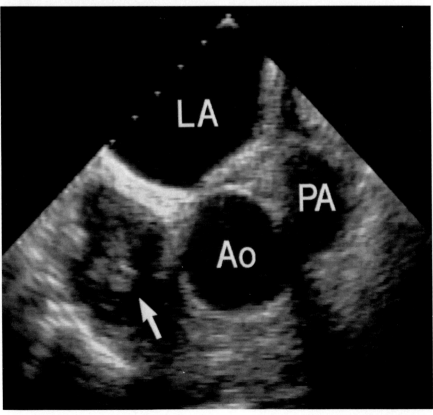

A

distinct advantage in the detection of associated thrombus within the superior vena cava [23] (Fig. 12-40).

Deep venous thromboembolism may be arrested within the right heart en route from the iliofemoral veins to the pulmonary arterial circulation [72,73] (see Chapter 15). On TEE imaging, a highly mobile and tubular thrombus cast can be seen within the right atrium, often with prolapse into the right ventricular inflow tract (Fig. 12-41).

A swirling serpentine and continuously changing appearance (likened by some to popcorn popping) is characteristic of right atrial thromboembolism in transit (see Chapter 15, Fig. 15-24) and readily differentiates this entity from a neoplastic process such as right atrial myxoma. Such a thrombus may become entrapped within the tricuspid valve apparatus or eustachian valve or across a patent foramen ovale, with paradoxical embolism [73] (see Chapter 15, Fig. 15-17). Usually the TEE findings are accompanied by significant completed pulmonary embolism, although the diagnosis may not be clinically apparent, hence prompting the indication for further evaluation by TEE. Proximal pulmonary artery thromboembolism itself may also be detected by TEE [74–76]. Most often, the thrombus can be de-

Fig. 12-40. Thrombus within superior vena cava; transverse TEE basal short-axis view. A. Thrombus *(arrow)* resulting from traumatic catheterization of the right heart causes subtotal occlusion of the proximal superior vena cava *(dashed circle)*. B. Thrombus extension into the superior right atrium *(arrow)* is also present.

B

Fig. 12-41. Deep venous thromboembolism in transit; transverse TEE plane, modified transgastric four-chamber view. A. During systole, a large serpentine thrombus *(arrowheads)* is seen just proximal to the closed tricuspid valve within the right atrium. B. During diastole, the thrombus *(arrowheads)* prolapses into the right ventricle. Both the right atrium and the right ventricle are enlarged, with deformation of the ventricular septum toward the left ventricle, consistent with acute cor pulmonale due to extensive pulmonary embolism completed by other thrombus not detained within the right heart.

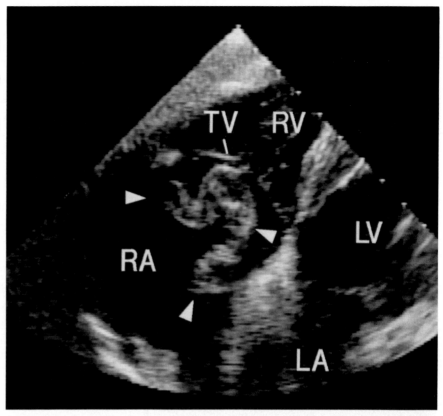

A

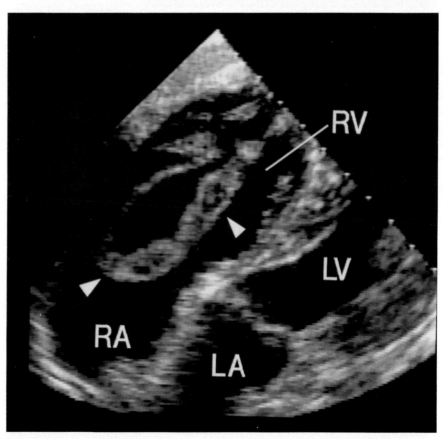

B

tected only within the proximal right and left pulmonary arteries. In acute or subacute pulmonary embolism, the thrombus may be partially mobile and is often coiled upon itself within the pulmonary artery (Fig. 12-42).

In a recent series of 60 patients with pulmonary thromboembolism associated with evidence of right ventricular pressure overload on transthoracic echocardiography, central pulmonary thromboemboli were detected by TEE in 58% of patients [76]. Long, tubular, and highly mobile thromboemboli within the central pulmonary arteries were associated with acute (especially initial) clinical events, whereas patients with chronic pulmonary hypertension due to

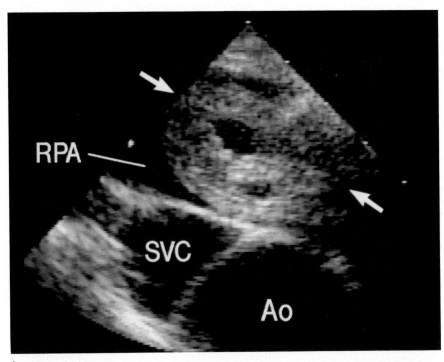

Fig. 12-42. Subacute pulmonary thromboembolism. A. Transverse plane, high basal short-axis view. A large tubular thromboembolism *(arrows)* is lodged within the proximal right pulmonary artery. Distal to-and-fro motion of the thrombus was seen on real-time examination. B. Longitudinal TEE plane. The thrombus *(arrows)*, which has coiled upon itself, is seen in transverse section within the right pulmonary artery.

A

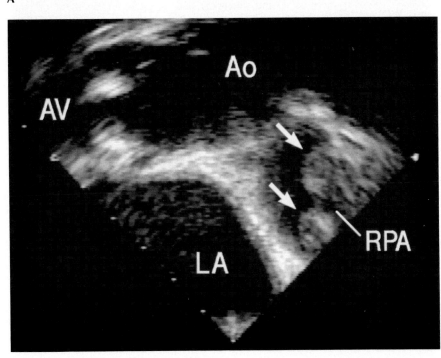

B

recurrent thromboembolic events had exclusively immobile thrombus densely adherent to the walls of the involved pulmonary artery. When compared with another imaging modality (pulmonary angiography or computed tomography) or anatomic confirmation (surgery or necropsy) or both, TEE was 97% sensitive and 88% specific in the detection of central pulmonary artery thromboemboli [76].

SUMMARY

Transesophageal echocardiography has greatly expedited the evaluation of intracardiac neoplasms and thrombi. By providing high-resolution images in multiple planes, TEE is usually far superior to transthoracic echocardiography or other imaging techniques in general for both the detection and the delineation of a broad spectrum of intracardiac mass lesions. Although isolated limitations exist, TEE is rapidly becoming accepted as the procedure of choice for the assessment of the patient in whom an intracardiac mass or thrombus is suspected.

REFERENCES

1. Salcedo EE, Adams KV, Lever HM, et al. Echocardiographic findings in 25 patients with left atrial myxoma. *J Am Coll Cardiol* 1983;1:1162–6.

2. Fyke FE III, Seward JB, Edwards WD, et al. Primary cardiac tumors: experience with 30 consecutive patients since the introduction of two-dimensional echocardiography. *J Am Coll Cardiol* 1985;5:1465–73.

3. Felner JM, Knopf WD. Echocardiographic recognition of intracardiac and extracardiac masses. *Echocardiography* 1985;2:3–55.

4. Seward JB, Khandheria BK, Oh JK, et al. Transesophageal echocardiography: technique, anatomic correlations, implementation, and clinical applications. *Mayo Clin Proc* 1988;63:649–80.

5. Seward JB, Khandheria BK, Edwards WD, et al. Biplanar transesophageal echocardiography: anatomic correlations, image orientation, and clinical applications. *Mayo Clin Proc* 1990;65:1193–213.

6. McAllister HA Jr, Fenoglio JJ Jr. Tumors of the cardiovascular system. In: *Atlas of Tumor Pathology.* Second Series, Fascicle 15. Washington DC: Armed Forces Institute of Pathology, 1978.

7. Salcedo EE, White RD, Cohen GI, Davison MB. Cardiac tumors: diagnosis and management. *Curr Probl Cardiol* 1992;17:75–137.

8. Cooley DA. Surgical treatment of cardiac neoplasms: 32–year experience. *Thorac Cardiovasc Surg* 1990;38 Special Issue:176–82.

9. Molina JE, Edwards JE, Ward HB. Primary cardiac tumors: experience at the University of Minnesota. *Thorac Cardiovasc Surg* 1990;38 Special Issue: 183–91.

10. Blondeau P. Primary cardiac tumors—French studies of 533 cases. *Thorac Cardiovasc Surg* 1990;38 Special Issue:192–5.

11. Sezai Y. Tumors of the heart: incidence and clinical importance of cardiac tumors in Japan and operative technique for large left atrial tumors. *Thorac Cardiovasc Surg* 1990;38 Special Issue:201–4.

12. Guang-ying L. Incidence and clinical importance of cardiac tumors in China—review of the literature. *Thorac Cardiovasc Surg* 1990;38 Special Issue: 205–7.

13. Nomeir A-M, Watts LE, Seagle R, et al. Intracardiac myxomas: twenty-year echocardiographic experience with review of the literature. *J Am Soc Echocardiogr* 1989;2:139–50.

14. Milano A, Dan M, Bortolotti U. Left atrial myxoma: excision guided by transesophageal cross-sectional echocardiography. *Int J Cardiol* 1990;27:125–7.

15. Turlapati RV, Jacobs LE, Kotler MN. Right atrial myxoma causing total destruction of the tricuspid valve leaflets. *Am Heart J* 1990;120:1227–31.

16. Smith ST, Hautamaki K, Lewis JW Jr, et al. Transthoracic and transesophageal echocardiography in the diagnosis and surgical management of right atrial myxoma. *Chest* 1991;100:575–6.

17. Wrisley D, Rosenberg J, Giambartolomei A, et al. Left ventricular myxoma discovered incidentally by echocardiography. *Am Heart J* 1991;121:1554–5.

18. Lyons SV, McCord J, Smith S. Asymptomatic giant right atrial myxoma: role of transesophageal echocardiography in management. *Am Heart J* 1991; 121: 1555–8.

19. Vargas-Barron J, Romero-Cardenas A, Villegas M, et al. Transthoracic and transesophageal echocardiographic diagnosis of myxomas in the four cardiac cavities. *Am Heart J* 1991;121:931–3.

20. Obeid AI, Marvasti M, Parker F, Rosenberg J. Comparison of transthoracic and transesophageal echocardiography in diagnosis of left atrial myxoma. *Am J Cardiol* 1989;63:1006–8.

21. Alam M, Sun I. Transesophageal echocardiographic evaluation of left atrial mass lesions. *J Am Soc Echocardiogr* 1991;4:323–30.

22. Reeder GS, Khandheria BK, Seward JB, Tajik AJ. Transesophageal echocardiography and cardiac masses. *Mayo Clin Proc* 1991;66:1101–9.

23. Mügge A, Daniel WG, Haverich A, Lichtlen PR. Diagnosis of noninfective cardiac mass lesions by two-dimensional echocardiography: comparison of the transthoracic and transesophageal approaches. *Circulation* 1991;83:70–8.

24. Vidaillet HJ Jr, Seward JB, Fyke FE III, et al. "Syndrome myxoma": a subset of patients with cardiac myxoma associated with pigmented skin lesions and peripheral and endocrine neoplasms. *Br Heart J* 1987;57:247–55.

25. Rahilly GT Jr, Nanda NC. Two-dimensional echographic identification of tumor hemorrhages in atrial myxomas. *Am Heart J* 1981;101:237–9.

26. Thier W, Schlüter M, Krebber H-J, et al. Cysts in left atrial myxomas identified by transesophageal cross-sectional echocardiography. *Am J Cardiol* 1983;51:1793–5.

27. Charuzi Y, Bolger A, Beeder C, Lew AS. A new echocardiographic classification of left atrial myxoma. *Am J Cardiol* 1985;55:614–5.

28. Rey M, Tuñon J, Compres H, et al. Prolapsing right atrial myxoma evaluated by transesophageal echocardiography. *Am Heart J* 1991;122:875–7.

29. Tuna IC, Julsrud PR, Click RL, et al. Tissue characterization of an unusual right atrial mass by magnetic resonance imaging. *Mayo Clin Proc* 1991;66:498–501.

30. Fyke FE III, Tajik AJ, Edwards WD, Seward JB. Diagnosis of lipomatous hypertrophy of the atrial septum by two-dimensional echocardiography. *J Am Coll Cardiol* 1983;1:1352–7.

31. Applegate PM, Tajik AJ, Ehman RL, et al. Two-dimensional echocardiographic and magnetic resonance imaging observations in massive lipomatous hypertrophy of the atrial septum. *Am J Cardiol* 1987;59:489–91.

32. Kindman LA, Wright A, Tye T, et al. Lipomatous hypertrophy of the interatrial septum: characterization by transesophageal and transthoracic echocardiography, magnetic resonance imaging, and computed tomography. *J Am Soc Echocardiogr* 1988;1:450–4.

33. Shub C, Tajik AJ, Seward JB, et al. Cardiac papillary fibroelastomas: two-dimensional echocardiographic recognition. *Mayo Clin Proc* 1981;56:629–33.

34. Topol EJ, Biern RO, Reitz BA. Cardiac papillary fibroelastoma and stroke: echocardiographic diagnosis and guide to excision. *Am J Med* 1986;80:129–32.

35. de Virgilio C, Dubrow TJ, Robertson JM, et al. Detection of multiple cardiac papillary fibroelastomas using transesophageal echocardiography. *Ann Thorac Surg* 1989;48:119–21.

36. Wolfe JT III, Finck SJ, Safford RE, Persellin ST. Tricuspid valve papillary fibroelastoma: echocardiographic characterization. *Ann Thorac Surg* 1991;51:116–8.

37. Bass JL, Breningstall GN, Swaiman KF. Echocardiographic incidence of cardiac rhabdomyoma in tuberous sclerosis. *Am J Cardiol* 1985;55:1379–82.

38. Freeman WK, Zellers TM, Taylor CL, et al. Echocardiographic findings in patients with tuberous sclerosis (abstract). *J Am Coll Cardiol* 1988;11:73A.

39. Parmley LF, Salley RK, Williams JP, Head GB. The clinical spectrum of cardiac fibroma with diagnostic and surgical considerations: noninvasive imaging enhances management. *Ann Thorac Surg* 1988;45:455–65.

40. Janigan DT, Husain A, Robinson NA. Cardiac angiosarcomas: a review and a case report. *Cancer* 1986;57:852–9.

41. Frohwein SC, Karalis DG, McQuillan JM, et al. Preoperative detection of pericardial angiosarcoma by transesophageal echocardiography. *Am Heart J* 1991;122:874–5.

42. Roberts WC, Glancy DL, DeVita VT Jr. Heart in malignant lymphoma (Hodgkin's disease, lymphosarcoma, reticulum cell sarcoma and mycosis fungoides): a study of 196 autopsy cases. *Am J Cardiol* 1968;22:85–107.

43. DeLoach JF, Haynes JW. Secondary tumors of heart and pericardium: review of the subject and report of one hundred thirty-seven cases. *Arch Intern Med* 1953;91:224–49.

44. Hanfling SM. Metastatic cancer to the heart: review of the literature and report of 127 cases. *Circulation* 1960;22:474–83.

45. Kutalek SP, Panidis IP, Kotler MN, et al. Metastatic tumors of the heart detected by two-dimensional echocardiography. *Am Heart J* 1985;109:343–9.

46. Hinds SW, Reisner SA, Amico AF, Meltzer RS. Diagnosis of pericardial abnormalities by 2–D echo: a pathology-echocardiography correlation in 85 patients. *Am Heart J* 1992;123:143–50.

47. Mancuso L, Pitrolo F, Bondi F, et al. Echocardiographic recognition of mediastinal masses. *Chest* 1988;93:144–8.

48. Schrem SS, Colvin SB, Weinreb JC, et al. Metastatic cardiac liposarcoma: diagnosis by transesophageal echocardiography and magnetic resonance imaging. *J Am Soc Echocardiogr* 1990;3:149–53.

49. Hsu T-L, Hsiung M-C, Lin S-L, et al. The value of transesophageal echocardiography in the diagnosis of cardiac metastasis. *Echocardiography* 1992;9:1–7.

50. Feigin DS, Fenoglio JJ, McAllister HA, Madewell JE. Pericardial cysts: a radiologic-pathologic correlation and review. *Radiology* 1977;125:15–20.

51. Page JE, Wilson AG, de Belder MA. The value of transoesophageal ultrasonography in the management of a mediastinal foregut cyst. *Br J Radiol* 1989;62:986–8.

52. Davis RD Jr, Oldham HN Jr, Sabiston DC Jr. The mediastinum. In: Sabiston DC Jr, Spencer FC, eds. *Surgery of the Chest*, Vol 1, 5th ed. Philadelphia: Saunders, 1990:498–535.

53. Faletra F, Ravini M, Moreo A, et al. Transesophageal echocardiography in the evaluation of mediastinal masses. *J Am Soc Echocardiogr* 1992;5:178–86.

54. von Schulthess GK, McMurdo K, Tscholakoff D, et al. Mediastinal masses: MR imaging. *Radiology* 1986;158:289–96.

55. Rienmüller R, Tiling R. MR and CT for detection of cardiac tumors. *Thorac Cardiovasc Surg* 1990;38 Special Issue:168–72.

56. Hatle LK, Appleton CP, Popp RL. Differentiation of constrictive pericarditis and restrictive cardiomyopathy by Doppler echocardiography. *Circulation* 1989;79:357–70.

57. Schweizer P, Bardos P, Erbel R, et al. Detection of left atrial thrombi by echocardiography. *Br Heart J* 1981;45:148–56.

58. Shrestha NK, Moreno FL, Narciso FV, et al. Two-dimensional echocardiographic diagnosis of left atrial thrombus in rheumatic heart disease: a clinicopathologic study. *Circulation* 1983;67:341–7.

59. Beppu S, Park Y-D, Sakakibara H, et al. Clinical features of intracardiac thrombosis based on echocardiographic observation. *Jpn Circ J* 1984;48:75–82.

60. Daniel WG, Nellessen U, Schröder E, et al. Left atrial spontaneous echo contrast in mitral valve disease: an indicator for an increased thromboembolic risk. *J Am Coll Cardiol* 1988;11:1204–11.

61. Bansal RC, Heywood JT, Applegate PM, Jutzy KR. Detection of left atrial thrombi by two-dimensional echocardiography and surgical correlation in 148 patients with mitral valve disease. *Am J Cardiol* 1989;64:243–6.

62. Herzog CA, Bass D, Kane M, Asinger R. Two-dimensional echocardiographic imaging of left atrial appendage thrombi. *J Am Coll Cardiol* 1984;3:1340–4.

63. Aschenberg W, Schlüter M, Kremer P, et al. Transesophageal two-dimensional echocardiography for the detection of left atrial appendage thrombus. *J Am Coll Cardiol* 1986;7:163–6.

64. Kuecherer HF, Lee E, Schiller NB. Enhanced detection of intracardiac masses by transesophageal echocardiography. *Am J Card Imaging* 1990;4:180–6.

65. Mügge A, Daniel WG, Hausmann D, et al. Diagnosis of left atrial appendage thrombi by transesophageal echocardiography: clinical implications and follow-up. *Am J Card Imaging* 1990;4:173–9.

66. Stratton JR, Lighty GW Jr, Pearlman AS, Ritchie JL. Detection of left ventricular thrombus by two-dimensional echocardiography: sensitivity, specificity, and causes of uncertainty. *Circulation* 1982;66:156–66.

67. Visser CA, Kan G, David GK, et al. Two dimensional echocardiography in the diagnosis of left ventricular thrombus: a prospective study of 67 patients with anatomic validation. *Chest* 1983;83:228–32.

68. Asinger RW, Mikell FL, Elsperger J, Hodges M. Incidence of left-ventricular thrombosis after acute transmural myocardial infarction: serial evaluation by two-dimensional echocardiography. *N Engl J Med* 1981;305:297–302.

69. Keren A, Goldberg S, Gottlieb S, et al. Natural history of left ventricular thrombi: their appearance and resolution in the posthospitalization period of acute myocardial infarction. *J Am Coll Cardiol* 1990;15:790–800.

70. Visser CA, Kan G, Meltzer RS, et al. Embolic potential of left ventricular thrombus after myocardial infarction: a two-dimensional echocardiographic study of 119 patients. *J Am Coll Cardiol* 1985;5:1276–80.

71. Jugdutt BI, Sivaram CA, Wortman C, et al. Prospective two-dimensional echocardiographic evaluation of left ventricular thrombus and embolism after acute myocardial infarction. *J Am Coll Cardiol* 1989;13:554–64.

72. Kasper W, Meinertz T, Henkel B, et al. Echocardiographic findings in patients with proved pulmonary embolism. *Am Heart J* 1986;112:1284–90.

73. Farfel Z, Shechter M, Vered Z, et al. Review of echocardiographically diagnosed right heart entrapment of pulmonary emboli-in-transit with emphasis on management. *Am Heart J* 1987;113:171–8.

74. Nixdorff U, Erbel R, Drexler M, Meyer J. Detection of thromboembolus of the right pulmonary artery by transesophageal two-dimensional echocardiography. *Am J Cardiol* 1988;61:488–9.

75. Klein AL, Stewart WC, Cosgrove DM III, et al. Visualization of acute pulmonary emboli by transesophageal echocardiography. *J Am Soc Echocardiogr* 1990;3:412–5.

76. Wittlich N, Erbel R, Eichler A, et al. Detection of central pulmonary artery thromboemboli by transesophageal echocardiography in patients with severe pulmonary embolism. *J Am Soc Echocardiogr* 1992;5:515–24.

13

Congenital Heart Disease

Transesophageal Echocardiography

James B. Seward

Congenital heart disease is a fascination as well as a challenge to the diagnostician. A sound understanding of normal and abnormal echocardiographic features of congenital heart disease is a prerequisite [1]. Transesophageal echocardiography (TEE) is the newest diagnostic modality to show great promise for high-resolution imaging of the heart [2–4]. This new window to the heart allows expanded anatomic and hemodynamic diagnoses in patients with congenital heart disease.

From the esophagus, details of the heart and great vessels are obtained in virtually every patient. Transesophageal echocardiography in the awake patient has been accepted as a logical extension of a comprehensive transthoracic echocardiographic examination [2]. Transesophageal echocardiography has also been used intraoperatively to monitor cardiac function and to monitor the repair of various acquired [5] and congenital [6–13] cardiac lesions. The purpose of this chapter is to familiarize the reader with the potential usefulness of TEE in the diagnosis and management of various congenital cardiovascular anomalies in adult patients and pediatric patients.

One should be intimately familiar with the TEE technique (see Chapter 3) and normal anatomic relationships (see Chapters 4 and 5) [2–4,14]. To date, most commercially available endoscopes have been predominantly adult-sized, with shafts of 9 to 15 mm in diameter. Investigators have avoided the use of these larger endoscopes in children younger than 7 years. However, an adult-sized 9-mm endoscope has been introduced into children with body weights as low as 10 kg. Pediatric probes with shafts of 5 mm or less are now available [15]. Experience is limited, however, and the transducer frequencies, focal length, and image quality are often not optimized for the pediatric patient.

Children younger than about 10 years usually have to undergo general anesthesia for an endoscopic examination. Because the transthoracic echocardiographic examination is diagnostic for most congenital anomalies in children [1] and having to use general anesthesia is a detraction, TEE has been used infrequently as a preoperative examination in children. However, in the adult patient with a more difficult or challenging transthoracic examination, TEE is considered a logical extension of a comprehensive echocardiographic examination, particularly in patients with poorly delineated congenital cardiovascular anatomy [10]. The atrial septum, cardiac crux [16], and adjacent vascular structures are the most relevant anatomic observations amenable to TEE.

This chapter is organized into a segmental approach to the assessment of various congenital anomalies [1]. The out-of-hospital patient population undergoing TEE typically ranges in age from 10 to 90 years and forms approximately 5% of the total TEE experience [2]. Pediatric TEE examinations are predominantly limited to patients under general anesthesia in the cardiac catheterization laboratory [12], operating room [7], or intensive care unit [17].

EXAMINATION OF CONGENITAL HEART DISEASE BY TEE

Cardiac Sidedness and Situs

We believe that the presentation of cardiac anatomy should comply with the recommendations of the American Society of Echocardiography [2,3] (see Chapter 4). The cardiac crux is one of the most constant anatomic landmarks for the assessment of congenital heart disease [16]. The right-sided atrioventricular valve (morphologic tricuspid) inserts lower at the crux than the left-sided atrioventricular valve (morphologic mitral) (Fig. 13-1). These relationships predictably designate valve and ventricular morphology [1,16]. A complete review of the anatomic correlations and image presentation of TEE has been reported from this laboratory [2]. For those unfamiliar with details of image orientation in congenital heart disease, more comprehensive descriptions should be consulted [1].

Great Veins

Superior and Inferior Venae Cavae

Normal caval anatomy as visualized has been described [2]. Anomalous connections of the superior and inferior venae cavae can best be appreciated by biplanar TEE [3]. The longitudinal and transverse imaging arrays are both utilized to visualize the cavae and their relationships to the atria (Fig. 13-2 and 13-3).

Persistent Left Superior Vena Cava

Enlarged coronary sinus and left-sided superior vena cava are common observations from the transthoracic approach. In TEE images, the left superior vena cava appears as a vascular structure within the sulcus between the left upper pulmonary vein and the left atrial appendage [10,19,20] (Fig. 13-4). Communication of the left superior vena cava with a dilated coronary sinus is the most common presentation. Left upper extremity venous contrast echocardiography can assist in these observations.

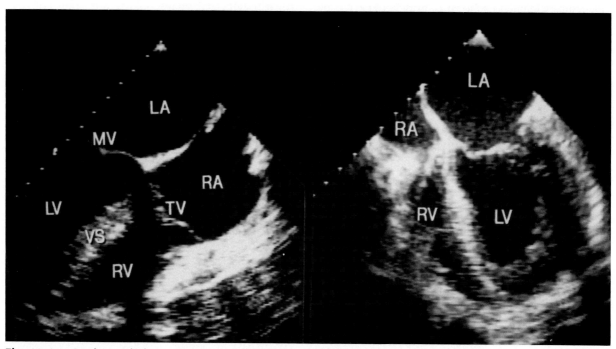

Fig. 13-1.   Cardiac sidedness (four-chamber view; transducer in midesophagus; transverse plane). *Left.* Dextrocardia (i.e., cardiac apex to the patient's right). Patient has situs inversus totalis (all structures are mirror-image). *Right.* Levocardia (i.e., cardiac apex to the patient's left). All structures are anatomically correct, with left-sided chambers to the patient's left and right-sided chambers to the patient's right.

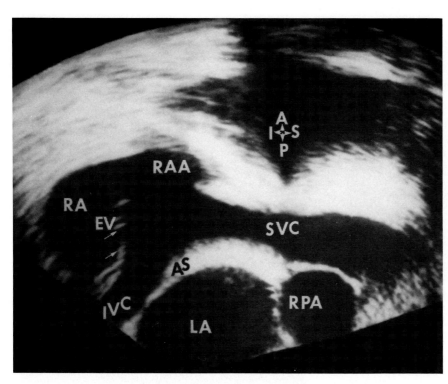

Fig. 13-2. Longitudinal scan of superior and inferior vena caval relationships. This is a long-axis scan from the midesophagus with the transducer shaft rotated to the patient's right to image the venae cavae. This particular image is a wide-field composite [18] designed to better illustrate contiguous anatomy. The posteriorly located esophageal transducer is adjacent to the left atrium. The atrial septum separates the left atrium and right atrium. The right pulmonary artery courses posterior to the superior vena cava and is cut in short axis with the longitudinal scan plane. The superior and inferior venae cavae enter the superior and inferior aspects of the right atrium, respectively. The eustachian valve *(arrows)* forms the anterior lip of the inferior vena cava and extends into the right atrium. The right atrial appendage is in the anterosuperior aspect of the right atrium. (*S* = superior)

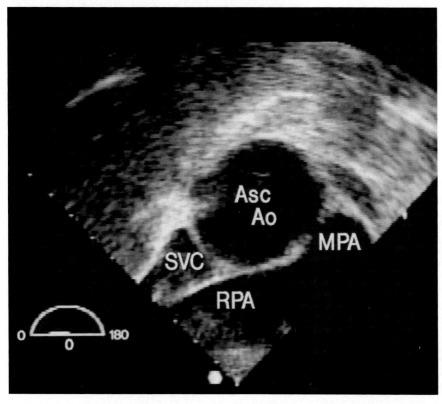

Fig. 13-3. Superior vena cava in short axis. Multiplane transducer is posterior, and the array is in the transverse plane (0 degrees). The endoscope is withdrawn superiorly to the level of the right pulmonary artery. The superior vena cava is visualized in the short axis anterior to the right pulmonary artery and adjacent to the ascending aorta.

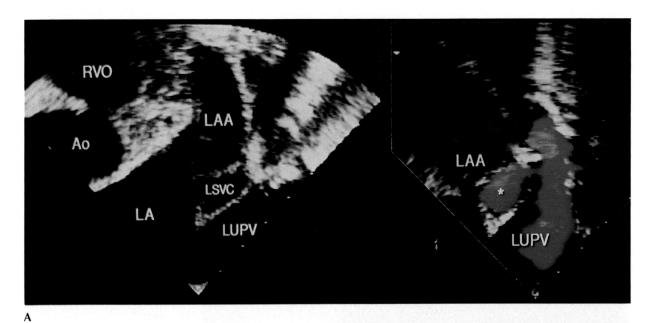

A

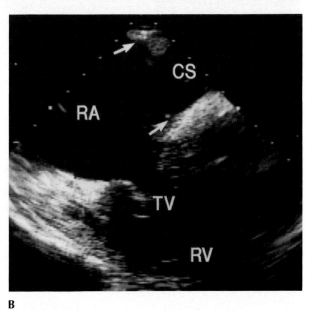

B

Fig. 13-4. Persistent left superior vena cava. A, Left. Short axis at the level of the aortic root (the transducer is in the transverse plane in midesophagus posterior to the left atrium). Note that interposed between the left atrial appendage and the left upper pulmonary vein is an echofree vascular structure, which is a persistent left superior vena cava. This vessel will usually connect to the coronary sinus. Right. The left superior vena cava *(asterisk)* and left upper pulmonary vein show blood movement, which confirms a vascular structure (i.e., left superior vena cava). Pericardial fluid can occasionally accumulate in this space but would not show blood flow. B. Four-chamber view with retroflexion of the transducer tip to visualize the coronary sinus. Note that the coronary sinus is dilated to 3 cm *(arrows)*, consistent with volume or pressure overload. A dilated coronary sinus is often the first indication of a persistent left superior vena cava.

In the longitudinal scan plane, the persistent left superior vena cava is visualized arching anteriorly over the left atrium and left pulmonary artery to enter the coronary sinus at the lateral aspect of the left atrium (Fig. 13-5).

Azygos Veins

Normal as well as abnormal dilated azygos or hemiazygos veins are visualized in the paravertebral retroperitoneal reflection, usually adjacent to the thoracic aorta [10,19] (Fig. 13-6). Azygos continuation of the inferior vena cava should be consistently recognized as a large paravertebral retrocardiac venous structure.

Anomalous Pulmonary Venous Connection

Normal pulmonary venous entry into the left atrium can be consistently imaged by comprehensive TEE examination [2,3,21] (see Chapter 4) (Fig. 13-7). These normal connections should be understood and sought with every complete TEE examination.

The most common form of partial anomalous connection is commitment of the right upper pulmonary vein to the right superior vena cava [10,22] (Fig. 13-8). This anomaly is best visualized by use of the horizontal transducer plane. The endoscope is withdrawn to the level of the right pulmonary artery to consistently image this anomaly. The anomalous

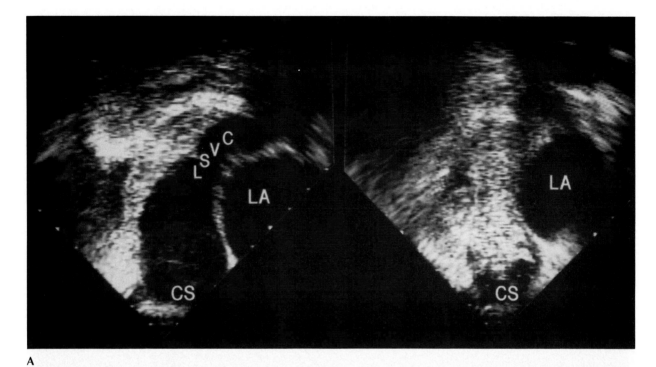

A

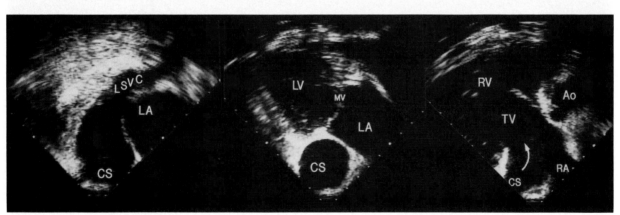

B

Fig. 13-5.   Longitudinal scan of a persistent left superior vena cava. A, Left. This long-axis scan is obtained from midesophagus with far leftward rotation of the endoscope shaft to the lateral wall of the heart. The left superior vena cava courses anteriorly over the left atrium and ultimately enters the coronary sinus, which then empties into the right atrium. Right. After left upper extremity venous injection of echocontrast material, the left superior vena cava becomes opacified. B. Longitudinal scan of left superior vena cava with slow rotation of the array from the lateral wall of the heart *(left panel)* rightward to the mitral atrioventricular groove and dilated coronary sinus *(middle panel)*, which finally empties *(curved arrow)* into the right atrium just superior to the tricuspid valve *(right panel)*.

vein appears as a vessel entering the medial wall of the superior vena cava (Fig. 13-9). Color-flow Doppler examination is very helpful in confirming the entry of turbulent blood into the medial superior vena cava.

The connection of an anomalous right inferior pulmonary vein can vary. The vein may enter the inferior vena cava, lateral wall of the right atrium, superior aspect of the right atrium, or directly into the superior vena cava. Biplanar TEE is usually necessary to completely elucidate this variable connection.

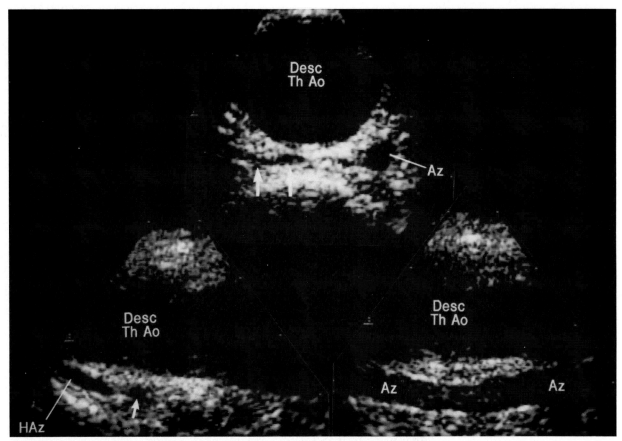

Fig. 13-6. Azygos veins. The azygos and hemiazygos veins course posterior and adjacent to the thoracic aorta. Top. Short axis of the thoracic aorta as though looking down the lumen (anterior, top; right, viewer's right). In the midthorax, the azygos vein is largest. Bridging veins *(arrows)* from the hemiazygos vein cross posterior to the descending thoracic aorta *(Desc Th Ao)* to communicate with the azygos vein. Bottom left. Long axis of the hemiazygos vein and a crossing vein *(large arrow)*. Bottom right. Long axis of the azygos vein posterior to the aorta. This image can be confused with an aortic dissection or hematoma.

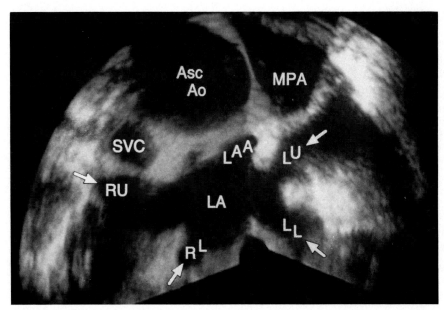

Fig. 13-7. Wide-field view [18] demonstration of all four pulmonary veins and the surrounding anatomy. This is a composite image acquired with the transverse plane. The esophageal transducer is posterior to the left atrium. All four pulmonary veins enter the left atrium *(arrows)*. Note the position of the left atrial appendage (i.e., leftward and anterior) relative to the left upper pulmonary vein. Anteriorly, the superior vena cava, ascending aorta, and main pulmonary artery are cut in short axis.

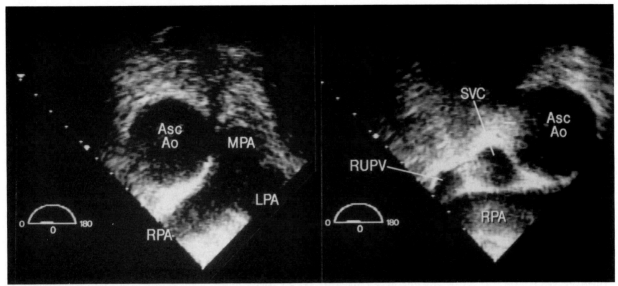

Fig. 13-8. Right upper pulmonary vein. The transducer array is in the transverse orientation (0 degrees multiplane array orientation). The endoscope shaft is withdrawn to the level of the pulmonary bifurcation *(left panel)*. The endoscope shaft is then rotated rightward to visualize the superior vena cava, which lies rightward and adjacent to the ascending aorta and anterior to the right pulmonary artery. Further to the right and adjacent to the superior vena cava is the hilar portion of the right upper pulmonary vein *(right panel)*. If the right upper pulmonary vein were connected anomalously to the superior vena cava, the abnormal communication would typically be visualized at this level.

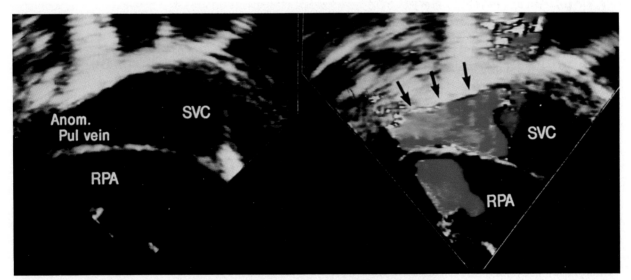

Fig. 13-9. Partial anomalous pulmonary venous connection of the right upper and middle pulmonary veins to the right superior vena cava. The scans are obtained with the transverse plane and the endoscope withdrawn to the level of the right pulmonary artery. Left. Short-axis scan of the superior vena cava, which lies to the right of the ascending aorta and anterior to the right pulmonary artery. Note that the anomalous right pulmonary vein *(Anom Pul vein)* enters the medial aspect of the superior vena cava. Right. Color-flow Doppler study (the polarity of the color signal has been reversed to improve appreciation) shows the pulmonary venous flow into the superior vena cava *(arrows)*. The patient also had a sinus venosus atrial septal defect (not shown).

Anomalous connection of the left pulmonary veins can be difficult to appreciate because of the proximity of the venous orifices to the left atrial wall and TEE transducer within the esophagus. Newer, high-frequency (7 MHz) transducers permit more accurate delineation of near-field anatomy. The anomalous connecting left upper pulmonary vein usually enters a vertical vein adjacent to the left atrial cavity. It is important to document a venous orifice into the left atrial cavity. If this cannot be demonstrated, further assessment may be necessary, including suprasternal surface echocardiography. If anomalously connected, the left inferior pulmonary vein is usually associated with an anomalous connection of the left upper pulmonary vein. Direct communication with other structures, such as the coronary sinus, should be delineated with biplane TEE.

Total anomalous pulmonary venous connection has been studied too infrequently to permit a confident discussion (Fig. 13-10). However, TEE can be an effective diagnostic modality by visualizing a venous confluence receiving pulmonary veins posterior to the left atrium.

Atrial Septum

The atrial septum is consistently visualized with TEE, but a complete examination is best performed with a biplanar instrument [3,4] (Fig. 13-11). With a single planar TEE instrument, it is estimated that 10% to 15% of the atrial septal defects are incompletely or inadequately visualized.

Common congenital anomalies confined to the atrial septum include patent valve of the fossa ovalis, atrial septal aneurysm, and atrial septal defect. The membrane of the fossa ovalis and potentially patent foramen ovale are most consistently imaged with the longitudinal plane [3] (Fig. 13-12, 13-13, and 13-14). In the longitudinal plane, the membrane of the fossa ovalis is visualized coursing posterior to the superior fatty limbus of the atrial septum, which is just posterior to the orifice of the superior vena cava [3]. When the valve of the fossa ovalis is patent, the fossal membrane is separated from the superior fatty limbus (Fig. 13-15). Color-flow Doppler examination is best suited for detection of left-to-right shunt, and contrast echocardiography is best suited

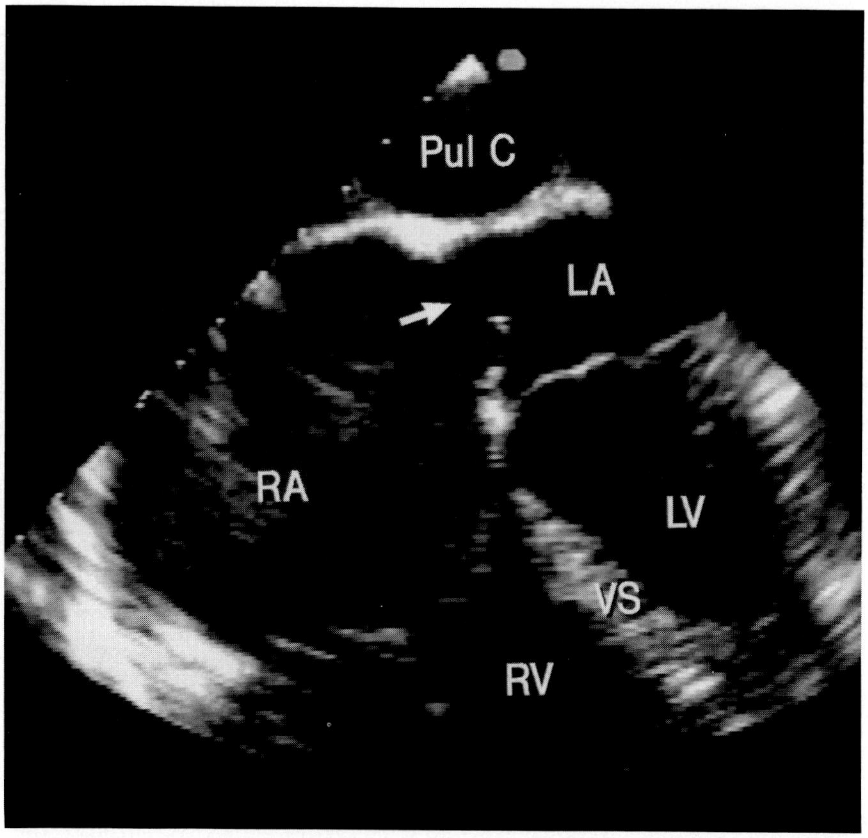

Fig. 13-10. Total anomalous pulmonary venous connection. Four-chamber view is obtained from midesophagus with retroflexion of the transverse plane. The cardiac chamber adjacent to the esophageal transducer (i.e., posterior) represents the pulmonary venous confluence *(Pul C)*. This confluence is connected to an extracardiac left vertical vein, which ultimately communicates with the right superior vena cava and right atrium. The dilated right atrium communicates with the left atrium through an atrial septal defect *(arrow)*. Chest radiographs in such patients often have a "snowman" appearance.

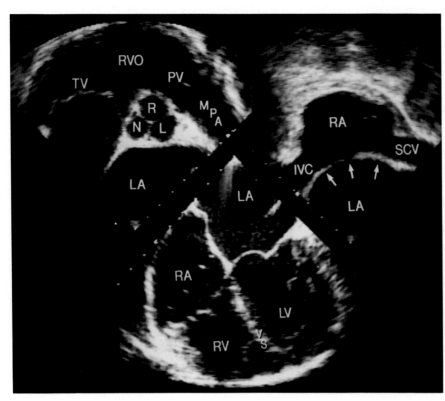

Fig. 13-11. Atrial septum. The atrial septum can be imaged in all three primary planes. Top left. Short axis. This image was obtained by multiplane TEE with the transverse array oriented to 45 degrees, which is short axis to the aortic valve. The esophageal transducer is posterior to the left atrium. The atrial septum originates just inferior to the noncoronary cusp of the aortic valve. Anteriorly, the tricuspid valve, right ventricular outflow, pulmonary valve *(PV)*, and main pulmonary artery encircle the aortic valve. Top right. Longitudinal scan of the atrial septum *(arrows)*. Note the central membranous portion of the atrial septum and the more fatty (thicker) superior and inferior limbus. The right atrium receives the superior and inferior venae cavae. Bottom. Four-chamber plane. Image is obtained from midesophagus with the transverse plane retroflexed. The atrial septum separates the right and left atria. (*L = left coronary cusp; N = noncoronary cusp; R =* right coronary cusp.)

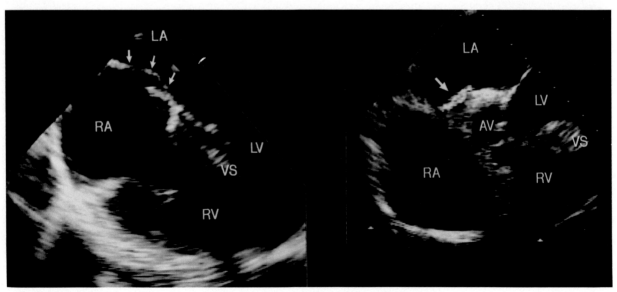

Fig. 13-12. Patent foramen ovale with color-flow Doppler demonstration of left-to-right shunt. Left. Four-chamber view showing a thin, mobile, membranous portion of the atrial septum *(arrows)*. Right. Color-flow Doppler image shows a mosaic signal *(arrow)* in the superior atrial septum. This is consistent with a small left-to-right shunt across a patent foramen ovale.

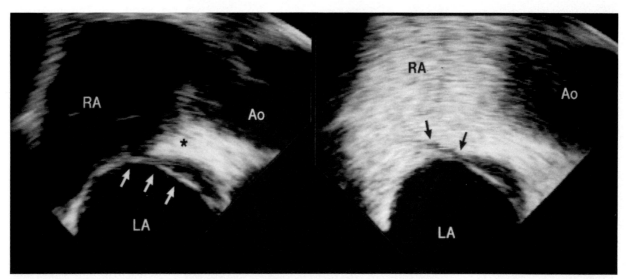

Fig. 13-13. Patent foramen ovale with small left-to-right shunt demonstrated with contrast echocardiography. Left. Longitudinal scan of the atrial septum and the thin valve of the fossa ovalis *(arrows)*. Superiorly, the valve courses posterior to the fatty tissue *(asterisk)* beneath the aortic root (i.e., fatty limbus of the atrial septum). The atrial septum separates right and left atria. Right. After an upper extremity venous injection of echocontrast material, the right atrium becomes densely opacified. Through a patent foramen ovale (the communication bounded by the membrane of the fossa ovalis posteriorly and fatty limbus anteriorly), there is a small left-to-right shunt with a resultant negative contrast effect *(arrows)* in the opacified right atrium.

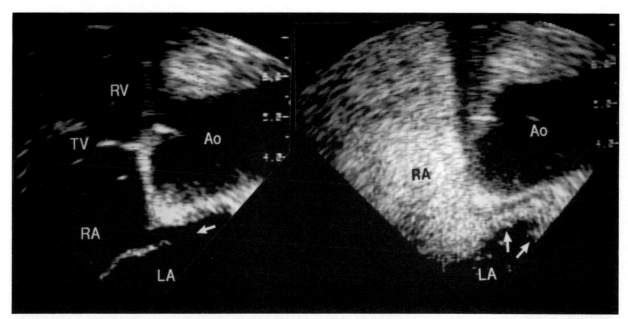

Fig. 13-14. Patent foramen ovale with right-to-left shunt in a desaturated patient with pulmonary hypertension. Left. Longitudinal scan of the atrial septum and a patent foramen ovale *(arrow)*, which allows free communication between right and left atria. The patent foramen ovale is just posterior to the aortic root. Right. After an upper extremity injection of echocontrast medium, the right atrium is densely opacified. Right-to-left shunting *(arrows)* occurs through the patent foramen ovale into the left atrium.

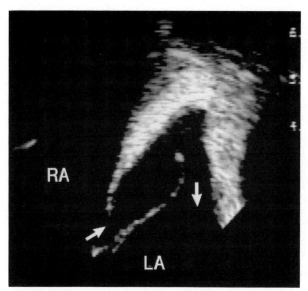

Fig. 13-15. Widely patent foramen ovale *(arrows)* in a cyanotic patient with primary pulmonary hypertension and secondary opening of the foramen. (This is a longitudinal scan of the atrial septum with the endoscope tip in the midesophagus.)

for right-to-left shunt detection across the atrial septum (Fig. 13-16).

Aneurysm of the atrial septum is defined as an excursion of the membrane of the fossa ovalis in excess of 1.5 cm [23] (Fig. 13-17 and 13-18). Frequently, an atrial septal defect or a patent foramen ovale is associated.

Atrial Septal Defect

In the adult patient, most atrial septal defects [24–29] are either imaged or suspected by transthoracic echocardiographic examination [30,31]. The sinus venosus atrial septal defect is the most commonly missed or incompletely elucidated atrial septal defect by transthoracic echocardiographic examination. Doppler and contrast echocardiography, as well as color-flow imaging, have helped considerably in the diagnosis of the sinus venosus defect [31].

Sinus Venosus Atrial Septal Defect

Approximately 30% of sinus venosus defects are undetected or incompletely assessed by precordial examination. Transesophageal echocardiography is extremely effective as a diagnostic procedure and in our experience has confidently diagnosed sinus venosus defect in 100% of patients [26,32]. Additionally, the associated partial anomalous pulmonary venous connections are usually fully elucidated (see

Fig. 13-9). The defect is best appreciated with the longitudinal imaging plane as an absence of the superior fatty limbus of the atrial septum just beneath the orifice of the superior vena cava and just inferior to the right pulmonary artery (Fig. 13-19). Conversely, the associated anomalous pulmonary venous connection of the right pulmonary veins is best imaged with the transverse plane at the level of the right pulmonary artery (see Fig. 13-9).

The sinus venosus atrial septal defect can also be visualized in basal short-axis scans (Fig. 13-20 and 13-21). In the transverse plane, the right atrial wall and orifice of the superior vena cava are centered. The endoscope is slowly withdrawn while the cava is kept continuously in view. Withdrawal continues until the right pulmonary artery is fully in view. The medial wall of the superior vena cava is observed to be incomplete; with color-flow Doppler technique, the flow of the anomalous pulmonary vein into the superior vena cava can be appreciated. This is the typical entry of an anomalous right middle and upper lobe pulmonary vein. Lower pulmonary veins usually enter at a lower level at the caval atrial junction or posterolateral wall of the right atrium. These anomalous pulmonary venous connections usually can be recognized by a thorough TEE examination.

Secundum and Primum Atrial Septal Defects

The secundum atrial septal defect and primum atrial septal defect are usually diagnosed confidently by transthoracic examination [30]. However, TEE is an excellent complement if the diagnosis is incomplete or further anatomic or hemodynamic assessment is deemed necessary. The anatomic details of both secundum (Fig. 13-22 through 13-26) and primum (Fig. 13-27 and 13-28) atrial septal defect are uniformly visualized by TEE. In a large prospective series at the Mayo Clinic, biplane TEE was diagnostic for atrial septal defect in virtually 100% of patients and reduced the incidence of needed cardiac catheterization to nearly zero [32]. Because the pulmonary artery pressure can be measured noninvasively by Doppler imaging [33], a complete hemodynamic and anatomic evaluation of atrial septal defect by precordial echocardiography and complementary TEE can be obtained in nearly every patient. Cardiac catheterization for diagnosis and hemodynamic assessment of atrial septal defect is now deemed unnecessary in most patients.

Fig. 13-16. Color-flow Doppler image of a patent foramen ovale with small left-to-right shunt. A. Longitudinal scan plane in mid-esophagus with rightward rotation of the endoscope shaft to view the long axis of the atrial septum. The membrane of the fossa ovalis *(arrows)* courses posterior to the superior fatty limbus of the atrial septum. The superior vena cava, right atrium, and right atrial appendage are cut in long axis. The eustachian valve *(arrowhead)* is near the orifice of the inferior vena cava. The right pulmonary artery, cut in short axis, courses posterior to the superior vena cava. B. A color-flow Doppler jet *(arrows)* shows a left-to-right shunt across the patent foramen ovale.

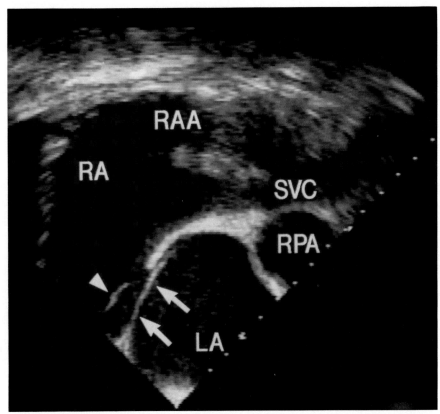

A

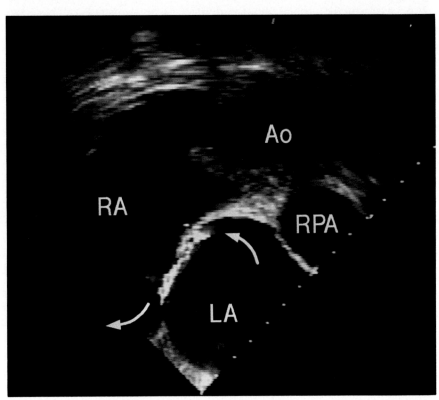

B

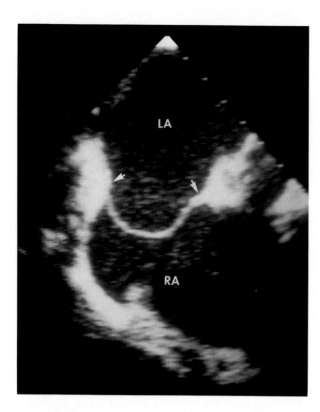

Fig. 13-17. Aneurysm of the atrial septum. This is a four-chamber view of the left and right atria with the cardiac apex down (and to the viewer's right). The transverse scan plane from midesophagus was used. The atrial septal aneurysm *(arrows)* bulges into the right atrial cavity.

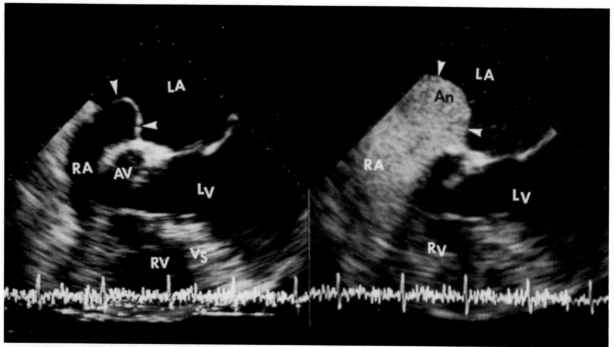

Fig. 13-18. Atrial septal aneurysm bulging into the left atrial cavity. This is a transverse scan plane with the tip retroflexed into the four-chamber view and the cardiac apex oriented downward (to the viewer's right). Left. An aneurysm of the membranous atrial septum *(arrowheads)*. Right. After an upper extremity injection of echocontrast material, the right atrium and aneurysm *(arrowheads)* become densely opacified. This patient did not have a shunt at the atrial level.

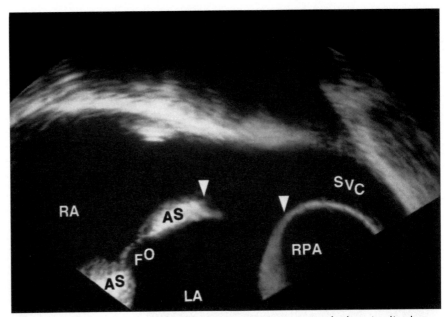

Fig. 13-19. Sinus venosus atrial septal defect. This is a wide-field composite image [18] of a longitudinal scan along the axis of the superior and inferior venae cavae. The esophageal transducer is adjacent to the posterior wall of the left atrium. Note the large atrial septal defect *(arrowheads)* in the superior fatty limbus of the atrial septum. The superior margin of the defect is the right pulmonary artery, which in this patient shows marked volume overload (dilated). There is no fatty limbus beneath the orifice of the superior vena cava. The inferior margin of the defect is the atrial septum. The membranous atrial septum (i.e., fossa ovalis) and superior and inferior fatty atrial septum remain intact and contiguous. The anterior right atrium is dilated (i.e., volume overload).

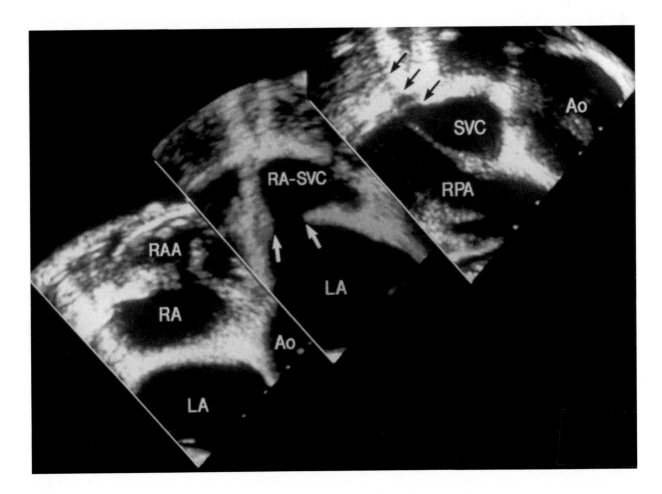

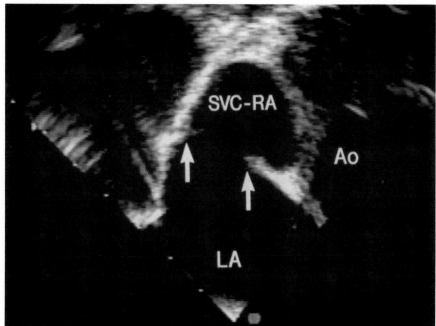

Fig. 13-21. Sinus venosus atrial septal defect. Short axis scan (midesophageal transducer, horizontal plane, withdrawn to the high atrial level just below the superior vena cava at the caval-atrial junction [*SVC-RA*]). A. The transducer is posterior to the left atrium. Note the typical sinus venosus atrial septal defect *(arrows)* between the left atrium and the right atrial caval-atrial junction. B. Color-flow Doppler study (the color polarity has been reversed to better illustrate the atrial septal defect left-to-right shunt) (i.e., left atrium to caval-atrial junction). (*Ao* = ascending aorta)

A

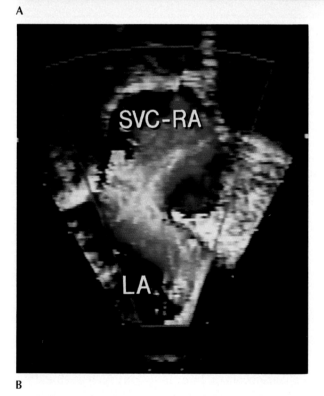

B

◀ **Fig. 13-20.** Short-axis scan to a sinus venosus atrial septal defect and partial anomalous pulmonary venous connection (view from left to right). These images were obtained with the transverse image plane, gentle anteflexion of the endoscope tip for improved esophageal contact, and slow withdrawal of the endoscope from the right atrial level *(lower left)* to the right pulmonary artery level *(upper right)*. Lower left. The esophageal transducer is posterior to the left atrium. The upper atrial septum and right atrium are imaged just beneath the caval-atrial junction. The right atrial appendage is anterior, and the short axis of the aorta is to the patient's left. Middle. In the high right atrium at the caval-atrial junction, there is a sinus venosus atrial septal defect *(arrows)*. This is the typical position of a sinus venosus atrial septal defect (i.e., high in the atrial septum just beneath the superior vena cava). Upper right. The endoscope has been further withdrawn to the level of the right pulmonary artery (imaged in its long axis). The superior vena cava, instead of being round, has a vascular structure entering its upper medial aspect *(arrows)*. This is the entry of the right upper and, probably, middle pulmonary veins into the superior vena cava (i.e., anomalous pulmonary venous connection).

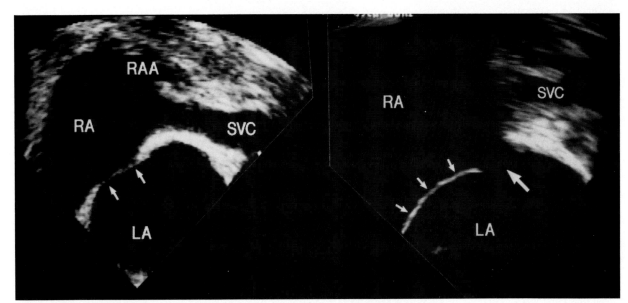

Fig. 13-22. Longitudinal scans of the intact atrial septum *(left)* and secundum atrial septal defect *(right)*. Left. Long-axis scan of the atrial septum is obtained from midesophagus with the longitudinal scan plane. The esophageal transducer is posterior and adjacent to the left atrium. The right atrium, right atrial appendage, and superior vena cava are anterior. The atrial septum has a central membranous portion (i.e., membrane of the fossa ovalis) *(arrows)* and a superior and inferior thicker (refractile) fatty limbus. Right. Secundum atrial septal defect *(large arrow)* in the superior membranous *(small arrows)* atrial septum. A small portion of the superior fatty limbus persists below the superior vena cava. This observation rules out a sinus venosus atrial septal defect.

Coronary Sinus Atrial Septal Defect

The infrequently encountered coronary sinus atrial septal defect [1] can be diagnosed by TEE (Fig. 13-29). The typical feature is an unroofed coronary sinus. The unroofed portion of the coronary sinus creates a communication between the left atrium and the coronary sinus. Blood then shunts into the right atrium through the orifice of the coronary sinus.

Atrial Cavity Membranes

Membranous structures within either the right or the left atrium are often incompletely assessed or missed by precordial echocardiographic examination. Transesophageal echocardiography has been shown to be a superior diagnostic modality for the morphologic assessment of cor triatriatum (Fig. 13-30 and 13-31), redundant or obstructing eustachian valve (Fig. 13-32), and supravalvular mitral ring [10].

Atrioventricular Valves

Many congenital anomalies of the atrioventricular valves can be diagnosed or further clarified by TEE (Fig. 13-33). Detailed crux anatomy, chordal insertions, and degree of regurgitation have been added enhancements of TEE. In lesions such as straddling atrioventricular valve [35] (Fig. 13-34) and Ebstein's anomaly [36] (Fig. 13-35), knowledge of chordal and atrioventricular valve anatomy is essential to surgical decisions. Transesophageal echocardiography is ideally suited for detailed anatomic delineation of these anomalies. When combined with continuous- and pulsed-wave Doppler hemodynamic assessment, TEE becomes an excellent extension of a comprehensive surface echocardiographic examination.

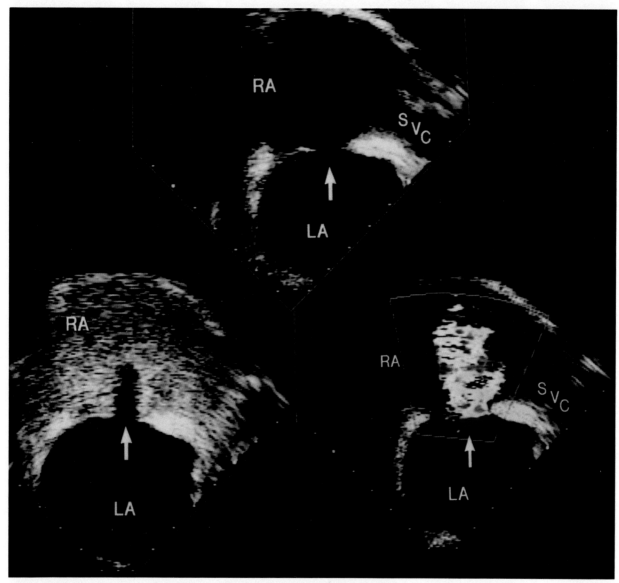

Fig. 13-23. Secundum atrial septal defect with contrast and color-flow echocardiographic study. These are longitudinal scans of the atrial septum from midesophagus. Top. Long-axis view of the atrial septum with a 1-cm atrial septal defect *(arrow)*. The transducer within the esophagus posterior and adjacent to the left atrium. Anteriorly, the right atrium and superior vena cava are visualized. Bottom left. After an upper extremity venous injection, the right atrium is densely opacified. Left-to-right shunt *(arrow)* across the atrial septal defect appears as a negative contrast effect in the right atrium. Bottom right. Color-flow Doppler study shows left-to-right shunt *(arrow)* across the same atrial septal defect.

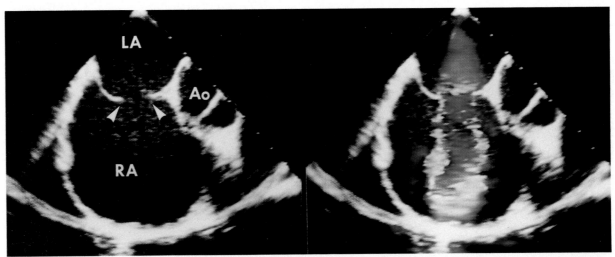

Fig. 13-24. Secundum atrial septal defect visualized in the four-chamber plane with cardiac apex down (apex is to the viewer's right). These views were obtained in the transverse plane, and the endoscope tip was retroflexed in the midesophagus to obtain a four-chamber view. Left. A secundum atrial septal defect *(arrowheads)* in the middle of the atrial septum permits communication between left and right atria. A portion of the ascending aorta is also visualized. Right. Color-flow Doppler image. The color polarity has been reversed (i.e., red away) to permit a more vivid appearance of the shunt from left atrium to right atrium (i.e., left-to-right shunt).

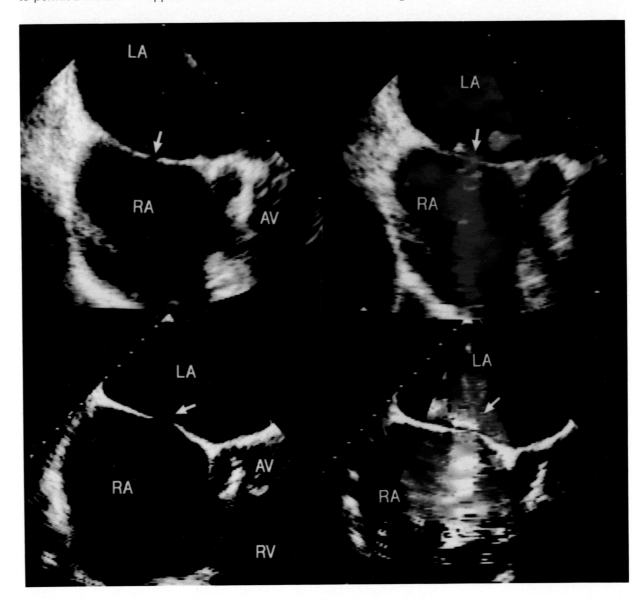

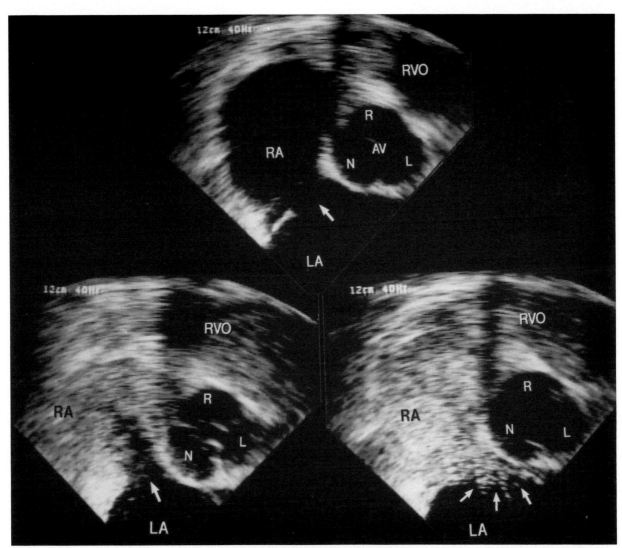

Fig. 13-26. Secundum atrial septal defect with left-to-right and right-to-left shunt. Short-axis scans of the aortic valve obtained by medial flexion of the longitudinal plane from midesophagus. Top. A large secundum atrial septal defect *(arrow)* is visualized in the middle of the atrial septum. Centrally, the aortic valve is visualized in short axis. Bottom left. After an upper extremity venous injection, the right atrium becomes densely opacified. Left-to-right shunt *(arrow)* appears as a negative effect in the right atrium. Bottom right. Transient right-to-left shunt *(arrows)* across the defect was intermittently associated with inspiration. (*L* = left coronary cusp; *N* = noncoronary cusp; *R* = right coronary cusp.)

◀ **Fig. 13-25.** Small secundum atrial septal defects. Two examinations were obtained in the four-chamber plane with the transverse array and retroflexion from the midesophagus. Top left. A 3-mm atrial septal defect *(arrow)* in the center of the membrane of the fossa ovalis. Top right. A small left-to-right shunt *(arrow)* is demonstrated with color-flow Doppler examination. Bottom left. A 15-mm atrial septal defect *(arrow)* in a patient with severe ischemic heart disease and dilated atria (this appearance could represent a stretched and patent foramen ovale). Bottom right. Color-flow Doppler study shows left-to-right shunting *(arrow)*. Transesophageal echocardiography is extremely sensitive for the diagnosis of even small atrial septal defects.

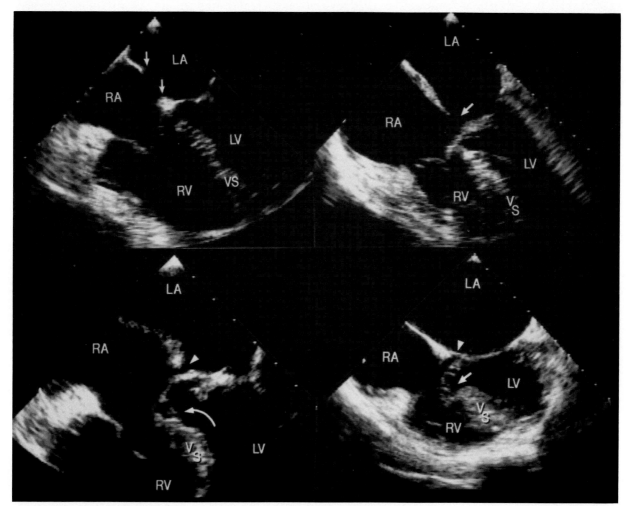

Fig. 13-27.   Primum atrial septal defect. All images are in the four-chamber plane; the midesophageal transducer position is used in the transverse plane. Top left. Low-lying atrial septal defect *(arrows)*. Because a small portion of the inferior fatty limbus is present, the defect might be called a secundum defect. However, the heart had other anatomic features consistent with atrioventricular canal (e.g., cleft mitral valve). Top right. Typical low-lying atrial septal defect *(arrow)* of the atrioventricular canal type (i.e., primum). Note that both septal portions of the atrioventricular valves insert at the same level to the crest of the ventricular septum. Bottom left. Primum atrial septal defect *(arrowhead)* with an inflow ventricular septal aneurysm *(arrow)*. There was no ventricular septal defect. This anatomy is typical of what has been called a transitional type of primum atrial septal defect. Bottom right. A more dramatic example of a transitional primum atrial septal defect *(arrowhead)* with associated inflow ventricular septal aneurysm *(arrow)*.

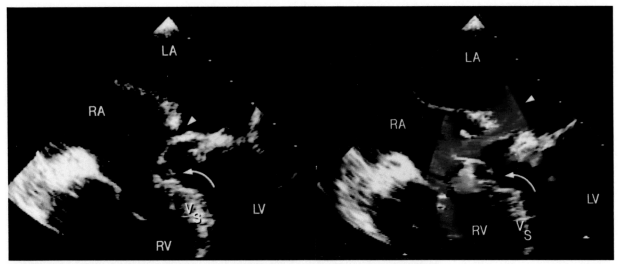

Fig. 13-28. Primum atrial septal defect with color-flow Doppler demonstration of left-to-right shunt (four-chamber plane). Left. Primum defect *(arrowhead)* in the low atrial septum. Note the inflow ventricular septal aneurysm *(arrow)*, which is typical of a transitional atrioventricular canal defect. Right. Color-flow Doppler image showing left-to-right shunt *(arrowhead; blue color)* across the primum atrial septal defect. Note that the ventricular septal aneurysm *(arrow)* has no color flow, a finding consistent with absence of a ventricular septal defect.

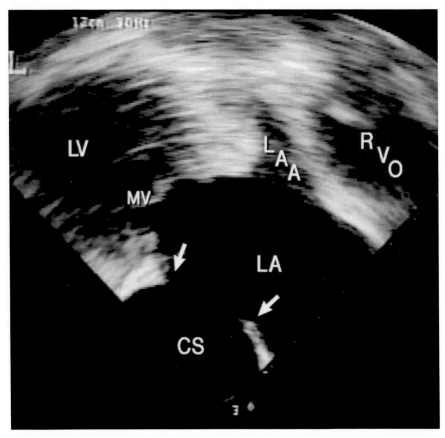

Fig. 13-29. Coronary sinus atrial septal defect. Longitudinal scan from midesophagus (i.e., two-chamber view of left ventricle and left atrium). Note the dilated coronary sinus posteriorly, adjacent to the esophageal transducer. The roof of the dilated coronary sinus has a large defect *(arrows)* that allows left atrial blood to enter the coronary sinus and subsequently cross into the right atrium (i.e., coronary sinus atrial septal defect).

Fig. 13-30. Cor triatriatum.
A. Four-chamber view. Within
the left atrium, a partially
obstructing membrane has an
orifice *(arrow)* connecting the
partitioned left atrial cavity.
B. Color-flow Doppler
examination shows
accelerated mosaic blood
(arrow) crossing the obstructing
membrane. The patient, a
young adult, has mild to
moderate atrial obstruction.

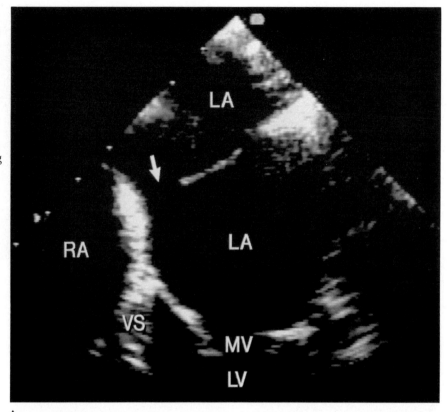

A

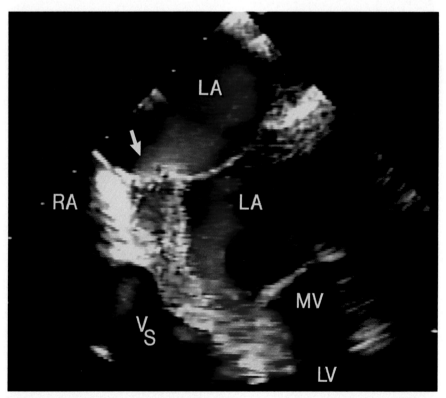

B

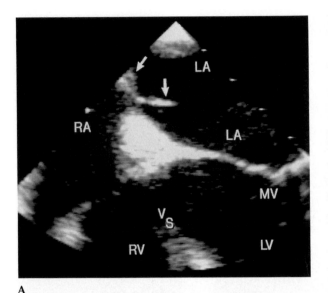

A

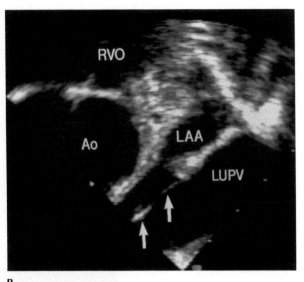

B

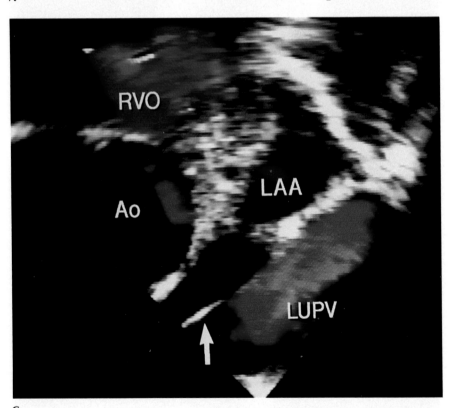

C

Fig. 13-31.   Forme fruste of cor triatriatum. A membranous remnant in the left atrium has been found in approximately 1 of 1,000 TEE examinations. The transverse plane is used with the transducer positioned in midesophagus. A. Retroflexion of the endoscope tip with an apex-down four-chamber view. Note that a small membrane *(arrows)* originates at the superior limbus of the fossa ovalis on the atrial septum. B. Short-axis scan at the base of the heart (anteflexion of the midesophageal transducer). Note that the esophageal transducer is posterior and adjacent to the left atrium. A membrane *(arrows)* crosses the left atrial cavity, originating from the common wall between the left upper pulmonary vein and the left atrial appendage. The membrane, if complete, would isolate the pulmonary veins posteriorly and the left atrial appendage and mitral valve inferoanteriorly (i.e., cor triatriatum). C. Color-flow Doppler study confirms blood flow from the left upper pulmonary vein into the posterior portion of the left atrial cavity. The membrane *(arrow)* at this level partitions the left atrial appendage from the left upper pulmonary vein. *(Ao* = ascending aorta)

Fig. 13-32.   Right atrial eustachian valve. The easiest and most confident means of visualizing and correctly recognizing a eustachian valve is with a longitudinal scan of the inferior and superior venae cavae. The valve originates from the anterior lip of the inferior vena cava. A. Longitudinal scan from midesophagus. From the anterior lip of the inferior vena cava is a small eustachian valve. This valve frequently has an undulating motion and may be confused with thrombus or tumor [34]. B. Another example of a longitudinal scan of superior and inferior venae cavae. Note the very long thin structure (eustachian valve, *arrows*) in the right atrial cavity. This membrane had a large excursion and by precordial examination could not be differentiated from thrombus. (*S* = superior)

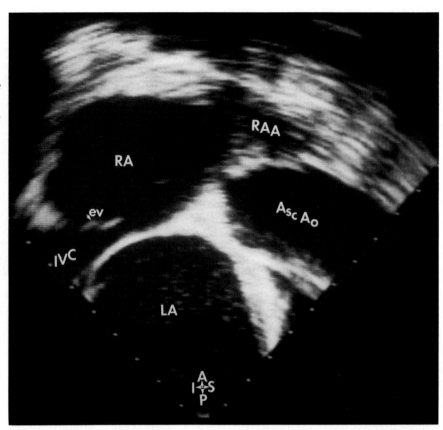

A

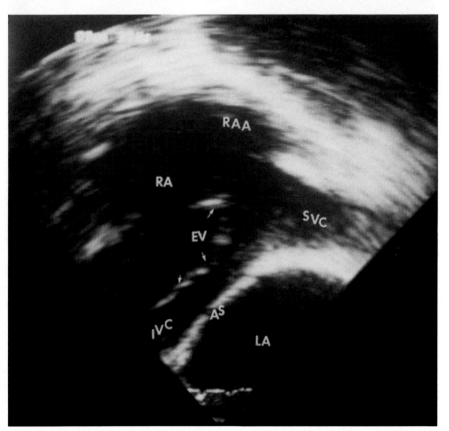

B

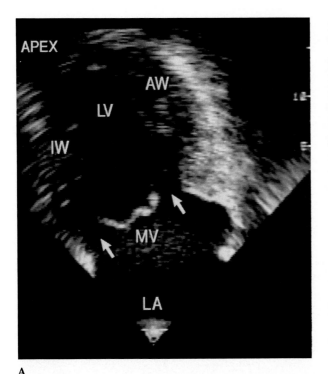
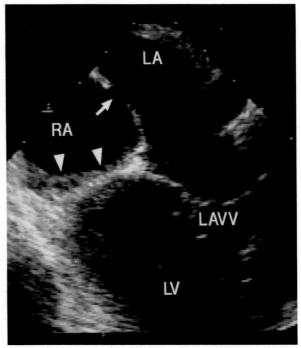

A **B**

Fig. 13-33. A. Double-orificed mitral valve. Transesophageal two-chamber view of left ventricle (longitudinal plane with leftward rotation of the endoscope shaft). Note the two orifices *(arrows)* of the mitral valve. This is a rare isolated congenital abnormality and is more commonly associated with atrioventricular canal defect. This patient had no other associations. B. Tricuspid valve atresia. Transesophageal four-chamber plane. In the floor of the right atrium, a band of tissue *(arrowheads)* represents an atretic tricuspid valve. An atrial septal defect *(arrow)* communicates from right atrium to left atrium. A single left atrioventricular valve *(LAVV)* empties the left atrium into a large left-sided ventricle. *(APEX* = left ventricular apex)

Ventricles and Ventricular Septum

The ventricular septum is consistently imaged; however, it has been stated that searching for the typical membranous ventricular septal defect can be one of the more challenging TEE examinations (Fig. 13-36 and 13-37). Multiplanar, high-frequency transducers and color-flow and contrast echocardiography all complement a complete anatomic assessment of ventricular septal defect (Fig. 13-38, 13-39, and 13-40). Most inflow and membranous ventricular septal defects are easily visualized. Small defects, particularly muscular defects in the body of the ventricle, are more difficult to image. Certainly, biplanar and multiplanar TEE devices greatly assist in the overall examination of the ventricular myocardium.

Semilunar Valves and Great Arteries

Both the aortic and the pulmonary valves are consistently imaged by TEE [37–39]. Biplanar and multiplanar transducers enhance the ability to make detailed anatomic and functional assessments with TEE. Number of cusps and degree of stenosis can be assessed by direct visualization as well as simultaneous Doppler hemodynamics (Fig. 13-41 and 13-42). Subaortic and supra-aortic stenoses are also consistently visualized (Fig. 13-43, 13-44, and 13-45).

Coarctation of the aorta is usually difficult to confidently image with TEE (see Chapter 14). The segment of the aorta involved with coarctation lies immediately adjacent to the left bronchus and thus

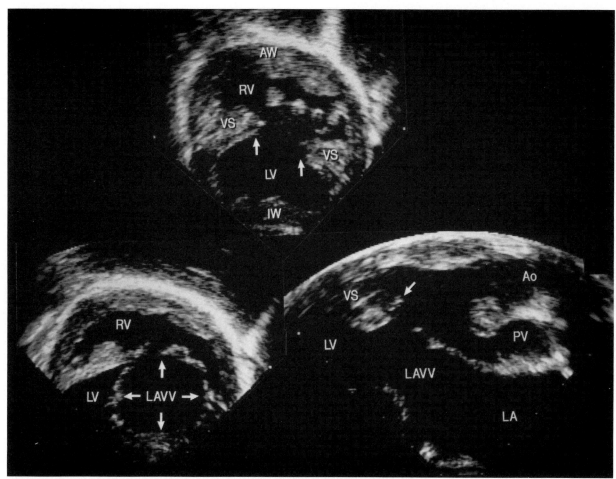

Fig. 13-34. Large ventricular septal defect and straddling atrioventricular valve. Top. Short-axis scan (transverse plane in low esophagus) at the midventricular level. A large ventricular septal defect *(arrows)* is visualized in the anterior ventricular septum. Only small lateral components of the ventricular septum remain. The two ventricles sit one above the other (i.e., over-under ventricles with the left ventricle posterior and the right ventricle anterior). Bottom left. A large left atrioventricular valve *(LAVV)* appears to cross the plane of the ventricular septum on this short-axis scan. Bottom right. The anterior leaflet or left atrioventricular valve clearly inserts into the ipsilateral ventricle *(arrow)*, a feature diagnostic of straddling atrioventricular valve. The great vessels are transposed (aorta, anterior, and pulmonary valve, posterior).

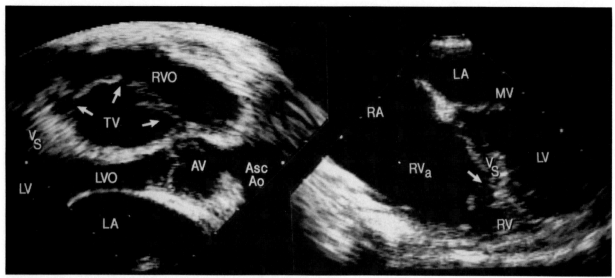

Fig. 13-35. Ebstein's anomaly. Left. Longitudinal long-axis scan of left ventricle. Note that the tricuspid valve *(arrows)* orifice is reoriented toward the dilated right ventricular outflow. The ventricular septum is pushed toward the left ventricular outflow. Right. Apex-down four-chamber view. The tricuspid valve septal leaflet *(arrow)* is displaced downward into the right ventricle. There is no evident anterior tricuspid valve leaflet, which is severely tethered to the underlying endocardium. The right atrium is markedly dilated. Note that most of the right ventricular cavity is atrialized *(RVa)*. Only a small apical remnant of right ventricle is evident in this projection.

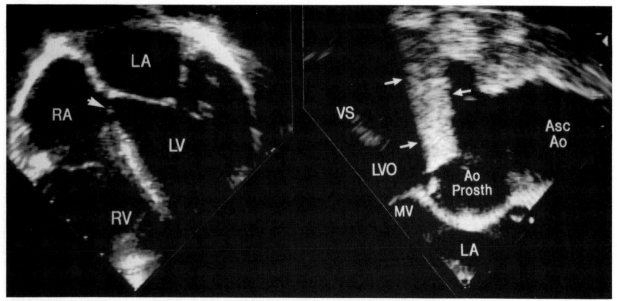

Fig. 13-36. Acoustic shadowing or reverberations across the ventricular septum can mimic a ventricular septal defect during a TEE examination. Left. Frequently in the four-chamber plane, the central fibrous body acoustically shadows the cardiac crux *(arrowhead)*, simulating a ventricular septal defect. Multiple scan projections and color-flow Doppler examination usually can resolve this common artifact. Right. Long-axis scan of the left ventricular outflow in a patient with an aortic prosthesis *(AoProsth)*. The prosthesis annulus can shadow *(arrows)* the anterior ventricular septum and either preclude the diagnosis or artifactually suggest the diagnosis of ventricular septal defect. Multiple off-axis and alternative scan planes usually can resolve this pitfall.

Fig. 13-37. Papillary muscle of the conus. The tricuspid valve normally inserts into the anterior ventricular septum (i.e., inserts onto the small papillary muscle of the conus *[arrows]*). With a ventricular septal defect and secondary hypertrophy of ventricular myocardium, this small papillary muscle can enlarge and confound a clear appreciation of a ventricular septal defect in the four-chamber plane. Using multiple imaging can alleviate this potential pitfall.

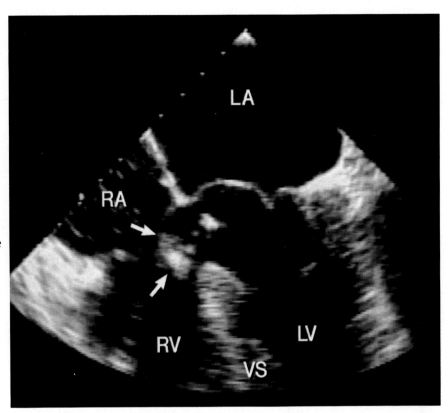

Fig 13-38. Membranous ventricular septum. Longitudinal array (90 degrees on a multiplane transducer) with the endoscope tip in the midesophagus. Medial (rightward) rotation of the endoscope shaft from the long-axis ascending aortic view toward the right ventricle. Just beneath the aortic valve cusp is the intact membranous ventricular septum *(arrow)*.

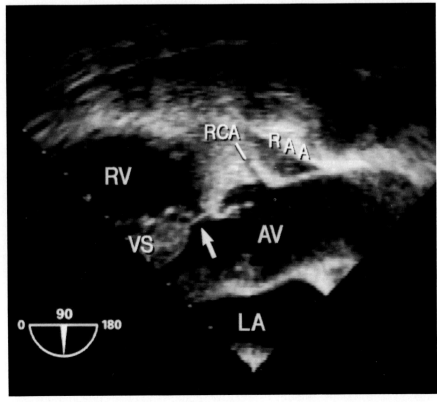

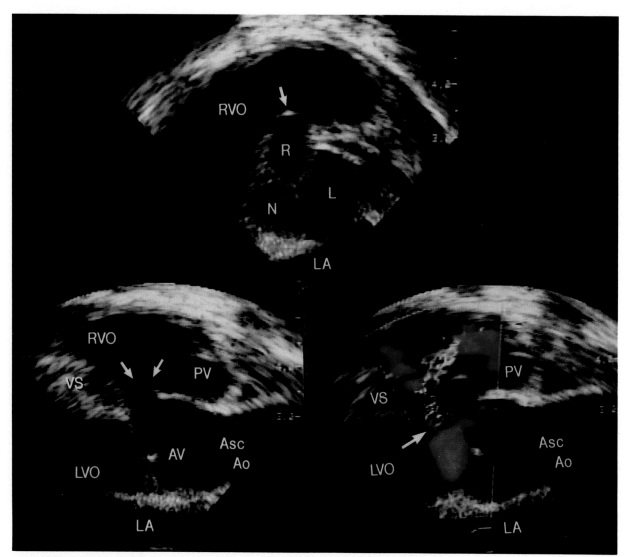

Fig. 13-39. Infundibular (subaortic) ventricular septal defect with prolapse of the right coronary aortic valve cusp. Top. Short-axis view of the aortic valve (transverse plane at midesophagus). The right coronary cusp *(R)* of the aortic valve prolapses into the right ventricular outflow *(arrow)*. Bottom left. Long-axis scan of the proximal ascending aorta (longitudinal plane). The right coronary aortic valve cusp prolapses *(arrows)* into the right ventricular outflow just beneath the pulmonary valve *(PV)*. Bottom right. Long-axis scan with color-flow Doppler imaging *(arrow)* demonstrates the associated small ventricular septal defect flow (the mosaic color represents flow through the defect) (L = left coronary cusp; N = noncoronary cusp.).

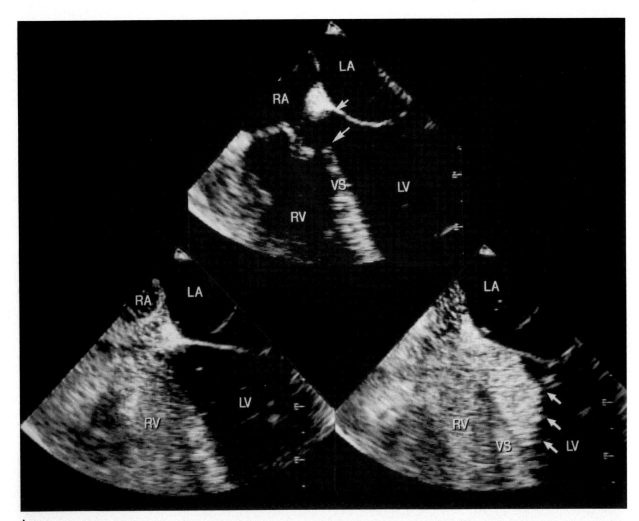

A

Fig. 13-40. Eisenmenger ventricular septal defect with right-to-left shunt. A. Four-chamber views (transverse plane with the TEE transducer in midesophagus) during a contrast echocardiographic study. Top. Questionable echo dropout *(arrows)* is seen at the crest of the ventricular septum. Bottom left. After an upper extremity echocontrast injection, the right-sided structures opacify. Bottom right. With the next diastole, the left ventricular outflow *(arrows)* opacifies, a result diagnostic of right-to-left shunt across a ventricular septal defect.

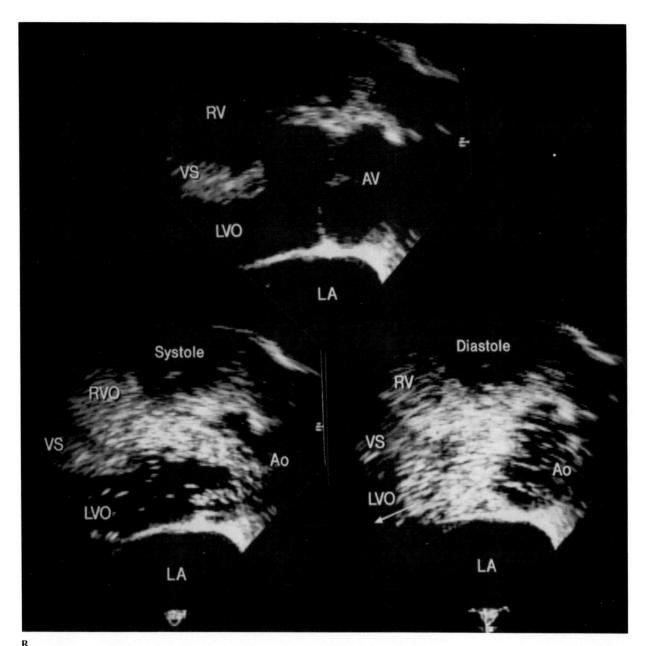

B

Fig. 13-40 (continued)   B, Top. Long-axis views of the left ventricular outflow (longitudinal scan plane with the transducer in midesophagus). Bottom left. During systole, the opacified right ventricular blood is ejected directly out the aorta (note that initially blood ejected from the right ventricle laminates along the anterior aortic wall). Bottom right. With the next diastole, blood captured beneath the aortic valve and in the right ventricular outflow crosses into the left ventricular outflow *(arrow)* (i.e., right-to-left shunt). This shunt pattern is diagnostic of a ventricular septal defect with significant increase in right heart pressures.

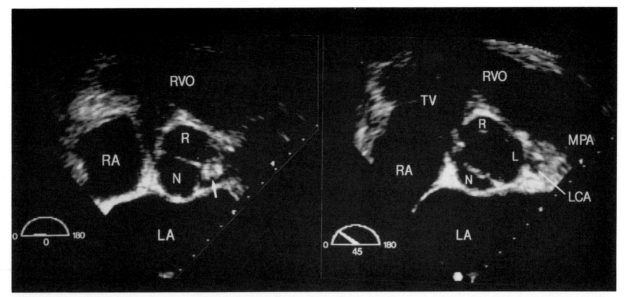

Fig. 13-41. Multiplane examination of aortic valve pseudomass. Left. Transducer array at 0 degrees results in an oblique view of the aortic valve. The left coronary cusp *(arrow)* of the aortic valve is cut in such a way that the belly of the sinus appears masslike. Right. The multiplane array is rotated to 45 degrees, a true short-axis orientation to the aortic valve. The left coronary cusp *(L)* and the proximal left coronary artery are normal. The multiplane examination permits a continuous visualization of contiguous anatomic structures, which helps avoid such potential misinterpretations of anatomy. (*N* = noncoronary cusp; *R* = right coronary cusp.)

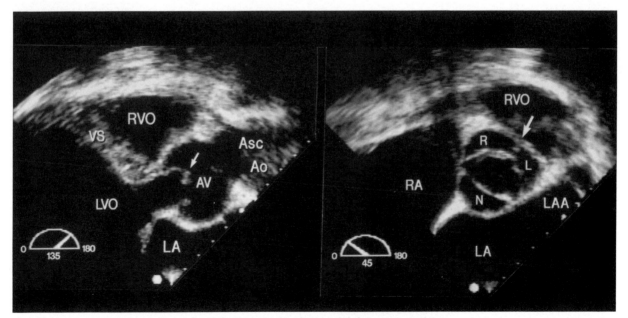

Fig. 13-42. Bicuspid aortic valve. Left. Longitudinal view of the aortic valve (135 degrees multiplane array orientation). Note that the valve is domed and thickened *(arrow)*. Right. Short-axis view of the aortic valve (45 degrees multiplane array orientation). There is fusion of the commissure between the right *(R)* and the left *(L)* aortic cusps *(arrow)*. The valve orifice extends from 10 o'clock to 5 o'clock, forming a typical bicuspid appearance. (*N* = noncoronary cusp)

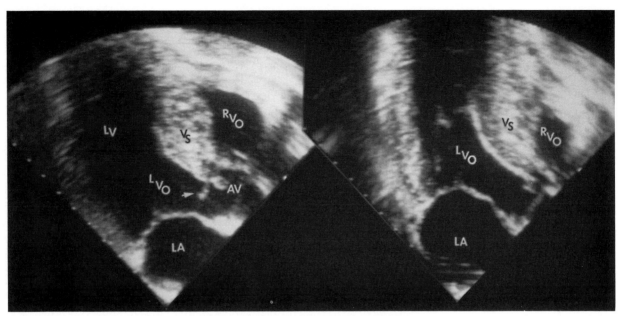

Fig. 13-43. Subaortic stenosis. Longitudinal scans of the left ventricular outflow. Scans were obtained with the transverse plane and lateral flexion of the endoscope tip (a maneuver that can be used to obtain long-axis views). Left. Long-axis scan of the left ventricular outflow. Note the discrete subaortic valve membrane *(arrow)*. The left ventricular myocardium is thickened, consistent with hypertrophy. Right. Postoperative echocardiographic view shows the successful surgical removal of the subaortic membrane.

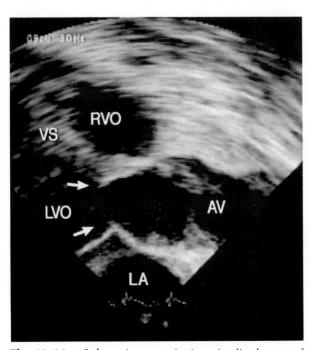

Fig. 13-44. Subaortic stenosis. Longitudinal scan of the left ventricular outflow. Note an encircling band *(arrows)* of tissue involving the ventricular septum and anterior leaflet of the mitral valve. This band produced moderately severe subaortic valve stenosis.

is often obscured by an air artifact. Similarly, patent ductus arteriosus, although it can frequently be imaged by TEE, can be a challenge because of the adjacent lung and bronchus.

Proximal pulmonary artery bifurcations can be consistently imaged by TEE examination. More distal pathologic features cannot be confidently imaged (see Chapter 4 for anatomic correlations).

INTRAOPERATIVE TEE FOR CONGENITAL HEART DISEASE

Transesophageal echocardiography, particularly in the pediatric population, has been predominantly limited to intraoperative (see Chapter 16) and immediate postoperative assessment of anatomic and functional details [11,40–43]. Transducers of smaller diameter and higher frequency have been used in the pediatric population [15,44]. Confirmation of anatomic detail has been markedly enhanced by simultaneous TEE examination (Fig. 13-46). Epicardial echocardiography has a still significant but decreasing role in the assessment of congenital heart

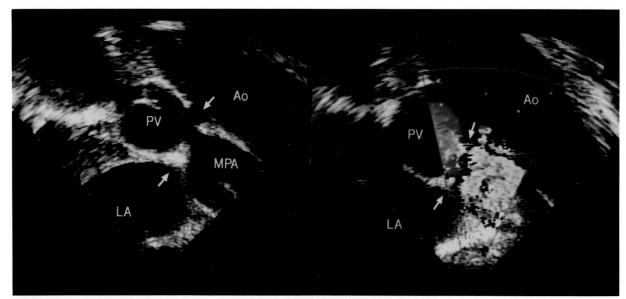

Fig. 13-45. Pulmonary artery band. Longitudinal scan in a patient with transposition of the great arteries (i.e., aorta is anterior to the pulmonary artery). Left. Within the main pulmonary artery just distal to the pulmonary valve *(PV)* is a constricting pulmonary artery band *(arrows)*. Right. Color-flow Doppler image shows acceleration of blood beginning at the pulmonary artery band *(arrows)*.

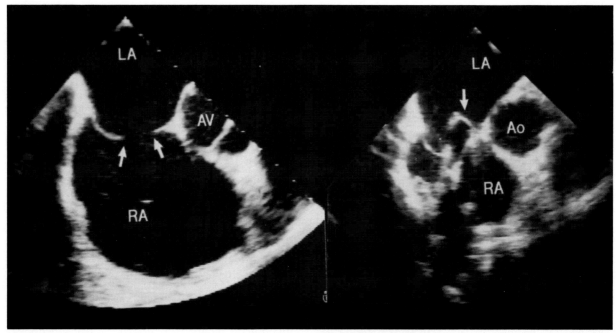

Fig. 13-46. Intraoperative TEE of an atrial septal defect. Left. Four-chamber view. Large secundum atrial septal defect *(arrows)* is visualized in the middle of the atrial septum. Right. At operation, the surgeon has placed a finger *(arrow)* across the defect to inspect its size and location.

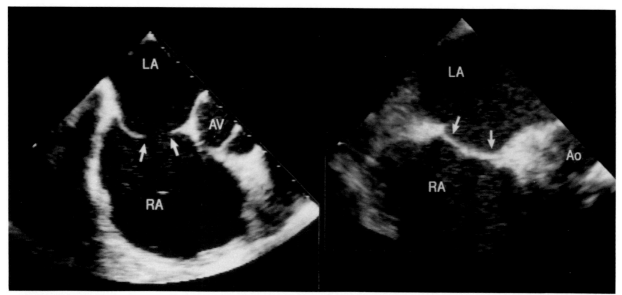

Fig. 13-47. Secundum atrial septal defect before *(left)* and after *(right)* operation. Left. Transverse plane in midesophagus in the four-chamber plane. A secundum atrial septal defect *(arrows)* in the middle of the atrial septum permits communication between left and right atria. Right. Postoperatively, the atrial septal defect has been closed by a patch *(arrows)*.

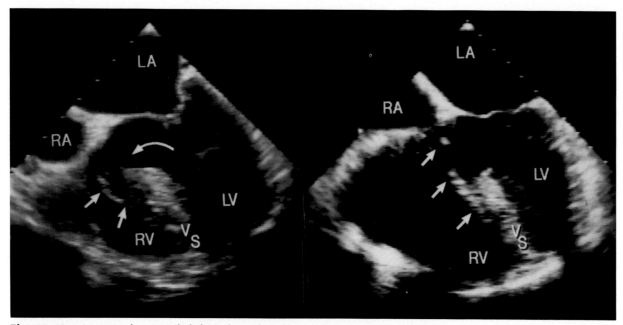

Fig. 13-48. Ventricular septal defect (four-chamber views, transverse plane). Left. Aneurysm of the membranous ventricular septum *(short arrows)*. Large aneurysm can appear as an undulating membrane beneath the aortic valve or in the high right ventricle. In the four-chamber plane, a deficiency of ventricular septal tissue *(curved arrow)* can often be appreciated. Right. Postoperative echocardiogram (different patient) in which a large ventricular septal defect has been closed with a patch *(arrows)*.

disease. Associated lesions that can easily be elucidated are residual atrial and ventricular septal defects, valvular regurgitation, structural or hemodynamic deterioration, and extraneous compression of cardiac structures causing hemodynamic compromise.

POSTOPERATIVE ASSESSMENT OF CONGENITAL HEART DISEASE

Transesophageal echocardiography can be used to excellent advantage in the postoperative period, both for immediate care and in long-term evaluation of congenital heart disease [40] (Fig. 13-47, 13-48, and 13-49). Because of the increased resolution of TEE, anatomy in and around prosthetic material is made clearer by the TEE examination. Residua and sequelae of congenital heart disease are frequent indications for TEE. In the critical care unit, TEE examination can be advantageous because the equipment can be brought to the bedside so that the patient need not be moved to an imaging or hemodynamic laboratory [17].

FUTURE

Transesophageal echocardiography has markedly expanded the role of diagnostic "comprehensive echocardiographic examination" of congenital heart disease. High-frequency, multiplanar endoscopes are becoming increasingly available [3,18,45,46]. Newer advances in digital technology will ultimately allow three-dimensional ultrasound reconstruction, which should enhance appreciation of congenital cardiovascular anomalies [47–49] (see Chapter 18) (Fig. 13-50). Increasingly, TEE is used for preoperative, intraoperative, and postoperative assessment of congenital heart disease. A comprehensive anatomic and hemodynamic examination includes a transthoracic echocardiographic examination and, if necessary (approximately 5% of patients), TEE. In

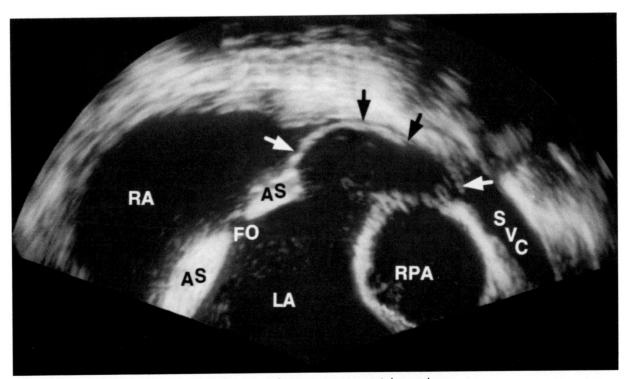

Fig. 13-49. Postoperative anatomy of corrected sinus venosus atrial septal defect and partial anomalous pulmonary venous connection. Wide-field [18] longitudinal scan. This long-axis scan of the superior vena cava is obtained from midesophagus in the longitudinal imaging plane. Note the surgical patch *(arrows)* that directs the blood from an anomalous right upper pulmonary vein (not shown) across the sinus venosus atrial septal defect. The superior vena cava is totally committed to the right atrium but must flow around the patch. *(FO = foramen ovale.)*

3D Image of Atrial Septal Defect from TEE Probe Rotation

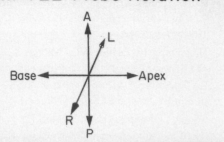

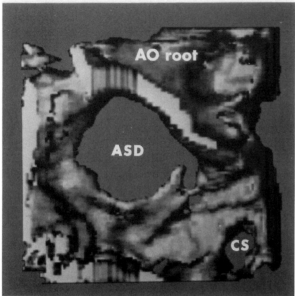

Fig. 13-50. Three-dimensional reconstruction of the atrial septum by TEE probe rotation in a patient with an atrial septal defect. The view is from the right atrial surface looking toward the left atrium. In the center of the atrial septum is a large ovoid secundum atrial septal defect. The orifice of the coronary sinus is visualized inferiorly, the aortic root anteriorly. Three-dimensional reconstruction is expected to enhance visualization of cardiovascular anatomy. Currently, TEE is an excellent means for obtaining appropriate sets of tomographic images that can be used to construct three-dimensional images. The example shown can help in the assessment of size, configuration, and anatomic relationships in planning closure. (*L* = left)

children younger than 10 to 12 years, general anesthesia is necessary. Thus, TEE examinations in children are preferably carried out in the cardiac catheterization laboratory, operating room, or intensive care unit. Application of TEE and other innovative ultrasound techniques is predicted to increasingly affect diagnosis and management in patients with congenital heart disease.

REFERENCES

1. Seward JB, Tajik AJ, Edwards WD, Hagler DJ. *Two-Dimensional Echocardiographic Atlas, Vol 1: Congenital Heart Disease.* New York: Springer-Verlag, 1987.

2. Seward JB, Khandheria BK, Oh JK, et al. Transesophageal echocardiography: technique, anatomic correlations, implementation, and clinical applications. *Mayo Clin Proc* 1988;63:649–80.

3. Seward JB, Khandheria BK, Edwards WD, et al. Biplanar transesophageal echocardiography: anatomic correlations, image orientation, and clinical applications. *Mayo Clin Proc* 1990;65:1193–213.

4. Seward JB, Khandheria BK, Freeman WK, et al. Multiplane transesophageal echocardiography: image orientation, examination technique, anatomic correlations, and clinical applications. *Mayo Clin Proc* 1993;68:523–51.

5. Currie PJ. Transesophageal echocardiography: intraoperative applications. *Echocardiography* 1989; 6:403–14.

6. Gussenhoven EJ, van Herwerden LA, Roelandt J, et al. Intraoperative two-dimensional echocardiography in congenital heart disease. *J Am Coll Cardiol* 1987;9:565–72.

7. Hsu Y-H, Santulli T Jr, Wong A-L, et al. Impact of intraoperative echocardiography on surgical management of congenital heart disease. *Am J Cardiol* 1991;67:1279–83.

8. Lam J, Neirotti RA, Nijveld A, et al. Transesophageal echocardiography in pediatric patients: preliminary results. *J Am Soc Echocardiogr* 1991;4:43–50.

9. Ritter SB. Transesophageal real-time echocardiography in infants and children with congenital heart disease. *J Am Coll Cardiol* 1991;18:569–80.

10. Seward JB, Tajik AJ. Transesophageal echocardiography in congenital heart disease. *Am J Card Imaging* 1990;4:215–22.

11. Stümper OFW, Elzenga NJ, Hess J, Sutherland GR. Transesophageal echocardiography in children with congenital heart disease: an initial experience. *J Am Coll Cardiol* 1990;16:433–41.

12. Weintraub R, Shiota T, Elkadi T, et al. Transesophageal echocardiography in infants and children with congenital heart disease. *Circulation* 1992;86: 711–22.

13. Santini F, Bonato R, Pittarello D, et al. Intraoperative transesophageal echocardiography during surgery for congenital heart disease. *Cardiovasc Imaging* 1992;4:127–32.

14. Fyfe DA, Ritter SB, Snider AR, et al. Guidelines for transesophageal echocardiography in children. *J Am Soc Echocardiogr* 1992;5:640–4.

15. Omoto R, Kyo S, Matsumura M, et al. Recent technological progress in transesophageal color Doppler flow imaging with special reference to newly developed biplane and pediatric probes. In: Erbel R, Khandheria BK, Brennecke R, et al. eds. *Transesophageal Echocardiography: A New Window to the Heart.* Berlin: Springer-Verlag, 1989;21–6.

16. Seward JB, Tajik AJ, Hagler DJ, Edwards WD. Internal cardiac crux: two-dimensional echocardiography of normal and congenitally abnormal hearts. *Ultrasound Med Biol* 1984;10:735–45.

17. Scott PJ, Blackburn ME, Wharton GA, et al. Transesophageal echocardiography in neonates, infants and children: applicability and diagnostic value in everyday practice of a cardiothoracic unit. *Br Heart J* 1992;68:488–92.

18. Seward JB, Khandheria BK, Tajik AJ. Wide-field transesophageal echocardiographic tomography: feasibility study. *Mayo Clin Proc* 1990;65:31–7.

19. Nanda NC, Pinheiro L, Sanyal R, et al. Transesophageal echocardiographic examination of left-sided superior vena cava and azygos and hemiazygos veins. *Echocardiography* 1991;8:731–40.

20. Podolsky LA, Jacobs LE, Schwartz M, et al. Transesophageal echocardiography in the diagnosis of the persistent left superior vena cava. *J Am Soc Echocardiogr* 1992;5:159–62.

21. Pinheiro L, Nanda NC, Jain H, Sanyal R. Transesophageal echocardiographic imaging of the pulmonary veins. *Echocardiography* 1991;8:741–8.

22. Weigel TJ, Seward JB, Hagler DJ. Transesophageal echocardiography in anomalous pulmonary and systemic venous connections (abstract). *Circulation* 1989;80 Suppl 2:II–339.

23. Hanley PC, Tajik AJ, Hynes JK, et al. Diagnosis and classification of atrial septal aneurysm by two-dimensional echocardiography: report of 80 consecutive cases. *J Am Coll Cardiol* 1985;6:1370–82.

24. Hanrath P, Schlüter M, Langenstein BA, et al. Detection of ostium secundum atrial septal defects by transesophageal cross-sectional echocardiography. *Br Heart J* 1983;49:350–8.

25. Morimoto K, Matsuzaki M, Tohma Y, et al. Diagnosis and quantitative evaluation of secundum-type atrial septal defect by transesophageal Doppler echocardiography. *Am J Cardiol* 1990;66:85–91.

26. Oh JK, Seward JB, Khandheria BK, Danielson GK, Tajik AJ. Visualization of sinus venosus atrial septal defect by transesophageal echocardiography. *J Am Soc Echocardiogr* 1988;1:275–7.

27. Mehta RH, Helmcke F, Nanda NC, et al. Transesophageal Doppler color flow mapping assessment of atrial septal defect. *J Am Coll Cardiol* 1990; 16:1010–6.

28. Kronzon I, Tunick PA, Freedberg RS, et al. Transesophageal echocardiography is superior to transthoracic echocardiography in the diagnosis of sinus venosus atrial septal defect. *J Am Coll Cardiol* 1991;17:537–42.

29. Hausmann D, Daniel WG, Mügge A, et al. Value of transesophageal color Doppler echocardiography for detection of different types of atrial septal defect in adults. *J Am Soc Echocardiogr* 1992;5:481–8.

30. Shub C, Dimopoulos IN, Seward JB, et al. Sensitivity of two-dimensional echocardiography in the direct visualization of atrial septal defect utilizing the subcostal approach: experience with 154 patients. *J Am Coll Cardiol* 1983;2:127–35.

31. Khandheria BK, Shub C, Tajik AJ, et al. Utility of color flow imaging for visualizing shunt flow in atrial septal defect. *Int J Cardiol* 1989;23:91–8.

32. Weigel TJ, Seward JB, Hagler DJ, et al. Transesophageal echocardiography in 21 atrial septal defect patients with incomplete precordial echocardiography (abstract). *Circulation* 1989;80 Suppl 2:II–474.

33. Currie PJ, Seward JB, Chan K-L, et al. Continuous wave Doppler determination of right ventricular pressure: a simultaneous Doppler-catheterization study in 127 patients. *J Am Coll Cardiol* 1985; 6:750–6.

34. Seward JB, Khandheria BK, Oh JK, et al. Critical appraisal of transesophageal echocardiography: limitations, pitfalls, and complications. *J Am Soc Echocardiogr* 1992;5:288–305.

35. Rice MJ, Seward JB, Edwards WD, et al. Straddling atrioventricular valve: two-dimensional echocardiographic diagnosis, classification and surgical implications. *Am J Cardiol* 1985;55:505–13.

36. Shiina A, Seward JB, Edwards WD, et al. Two-dimensional echocardiographic spectrum of Ebstein's anomaly: detailed anatomic assessment. *J Am Coll Cardiol* 1984;3:356–70.

37. Stümper O, Elzenga NJ, Sutherland GR. Obstruction of the left ventricular outflow tract in childhood—improved diagnosis by transoesophageal echocardiography. *Int J Cardiol* 1990;28:107–9.

38. Samdarshi TE, Morrow WR, Nanda NC, et al. Transesophageal echocardiography in aortopulmonary communications. *Echocardiography* 1991;8: 383–95.

39. Essop MR, Skudicky D, Sareli P. Diagnostic value of transesophageal versus transthoracic echocardiography in discrete subaortic stenosis. *Am J Cardiol* 1992;70:962–3.

40. Fyfe DA, Kline CH. Transesophageal echocardiography for congenital heart disease. *Echocardiography* 1991;8:573–84.

41. Cyran S, Kimball TR, Meyer RA, et al. Efficacy of intraoperative transesophageal echocardiography in children with congenital heart disease. *Am J Cardiol* 1989;63:594–8.

42. Muhiudeen IA, Roberson DA, Silverman NH, et al. Intraoperative echocardiography in infants and children with congenital cardiac shunt lesions: transesophageal versus epicardial echocardiography. *J Am Coll Cardiol* 1990;16:1687–95.

43. Stümper O, Fraser AG, Elzenga N, et al. Assessment of ventricular septal defect closure by intraoperative epicardial ultrasound. *J Am Coll Cardiol* 1990;16:1672–9.

44. Ritter SB, Thys D. Pediatric transesophageal color flow imaging: smaller probes for smaller hearts. *Echocardiography* 1989;6:431–40.

45. Flachskampf FA, Hoffman R, Hanrath P. Experience with a transesophageal echotransducer allowing full rotation of the viewing plane: the omniplane probe (abstract). *J Am Coll Cardiol* 1991;17:34A.

46. Hsu TL, Weintraub AR, Ritter SB, Pandian NG. Panoramic transesophageal echocardiography: clinical application of real-time, wide-angle, transesophageal two-dimensional echocardiography and color flow imaging. *Echocardiography* 1991;8:677–85.

47. Kuroda T, Kinter TM, Seward JB, et al. Accuracy of three-dimensional volume measurement using biplane transesophageal echocardiographic probe: in vitro experiment. *J Am Soc Echocardiogr* 1991;4:475–84.

48. Wollschläger H, Zeiher AM, Klein H-P, Kasper W, Wollschläger S, Just H. Transesophageal echo computer tomography: a new method for dynamic 3-D imaging of the heart (abstract). *J Am Coll Cardiol* 1989;13 Suppl A:68A.

49. Belohlavek M, Foley DA, Gerber TC, Kinter TM, Greenleaf JF, Seward JB. Three- and four-dimensional cardiovascular ultrasound imaging: a new era for echocardiography. *Mayo Clin Proc* 1993;68:221–40.

14

Diseases of the Thoracic Aorta

Assessment by Transesophageal Echocardiography

William K. Freeman

A vast spectrum of diseases of the thoracic aorta exists, ranging from aortic aneurysm with or without dissection to complications of atherosclerotic disease, such as intra-aortic debris or penetrating ulcer, to traumatic and congenital lesions. Traditionally, catheterization with contrast aortography has been used for the evaluation of many such aortic lesions, and more recently noninvasive imaging with computed tomography and magnetic resonance imaging has been used. Several diseases, in particular aortic dissection, are life-threatening, with acute clinical presentations that compel immediate diagnostic investigation. Transesophageal echocardiography (TEE) has emerged as a highly sensitive bedside modality to expedite such evaluation. In addition, TEE provides high-resolution delineation of numerous chronic thoracic aortic diseases.

Before the advent of TEE, transthoracic examination was the only means of ultrasound imaging of the thoracic aorta. The aortic root and proximal ascending aorta are usually readily visualized by transthoracic echocardiography through a variety of more cephalad left and occasionally right parasternal long- and short-axis windows [1,2]. Transthoracic delineation of the aortic arch, and especially of descending portions of the thoracic aorta, is generally much more challenging and may require painstaking two-dimensional imaging from multiple left and right high parasternal, infraclavicular, supraclavicular, and suprasternal windows [2–4], if they are available. Rarely, an excellent left posterolateral transthoracic window is opened by a significant left pleural effusion, allowing visualization of the descending thoracic aorta. Even with optimal windows, transthoracic echocardiography is usually limited to the gross detection of dissection, aneurysm, and, rarely, mural thrombus of the more distal thoracic aorta [5]. Because resolution is lost with far-field imaging, more subtle details of thoracic aortic disease are rarely visualized by the transthoracic approach.

Transesophageal echocardiography overcomes the multiple problems of acoustic impedance from the thoracic cage, lungs, and other mediastinal structures, vastly improving the resolution lost with far-field imaging, which typically limits transthoracic examination of the thoracic aorta.

ANATOMIC CORRELATIONS

Because the esophagus lies in close proximity to the thoracic aorta, especially the distal arch and the descending portion, imaging from this vantage point provides multiple outstanding echocardiographic windows for the delineation of aortic anatomy and abnormalities. The addition of the longitudinal plane [6,7] has markedly enhanced the imaging potential of earlier monoplane (transverse) TEE systems [8,9]. The multiple planes of the thoracic aorta available for transverse and longitudinal TEE imaging are shown in Figures 14-1 and 14-2, respectively (also see Chapter 3). The esophagus and aorta have an "intertwining" relationship within the mediastinum.

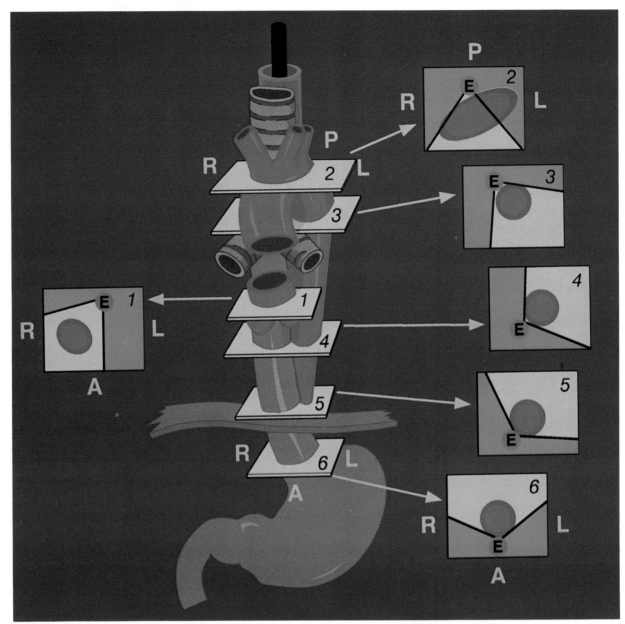

Fig.14-1. Transesophageal echocardiographic imaging of the thoracic aorta in the transverse plane. The proximal ascending aorta (plane 1), arch (plane 2), descending aorta (planes 3–5), and proximal abdominal aorta (plane 6) are shown in relation to the esophagus. The close, intertwining relationship of the aorta and esophagus is evident with orientation to the right of, to the left of, anterior to, and posterior to the patient, as shown.

Most proximally, the aortic arch is anterior to the upper esophagus; in the midthorax, these two structures are side-by-side; and in the lower chest, the distal esophagus is anterior to the distal thoracic aorta before they both traverse the diaphragm (Fig. 14-1). Depending on the patient's body habitus, approximate depths of TEE probe insertion from the incisors can be used to guide the localization of various portions of the aorta.

Aortic Root and Ascending Aorta

After introduction of the TEE probe into the esophagus, advancement to approximately 25 to 30 cm permits imaging of the aortic valve and root in transverse section (Fig. 14-3). Anteflexion and slow withdrawal of the TEE probe in the transverse plane allow visualization of the proximal ascending aorta, but images frequently become oblique and foreshort-

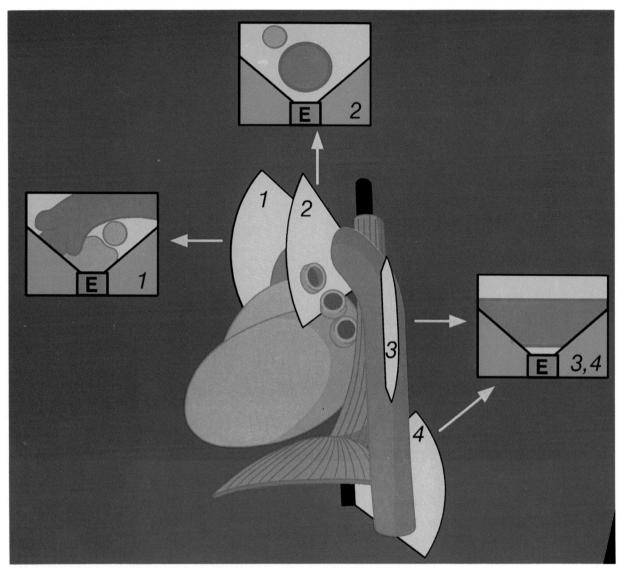

Fig. 14-2. Transesophageal echocardiographic imaging of the thoracic aorta in the longitudinal plane. The aortic valve, aortic root, and ascending aorta are visualized in continuum (plane 1), whereas the arch is viewed in short axis (plane 2) and the descending aorta in long axis (planes 3, 4) from the esophagus.

ened toward the middle portion of the ascending aorta. Longitudinal long-axis imaging at the same level significantly improves the delineation of nearly the entire ascending aorta [6]. This plane displays in continuum the aortic valve, aortic root, and sinuses of Valsalva and the ascending aorta several centimeters distal to its crossing anterior to the right pulmonary artery (Fig. 14-4A). Slight withdrawal of the probe in the same plane visualizes the more distal ascending aorta (Fig. 14-4B).

The far distal ascending aorta to the origin of the innominate artery is obscured within a TEE blind spot caused by interposition of the air-filled distal trachea and proximal mainstem bronchi between the esophagus and distal ascending aorta (Fig. 14-5). This blind spot is predominantly present during imaging in the transverse plane but is virtually eliminated by scanning in the longitudinal plane with varying degrees of probe anteflexion. In some patients, because of body habitus or anatomic orientation of the ascending aorta in relation to the esophagus and trachea, the blind spot cannot be totally eliminated even with the longitudinal approach [6,7,10].

Fig. 14-3. Transverse TEE imaging of the left ventricular outflow tract to aortic root and proximal ascending aorta *(Ao).* Long-axis visualization of the ascending aorta is often quite limited in this plane.

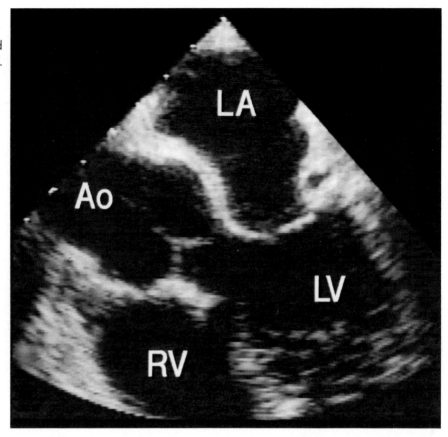

Aortic Arch

Further withdrawal and mild counterclockwise rotation of the TEE probe to 15 to 20 cm allows imaging of the aortic arch. In the transverse plane, the arch is seen in its long axis with the most proximal portion of the descending aorta oriented downward and to the left of the video screen display (Fig. 14-6). Longitudinal imaging in this location views the arch in its short axis; the arch is circular in the middle portion and tangentially ovoid more proximally and distally. The proximal portions of the left common carotid and left subclavian arteries may be seen [7]; full delineation of the brachiocephalic vessels, however, usually is not possible. Placement of the TEE probe at this level of the upper esophagus often evokes a significant gagging reaction and some discomfort to the patient. To improve patient tolerance, the examiner should not tarry in this position and preferably should perform this portion of the study while withdrawing the TEE probe at the conclusion of the examination.

Descending Thoracic Aorta

Short-axis views of the descending thoracic aorta in the transverse plane are obtained by rotating the TEE probe another 90 to 120 degrees counterclockwise toward the patient's left and posterior (Fig. 14-7). The descending thoracic aorta intertwines with the esophagus and progressively becomes more posterior to the esophagus distally toward the diaphragm. Hence, gentle counterclockwise rotation of the TEE probe during advancement into the esophagus is necessary to maintain centering of the cross-sectional image of the aorta on the video screen. While in this plane, it is important to keep the aorta completely round and centered within the sector to ensure a true transverse image. Often the descending aorta is examined as the next step after transgastric imaging of the heart, and slow withdrawal of the TEE probe with gradual clockwise rotation is done to maintain image centering (see Fig. 14-1). The proximal abdominal aorta is usually visible from the transgastric position. Slight posteroflexion of the

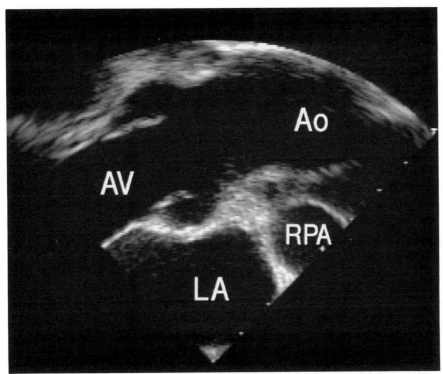

A

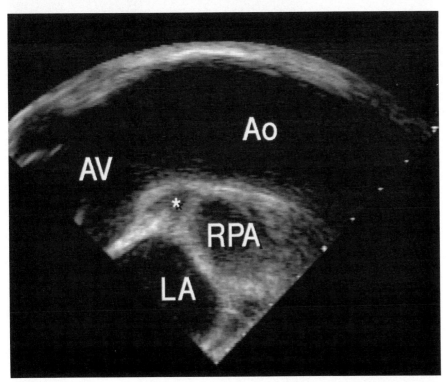

B

Fig. 14-4. A. Longitudinal TEE imaging of the aortic valve and proximal ascending aorta *(Ao)*. The left atrium is immediately anterior to the transducer at the downward apex of the sector, and the right pulmonary artery is to the far right of the sector. B. Slight withdrawal and anteflexion of the TEE probe permits visualization of nearly the entire ascending aorta, with the left atrium now off to the left of the sector and right pulmonary artery seen more centrally with the transverse sinus *(asterisk)*, the pericardial reflection between the aorta and the pulmonary artery.

TEE probe optimizes transducer-esophageal contact in this position.

Longitudinal imaging with the apex of the sector down displays the descending aorta in its long axis, with its more proximal aspect toward the right of the video screen (Fig. 14-8). Slight lateral rotation of the TEE probe is needed to sweep the entire aortic lumen for the exclusion of eccentric lesions. During withdrawal of the probe, mild clockwise rotation is used for continued visualization of the aorta.

AORTIC DISSECTION

Aortic dissection is a medical and often surgical emergency that mandates expeditious diagnosis [11]. Multiple diagnostic modalities have been described to this end. Conventional aortography, the initial standard of diagnosis, is invasive, has several limitations, and may be less sensitive than contemporary computed tomographic imaging [12–15]. With current-generation computed tomographic imaging equipment, noninvasive diagnostic accuracy generally exceeds 95% [13,16], but some time is required for image acquisition. Magnetic resonance imaging (MRI) has the ability to visualize the thoracic aorta in multiple planes with a high degree of sensitivity for detection of dissection [17,18]. However, MRI is not widely available and currently requires an inordinate amount of time for image processing, which is not suitable for potentially unstable patients. Despite continuing technologic advances,

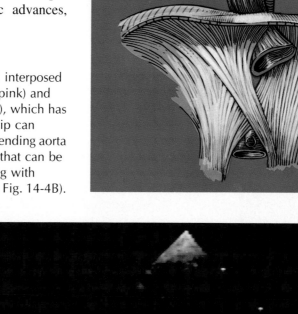

Fig. 14-5. Schema of the trachea (gray) interposed between the more posterior esophagus (pink) and more anterior distal ascending aorta (red), which has been cut away. This anatomic relationship can obscure the visualization of the distal ascending aorta in the transverse TEE plane, a limitation that can be largely overcome by longitudinal imaging with various degrees of probe anteflexion (see Fig. 14-4B).

Fig. 14-6. Transverse TEE imaging of the normal aortic arch. The more proximal portion of the arch is located downward to the left, and the distal arch is directed near the apex of the sector.

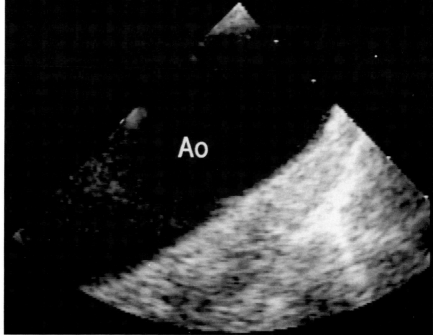

both computed tomography [19] and MRI [20] have potential pitfalls in the diagnosis of aortic dissection.

Multiple investigators have described experience in the diagnosis of aortic dissection with transthoracic two-dimensional [4,5,21–24] and color Doppler [24] echocardiography. Although this approach greatly facilitates a rapid noninvasive bedside evaluation for aortic dissection, its reported sensitivity has been variable, usually limited to a range of 75 to 85% [5,15,23] and even lower for distal type B dissections [25].

Of all thoracic aortic lesions evaluated by TEE, aortic dissection has been by far the most extensively described in the literature [26,27].

Two-Dimensional TEE Examination

The hallmark of two-dimensional TEE diagnosis of aortic dissection is the demonstration of an intraluminal intimal flap [28–30]. According to the Stanford classification [31], type A dissections (surgical lesions) involve the ascending aorta, typically arising near the sinutubular junction, with variable distal extension. Type B dissections (treated medically if stable and uncomplicated) originate at or distal to the orifice of the left subclavian artery and do not extend proximally.

The ultrasonic characteristics of the intimal flap closely resemble those of the aortic wall from whence it originates. The appearance of a uniform,

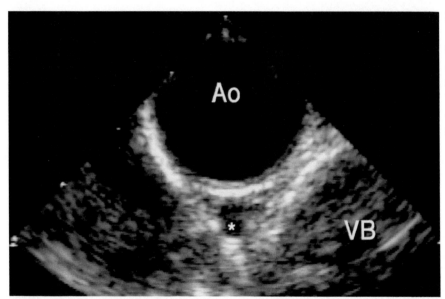

Fig. 14-7. Transverse TEE imaging of the descending thoracic aorta in short axis. The adjacent vertebral body of the spinal column is seen; vertebrae are frequently noted at multiple imaging levels. Also seen is the hemiazygous vein *(asterisk).*

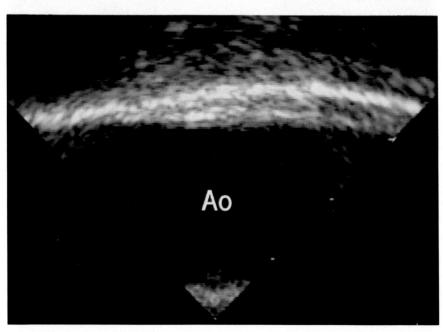

Fig. 14-8. Longitudinal TEE imaging of the descending thoracic aorta in long axis with downward projection of the sector apex. The more proximal aspect of the aorta is located to the right of the sector.

Fig. 14-9. Transverse TEE imaging of the aortic arch in type A aortic dissection. A. Systolic expansion of the perfused true lumen causes compression of the false lumen by the intimal flap *(arrow)*. B. Color-flow Doppler image during systole. Normal antegrade flow (orange) with central aliasing (blue) is observed within the true lumen *(arrow)*, with lower velocity retrograde flow in the false lumen *(arrow)* producing a double-barreled appearance to intraluminal flow, separated by the intimal flap *(arrowhead)*. C. Two-dimensional imaging during diastole; the undulating intimal flap *(arrow)* has moved centrally between the true and false lumens. D. Color-flow Doppler image reveals low-velocity flow in both lumens separated by the intimal flap *(arrowhead)*.

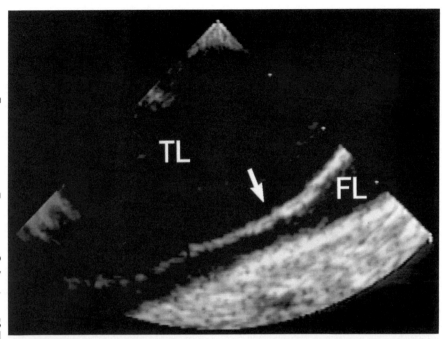

A

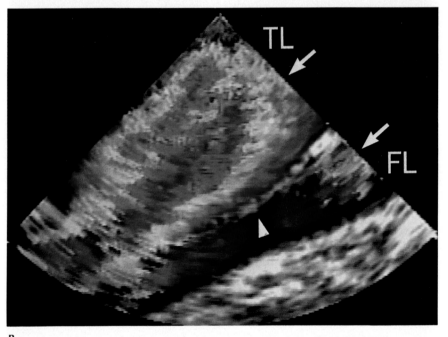

B

dense, and hyperrefractile intimal flap contrasts sharply with the more nebulous characteristics of linear reverberation artifacts that may mimic dissection (see "Potential Limitations and Pitfalls," below). On long-axis imaging, typically there is undulating motion of the intimal flap throughout the cardiac cycle; it often nearly parallels the aortic walls but clearly is independent (Fig. 14-9). In both imaging planes, there are systolic expansion of the perfused true lumen and variable compression of

the adjacent false lumen. In type A dissections, the proximal course of the flap is best delineated in longitudinal plane imaging; the flap is traced from its origin near the aortic root to the distal ascending arch in one imaging plane. Commonly, spiraling of the flap throughout the course of dissection more distally is evident on short-axis transverse imaging. Occasionally, the intimal flap is folded on itself, so that the false lumen is encompassed by the true lumen (Fig. 14-10). The false lumen usually contains

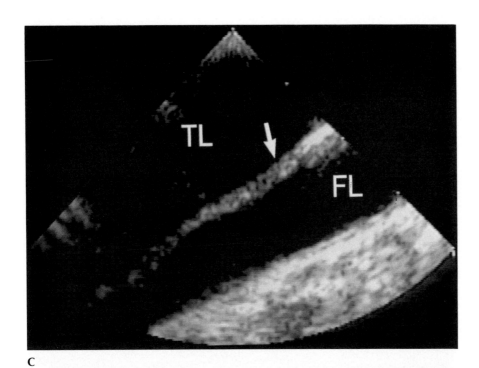

C

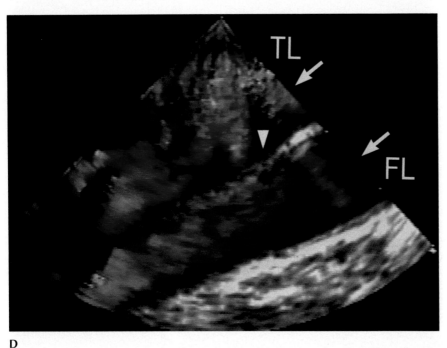

D

some degree of spontaneous echocontrast (typical of low-velocity blood flow), and various amounts of thrombus are present (Fig. 14-11). In a report by Ballal et al. [27], thrombus within the false lumen was detected by TEE in 41% of 34 patients with aortic dissection; similar distribution of thrombus was noted between proximal and distal dissections.

Depending on the acuity of presentation, there is mild to moderate fusiform dilatation of the dissected portion of the thoracic aorta. Massive enlargement of the aorta may occur in chronic dissections (Fig. 14-12). In type A dissections, the degree of aortoannular dilatation, dissecting hematoma, and resultant aortic regurgitation can be readily assessed by short-axis imaging of the aortic root and valve in both transverse and longitudinal planes. Examination of the aortic valve and root is also greatly facilitated by longitudinal long-axis imaging, which allows simultaneous comparison of aortoannular and ascending aortic involvement.

Fig. 14-10. Type B aortic dissection. A. Transverse imaging reveals the true lumen to be enclosed by the much larger false lumen, which contains dense spontaneous echocardiographic contrast *(arrowheads)*, indicative of the low-velocity flow within this channel. B. In the longitudinal plane, low-velocity color-flow signals are seen within the slitlike true lumen *(arrow)*, whereas the velocity of sluggish flow within the false lumen is below even the low-velocity color-flow map limits, and color signals fail to register within these two channels *(arrowheads)*.

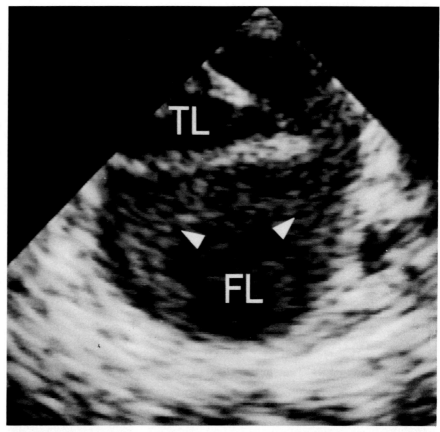

A

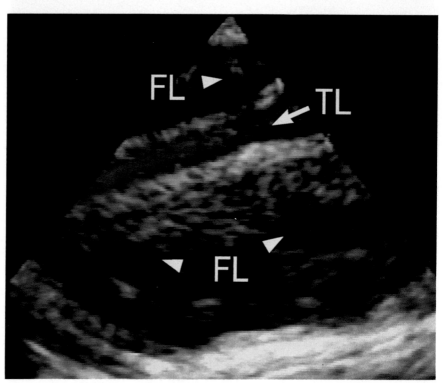

B

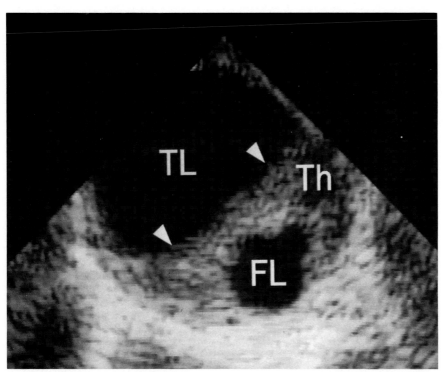

Fig. 14-11. Transverse TEE imaging of partial thrombotic obliteration of the false lumen. The intimal flap *(arrowheads)* separating this lumen from the true aortic lumen is partially obscured by thrombus.

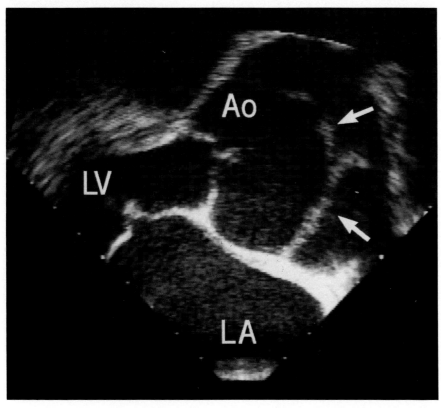

Fig. 14-12. Severe enlargement of the ascending aorta *(Ao)* in chronic type A aortic dissection. A transverse intimal flap *(arrows)* arises near the sinotubular junction; the very proximal ascending aorta is nearly 7 cm in diameter (1 cm distance between calibration dots).

Fig. 14-13. Severe aortic regurgitation complicating type A aortic dissection; evaluation by intraoperative monoplane TEE before and after surgical repair. A. Aortic dissection is present with a transverse intimal flap *(arrowheads)* within the aortic root; dilatation of the aortic annulus has precipitated diastolic prolapse and gross malcoaptation of the right coronary cusp *(arrow)*. B. Severe aortic regurgitation fills the entire left ventricular outflow tract *(arrow)* on color Doppler image; the intimal flap is noted by *arrowheads*. C. After conduit (not seen) repair of the aortic dissection, the intimal flap *(arrowheads)* has been oversewn and the aortic valve cusps now have normal diastolic coaptation *(arrow)* after aortic valve repair with resuspension. D. Mild aortic regurgitation *(arrow)* is detected by color Doppler imaging after aortic valve repair. The intimal flap *(arrowhead)* is no longer mobile after suture repair.

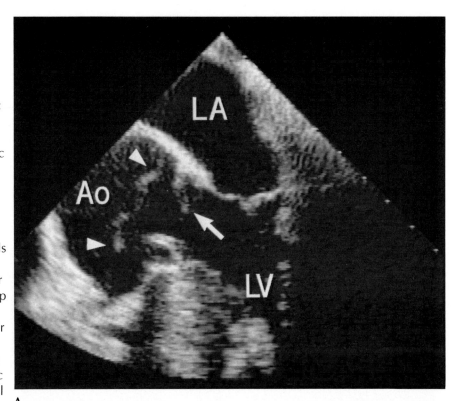

A

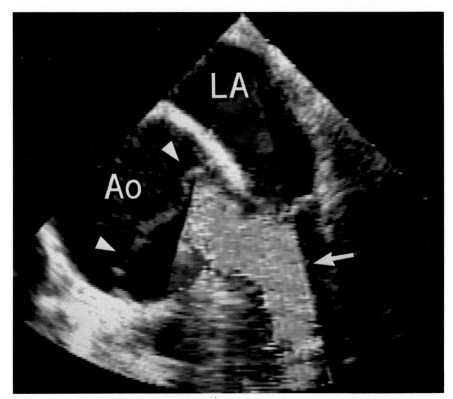

B

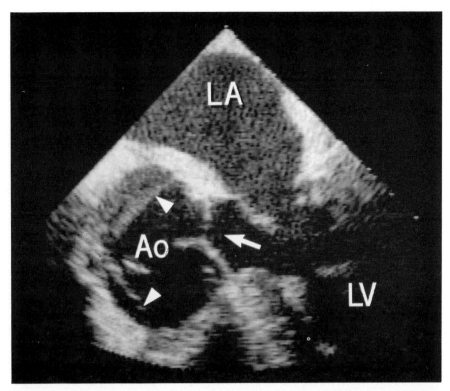

C

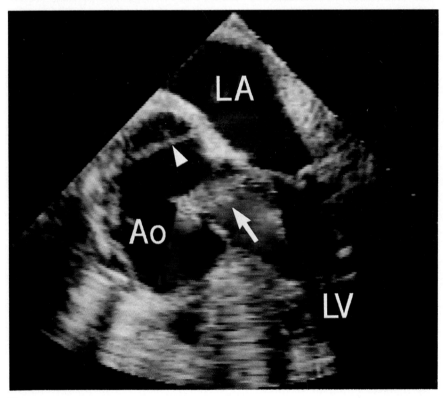

D

Fig. 14-14. Coronary artery dissection associated with Marfan's syndrome. There is massive enlargement of the aortic root, with compression of the superior vena cava *(asterisk),* as viewed from the transverse plane. The intimal flap *(arrowheads)* of a localized type A dissection extends into the proximal left main coronary artery *(arrow).* These findings were confirmed at the time of surgical repair.

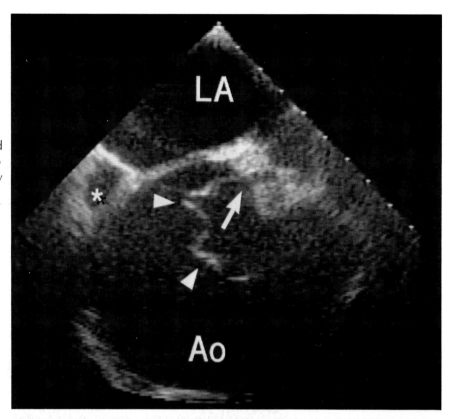

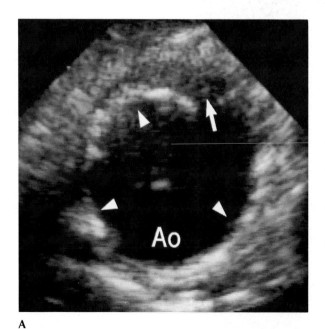

A

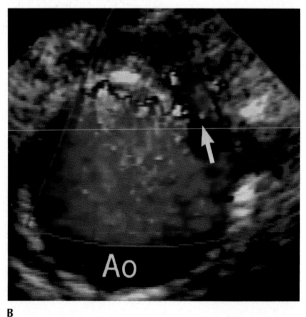

B

Fig. 14-15. Localized dissection and intramural hematoma of the descending aorta; transverse TEE plane. A. Disruption and displacement *(arrow)* of the calcified intima *(arrowheads)* are present. B. Localized low-velocity flow disturbance is demonstrated by color Doppler imaging at the point of intimal disruption *(arrow).* C. Intramural hematoma extends from the site of intimal disruption *(large arrow),* causing approximately 10 mm of intraluminal displacement of the calcified intima *(arrowhead* pointing toward top of sector) from the adventitial margin *(small arrows)* of the aorta.

Details of aortic cusp malcoaptation as a result of aortic annular dissection and expansion are obtainable with TEE. Significant aortic regurgitation may result from symmetrical dilatation of the root and incomplete central cusp coaptation or from asymmetrical involvement precipitating diastolic prolapse or even flail of one or more aortic cusps (Fig. 14-13). Such information about the aortic valve is vital to the surgical management of aortic dissection, as aortic valve repair or replacement may be needed for accompanying aortic regurgitation. Impingement of the intimal flap on the aortic valve or even frank diastolic prolapse of the flap into the left ventricular outflow tract also have been found to precipitate severe aortic regurgitation in patients with type A aortic dissection [27].

Two-dimensional TEE imaging is also a sensitive means of detecting coronary artery dissection associated with aortic dissection (Fig. 14-14). Of the 34 patients with aortic dissection reported by Ballal et al. [27], seven (21%) were found to have coronary artery involvement at the time of surgery. Extension of the dissecting intimal flap into the ostium and lumen of the involved coronary artery was detected by TEE in six (86%) of these patients. The right

coronary artery was visualized by TEE in 50% of this population (compared with visualization of the left main artery in 88%), and right coronary dissection was undetected by TEE in the seventh patient because this artery could not be visualized. Right and left coronary artery dissection occurred in nearly equal frequency, 57% and 43%, respectively; however, only two (29%) patients had clinical evidence of associated myocardial infarction [27].

A mobile, well-defined intimal flap with clear definition of true and false lumens may not always be identified by TEE in aortic dissection. Localized intramural aortic hematoma, an early sign of aortic dissection, may instead be seen in nearly 20% of patients, typically in the descending thoracic aorta [15,32]. Intramural hematoma on TEE may be manifested by central displacement of a locally disrupted intimal boundary (Fig. 14-15) or complicate extensive atherosclerotic disease. As observed by Mohr-Kahaly et al. [32], intramural hematoma may increase the aortic wall thickness from 5 to 40 mm, with longitudinal extension averaging from 7 to 11 cm. The same investigators reported the prognostic implications of aortic intramural hematoma [33]. Of 15 patients with follow-up of ten months after initial TEE examination, 27% had progressive aortic dissection, of whom three-fourths had aortic rupture; 40% of patients remained stable on medical therapy, but in only one patient (7%) was complete healing of the intramural hematoma observed on follow-up TEE [33].

Extracardiac complications of aortic dissection can also be detected by two-dimensional TEE. Pericardial effusion can be readily identified, being detected in generally 20% to 25% of patients with aortic dissection studied by this technique [27,34]. Modified anteflexed four-chamber and transgastric imaging is useful for delineation of right atrial or ventricular diastolic free-wall compression. Cardiac tamponade can also be diagnosed from characteristic respiratory changes in pulmonary venous and mitral inflow signals by pulsed-wave Doppler [35] (see Chapter 17, Fig. 17–7). Left pleural effusion is easily visualized in the left medial costophrenic angle adjacent to the descending thoracic aorta (Fig. 14-16). Extravasated blood with or without hematoma formation can also be identified extrinsic to the aorta in patients with dissection complicated by aortic rupture. Of the 34 patients with aortic dissection reported by Ballal et al. [27], two (6%) were found

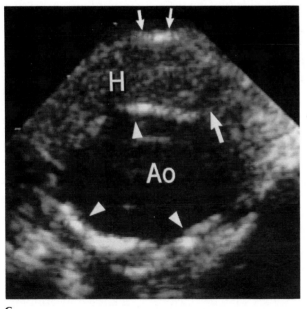

C

Fig. 14-16. Acute aortic dissection complicated by pleural effusion. A left pleural effusion within the posteromedial costophrenic angle highlights the dissected *(arrow)* descending thoracic aorta; a portion of the left lung *(L)* is also noted within the effusion.

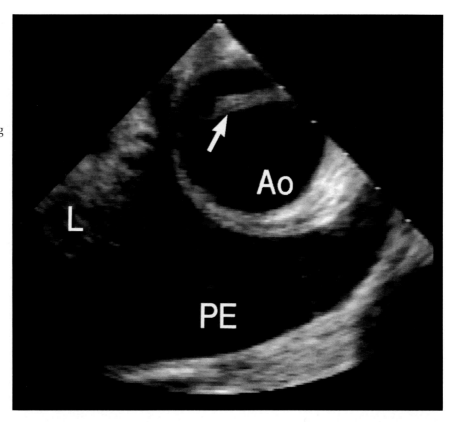

to have large aortic false aneurysms with thrombus by TEE; both of these instances of aortic rupture were missed on aortography.

Doppler TEE Examination

Transesophageal color Doppler echocardiography vividly characterizes the abnormal flow dynamics in aortic dissection [36–39]. When dissection is present, the normal pulsatile, homogeneous laminar flow within the aorta is disrupted. Aliased, higher velocity flow patterns are seen within the true lumen, becoming more turbulent and mosaic with decreasing caliber of this channel. Depending on the size of the entry site, turbulent, high-velocity color Doppler jets are visualized at the points of communication between the true and false lumens. Typically, flow from the true into the false lumen is visualized during systole, with flow reversal of lower velocity occurring through the entry site and back into the true lumen during diastole [36,39] (Fig. 14-17). Proximally, unidirectional flow from true to false lumen may also be seen, with to-and-fro bidirectional flow occurring more distally [36].

The detection rate of entry sites has been reported to be 87% for transverse monoplane and 89% for biplane TEE [38]. Slow, swirling color-flow patterns are noted in the false lumen (Fig. 14-18), consistent with the spontaneous echocontrast often present on two-dimensional imaging. Usually, low-velocity color filter maps are required for recognition of this characteristic finding. On long-axis imaging, bidirectional flow within the true and false lumens can be seen (see Fig. 14-9). Longitudinal color Doppler imaging often can identify multiple entry sites into the false lumen (Fig. 14-19). Entry site localization by TEE correlated with surgical findings in nearly 90% of patients studied by Adachi et al. [38]. Ballal et al. [27] found lesser agreement among TEE, angiography, and surgical exploration. In their study, only 13 (52%) of 25 communications noted at aortography or surgery were identified by TEE, but only 36% of patients in this study had biplane TEE evaluation. In addition, 27 communications in 18 patients were detected by TEE but not by aortography or surgery [27]. It is suspected that the latter communications were quite small, and although highlighted by the very sensitive technique of color Doppler imaging, they were missed by other imaging modalities and were not conspicuous at the time of surgery. Other investigators have noted that TEE has significantly enhanced the delineation of flow abnormalities and entry sites compared with computed tomography or angiography [36,37].

Aortic regurgitation, which may also complicate type A aortic dissections (see Fig. 14-13), can be semiquantitated by composite TEE Doppler examination (see Chapter 9). Comparison of transthoracic color flow mapping of the subvalvular aortic regurgitant width with left ventricular outflow tract diameter correlates with angiographic grade of aortic regurgitation [40] and is currently undergoing validation for TEE. Longitudinal long-axis imaging augments visualization of the left ventricular outflow tract and estimation of aortic regurgitation. Pulsed-wave Doppler [41] and color M-mode examinations complement the color Doppler examination, and holodiastolic flow reversal within the true aortic lumen is detectable with hemodynamically severe aortic regurgitation.

Aortic regurgitation of moderate or severe degree has been detected by TEE color Doppler imaging in approximately one-third of patients with proximal aortic dissection; the most common mechanisms are aortic root dilatation causing aortic cusp malcoaptation and impingement of the aortic valve by the intimal flap [27]. Aortic regurgitation may also be incidentally noted in patients because of intrinsic valvular lesions, such as congenitally bicuspid or calcific aortic valve disease.

Diagnostic Accuracy and Utility of TEE

Transesophageal echocardiography has been shown by multiple investigators to have a very high rate, generally approaching 100%, of correct diagnosis of aortic dissection detected by other imaging methods or at surgery [15,29,34,37,38].

A multicenter study with TEE was performed by Erbel et al. [34] of the European Cooperative Study Group for Echocardiography in 164 patients with clinically suspected aortic dissection, 82 of whom had the diagnosis proved anatomically or confirmed by at least two imaging methods. Transesophageal echocardiography (performed with monoplane instruments, usually without availability of color Doppler imaging) identified aortic dissection in all but one patient with this diagnosis proved by either surgery or autopsy; two patients had a false-positive

study. For anatomically proven dissection, these investigators found that TEE had a sensitivity of 98% and a specificity of 98%, with positive and negative predictive values of 97% and 93%, respectively [34]. When all aortic dissections diagnosed anatomically or by at least two imaging modalities were considered, TEE compared very favorably with computed tomography and aortic angiography in diagnostic accuracy (Table 14-1). The relatively low sensitivity of computed tomography in this study likely depends to some degree on the generation of imaging instruments used. Interestingly, one study [27] noted an even lower sensitivity (67%) for computed tomography but a similar sensitivity for aortography (93%) in the detection of aortic dissection. Similar results have been noted by other investigators [26,38,42].

Erbel et al. [15,34,43] advocated that TEE be used as the diagnostic method of choice to evaluate suspected aortic dissection (Fig. 14-20). When the diagnosis of aortic dissection is clear by TEE, other investigators who also have reported high diagnostic accuracy of TEE for aortic dissection advise proceeding directly to surgery, if indicated, without routine aortography or other noninvasive imaging [44]. Further investigation with computed tomography or angiography is indicated if the diagnosis is unclear or if additional information, such as that obtained by investigation of branch vessel deficit, is required.

One study used a dual, randomized, noninvasive imaging protocol with both monoplane TEE and magnetic resonance imaging (MRI) in the evaluation of patients with clinically suspected aortic dissection [45]. In comparison with intraoperative, postmortem, or angiographic findings in the same patients, the sensitivity of both TEE and MRI for the detection of aortic dissection was 100%. Primarily because of a number of false-positive TEE findings in the ascending aorta, the specificity for TEE was reported to be 68%, whereas that for MRI was 100%. Most of these findings were likely due to reverberation artifacts within an ectatic vessel with extensive mural plaque and calcification; these were not evaluated with the clearly superior longitudinal TEE imaging plane or systematically examined with color-flow Doppler technique to confirm or exclude double-lumen intra-aortic flow patterns (see "Potential Limitations and Pitfalls," below). In this study [45], the overall diagnostic accuracy of TEE was 87% for type A aortic dissection and 96% for type B dissection (compared with 100% for MRI in both

Fig. 14-17. Color-flow Doppler imaging in dissection of the descending aorta; transverse TEE plane. A. An exit jet *(arrow)* of flow leaves the true lumen *(arrowhead)* and enters the false lumen during systole. B. Diastolic flow reversal traverses the same defect *(arrow)* within the intimal flap and reenters the true lumen during diastole. C. At a different level of the descending aorta, two systolic exit jets *(arrowheads)* are detected entering the false lumen during systolic expansion of the perfused true lumen *(arrow)*. D. Lower velocity diastolic flow *(arrows)* returns from the false lumen into the contracted true lumen.

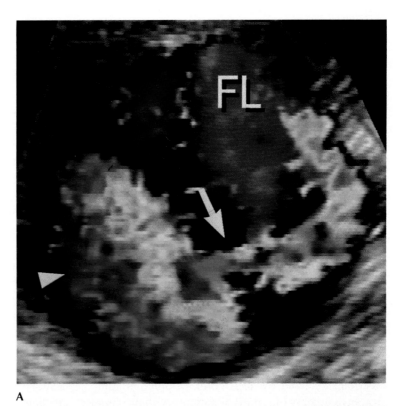

A

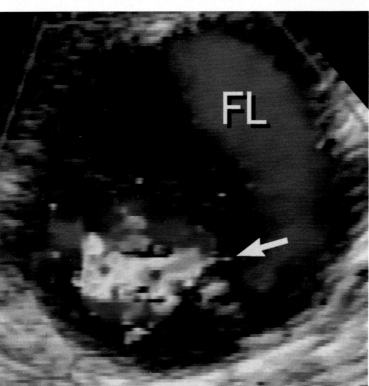

B

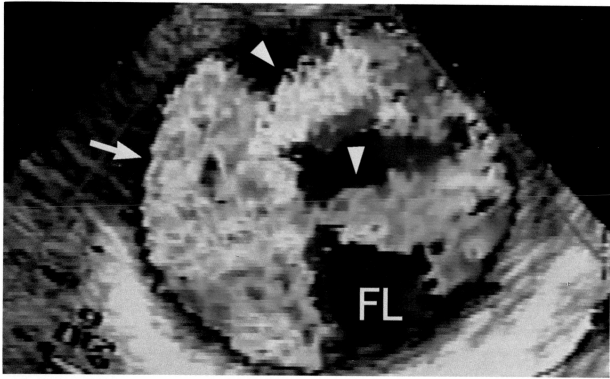

C

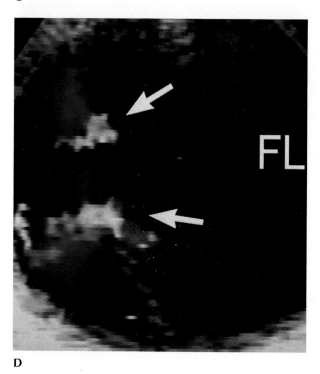

D

in patients studied by both computed tomography and MRI compared with TEE (Table 14-2).

Transesophageal echocardiography is also useful for the delineation of conditions that mimic acute aortic dissection. In a report by Chan [46], 40 patients with clinically suspected aortic dissection were referred for TEE, which confirmed this diagnosis in 18 (45%). Five patients were found instead to have ischemic coronary syndromes; ten of the remaining 17 patients had mild to aneurysmal dilatation of the thoracic aorta. Two patients had extrinsic masses adjacent to the aorta, one of which proved to be a small cell carcinoma and the other, a postoperative hematoma. One patient had mobile intra-aortic thrombus after blunt chest trauma, and another had a para-aortic hematoma and leaking coronary anastomosis after Bentall repair of the aortic root [46]. Acute pulmonary embolism may also clinically mimic aortic dissection. Transesophageal echocardiography may reveal venous thromboembolism in transit within the right heart or within the proximal pulmonary arteries (see Chapters 12 and 15).

Procedural Considerations for TEE in Acute Aortic Dissection

types) but should be considerably higher for type A aortic dissections with the use of contemporary biplane TEE systems supplemented by color Doppler analysis of intraluminal flow patterns. Similar findings were noted by the same investigators [45a]

Despite the life-threatening nature of acute aortic dissection, TEE performed in this condition has been

Fig. 14-18. Dissection of the descending aorta; transverse TEE imaging plane. A. The intimal flap *(arrowheads,* the lower of which points to a clear defect within the flap) demarcates the true lumen from the much larger false lumen, which contains speckled spontaneous echocardiographic contrast. B. The true lumen exhibits a homogeneous flow pattern *(arrow)* during systole, with two turbulent exit jets *(arrowheads)* entering the false lumen. C. Low-velocity swirling flow *(curved arrows)* directed toward the TEE transducer (red) and away (blue) is present in the false lumen.

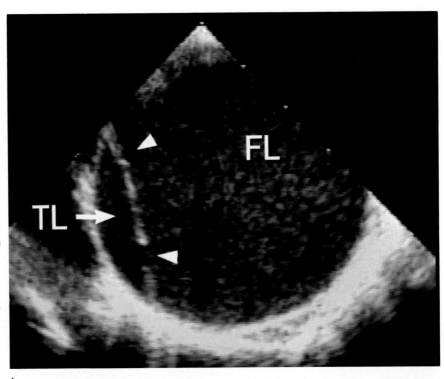

A

B

found to be safe and without significant complications [15,26,29,34,37,38,44,45]. As discussed in Chapter 17, TEE in the critically ill patient is generally very safe and often expedites immediate bedside diagnosis, prompting potentially lifesaving intervention.

In general, patients with suspected acute aortic dissection should be immediately treated with combined intravenous infusions of an arterial vasodilator (often nitroprusside) and beta-antagonist to maintain the mean arterial blood pressure around 70 to 80 mm Hg and pulse at about 60 beats per minute.

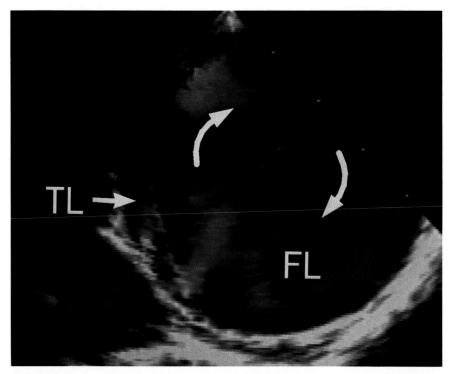

C

Liberal local oropharyngeal anesthesia with lido-caine spray is administered to minimize potential gagging. Generous short-acting intravenous seda-tion with midazolam is also given to maximize patient comfort. The anticholinergic effects of glyco-pyrrolate uncommonly may cause a significant in-crease in heart rate; however, this should be precluded by concomitant beta-antagonist infusion. Provided that the patient is adequately premedicated, any increase in blood pressure during TEE examina-tion is usually mild and well tolerated [44].

Chronic Aortic Dissection and Follow-Up TEE

Serial examinations by TEE have provided useful information about the pathoanatomic changes in chronic aortic dissection. In patients with medically treated dissection, obliteration of the false lumen by thrombus may be observed [47]; however, this has been noted in only about 20% of patients at a mean of 15 months after initial TEE [36]. Most patients have some nonobliterative thrombus within a patent false lumen, which is usually larger than the true lumen. Persistent flow within the false lumen is detectable by color Doppler imaging in nearly 80% of patients on follow-up. In the small series reported by Mohr-Kahaly et al. [36], extension of dissection at follow-up (6%) and localized expansion of the chronically dissected aorta (11%) were uncommon.

In a preliminary report, Erbel et al. [48] of the European Cooperative Study Group proposed a new classification of aortic dissection based on TEE find-ings to further aid prognostication. In prospective TEE studies of 70 patients with aortic dissection, follow-up mortality was relatively low (13%) in pa-tients without a demonstrable communication be-tween true and false lumens, especially in those with complete thrombosis of the false lumen. Patients having detectable communications through an inti-mal tear with either antegrade or retrograde dissec-tion had higher mortality (approximately 30%); patients without partial or complete thrombosis of the false lumen in this group were at higher risk (50% mortality). A separate small subgroup of this study population who had mediastinal hematoma (caused by aortic rupture) documented by TEE had the highest mortality (89%) [48].

NONDISSECTING THORACIC AORTIC ANEURYSMS

Transesophageal echocardiography likewise facili-tates examination of nondissecting thoracic aortic aneurysms [26,49].

Various degrees of fusiform aneurysmal dilatation may be observed in the ascending aorta, aortic arch,

Fig. 14-19. Dissection of the descending aorta; longitudinal TEE plane with sector apex-up orientation. A. The double-channel aorta is seen in long axis with the intimal flap *(arrowheads)* separating the true and false lumens. B. Color Doppler imaging demonstrates two of multiple systolic exit sites *(arrows)* into the false lumen. By conventional color Doppler mapping, laminar flow within the true lumen is orange-red when directed toward the transducer and blue when directed away from the transducer.

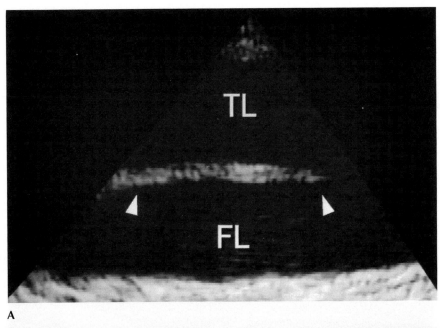

A

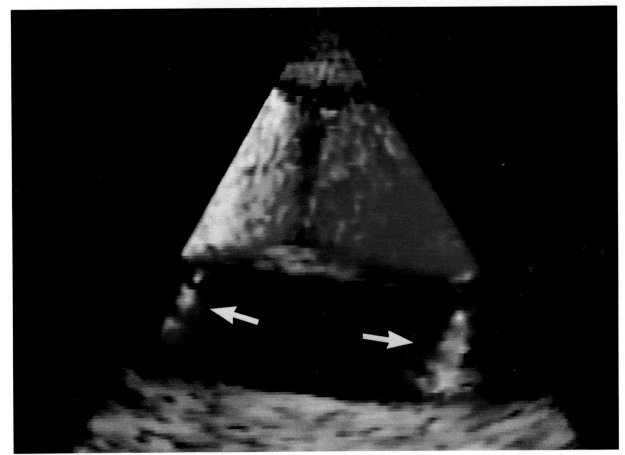

B

Table 14-1. European Cooperative Study Group for Echocardiography: Cumulative results of transesophageal echocardiography, computed tomography, and angiography in aortic dissection (82 patients)

	Percent		
	Transesophageal echocardiography	**Computed tomography**	**Aortic angiography**
Sensitivity	99	83	88
Specificity	98	100	94
Positive predictive value	98	100	96
Negative predictive value	99	86	84

Source: Data from R Erbel, R Engberding, W Daniel, et al. Echocardiography in diagnosis of aortic dissection. *Lancet* 1989; 1:457–61.

Table 14-2. Diagnosis of thoracic aortic dissection: Transesophageal echocardiography compared with computed tomography and magnetic resonance imaging (110 patients)

	Percent		
	Transesophageal echocardiography	**Computed tomography**	**Magnetic resonance imaging**
Sensitivity	98	94	98
Specificity	77	87	98
Accuracy	90	91	98
Positive predictive value	88	92	98
Negative predictive value	95	90	98

Source: Data from CA Nienaber, Y von Kodolitsch, V Nicolas, et al. The diagnosis of thoracic aortic dissection by noninvasive imaging procedures. *N Engl J Med* 1993;328:1–9.

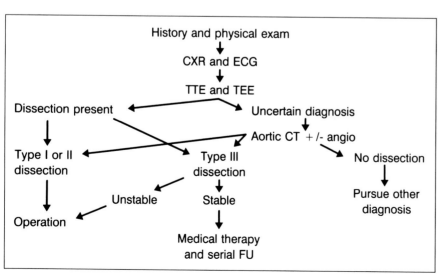

Fig. 14-20. Algorithm for the evaluation of suspected aortic dissection. (Modified from R Erbel, S Mohr-Kahaly, H Rennollet, et al. Diagnosis of aortic dissection: the value of transesophageal echocardiography. *Thorac Cardiovasc Surg* 1987; 35 [Special Issue 1]:126–33.)

and descending thoracic aorta. With increasing aneurysmal caliber, the velocity of intraluminal blood flow decreases, and frequently spontaneous echocontrast, reflective of sluggish flow, is visualized. Laminated mural thrombus is commonly seen accompanying this finding (Fig. 14-21), generally confined to more distal descending thoracic aneurysms [26]. By high-resolution tissue characterization, TEE confers the important ability to differentiate three abnormalities from one another: extensive aortic intimal calcification, irregularly calcified interfaces of intraluminal thrombus, and aortic dissection with a linear hyperrefractile intimal flap separating a thrombosed false lumen from the true lumen [26].

Localized aneurysmal dilatation of the aortic root and sinuses associated with Marfan's syndrome and annuloaortic ectasia is evident from a variety of transverse (see Fig. 14-14) and longitudinal (Fig. 14-22) planes. Fusiform aneurysms of the ascending aorta are best visualized in the longitudinal long-axis plane (Fig. 14-23). Sinus of Valsalva aneurysms are also readily identified by TEE, along with sur-

rounding anatomic derangement as a result of aneurysm impingement [50]. Complications of sinus of Valsalva aneurysm, such as rupture into another cardiac chamber and aortic regurgitation, can be delineated by color Doppler mapping (Fig. 14-24).

Saccular aneurysm may complicate a variety of thoracic aortic lesions and may be associated with dissection, atherosclerosis, trauma, or infection. These aneurysms are localized and often have relatively narrow necks communicating to the aortic lumen. The fundus of saccular aneurysms may be globular or eccentric and often contains thrombus [26,51] (Fig. 14-25).

Pseudoaneurysm of the aorta (Fig. 14-26) represents a contained transmural rupture of the aorta and may be post-traumatic, mycotic, or associated with aortic dissection or penetrating aortic ulcer [52]. The defect in the aorta often is small and may not be readily evident by two-dimensional TEE imaging alone. Color Doppler echocardiography greatly aids in the diagnosis by demonstrating a narrow low-velocity jet exiting the aortic lumen into the pseudoaneurysm cavity; to-and-fro flow is redirected back into the aorta during diastole. These cavities are of various sizes and configurations and, like saccular aneurysms, frequently contain thrombus.

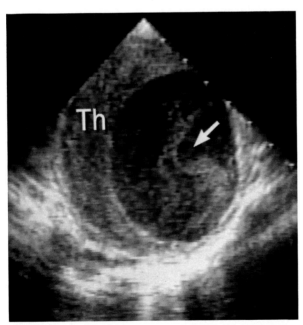

Fig. 14-21. Large nondissecting aneurysm of the descending thoracic aorta; transverse short-axis image. The aneurysm measures approximately 7 cm in diameter (1 cm per calibration) and contains laminated thrombus along the majority of its circumference. Dense, swirling spontaneous echocontrast *(arrow)* is consistent with very low-velocity blood flow within the aneurysm.

ATHEROSCLEROTIC THORACIC AORTIC DISEASE

In addition to both dissecting and nondissecting aortic aneurysms, a broad spectrum of atherosclerotic disease can affect the thoracic aorta. After the abdominal portion of the aorta, involvement is most common in the descending thoracic aorta, less common in the arch, and least common in the ascending aorta [53,54]. In general, significant atherosclerotic disease within the thoracic aorta is a marker for a diffuse atherosclerotic process involving both the coronary and the cerebrovascular circulation [53–55].

An extensive array of thoracic aortic atherosclerotic lesions can be vividly demonstrated by TEE. Simple atherosclerotic plaques may appear as focal, smooth, and hyperrefractile echodensities with minimal protrusion into the aortic lumen. Extensive atherosclerotic disease may give a geographic contouring of the aortic lumen, which is best delineated

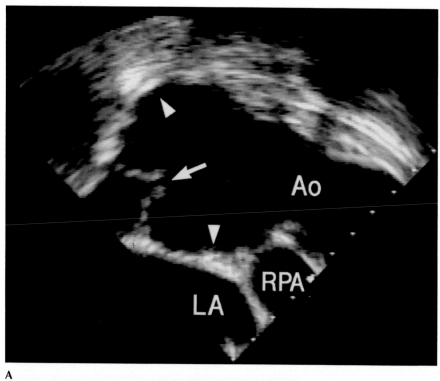

Fig. 14-22. Annuloaortic ectasia of the aortic root; longitudinal TEE plane. A. Severe dilatation of the sinuses of Valsalva *(arrowheads)* with incomplete diastolic coaptation of the cusps of the aortic valve *(arrow)*; the ascending aorta is otherwise only mildly enlarged. B. Color Doppler examination reveals a broad central jet of aortic regurgitation *(arrows)* emanating from the site of incomplete cusp coaptation.

A

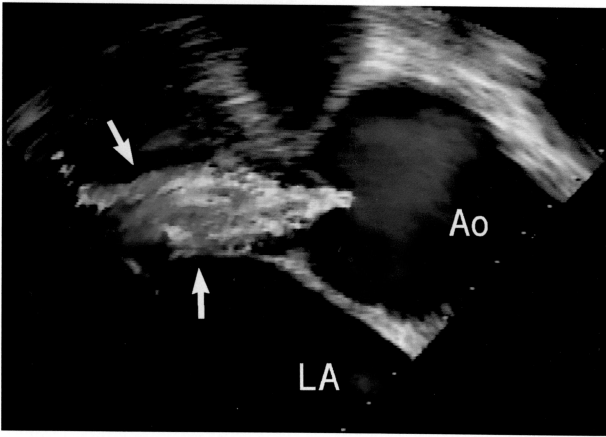

B

Fig. 14-23. Massive ascending aortic aneurysm; longitudinal TEE plane. The aortic aneurysm measures 8.5 cm (1.0 cm per calibration) and dwarfs the normal-sized right pulmonary artery and left atrium. The aortic valve and annulus are also visualized.

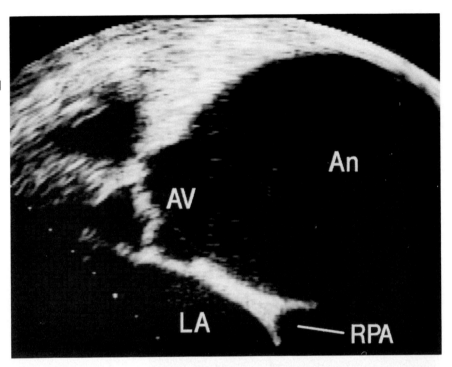

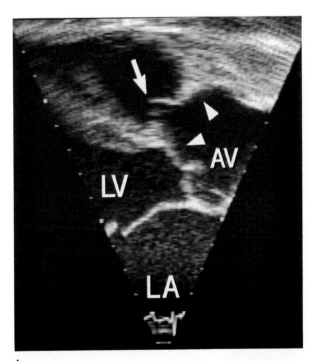

A

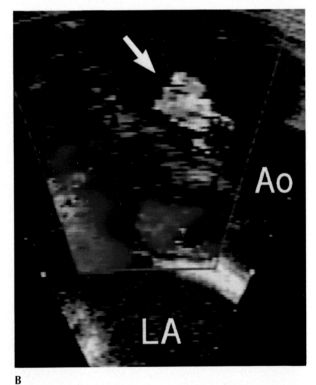

B

Fig. 14-24. Ruptured sinus of Valsalva aneurysm; longitudinal TEE plane. A. Asymmetrical aneurysmal enlargement of the right sinus of Valsalva *(arrowheads)* with rupture into the right ventricular outflow tract *(arrow)*; the typical "windsock" appearance of the communication *(arrow)* is evident. B. Color Doppler study confirms shunting from the aortic root into the right ventricular outflow tract *(arrow)*.

in the longitudinal plane (Fig. 14-27). Complex atherosclerotic lesions have grossly irregular and heaped-up margins, often with significant intraluminal protrusion. Pedunculated and mobile echodensities commonly extend from such complicated lesions, representing a combination of atherosclerotic debris and thrombus (Fig. 14-28). Such athero-

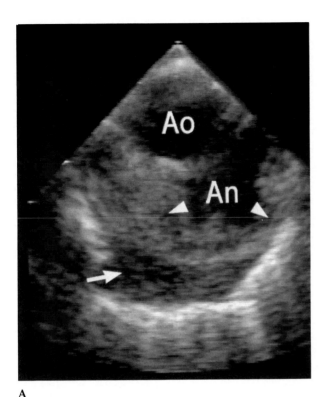
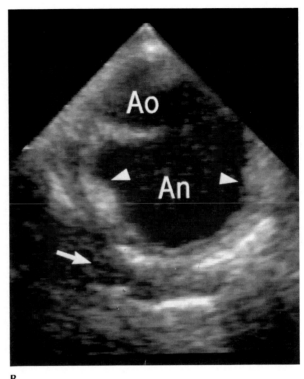

A   **B**

Fig. 14-25. Saccular aneurysm of the distal descending thoracic aorta; transverse TEE plane. A. A globular saccular aneurysm cavity extends from the lumen of the aorta, and contains laminated thrombus *(arrowheads)*. An echo-lucent area *(arrow)* adjacent to the aneurysm was found to be an aseptic inflammatory mass at the time of surgery. B. Slight advancement of the TEE probe distally reveals the extent of the saccular aneurysm; the diameter of the aneurysm *(arrowheads)* is nearly three times greater than that of the neck communicating to the aorta. The inflammatory mass *(arrow)* is again seen.

sclerotic disease can be diffuse, producing a "shaggy" appearance of the aorta (Fig. 14-29).

Intra-aortic atherosclerotic debris has been observed by TEE, with an incidence of 7% in a series of 556 unselected patients studied by Karalis et al. [56]. These investigators observed that atherosclerotic debris involved both the arch and the descending aorta in 70% of patients and was confined to the descending thoracic aorta in the remaining 30%. Atheroembolism is a recognized complication of atherosclerotic disease of this nature [55,57–59] (see Chapter 15). In the study by Karalis et al. [56], the risk of systemic embolic events was greater with pedunculated and mobile intra-aortic debris (73%) than with laminated, lower profile, and immobile disease (12%).

Rarely, exuberant atherosclerotic disease forms a "coral reef" atheroma that may even produce significant thoracic aortic obstruction. One severely hypertensive patient studied in our laboratory was found to have a massive atheroma in the distal arch and proximal descending thoracic aorta (Fig. 14-30). This lesion had the pathophysiology of

severe coarctation, producing a pressure gradient in excess of 100 mm Hg; surgical correction was necessary.

Penetrating aortic atherosclerotic ulcer warrants special attention because it is potentially life-threatening and often not considered or recognized. Penetrating aortic ulcers generally occur in patients with diffuse atherosclerotic vascular disease and are usually found in the distal arch or descending thoracic aorta [60]. The clinical presentation often mimics aortic dissection; however, signs and symptoms of aortic branch vessel compromise are not present [52,60]. Imaging by computed tomography or angiography (or both) in 16 patients (14 having aortic surgery) reported by Stanson et al. [60] found that penetrating ulcers range from 5 to 20 mm in diameter and 5 to 30 mm in depth.

Because of the relatively small size of penetrating aortic ulcers, meticulous two-dimensional, preferably biplanar, TEE examination is indicated. Located within usually extensive atheromatous disease, the punctate aortic ulcer crater interrupts the aortic wall (Fig. 14-31) and may extend outward as an adventi-

Fig. 14-26. Pseudoaneurysm of the aortic root; transverse TEE plane. A. A large pseudoaneurysm cavity containing laminated thrombus is present along the posterior aspect of the aortic root *(arrowheads)* and compresses the left atrium. The very narrow communication to the aortic root *(arrow)* is barely visible adjacent to the aortic valve. B. Color Doppler image demonstrates low-velocity flow from the aortic root *(arrow)* at the level of the aortic valve into the pseudoaneurysm *(arrowheads)* cavity.

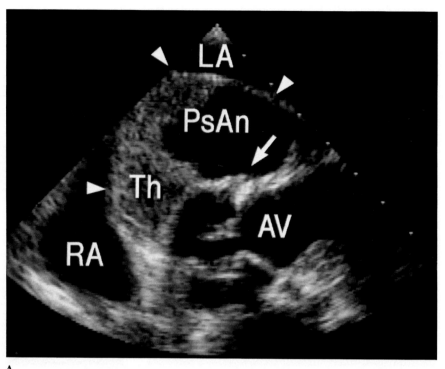

A

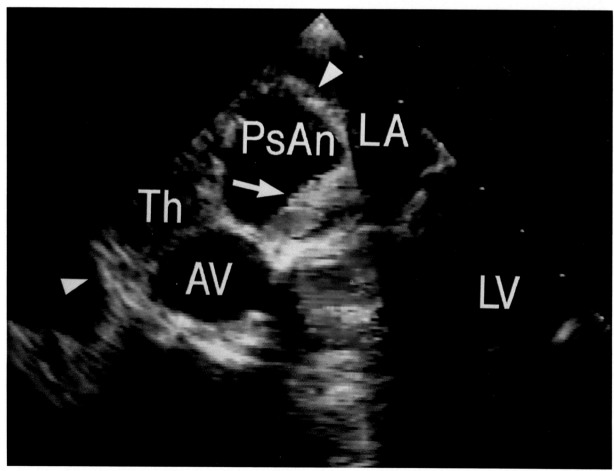

B

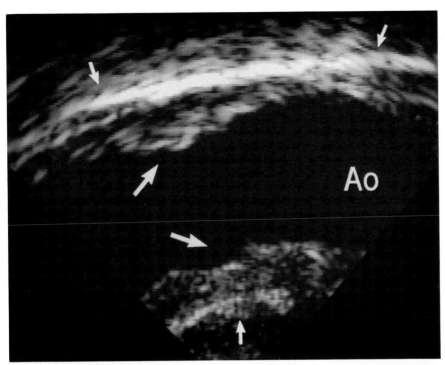

Fig. 14-27. Atherosclerotic disease of the descending thoracic aorta; longitudinal TEE plane. An irregular profile of the lumen of the aorta is caused by diffuse circumferential atherosclerotic disease *(large arrows)* contrasting with the linear outer margins *(small arrows)* of this vessel.

tial false aneurysm. A small aortic intramural hematoma may be present, as may a very localized intimal flap. Other features of aortic dissection, such as a false lumen and bidirectional flow on color Doppler imaging, are absent.

OTHER THORACIC AORTIC PATHOLOGIC CONDITIONS

Congenital Abnormalities

Coarctation of the aorta can be detected by TEE (Fig. 14-32), and a fair correlation of the minimal aortic isthmus diameter by TEE with that by contrast aortography has been observed [61]. Usually, exact delineation of the coarctation, even with biplanar TEE, is imperfect because of oblique imaging of this region, which is located in the very proximal portion of the descending aorta. Although steerable continuous-wave TEE Doppler systems are available, adequate alignment of the interrogating beam with the coarctation for accurate determination of pressure gradient is improbable. Detection by TEE of the anatomic effects of balloon angioplasty in coarctation, such as intimal and medial dissection, has been described [62].

Supravalvular aortic stenosis should be readily and fully visualized by longitudinal long-axis im-

aging of the proximal ascending aorta. Congenital anomalies of the aortic arch may be visible by TEE; however, further experience is necessary.

Traumatic Thoracic Aortic Disease

Experience with TEE in the evaluation of traumatic aortic disease has been limited. Detection of aortic thrombosis secondary to penetrating and nonpenetrating chest trauma has been reported [46,63]. Typically, the site of traumatic aortic rupture is the very proximal part of the descending aorta, or aortic isthmus, adjacent to the origin of the left subclavian artery and ligamentum arteriosum. In a study of 116 patients with traumatic rupture of the thoracic aorta documented by aortography, surgery, or necropsy, the site of disruption was the aortic isthmus in 90% of patients, the more distal thoracic aorta in 8%, and the aortic arch in 2% [64]. In a preliminary report [65], TEE correctly identified all aortic ruptures found at surgery (100% sensitivity and specificity) in 20 patients with severe blunt chest trauma, whereas aortography falsely diagnosed one case of rupture (100% sensitivity and 75% specificity). Right ventricular contusion was also detected by TEE in 35% of patients in this study [65]. Descending thoracic aortic rupture complicating a motor vehicle accident injury has been observed by TEE in our experience. In this patient, the large aortic disruption was readily

Fig. 14-28. Complex atherosclerotic plaque within the descending thoracic aorta. A. Transverse TEE plane; a pedunculated mass of atherosclerotic debris *(arrow)* is detected on short-axis imaging of the aorta. B. Longitudinal TEE imaging at the same level; the pedunculated mass *(arrow)* is seen to be attached to a large, complex atherosclerotic lesion *(arrowheads)*. C. The mobility of the pedunculated mass *(arrow)* is shown with respect to the sessile atherosclerotic lesion *(arrowheads)*. Most often, such mobile attachments are primarily thrombus complicating extensive atherosclerotic plaque and are associated with significant risk of distal embolism (see text).

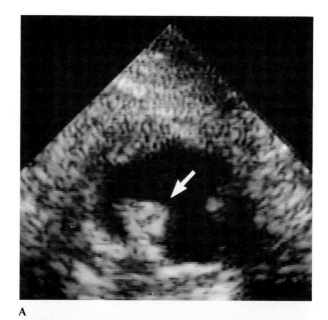

A

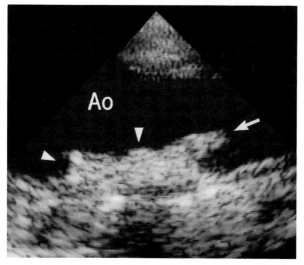

B

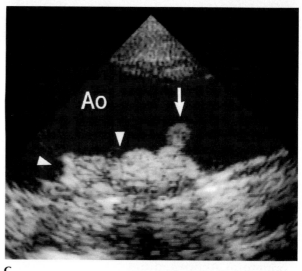

C

Fig. 14-29. Extensive atherosclerotic debris within the descending thoracic aorta; transverse TEE plane. A "shaggy" appearance of the lumen of the aorta is produced by several partially mobile lesions *(arrowheads)* projecting far into the aortic lumen. This patient presented with diffuse atheroembolic cutaneous infarcts of the feet and the "blue toe" syndrome.

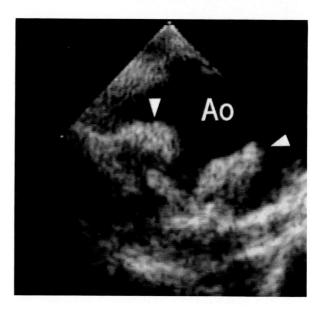

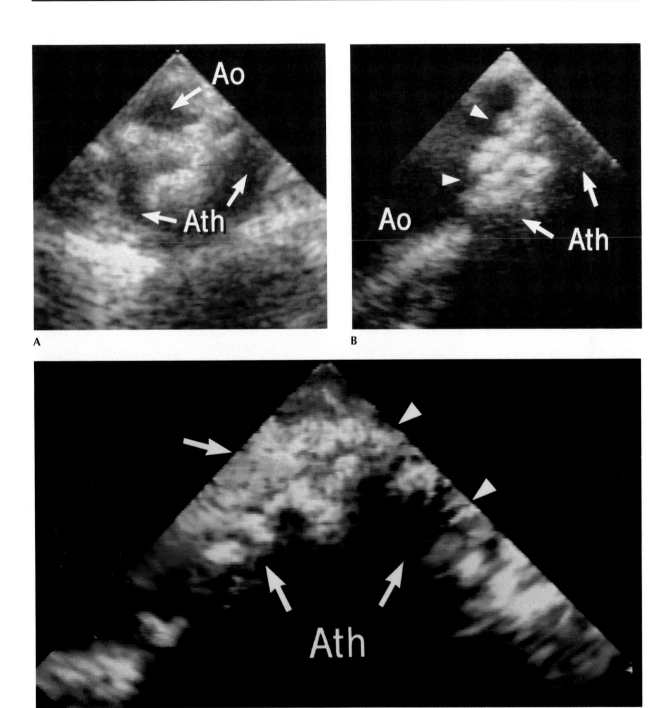

C

Fig. 14-30. Massive atheroma of the proximal descending aorta associated with the pathophysiologic features of severe coarctation. A. Transverse TEE short-axis imaging reveals near-obliteration (cross-sectional diameter, 6 mm) of the aortic lumen *(arrow)* by very extensive atherosclerotic disease. B. Transverse long-axis imaging of the distal aortic arch *(Ao)* and proximal descending aorta demonstrates an immense "coral reef" atheroma protruding into the entire aortic lumen *(arrowheads)* in this view (compare with normal aorta in the same view, Fig. 14-6). C. Off-axis transverse long-axis imaging of the atheroma *(lower arrows)*. A large acoustic shadow is cast away from the apex of the sector because of diffuse calcific disease within this lesion. Color Doppler imaging reveals normal flow (orange) proximal to this lesion *(upper arrow)* and turbulent high-velocity flow (blue-green) distally *(arrowheads)*, consistent with obstruction (see text).

Fig. 14-31. Penetrating atherosclerotic ulcer of the aorta; transverse long-axis TEE imaging of the distal aortic arch. A punctate ulcer channel *(arrow)* has burrowed through a complex atherosclerotic plaque *(arrowheads)*, forming an ulcer crater within the wall of the aorta.

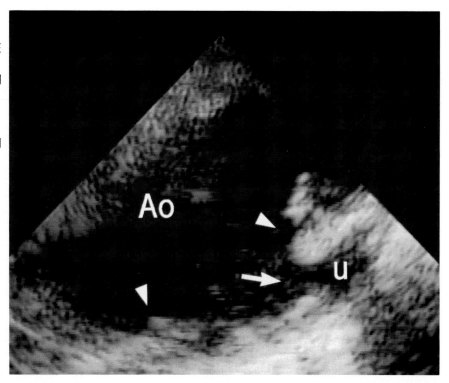

evident, and gross aortic extravasation contained by a large para-aortic hematoma was seen on color Doppler imaging (Fig. 14-33).

As in any patient being evaluated for severe trauma, manipulation of the head and neck for the purposes of TEE examination should not be done until instability of the cervical spine has been excluded.

Intra-Aortic Balloon Counterpulsation

Transesophageal echocardiography can aid in the placement of an intra-aortic balloon pump [66]. Characteristic diastolic flow reversals can be visualized by color Doppler imaging during balloon augmentation accompanied by increased diastolic velocities by pulsed-wave Doppler echocardiography within the coronary arteries. Complications from intra-aortic balloon pump insertion, such as thrombosis and iatrogenic dissection, can also be visualized by TEE (Fig. 14-34).

POTENTIAL LIMITATIONS AND PITFALLS

The assessment of thoracic aortic disease by TEE may be compromised by problems similar to those that limit the examination of the heart, such as a large diaphragmatic hernia or significant alterations of mediastinal anatomy that may occur after major thoracic surgery. Occasionally, massive ectasia and "unfolding" of the thoracic aorta can occur, displacing the aorta far from the esophagus at often oblique angles and limiting visualization of the aorta in conventional imaging planes.

The TEE blind spot encompassing the distal ascending aorta has been considerably narrowed by longitudinal biplane imaging but remains a potential hazard for imaging in the transverse plane only. Significant focal aortic disease, such as a penetrating aortic ulcer, may be concealed within this region. The author has examined a patient in whom aortic dissection localized to the distal ascending aorta

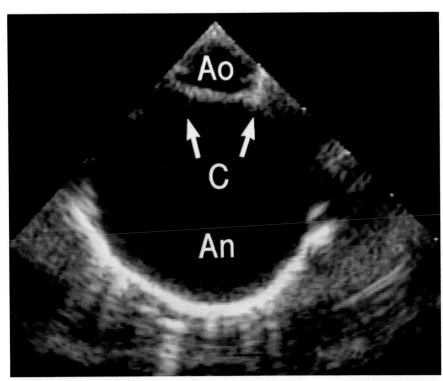

A

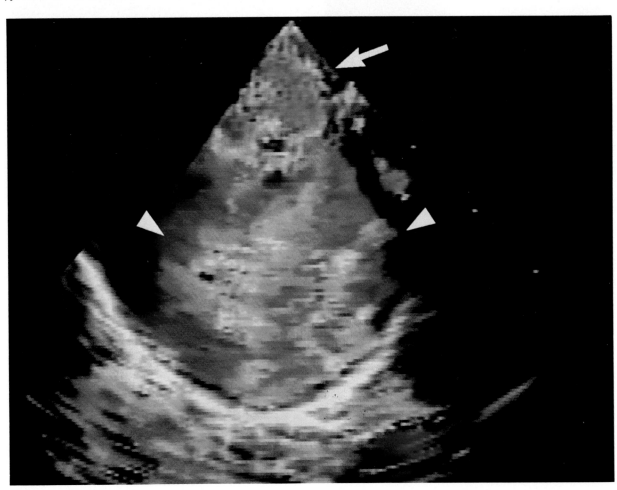

B

Fig. 14-32.   Coarctation of the aorta; transverse short-axis TEE plane. A. The coarctation *(arrows)* has severely compromised the aortic lumen *(Ao),* which has a diameter of approximately 8 mm in this adult patient. A large ductal diverticular aneurysm also is present. B. Turbulent flow across the coarctation *(arrow)* by color Doppler study is consistent with the severe obstruction documented by transthoracic continuous-wave Doppler echocardiography. Low-velocity flow is also noted in the communicating ductal diverticular aneurysm *(arrowheads).*

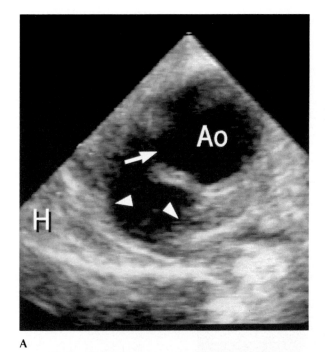

A

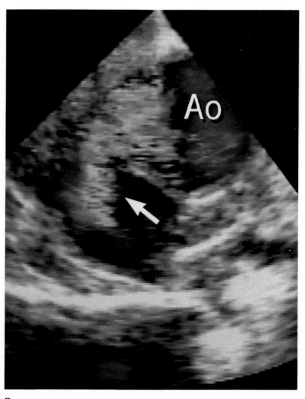

B

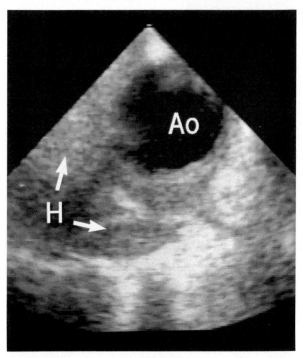

C

Fig. 14-33. Traumatic rupture of the descending thoracic aorta after a motor vehicle accident; transverse TEE plane. A. A large rent in the aorta is clearly visualized *(arrow)* communicating with an adjacent para-aortic space *(arrowheads)*; there is also hematoma formation. B. Color Doppler imaging confirms blood flow extravasation into the para-aortic space *(arrow)* from the aorta. C. More distal TEE imaging demonstrates extension of the large hematoma *(arrows)*, which nearly encircles the aorta at this level.

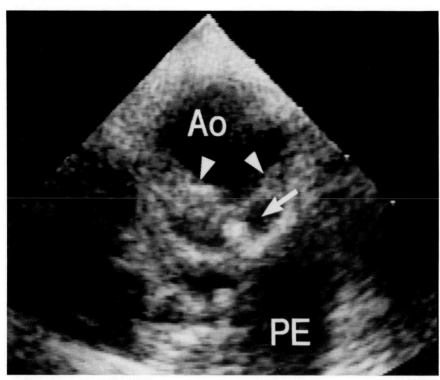

A

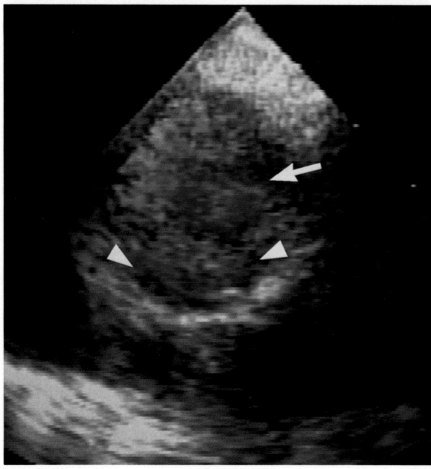

B

Fig. 14-34. Iatrogenic distal aortic dissection precipitated by intra-aortic balloon pump insertion; transverse TEE imaging. A. The tip of the balloon pump catheter *(arrow)* is visualized within a false lumen of the aorta, and the intimal flap *(arrowheads)* is shifted toward the false lumen during balloon deflation. A left pleural effusion is present. B. Double-channel systolic flow within the true lumen *(arrow)* and false lumen *(arrowheads)* is detected by color Doppler examination during systole.

Fig. 14-34 continued C. Inflation of the intra-aortic balloon *(arrow)* during diastolic counterpulsation causes the intimal flap *(arrowheads)* to compress the true aortic lumen. D. Turbulent diastolic flow *(arrows)* with considerable motion artifact is detected by color Doppler imaging during balloon *(arrowheads)* counterpulsation.

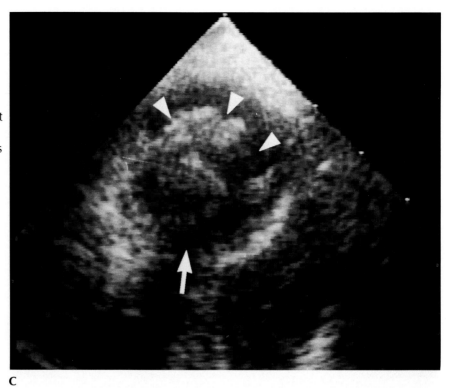

C

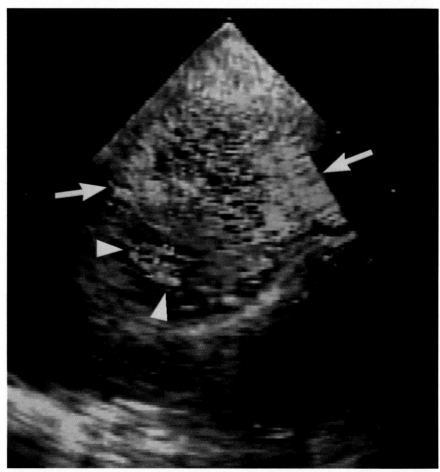

D

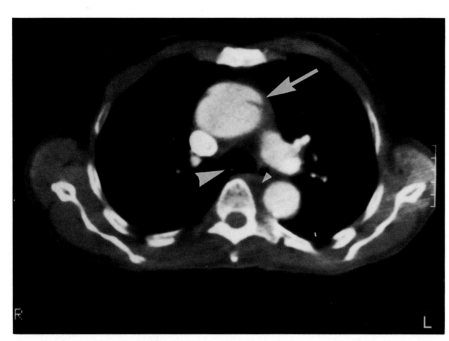

Fig. 14-35. Localized dissection of the aortic arch that was undetected by monoplane transverse TEE imaging. Computed tomographic imaging reveals a focal intimal flap *(arrow)* within the aorta that was obscured by the air-filled, interposed distal trachea and proximal mainstem bronchi *(large arrowhead)* during TEE imaging from the esophagus *(small arrowhead)*. Biplane TEE was not available at the time of this evaluation.

was totally obscured by the interposed airways on monoplane TEE imaging and was discovered later only by computed tomographic scanning (Fig. 14-35).

Several ultrasonic phenomena can lead to potential pitfalls in interpretation despite the high-resolution imaging capabilities of TEE (see Chapter 6). Crescentic, mobile reverberation artifacts or even stationary side lobe artifacts may be seen. These are most commonly present within the ascending aorta imaged with excessive gain settings. Such artifacts may be seen in more than one imaging plane and can mimic the appearance of an intimal flap. These artifacts are distinguished from true intra-aortic disease because they cross the anatomic boundaries of the aorta and have no influence on the intraluminal flow patterns visualized by color Doppler mapping (Fig. 14-36).

The left lung adjacent to the descending thoracic aorta produces a highly reflective interface to ultrasound and commonly causes a mirror-image reflection artifact of the aorta. On two-dimensional imaging, the appearance may be mistaken for a para-aortic aneurysm, fluid collection, or even the double lumen of aortic dissection. The artifactual nature of this finding is revealed by the reflected color Doppler flow signals, which are identical to those within the actual aortic lumen. Such mirror-image color Doppler findings, which can be displayed in either transverse or longitudinal planes (Fig. 14-37), are

not seen with any pathologic condition of the thoracic aorta.

Extra-aortic structures should be recognized and not be confused with pathologic conditions. The transverse sinus may appear as an echolucent aortic periannular abscess or the vertebral body as a peri-aortic mass or hematoma (see Fig. 14-7). Collapse of the posteromedial portion of the left lung, highlighted by an adjacent localized left pleural effusion, has been reported to mimic the appearance of a descending thoracic aortic aneurysm with thrombus [67].

SUMMARY

High-resolution delineation of a broad spectrum of thoracic aortic pathologic conditions is possible by TEE. This technique allows expeditious bedside diagnosis and is safe and well tolerated, even in life-threatening conditions. Transesophageal color Doppler flow imaging has contributed significantly to the understanding of the pathophysiology of various lesions, notably aortic dissection. Transesophageal echocardiographic windows for the investigation of thoracic aortic disease have broadened with development of biplanar longitudinal imaging and should further expand with the improvement of multiplanar imaging systems in the future.

Fig. 14-36. Reverberation artifact mimicking aortic dissection; longitudinal TEE plane. A. A linear, hyperrefractile echodensity *(arrows)* is visualized within the ascending aorta. The artifactual nature of this finding is revealed as it crosses anatomic boundaries into the right pulmonary artery *(lower arrow)*. B. Color-flow Doppler imaging demonstrates undisturbed laminar flow within the aorta *(arrow)*, confirming the absence of an intimal flap. Normal flow aliasing is seen just distal to the aortic valve (yellow-orange).

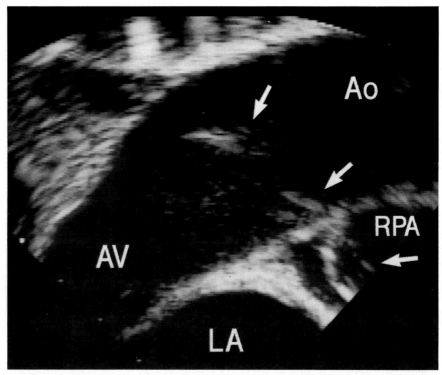

A

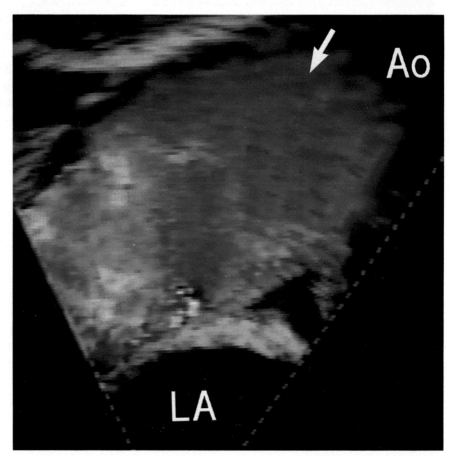

B

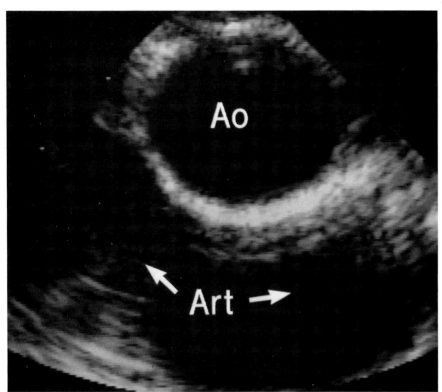

A

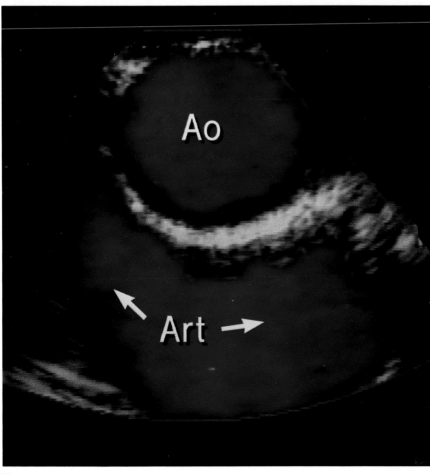

B

Fig. 14-37. Para-aortic artifact caused by ultrasound reflection by the left lung interface with the aorta. A. A large reflection artifact *(Art)* encompasses the transverse short-axis image of the aorta, potentially mimicking an effusion or a para-aortic cavity. B. Color Doppler signals of aortic flow are also reflected within the artifact.

Fig. 14-37 (continued)   C. The same reflection artifact is present in the longitudinal plane. The wall of the aorta adjacent to the artifact must not be mistaken for an intimal flap. D. Characteristic mirror image reflection of color signals within the aorta occurs in the artifact. Such color Doppler findings exclude a separate flow pattern such as that seen with aortic dissection.

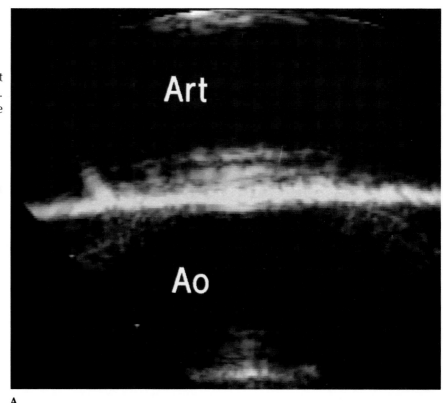

A

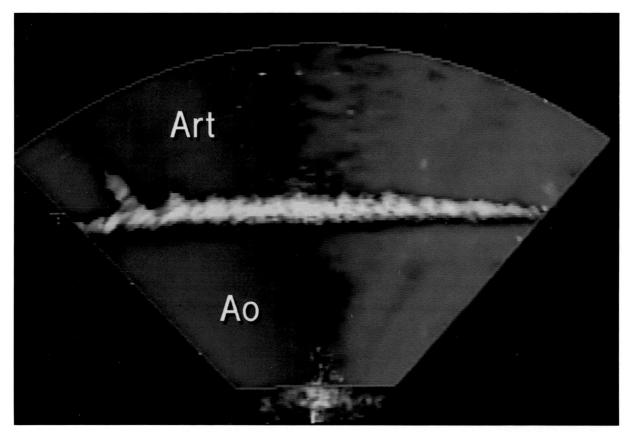

B

REFERENCES

1. Tajik AJ, Seward JB, Hagler DJ, et al. Two-dimensional real-time ultrasonic imaging of the heart and great vessels: technique, image orientation, structure identification, and validation. *Mayo Clin Proc* 1978;53:271–303.

2. Bansal RC, Tajik AJ, Seward JB, Offord KP. Feasibility of detailed two-dimensional echocardiographic examination in adults: prospective study of 200 patients. *Mayo Clin Proc* 1980;55:291–308.

3. Iliceto S, Antonelli G, Biasco G, Rizzon P. Two-dimensional echocardiographic evaluation of aneurysms of the descending thoracic aorta. *Circulation* 1982;66:1045–9.

4. Mathew T, Nanda NC. Two-dimensional and Doppler echocardiographic evaluation of aortic aneurysm and dissection. *Am J Cardiol* 1984;54:379–85.

5. Khandheria BK, Tajik AJ, Taylor CL, et al. Aortic dissection: review of value and limitations of two-dimensional echocardiography in a six-year experience. *J Am Soc Echocardiogr* 1989;2:17–24.

6. Seward JB, Khandheria BK, Edwards WD, et al. Biplanar transesophageal echocardiography: anatomic correlations, image orientation, and clinical applications. *Mayo Clin Proc* 1990;65:1193–213.

7. Bansal RC, Shakudo M, Shah PM, Shah PM. Biplane transesophageal echocardiography: technique, image orientation, and preliminary experience in 131 patients. *J Am Soc Echocardiogr* 1990;3:348–66.

8. Seward JB, Khandheria BK, Oh JK, et al. Transesophageal echocardiography: technique, anatomic correlations, implementation, and clinical applications. *Mayo Clin Proc* 1988;63:649–80.

9. Schlüter M, Hinrichs A, Thier W, et al. Transesophageal two-dimensional echocardiography: comparison of ultrasonic and anatomic sections. *Am J Cardiol* 1984;53:1173–8.

10. Stümper O, Fraser AG, Ho SY, et al. Transoesophageal echocardiography in the longitudinal axis: correlation between anatomy and images and its clinical implications. *Br Heart J* 1990;64:282–8.

11. DeSanctis RW, Doroghazi RM, Austen WG, Buckley MJ. Aortic dissection. *N Engl J Med* 1987;317:1060–7.

12. Singh H, Fitzgerald E, Ruttley MST. Computed tomography: the investigation of choice for aortic dissection? *Br Heart J* 1986;56:171–5.

13. White RD, Lipton MJ, Higgins CB, et al. Noninvasive evaluation of suspected thoracic aortic disease by contrast-enhanced computed tomography. *Am J Cardiol* 1986;57:282–90.

14. Morgan JM, Oldershaw PJ, Gray HH. Use of computed tomographic scanning and aortography in the diagnosis of acute dissection of the thoracic aorta. *Br Heart J* 1990;64:261–5.

15. Erbel R, Mohr-Kahaly S, Oelert H, et al. Diagnostic strategies in suspected aortic dissection: comparison of computed tomography, aortography, and transesophageal echocardiography. *Am J Cardiac Imaging* 1990;4:157–72.

16. Vasile N, Mathieu D, Keita K, et al. Computed tomography of thoracic aortic dissection: accuracy and pitfalls. *J Comput Assist Tomogr* 1986;10:211–5.

17. Amparo EG, Higgins CB, Hricak H, Sollitto R. Aortic dissection: magnetic resonance imaging. *Radiology* 1985;155:399–406.

18. Kersting-Sommerhoff BA, Higgins CB, White RD, et al. Aortic dissection: sensitivity and specificity of MR imaging. *Radiology* 1988;166:651–5.

19. Godwin JD, Breiman RS, Speckman JM. Problems and pitfalls in the evaluation of thoracic aortic dissection by computed tomography. *J Comput Assist Tomogr* 1982;6:750–6.

20. Solomon SL, Brown JJ, Glazer HS, et al. Thoracic aortic dissection: pitfalls and artifacts in MR imaging. *Radiology* 1990;177:223–8.

21. Victor MF, Mintz GS, Kotler MN, et al. Two dimensional echocardiographic diagnosis of aortic dissection. *Am J Cardiol* 1981;48:1155–9.

22. Granato JE, Dee P, Gibson RS. Utility of two-dimensional echocardiography in suspected ascending aortic dissection. *Am J Cardiol* 1985;56:123–9.

23. McLeod AA, Monaghan MJ, Richardson PJ, et al. Diagnosis of acute aortic dissection by M-mode and cross-sectional echocardiography: a five-year experience. *Eur Heart J* 1983;4:196–202.

24. Iliceto S, Nanda NC, Rizzon P, et al. Color Doppler evaluation of aortic dissection. *Circulation* 1987;75:748–55.

25. Iliceto S, Ettorre G, Francioso G, et al. Diagnosis of aneurysm of the thoracic aorta. Comparison between two non invasive techniques: two-dimensional echocardiography and computed tomography. *Eur Heart J* 1984;5:545–5.

26. Taams MA, Gussenhoven WJ, Schippers LA, et al. The value of transesophageal echocardiography for diagnosis of thoracic aorta pathology. *Eur Heart J* 1988;9:1308–16.

27. Ballal RS, Nanda NC, Gatewood R, et al. Usefulness of transesophageal echocardiography in assessment of aortic dissection. *Circulation* 1991;84:1903–14.

28. Börner N, Erbel R, Braun B, et al. Diagnosis of aortic dissection by transesophageal echocardiography. *Am J Cardiol* 1984;54:1157–8.

29. Erbel R, Börner N, Steller D, et al. Detection of aortic dissection by transoesophageal echocardiography. *Br Heart J* 1987;58:45–51.

30. Engberding R, Bender F, Grosse-Heitmeyer W, et al. Identification of dissection or aneurysm of the descending thoracic aorta by conventional and transesophageal two-dimensional echocardiography. *Am J Cardiol* 1987;59:717–9.

31. Miller DC, Mitchell RC, Oyer PE, et al. Independent determinants of operative mortality for patients with aortic dissections. *Circulation* 1984;70 Suppl 1:I–153-I–64.

32. Mohr-Kahaly S, Puth M, Erbel R, Meyer J. Intramural hematoma visualized by transesophageal echocardiography: an early sign of aortic dissection (abstract). *J Am Coll Cardiol* 1991;17 Suppl A:20A.

33. Mohr-Kahaly S, Erbel R, Puth M, et al. Aortic intramural hematoma visualized by transesophageal echocardiography (abstract). *Circulation* 1991;84 Suppl 2:II–128.

34. Erbel R, Engberding R, Daniel W, et al. Echocardiography in diagnosis of aortic dissection. *Lancet* 1989;1:457–61.

35. Burstow DJ, Oh JK, Bailey KR, et al. Cardiac tamponade: characteristic Doppler observations. *Mayo Clin Proc* 1989;64:312–24.

36. Mohr-Kahaly S, Erbel R, Rennollet H, et al. Ambulatory follow-up of aortic dissection by transesophageal two-dimensional and color-coded Doppler echocardiography. *Circulation* 1989;80:24–33.

37. Hashimoto S, Kumada T, Osakada G, et al. Assessment of transesophageal Doppler echography in dissecting aortic aneurysm. *J Am Coll Cardiol* 1989;14:1253–62.

38. Adachi H, Kyo S, Takamoto S, et al. Early diagnosis and surgical intervention of acute aortic dissection by transesophageal color flow mapping. *Circulation* 1990;82 Suppl 4:IV–19-IV–23.

39. Takamoto S, Omoto R. Visualization of thoracic dissecting aortic aneurysm by transesophageal Doppler color flow mapping. *Herz* 1987;12:187–93.

40. Perry GL, Helmcke F, Nanda NC, et al. Evaluation of aortic insufficiency by Doppler color flow mapping. *J Am Coll Cardiol* 1987;9:952–9.

41. Touche T, Prasquier R, Nitenberg A, et al. Assessment and follow-up of patients with aortic regurgitation by an updated Doppler echocardiographic measurement of the regurgitant fraction in the aortic arch. *Circulation* 1985;72:819–24.

42. Mügge A, Daniel WG, Laas J, et al. False-negative diagnosis of proximal aortic dissection by computed tomography or angiography and possible explanations based on transesophageal echocardiographic findings. *Am J Cardiol* 1990;65:527–9.

43. Erbel R, Mohr-Kahaly S, Rennollet H, et al. Diagnosis of aortic dissection: the value of transesophageal echocardiography. *Thorac Cardiovasc Surg* 1987;-35 (Special Issue 1):126–33.

44. Adachi H, Omoto R, Kyo S, et al. Emergency surgical intervention of acute aortic dissection with the rapid diagnosis by transesophageal echocardiography. *Circulation* 1991;84 Suppl 3:III–14-III–9.

45. Nienaber CA, Spielmann RP, von Kodolitsch Y, et al. Diagnosis of thoracic aortic dissection: magnetic resonance imaging versus transesophageal echocardiography. *Circulation* 1992;85:434–47.

45a. Nienaber CA, von Kodolitsch Y, Nicolas V, et al. The diagnosis of thoracic aortic dissection by non-invasive imaging procedures. *N Engl J Med* 1993;328:1–9.

46. Chan K-L. Usefulness of transesophageal echocardiography in the diagnosis of conditions mimicking aortic dissection. *Am Heart J* 1991;122:495–504.

47. Hixson CS, Cater A, Smith MD. Diagnosis and documentation of healing in descending thoracic aortic dissection by transesophageal echocardiography and Doppler color flow imaging. *Am Heart J* 1990;119:1432–5.

48. Erbel R, Oelert H, Meyer J, et al. New classification of aortic dissection by transesophageal echocardiography (abstract). *Circulation* 1991;84 Suppl 2:II–23.

49. Schippers OA, Gussenhoven WJ, van Herwerden LA, et al. The role of intraoperative two-dimensional echocardiography in the assessment of thoracic aorta pathology. *Thorac Cardiovasc Surg* 1988;36:208–13.

50. Blackshear JL, Safford RE, Lane GE, et al. Unruptured noncoronary sinus of Valsalva aneurysm: preoperative characterization by transesophageal echocardiography. *J Am Soc Echocardiogr* 1991;4:485–90.

51. Taams MA, Gussenhoven WJ, Bos E, Roelandt J. Saccular aneurysm of the transverse thoracic aorta detected by transesophageal echocardiography. *Chest* 1988;93:436–7.

52. Cooke JP, Kazmier FJ, Orszulak TA. The penetrating aortic ulcer: pathologic manifestations, diagnosis, and management. *Mayo Clin Proc* 1988;63:718–25.

53. Wissler RW. Principles of the pathogenesis of atherosclerosis. In: Braunwald E, ed. *Heart Disease: A Textbook of Cardiovascular Medicine,* 2nd ed. Philadelphia: Saunders, 1984:1185–6.

54. Tobler HG, Edwards JE. Frequency and location of atherosclerotic plaques in the ascending aorta. *J Thorac Cardiovasc Surg* 1988;96:304–6.

55. Dahlberg PJ, Frecentese DF, Cogbill TH. Cholesterol embolism: experience with 22 histologically proven cases. *Surgery* 1989;105:737–46.

56. Karalis DG, Chandrasekaran K, Victor MF, et al. Recognition and embolic potential of intraaortic atherosclerotic debris. *J Am Coll Cardiol* 1991; 17:73–8.

57. Fine MJ, Kapoor W, Falanga V. Cholesterol crystal embolization: a review of 221 cases in the English literature. *Angiology* 1987;38:769–84.

58. Tunick PA, Kronzon I. Protruding atherosclerotic plaque in the aortic arch of patients with systemic embolization: a new finding seen by transesophageal echocardiography. *Am Heart J* 1990;120: 658–60.

59. Tunick PA, Culliford AT, Lamparello PJ, Kronzon I. Atheromatosis of the aortic arch as an occult source of multiple systemic emboli. *Ann Intern Med* 1991;114:391–2.

60. Stanson AW, Kazmier FJ, Hollier LH, et al. Penetrating atherosclerotic ulcers of the thoracic aorta: natural history and clinicopathologic correlations. *Ann Vasc Surg* 1986;1:15–23.

61. Stern H, Erbel R, Schreiner G, et al. Coarctation of the aorta: quantitative analysis by transesophageal echocardiography. *Echocardiography* 1987;4: 387–95.

62. Erbel R, Bednarczyk I, Pop T, et al. Detection of dissection of the aortic intima and media after angioplasty of coarctation of the aorta: an angiographic, computer tomographic, and echocardiographic comparative study. *Circulation* 1990;81:805–14.

63. Bergin PJ. Aortic thrombosis and peripheral embolization after thoracic gunshot wound diagnosed by transesophageal echocardiography. *Am Heart J* 1990;119:688–90.

64. Kodali S, Jamieson WRE, Leia-Stephens M, et al. Traumatic rupture of the thoracic aorta: a 20–year review: 1969–1989. *Circulation* 1991;84 Suppl 3:III–40-III–6.

65. Moloney JF, Duffy CI, Plehn JF. Transesophageal echocardiographic findings in severe blunt chest trauma (abstract). *Circulation* 1991;84 Suppl 2:II–128.

66. Nakatani S, Beppu S, Tanaka N, et al. Application of abdominal and transesophageal echocardiography as a guide for insertion of intraaortic balloon pump in aortic dissection. *Am J Cardiol* 1989;64: 1082–3.

67. Kronzon I, Demopoulos L, Schrem SS, et al. Pitfalls in the diagnosis of thoracic aortic aneurysm by transesophageal echocardiography. *J Am Soc Echocardiogr* 1990;3:145–8.

15

Source of Embolism

Utility of Transesophageal Echocardiography

Roger L. Click • Raúl Emilio Espinosa • Bijoy K. Khandheria

Embolic events and source of embolism have become major indications for transesophageal echocardiography (TEE). In the initial Mayo Clinic series of patients undergoing TEE, 16% were referred for a source of embolism [1]. With the realization that TEE can demonstrate possible sources of emboli such as patent foramen ovale and slow, swirling blood flow in the left atrium (spontaneous echocardiographic contrast), referrals for source of embolism increased, now averaging more than 30% of our TEE practice [2]. By far, the largest proportion of studies of and experience with source of embolism has been with central embolic events, stroke, and transient ischemic attack. Referrals for peripheral embolism make up a smaller number, but the principles of evaluation and the echocardiographic approach are the same.

It has been estimated that 75% of cardiac emboli lodge in the brain [3]; the remainder embolize peripherally, and many may be silent. The number of cerebrovascular events that can be attributed to a cardiac source of embolism varies and depends on the population studied. In clinical studies, cardiogenic embolism accounts for approximately 15% (range, 6 to 23%) of all ischemic strokes [4–6]. Autopsy studies have shown that cardiogenic emboli may be even more frequent. Nonvalvular atrial fibrillation is the underlying cause in an estimated 45%, the remainder nearly equally divided among patients with acute myocardial infarction, left ventricular aneurysm, rheumatic heart disease, prosthetic valves, and a variety of other causes [4] (Table 15-1).

With the superiority of TEE for visualization of intracardiac structures, it has become a procedure widely used by physicians in examining patients who present with an embolic event. In this chapter, we review the role of TEE in assessing this group of patients.

Table 15-1. Cardiac sources of embolism

Source	Percentage of all embolic events
Nonvalvular atrial fibrillation	45
Acute myocardial infarction	15
Ventricular aneurysm	10
Rheumatic heart disease	10
Prosthetic cardiac valves	10
Other	10
Mitral valve prolapse	
Mitral annulus calcification	
Infectious endocarditis	
Nonbacterial thrombotic endocarditis	
Calcific aortic stenosis	
Cardiac myxoma	
Paradoxical embolism and congenital heart disease	
Nonischemic dilated cardiomyopathy	
Atrial septal aneurysm	
Patent foramen ovale	
Aortic atheroma	

Source: Modified from Cerebral Embolism Task Force. Cardiogenic brain embolism. *Arch Neurol* 1986; 43:71–84.

ETIOLOGY

A direct cause and effect relationship is often difficult to establish when attempting to find the source of an embolic event. Dividing this discussion into direct and indirect sources of emboli is helpful (Table 15-2). If the echocardiographic findings show that the cause and effect relationship is almost certain, the source of embolism is *direct*. Lesions in this category are an intracardiac thrombus in the ventricles, atria, or atrial appendages; intracardiac tumors, especially atrial myxomas; valvular vegetations; and bulky, mobile aortic plaques. If the echocardiographic findings show a less certain cause and effect relationship, the source of embolism is *indirect*. These findings may represent potential intracardiac sources of emboli. They include valvular abnormalities, such as mitral valve prolapse, mitral annulus calcification, and aortic valve calcification; cardiomyopathy; spontaneous echocardiographic contrast; atrial septal aneurysm; and atrial septal defect or patent foramen ovale with the potential for paradoxical embolism.

ROLE OF TRANSTHORACIC ECHOCARDIOGRAPHY

After the development of two-dimensional (2-D) transthoracic imaging, which had obvious advantages over M-mode echocardiography for defining intracardiac anatomy, there was much enthusiasm for its use in identifying intracardiac sources of embolism. Unfortunately, most studies showed the yield to be low and the imaging beneficial only in the subgroup of patients with identifiable cardiovascular disease by physical examination, electrocardiography, or chest radiography. Lovett et al. [7], using 2-D transthoracic echocardiography in patients with episodes of focal cerebral ischemia, found a direct cause in 6.5% and an indirect (potential) source in 23%. The yield was higher in patients with clinically identifiable cardiac disease, hypertension, and, especially, atrial fibrillation. The overall low yield for a direct embolic source did not warrant routine use of 2-D echocardiography in all patients with unexplained cerebral ischemic events. Similarly, others found a low yield for 2-D transthoracic echocardiography in the routine evaluation for intracardiac sources of embolism [8–10]. However, in patients younger than 45 years with clinically evident cardiovascular disease, the potential yield was higher. In

Table 15-2. Classification of sources of emboli

Direct source
  Thrombus
  Tumor
  Vegetation
  Aortic atheroma
Indirect source
  Valvular disease
  Dilated cardiomyopathy
  Atrial septal aneurysm
  Atrial septal defect
  Patent foramen ovale
  Spontaneous echocardiographic contrast

elderly persons, among whom strokes are more prevalent, the yield was low.

Larson et al. [11] addressed the problem of applying 2-D echocardiography to a population with a low prevalance of intracardiac sources of embolism. They reemphasized that low predictive value and low yield have a major impact on the healthcare dollar and patient management. They suggested that 2-D echocardiography should not be routinely performed in all patients with an embolic event. Despite this overwhelming evidence, 2-D echocardiography continued to be frequently performed for this purpose.

With improved technology in 2-D imaging over the past decade, the temptation to continue referring and evaluating patients with an embolic event who are at low risk for cardiovascular disease has persisted despite earlier studies. An article on transient ischemic attacks emphasized the low yield of diagnostic evaluation, part of which was done by echocardiography [12].

ROLE OF TEE

Transesophageal echocardiography has opened a new era for assessment of patients with embolic events. Many of the limitations of transthoracic echocardiography have been overcome. The gains include ability to image in patients presenting technical difficulties and improvement in visualization of the left atrium, left atrial appendage, atrial septum, and thoracic aortic, native, and prosthetic valves. In addition, the sensitivity for detecting potential sources of emboli, patent foramen ovale, and spontaneous echocardiographic contrast has increased considerably with the use of TEE. However, the yield in various patient populations is still uncertain, the cause and effect relationship for indirect or potential sources of embolism remains unclear, and the impact on therapeutic decisions has not been clearly defined. In the remaining sections, we address the role of TEE in defining specific causes of embolism and, finally, summarize the overall role of TEE in this patient population.

Left Atrial Contents

One of the major advantages of TEE in the evaluation of a suspected cardiac source of embolism is the ability to better visualize the left atrium and atrial appendage contents.

Although 2-D transthoracic echocardiography has been valuable for the assessment of left atrial masses, there are limitations in visualizing small left atrial thrombi and the left atrial appendage [13,14]. In a study by Shrestha et al. [15], 293 patients with rheumatic heart disease had a 2-D transthoracic echocardiogram for assessment of left atrial thrombus before open heart surgery. In comparison with the findings at surgery, the specificity was 98.8%. However, the sensitivity was only 58.8%. In 21 patients, left atrial thrombi were missed by 2-D trans-

thoracic echocardiography. Eleven of these were in the left atrial appendage, and all were missed by this procedure. In another study, only one-third of surgically proven left atrial thrombi were detected by transthoracic 2-D echocardiography [16]. In contrast, Aschenberg et al. [17] reported results with TEE in patients with mitral valve stenosis. In six of 21 patients, a left atrial appendage thrombus was diagnosed by TEE. All thrombi were confirmed at surgery, and none were diagnosed by transthoracic echocardiography. In a study looking specifically at a population with embolic events, Pop et al. [18] evaluated 72 patients by transthoracic echocardiography and TEE; three had left atrial appendage thrombi by TEE, none of which were detected by transthoracic echocardiography.

In patients referred for source of embolism, one of the most common positive findings is thrombus in the left atrium or left atrial appendage. Visualization of the left atrium and left atrial appendage is described in Chapters 4 and 5. It is important to scan the entire left atrium for thrombus and, particularly, the dome of the left atrium. Frequently, after a thrombus is seen in the left atrial appendage, other thrombi are found hiding within the body of the left atrium (Figs. 15-1, 15-2, and 15-3).

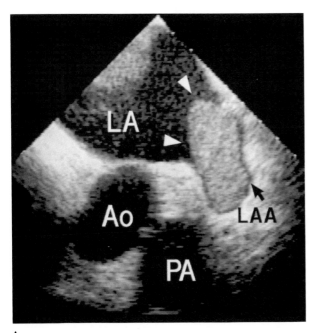
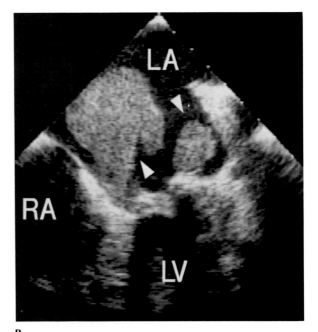

A
B

Fig. 15-1. A. Horizontal plane, short-axis view of the base of the heart visualizes the left atrial appendage *(black arrow)* and left atrium. Optimal view of left atrial appendage shows large thrombus *(white arrowheads)*. B. After the scan beam is moved back across the left atrium, more thrombus *(arrowheads)* is seen.

Fig. 15-2. A. Thrombus *(arrow)* is seen only in the left atrial appendage with spontaneous echocardiographic contrast in the body of the left atrium. B. Inspection of the dome of the left atrium reveals a much larger thrombus *(arrows)*.

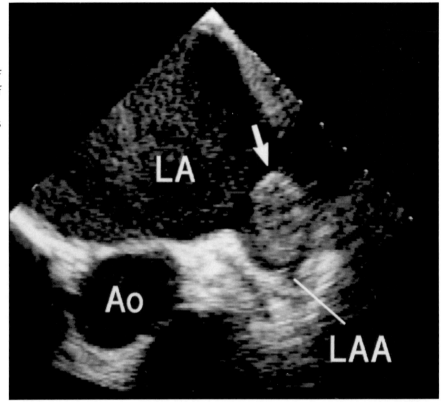

A

B

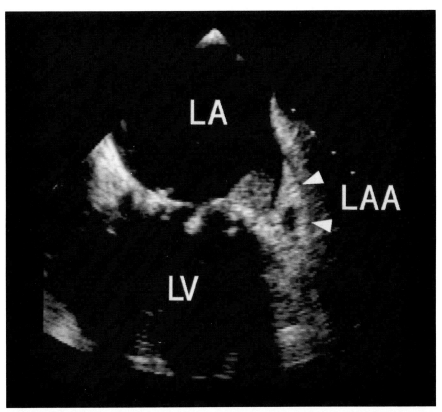

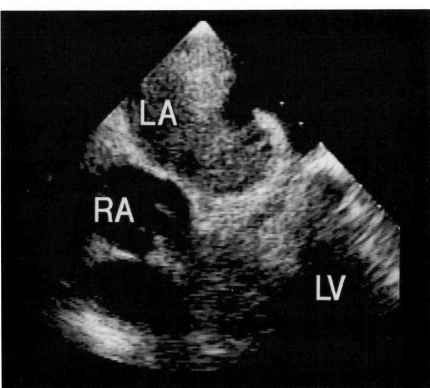

Fig. 15-3.   A. Only a small thrombus is initially seen in the proximal left atrial appendage *(arrowheads)*. B. Further inspection of the left atrium revealed much more thrombus.

Often, well-defined thrombi are not seen in the left atrium or left atrial appendage, but instead "string" thrombus or "sludge" is found, especially in the left atrial appendage (Fig. 15-4). Biplane TEE may be helpful in visualizing the left atrial appendage. Figure 15-5 demonstrates thrombus in the left atrial appendage in the longitudinal plane that was missed in the horizontal plane.

The left atrium may also contain other types of masses that may have embolic potential, such as myxoma. Often these are easily seen on transthoracic echocardiography, but TEE helps to clarify the location and attachment site (Fig. 15-6). Other unusual sources of emboli in the left atrium include foreign bodies (Fig. 15-7).

Because of the unique position of the probe behind the left atrium, TEE is the procedure of choice for assessment of left atrial and left atrial appendage contents. However, the overall yield of finding a direct source of embolism remains low.

Spontaneous Echocardiographic Contrast

Spontaneous echocardiographic contrast (or echo-contrast) is the smokelike appearance of swirling blood seen in low blood flow states (Fig. 15-8). It is not a common finding by transthoracic echocardiography and is seen most commonly in the left ventricle in dilated cardiomyopathy and severely reduced left ventricular function. By transthoracic echocardiography, spontaneous echocardiographic contrast is rarely seen in the left atrium. With TEE, the close proximity of the probe to the left atrium improves resolution, and spontaneous echocardiographic contrast is a more frequent finding, especially in patients with atrial fibrillation or mitral valve disease.

Several studies have found an association between spontaneous echocardiographic contrast and embolic events. Daniel et al. [19] evaluated 50 patients

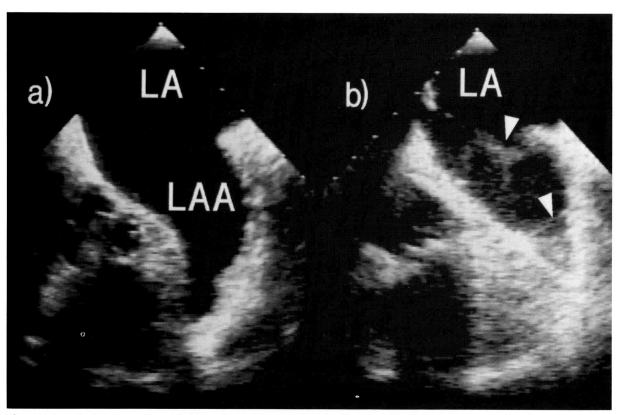

Fig. 15-4. a). Left atrium and left atrial appendage shortly after mitral valve replacement. b). Six months later, during evaluation for the source of the embolism, the same left atrium and left atrial appendage view now shows "sludge" thrombus *(arrowheads)* in the left atrial appendage. Note that anticoagulation in the six-month interim had been suboptimal.

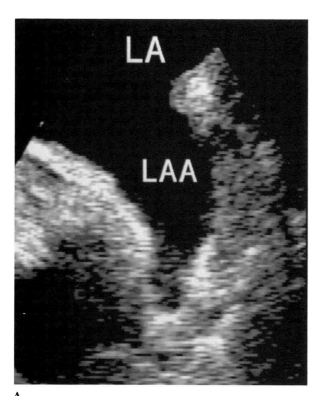

A

Fig. 15-5.   A. View of the left atrial appendage in the horizontal plane shows only haziness in the tip. B. In the longitudinal plane of the left atrial appendage in the same patient, thrombus *(arrowheads)* in the left atrial appendage is clearly shown.

B

with mitral stenosis and 70 patients after mitral valve replacement. Spontaneous echocardiographic contrast was found in 61 patients (50%). Most of the patients were in atrial fibrillation, but seven were in sinus rhythm. Transthoracic echocardiography revealed spontaneous echocardiographic contrast in only one patient. Twenty-nine of the 61 patients with spontaneous echocardiographic contrast had atrial thrombi or a history of documented arterial embolization or both. Only four of 61 patients without spontaneous echocardiographic contrast had evidence of thrombi or embolic events. However, spontaneous echocardiographic contrast was not related to whether patients did or did not have treatment with anticoagulants. Similar studies have also shown an association between spontaneous echocardiographic contrast and embolic events [20–22]. In one report, Black et al. [22] reported on 400 consecutive patients undergoing TEE for a variety of reasons. Spontaneous echocardiographic contrast was seen in 75 patients (19%) and was significantly associated

with atrial fibrillation, mitral stenosis, absence of mitral regurgitation, increased left atrial dimension, and a history of suspected embolism. Multivariate analysis in 89 patients with mitral stenosis or mitral valve replacement showed that spontaneous echocardiographic contrast was the only independent predictor of left atrial thrombus or suspected embolism. In 60 patients with nonvalvular atrial fibrillation, spontaneous echocardiographic contrast and age were independent predictors of left atrial thrombus or suspected embolic event, or both. The factors contributing to left atrial spontaneous echocardiographic contrast are mitral valve disease, mitral valve prosthesis, enlarged left atrium, and atrial fibrillation [21–25].

Spontaneous echocardiographic contrast is not an unusual finding by TEE, especially in the left atrium. An increased embolic risk appears to be associated with this finding. The magnitude of the risk is uncertain, and the effect of this finding on patient management and outcome is unclear.

Fig. 15-6. A. In the horizontal plane, a myxoma *(arrows)* is shown in the left atrium. B. In the longitudinal plane, the same myxoma *(arrows)* is positioned near the interatrial septum.

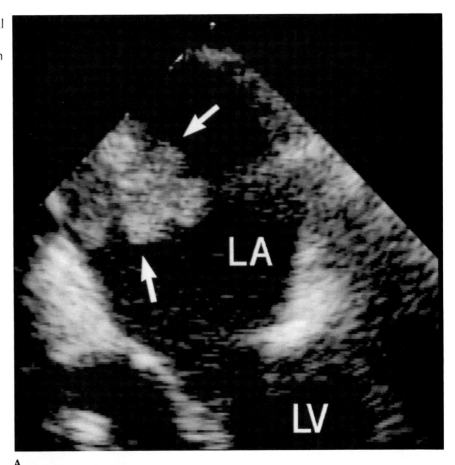

A

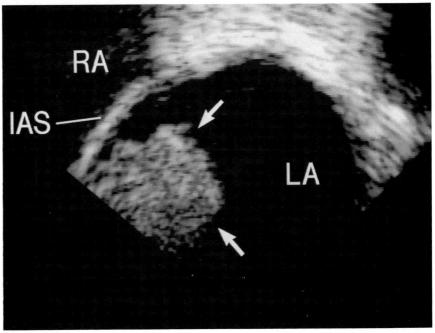

B

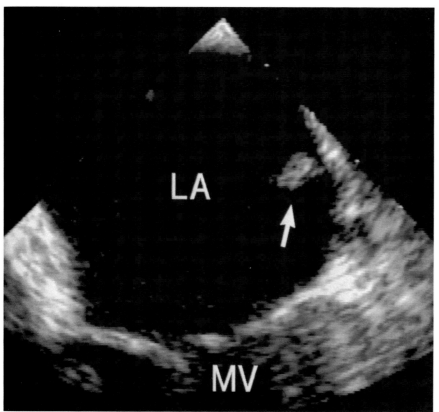

A

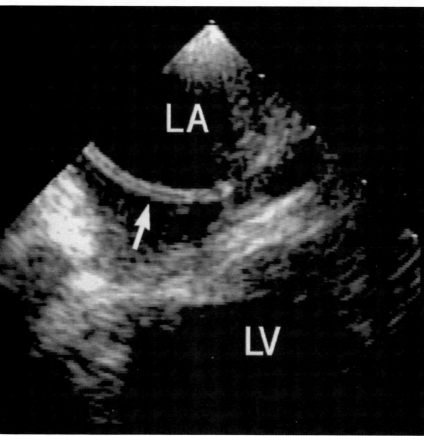

B

Fig. 15-7. A. Small thrombus *(arrow)* is identified in horizontal plane view of left atrium. B. In another frame focusing on the left atrium, a retained left atrium monitoring catheter *(arrow)* from a previous coronary artery bypass graft operation is visualized. A thrombus was attached to the end of the catheter.

Fig. 15-8. Dense spontaneous echocardiographic contrast swirling *(arrows)* in the left atrium.

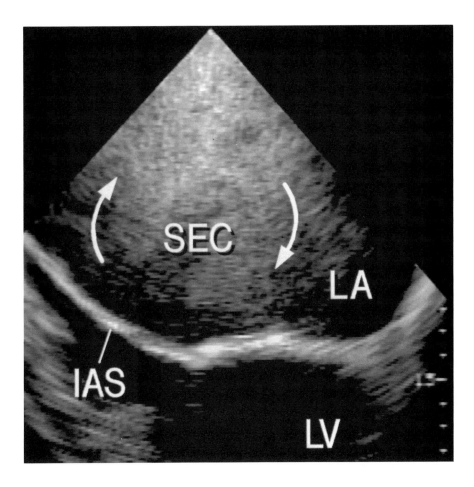

Atrial Septum

The atrial septum is implicated in two ways as a source of embolism: (1) patent foramen ovale with the potential for a paradoxical embolism and (2) atrial septal aneurysm with the potential for thrombus formation within the aneurysm.

A patent foramen ovale is found at autopsy in 25% to 34% of patients of all ages [26]. The vast majority of these abnormalities remain clinically silent and undetected; however, they have the potential for paradoxical embolism, albeit rare. The presumptive diagnosis of paradoxical embolism can be made if venous thrombosis, intracardiac right-to-left shunt, and arterial embolism are present without a cardiac source being identified in the left heart [27]. Echocardiography has been used primarily to detect a right-to-left shunt, most commonly at the atrial level and through a patent foramen ovale. The absolute diagnosis of paradoxical embolism requires that a thrombus crossing the atrial septum be visualized by echocardiography or at autopsy [28].

Transthoracic echocardiography can in many cases adequately visualize the atrial septum, and with color-flow Doppler imaging or contrast medium injection with provocative measures (Valsalva's maneuver, cough), a patent foramen ovale and a shunt can be detected. This finding establishes the potential for paradoxical embolism. Lechat et al. [29], using transthoracic echocardiography with contrast medium and provocative maneuvers, found a higher prevalence of patent foramen ovale in patients with ischemic stroke, especially if no other cause was identified.

Transesophageal echocardiography has the advantage of far superior visualization of the atrial septum and the fossa ovalis membrane, especially with biplane examination. A patent foramen ovale is usually best seen from the longitudinal plane (Fig. 15-9). In addition, with contrast medium injection and color-flow Doppler imaging [30], right-to-left shunt detection is superior with TEE [31–33]. Often, a patent foramen ovale can be diagnosed simply by visualizing the channel through or interruption of

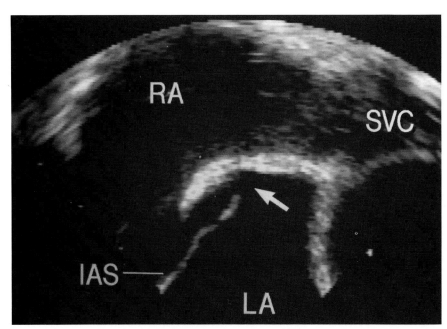

A

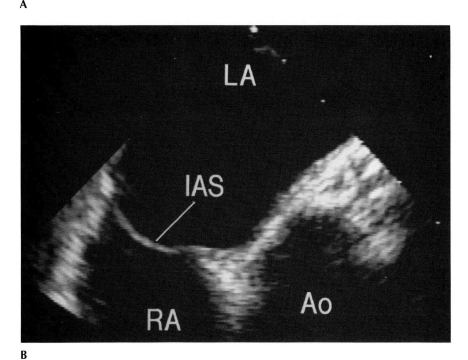

B

Fig. 15-9. A. In this view of the fossa ovalis membrane in the longitudinal plane, the fossa ovalis *(arrow)* is clearly interrupted. B. This defect was not well seen from the horizontal plane.

the superior portion of the fossa ovalis membrane and the atrial septum. This channel may be large (Fig. 15-10) or just a barely detectable slit (Fig. 15-11). The size of the patent foramen ovale often varies throughout the respiratory cycle, with increased right atrial blood flow during inspiration increasing not only the size of the defect but also the degree of right-to-left shunting. In both cases, injection of contrast medium clarifies the presence of a shunt. Other ex-amples of contrast studies and color-flow imaging to help define the integrity of the atrial septum are shown in Figures 15-12, 15-13, and 15-14. It has been demonstrated that contrast injection with the Valsalva maneuver is necessary to optimally visual-ize a patent foramen ovale and right-to-left shunt [31]. If the atrial septum is redundant, the septum bulges toward the left atrium after the release phase of the Valsalva maneuver because of the transient

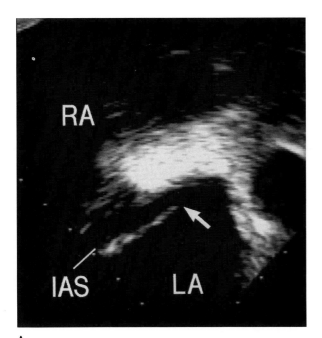
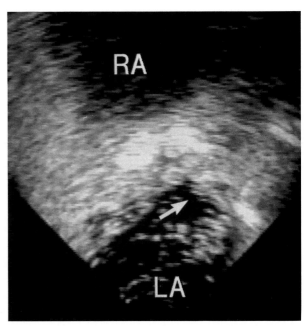

A   B

Fig. 15-10. A. View of atrial septum in the longitudinal plane shows fossa ovalis membrane and wide-open patent foramen ovale *(arrow)*. B. After injection of contrast medium, right-to-left shunt *(arrow)* is seen.

right greater than left atrial pressure differential. Injection of contrast medium at that point shows a right-to-left shunt if the foramen ovale is patent (Fig. 15-15). This may be the only way a patent foramen ovale is demonstrated (Fig. 15-16).

Whether a systemic embolic event and presence or absence of a patent foramen ovale by TEE are related is very controversial. Some investigators maintain that the incidence is not increased [31,34], whereas others suggest that thromboembolic events and a patent foramen ovale found by TEE are related [32,33].

Using contrast TEE, we studied the prevalence of patent foramen ovale and its association with embolic events in 802 patients [35]. Source of embolism was the referral in 437 patients, and 365 patients were referred for other reasons. The overall prevalence of a patent foramen ovale was 17.8% at rest and 35.9% with the Valsalva maneuver. The prevalence was not significantly different between patients with and those without embolic events before and after adjustment for cardiovascular risk factors and cerebrovascular disease. In a subset of patients who had no identifiable risk factors and who were 40 years old or younger, there was no significant difference in the prevalence of patent foramen ovale between those with and those without systemic embolic events [35].

In an editorial by Falk [36], the significance of finding a patent foramen ovale and attributing an ischemic event to paradoxical embolism was questioned. It was noted that, historically, paradoxical embolism has occurred in association with significant concomitant deep venous thrombi or pulmonary embolism and pulmonary hypertension. None of the studies suggesting an increased incidence of embolic events in patients with patent foramen ovale have addressed this association. Furthermore, the likelihood of a venous thrombus passing preferentially through a small patent foramen ovale without pulmonary embolism in an otherwise normal subject would be extremely small. Rarely with TEE, the diagnosis of paradoxical embolism can be made with certainty when a thrombus is "caught in the act" crossing a patent foramen ovale (Fig. 15-17).

Although a controversial point, the weight of the evidence suggests that even though a patent foramen ovale is a potential indirect source or, more appropriately, an avenue for embolic events, the overall actual incidence of true paradoxical embolism is probably very low. In the young patient with a clear-cut embolic event, evidence of deep venous thrombosis, and a patent foramen ovale, one can make a case for aggressive management with anticoagulation or surgical closure of the patent foramen ovale. Certainly, this relationship needs further evaluation

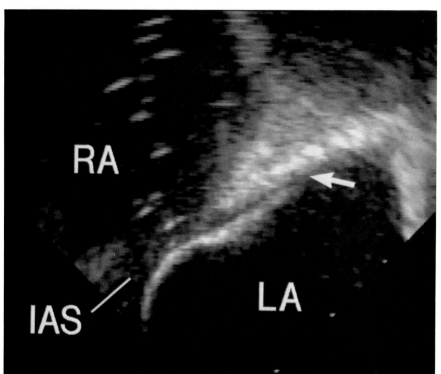

Fig. 15-11. A. View of atrial septum in the longitudinal plane shows "slitlike" patent foramen ovale channel *(arrow).* B. Injection of contrast medium reveals right-to-left shunt. Note bubbles *(arrow)* in the left atrium.

A

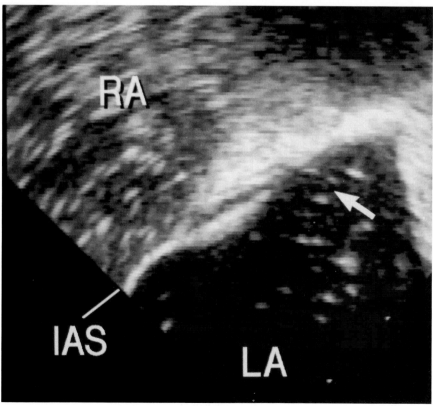

B

Fig. 15-12. View of atrial septum and patent foramen ovale *(arrow)* in longitudinal plane before (A) and after (B) injection of contrast medium. In B, *arrows* point to contrast medium spilling into the left atrium from the right atrium.

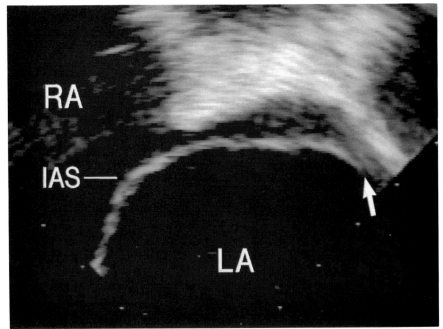

A

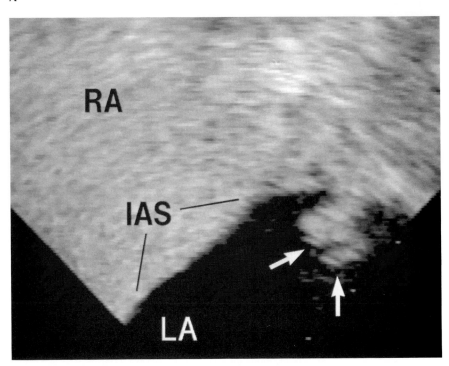

B

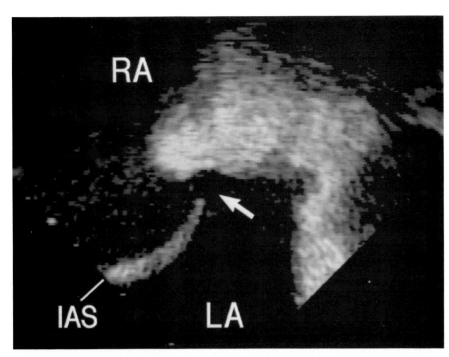

Fig. 15-13. A. View of atrial septum and patent foramen ovale *(arrow)* in the longitudinal plane with two-dimensional imaging only. B. Addition of color-flow to two-dimensional imaging demonstrates shunt *(arrow)*.

A

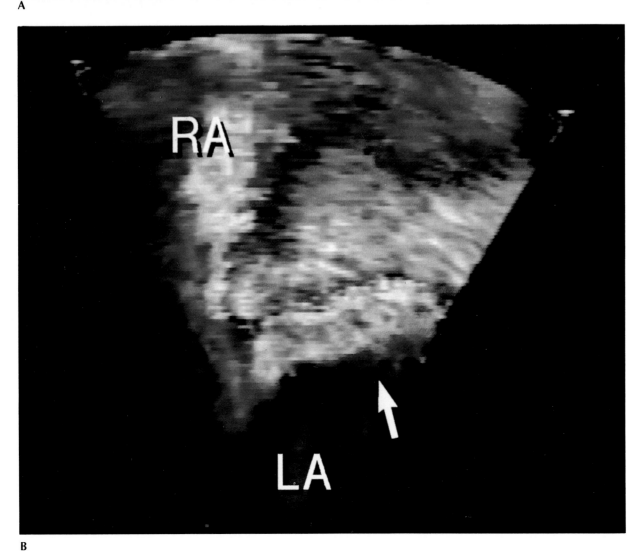

B

Fig. 15-14. View of atrial septum in the longitudinal plane without (A) and with (B) color-flow imaging. Discrete left-to-right shunt *(arrowheads)* is demonstrated on color-flow study.

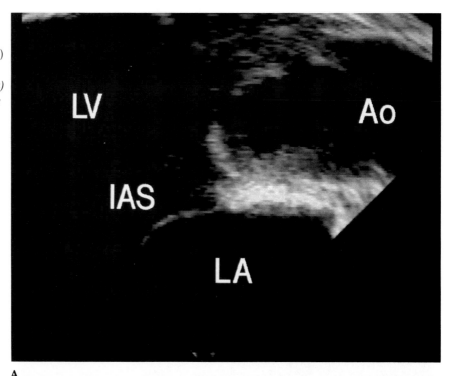

A

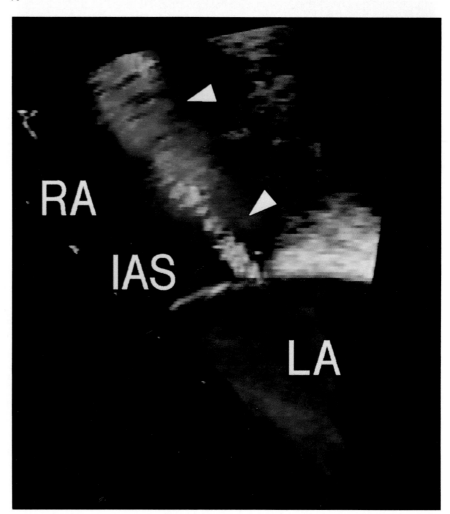

B

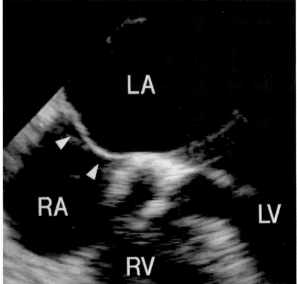

A

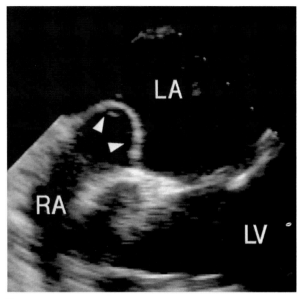

B

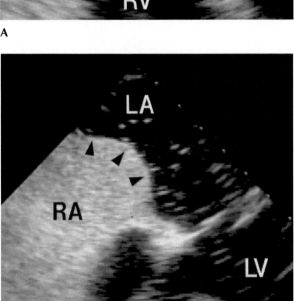

C

Fig. 15-15. A. Atrial septum *(arrowheads)* at rest in the horizontal plane. B. After Valsalva release, the atrial septum *(arrowheads)* bulges toward the left atrium. C. Injection of contrast medium at the time of Valsalva release shows right-to-left shunt *(arrowheads).*

and a more clearly defined cause and effect so that therapeutic options can be maximized and tailored to a given person with an embolic event.

The second abnormality in which the atrial septum is important in the assessment of source of embolism is atrial septal aneurysm (Fig. 15-18). This has double the potential for source of embolism. Atrial septal aneurysms are commonly perforated or fenestrated and have potential for right-to-left flow and paradoxical embolism [37,38]. Likewise, the aneurysm itself may be a site of thrombus formation [39,40]. Transthoracic echocardiographic studies have suggested an association between atrial septal aneurysm and embolic events [38,41].

More recently, TEE recognition of atrial septal aneurysms and association with embolic events have been described [42,43]. Interatrial shunting was seen in 83% of 23 patients with atrial septal aneurysms on TEE. Multiple fenestrations and thrombi were identified within the aneurysm in four and two patients, respectively. Cerebrovascular events occurred in 52% of the patients, and in one patient, no source other than mitral valve prolapse could be found [42]. In a larger series of 78 patients who had transthoracic echocardiography and TEE, the atrial septal aneurysm was missed by transthoracic echocardiography in 56%. Forty percent had a history of an embolic event [43]. Pearson et al. [44] described their experience in 410 consecutive patients. Transesophageal echocardiography found an atrial septal aneurysm in 8%, and only 3% of aneurysms were detected by transthoracic echocardiography. In patients referred for source of embolism, 15% had atrial septal aneurysm, a significant difference from the 4% incidence of atrial septal aneurysm in patients referred for other reasons. These data support the conclusions that atrial septal aneurysms have embolic potential and that TEE is the method of choice to diagnose atrial septal aneurysms and the potential for either

Fig. 15-16. View of atrial septum in the longitudinal plane. A. Fossa ovalis membrane *(arrows)* at rest. B. Injection of contrast medium during rest; no shunt. C. Injection of contrast medium with the Valsalva maneuver demonstrates right-to-left shunt *(arrow)*.

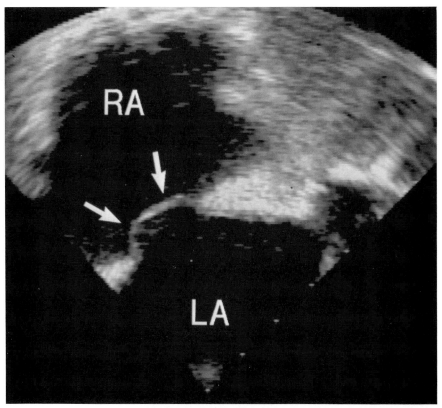

A

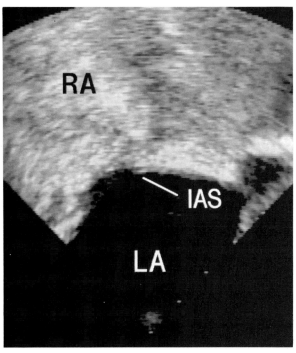

B

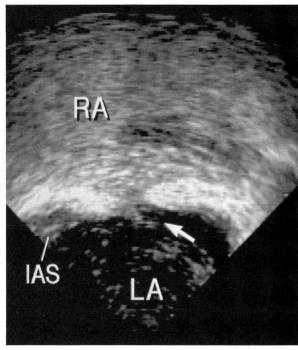

C

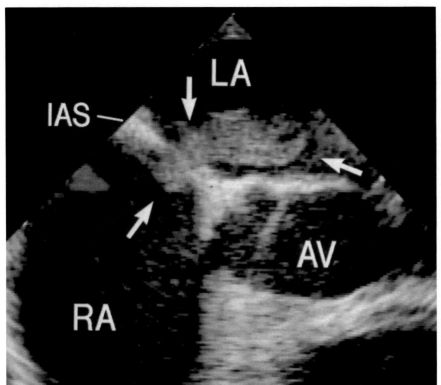

A

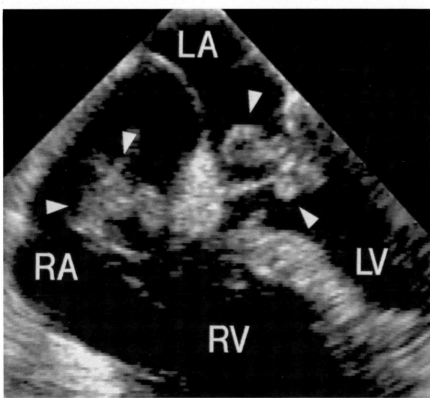

B

Fig. 15-17. Examples of transesophageal echocardiographic findings in patients with paradoxical embolism. In each case, a thrombus *(arrows or arrowheads)* is crossing through a patent foramen ovale.

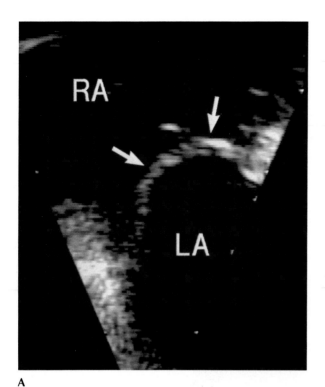

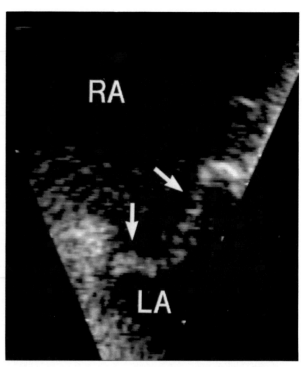

A   B

Fig. 15-18. Atrial septal aneurysm *(arrows)* has typical "jump rope"
appearance, with bulging toward right atrium (A) and then to left atrium (B).

direct or paradoxical emboli. The overall impact that
discovery of an atrial septal aneurysm has on the
individual patient and on clinical management decisions remains to be clarified.

Endocarditis

One of the major complications of bacterial endocarditis is the embolic event. Sanfilippo et al. [45]
described the risk of complication from infective
endocarditis on the basis of transthoracic echocardiographic characteristics in 204 patients. The overall
incidence of complications was 55%. There were
significantly fewer complications (27%) in patients
without discernible valvular abnormalities. In this
study, the incidence of central nervous system embolization was 19%. Vegetation size, extent, and mobility were predictors of complications, including
embolization.

A number of studies have shown that TEE is
superior to transthoracic echocardiography in detecting vegetative endocarditis [46–49] (see Chapter
11). Erbel et al. [46] demonstrated that the rate of
embolization in patients with vegetations on TEE

and negative blood cultures was just as high as that
in patients with positive blood cultures; however, in
patients without vegetations, the rate of embolism
was lower, independent of whether blood cultures
were positive or not. The rate of embolization seems
to be related to the size of vegetations. Most authors
recommend TEE in all patients with suspected endocarditis. Figure 15-19 shows the typical transesophageal appearance of aortic and mitral valve
endocarditis in a patient with a cerebral embolic
event.

Aortic Atheroma

Assessment of aortic disease by TEE is reviewed in
Chapter 14. Aortic atheromatous disease, especially
with mobile intra-aortic debris, appears to have a
clear embolic potential. In our experience [50], there
was a surprisingly high yield of thoracic aortic disease (44% of direct sources of emboli) unrecognized
by transthoracic echocardiography. Likewise, Karalis et al. [51] and Pop et al. [18] found a higher
incidence of thoracic aortic disease by TEE in patients with embolic events. Peripheral emboli from

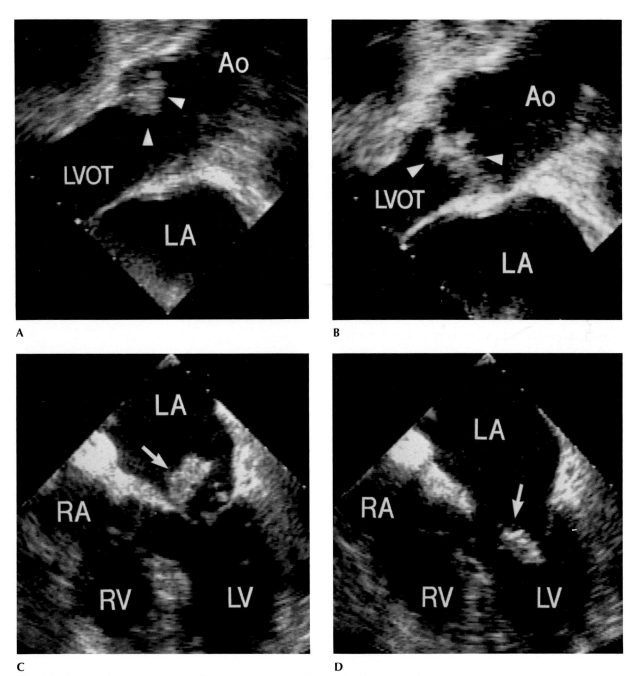

Fig. 15-19.   In the longitudinal plane, aortic vegetation *(arrowheads)* is shown during systole (A) and diastole (B). In the horizontal plane, mitral valve vegetation *(arrows)* is shown during systole (C) and diastole (D)

descending aortic atheromas can be more easily explained than central emboli. However, there is normally a small amount of diastolic flow reversal in the descending aorta, and debris from an aortic atheroma just below the brachiocephalic vessels could, in retrograde fashion, embolize centrally. How far distally in the descending aorta an atheroma can pose a risk for central embolization is not known. Figures 15-20, 15-21, and 15-22 show representative examples of aortic atheroma in the descending aorta.

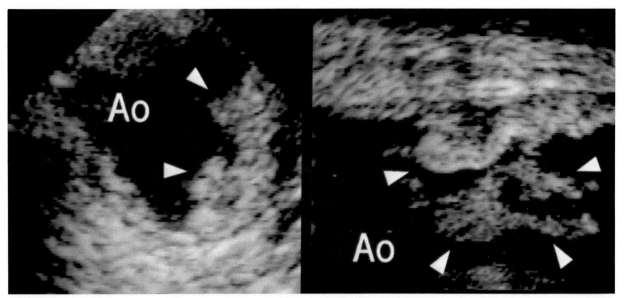

Fig. 15-20. Views in horizontal *(left)* and longitudinal *(right)* planes of aortic atheroma *(arrowheads)* in the descending thoracic aorta.

Valvular Disease

A number of valvular abnormalities, including mitral valve prolapse, aortic sclerosis, and papilloma of aortic or mitral valves, are implicated in embolic events. Transesophageal echocardiography has been shown to be superior in detecting these abnormalities. The cause and effect relationship between these types of valvular abnormalities and embolic events requires further clarification.

OVERALL ROLE OF TEE

A number of reports have compared the overall usefulness of TEE with that of transthoracic echocardiography in assessment of source of embolism [18,52–59]. In all studies, TEE has proved to be significantly more sensitive than transthoracic echocardiography in visualizing potential sources of intracardiac emboli, both direct and indirect.

Daniel et al. [52] reported the European experience in 479 patients evaluated by transthoracic echocardiography and TEE for central (327 patients) and peripheral (152 patients) emboli. Potential sources of emboli were found in 37% of the patients by transthoracic echocardiography and 65% of the patients by TEE. Both direct and indirect sources of emboli were included. Transesophageal echocardi-

ography yielded significantly higher detection rates of mitral valve prolapse, patent foramen ovale, left atrial and appendage thrombi, spontaneous echo contrast, vegetations, and atrial septal aneurysm [52].

In a study by Pearson et al. [54] of 79 patients with unexplained stroke or transient ischemic attack, TEE identified a potential cardiac source in 57%, whereas only 15% were identified by transthoracic echocardiography. As with other studies, TEE was more sensitive in identifying atrial septal aneurysm and patent foramen ovale, left atrial thrombus or tumor, and left atrial spontaneous echocardiographic contrast. Additionally, TEE identified abnormalities in 39% of patients without other evidence of cardiac disease, whereas transthoracic echocardiography did so in only 19%.

We performed a retrospective analysis of 184 patients who underwent both transthoracic echocardiography and TEE during an 18–month period for investigation of source of embolism [50]. The average age of this population was 64 years, with a range of 27 to 88 years. Stroke or a transient cerebral ischemic event prompted the search for source of embolism in 86% of patients; retinal emboli occurred in 7%, upper or lower extremity emboli in 4%, and visceral emboli in 3%.

To more precisely define the additional yield of TEE over transthoracic echocardiography, findings

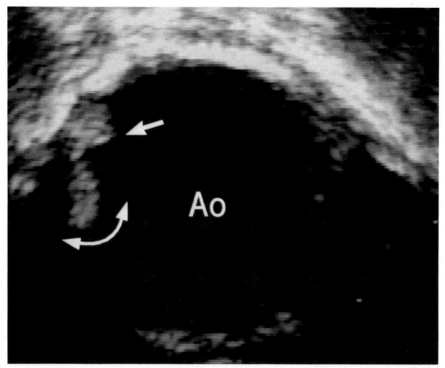

A

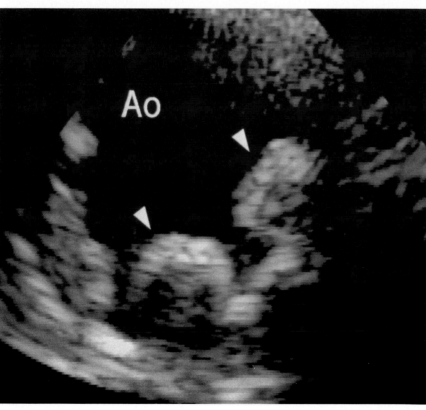

B

Fig. 15-21. Examples of descending thoracic and aortic atheromas *(arrows* or *arrowheads)*, both in the horizontal plane. The atheroma in A is just below the arch and is mobile, swinging back and forth *(curved arrow)* during systole and diastole.

Fig. 15-22. Descending aortic atheroma *(arrowheads)* in horizontal (A) and longitudinal (B) planes.

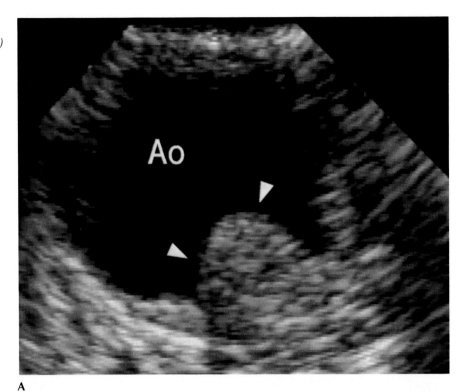

A

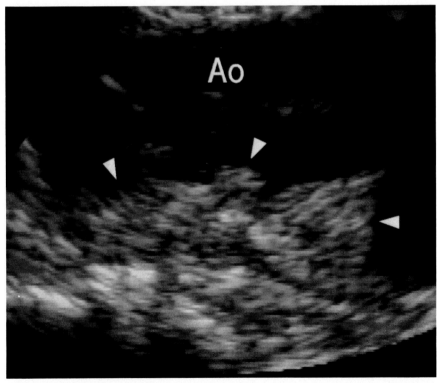

B

were categorized as direct or indirect sources of embolism, as explained above. Clearly, the identification by TEE of a direct source of embolism (e.g., left atrial thrombus) unrecognized by transthoracic echocardiography would strongly support the diagnosis of cardiogenic embolism and likely have a significant effect on patient management. In contrast, the discovery by TEE of an unrecognized indirect source of embolism (e.g., mitral valve prolapse), although important, would leave the diagnosis of cardiogenic embolism ambiguous. Thus, we considered it important to establish the incremental benefit of TEE in both of these disease categories.

Our study demonstrated that TEE reveals a direct source of embolism in considerably more cases than does transthoracic echocardiography. Transesophageal echocardiography identified a direct source of embolism in 18.5% of patients, compared with only 4.3% on transthoracic echocardiography. This incremental yield of TEE resulted primarily from the discovery of unrecognized intracavitary thrombus or bulky aortic atheroma. Furthermore, in 3.9% of patients, transthoracic echocardiography mistakenly identified a direct source of embolism, which was subsequently refuted on TEE.

For indirect source of embolism, TEE also was superior to transthoracic echocardiography. Among the 88 patients with an indirect source of embolism on TEE, the abnormality was unrecognized by transthoracic echocardiography in 50 (57%). Transesophageal echocardiography identified left atrial spontaneous echocardiographic contrast and patent foramen ovale in 46% and 44% of these 50 patients, respectively. The remaining patients had an atrial septal aneurysm or additional valvular disease.

Interestingly, TEE provided a significant yield even when the transthoracic study was considered entirely negative for source of embolism. Nine percent of these patients had a direct source of embolism on TEE. It should be emphasized that the aortic arch was the embolic source in most of them (71%), and the embolism was related to bulky aortic atheroma with or without intraluminal thrombus. Studies by Karalis et al. [51] and Pop et al. [18] also observed this finding. Twenty-three percent of our study patients with a normal transthoracic echocardiogram had an indirect source of embolism by TEE. Again, spontaneous left atrial echocardiographic contrast and patent foramen ovale were the primary findings in most of these cases.

As previously demonstrated for transthoracic echocardiography, our study indicated that TEE provides an increased yield when the clinical suspicion for cardiogenic embolism is high and there is evidence for underlying cardiac disease. Figure 15-23 illustrates that identification by TEE of a source of embolism (direct or indirect), in addition to that found by transthoracic echocardiography, increased as the clinical suspicion for cardiac source of embolism increased: 21% for low, 42% for equivocal, and 56% for high suspicion. For direct source of embolism, these differences reached statistical significance. Table 15-3 summarizes the results of the most comprehensive studies comparing TEE with transthoracic echocardiography. In this table, the most impressive TEE findings missed by transthoracic echocardiography are left atrial appendage thrombus, aortic atheroma, patent foramen ovale, and spontaneous echocardiographic contrast. For these abnormalities, there were 325

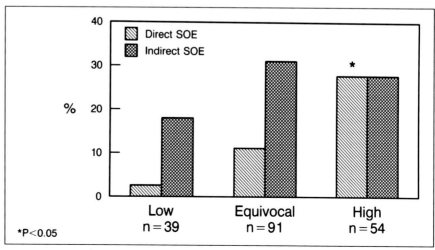

Fig. 15-23. Percentage of positive findings for source of embolism *(SOE)* in patients with a low, equivocal, or high degree of suspicion for embolism. The asterisk indicates that a significantly greater percentage of patients with high clinical suspicion of embolism are found to have a direct source of emboli.

Table 15-3. Summary of studies comparing transesophageal echocardiography (TEE) with transthoracic echocardiography (TTE) for source of embolism

Study (first author)	No. of patients	LAT	LAAT	VV	AA	MVP, AC	PFO	SEC	ASA
Daniel [52]	479	49/30	68/1	73/43		63/44	29/4	96/2	6/2
Espinosa [50]	184	7/2	6/0	4/3	11/0	67/61	25/1	33/0	7/3
Hofmann [59]	153	22/2		6/2	9/0	47/46			23/5
Pop [18]	72		3/0	1/0	2/0	1/0		4/0	
Zenker [53]	40					24/20	2/0		
Jacobs [57]	60	0/0				1/0	7/0	4/0	
Pearson [54]	79	6/0				5/3	13/4	13/0	4/1

Key: LAT = left atrial thrombus; LAAT = left atrial appendage thrombus; VV = valvular vegetation; AA = aortic atheroma; MVP, AC = mitral valve prolapse, aortic calcification; PFO = patent foramen ovale; SEC = spontaneous echocardiographic contrast; ASA = atrial septal aneurysm.

positive findings by TEE but only 12 on transthoracic echocardiography.

The overall impact of TEE findings on patient management must now be considered. There is limited available information. In one report, Hata et al. [60] evaluated the overall impact of TEE on the management of patients with cerebral ischemic events. They found that in 16% of patients, TEE findings strongly influenced the decision to anticoagulate. Further studies with this result as an end point need to be done.

Pulmonary Emboli

Thus far, left-sided source of emboli and potential causes of systemic central or peripheral emboli have been discussed. Emboli within the right-sided circulation are also important, because pulmonary embolism is a major cause of morbidity and mortality in general patient populations.

The diagnosis of pulmonary embolism presents two problems. First, the signs and symptoms of acute pulmonary embolism are widely varying and nonspecific and may be similar to those from a variety of other cardiovascular or pulmonary diseases [61–63]. Second, the usual noninvasive diagnostic tests are far from perfect. Ventilation-perfusion scans are helpful if the results are entirely negative or show a high probability for pulmonary embolism. Pulmonary angiography remains the definitive test for the diagnosis of pulmonary embolism. However, it is invasive, costly, and not always available, and up to 20% of patients cannot have pulmonary angiography because of life-threatening cardiac or respiratory illness [64].

The most important role of echocardiography in the evaluation of the patient with suspected pulmonary embolism is in expediting and clarifying the diagnosis. Noninvasiveness, portability of the equipment, ease and expediency of obtaining an image, and immediate availability of the results make echocardiography a valuable imaging technique in sorting out possible etiologies during emergency situations. Echocardiography can help define whether the problem is cardiac or noncardiac and focus further testing. In acute pulmonary embolism, specific echocardiographic features help establish or suggest the diagnosis [65]. These include dilated right heart chambers and pulmonary artery, small left ventricular cavity, and paradoxical septal motion.

The other important echocardiographic finding is evidence of a right heart embolic source, in most cases, thrombus. Thromboembolism from the lower extremity venous system in transit through the right heart has a very characteristic appearance echocardiographically that, in the proper clinical setting, strongly corroborates the diagnosis of pulmonary embolism (Fig. 15-24).

Transesophageal echocardiography can be easily and quickly performed at the bedside in unstable patients. Often, acutely ill patients are supported by a ventilator and transthoracic echocardiographic images may be technically difficult to obtain; TEE is superior to transthoracic echocardiography in these clinical situations [66]. The intracardiac anatomy is much better delineated for identification of thrombus, assessment of the atrial septum (to rule out shunting), and visualization of the pulmonary arteries, especially the main artery and the proximal branches (Fig. 15-25). A few reports on the role

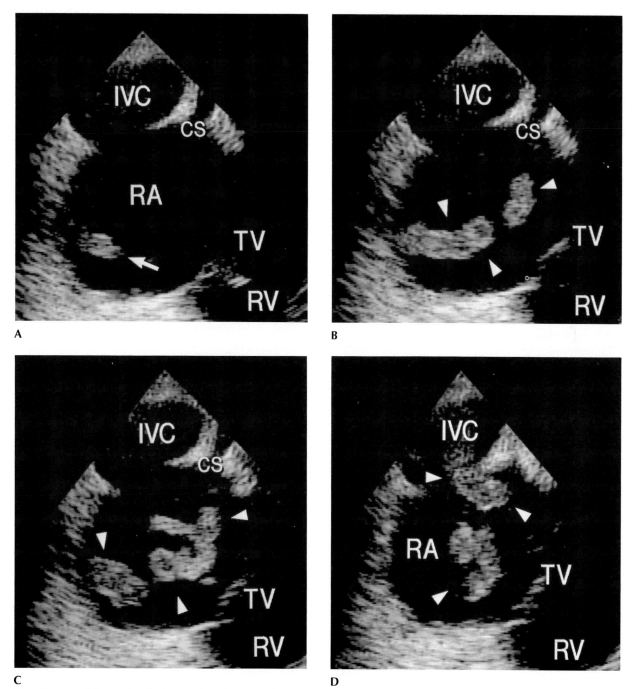

Fig. 15-24. View of right heart chambers in the horizontal plane. Successive frames (A–D) show the changing "snakelike" appearance of a deep venous thrombosis *(arrow* or *arrowheads)* entrapped in the right atrium. In D, thrombus is seen emerging from the inferior vena cava.

of TEE have specifically evaluated patients with suspected pulmonary embolus [67–69]. Wittlich et al. [69] described TEE evaluation of 60 patients with evidence of hemodynamically significant pulmonary embolism demonstrated by signs of right ventricular pressure overload on transthoracic echocardiography. Central pulmonary artery thromboemboli were detected in 58% of these patients by

TEE, with 97% sensitivity and 88% specificity when compared with pulmonary angiography, computed tomography, or anatomic confirmation [69] (see Chapter 12).

One other area in which TEE can help assess suspected or proven pulmonary embolism is evaluation of the atrial septum and presence of right-to-left shunting. In autopsy studies, approximately 30%

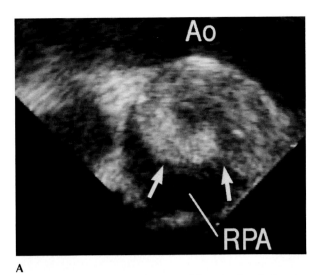
A

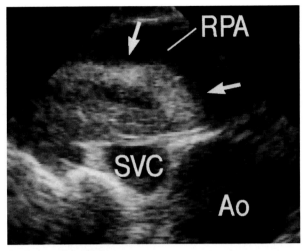
B

Fig. 15-25. Horizontal (A) and longitudinal (B) planes with a view of a large pulmonary embolism *(arrows)* in the right pulmonary artery.

Fig. 15-26. Algorithm for workup of source of embolism *(SOE)* referral. *(AF = atrial fibrillation.)*

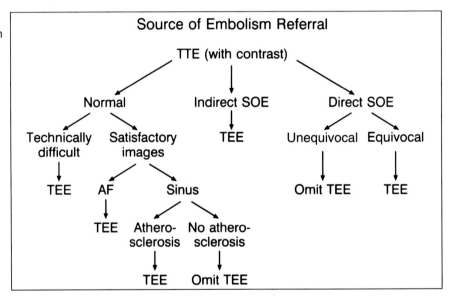

of patients have a patent foramen ovale [26]. With increased right heart pressures secondary to a pulmonary embolism, the potential for right-to-left shunting through a patent foramen ovale increases. This certainly complicates the already tenuous clinical problem and may explain less than expected improvement in a patient receiving maximal therapy. With TEE and venous contrast injection (saline or indocyanine green), shunting can be easily detected and semiquantitated.

WHO SHOULD HAVE TEE?

Transesophageal echocardiography in every patient with a suspected embolic event is neither practical nor indicated. Furthermore, because of the risk, al-

beit very small, of complication in performance of TEE, the yield and impact of findings on patient management should be considered in each patient beforehand. We have formulated an algorithm (Fig. 15-26) for echocardiographic assessment in patients referred for source of embolism. In patients with normal results of transthoracic echocardiography who are 40 or younger, are in sinus rhythm, have no clinical history of cardiovascular disease, and have no evidence of atherosclerotic disease (carotid bruits, atherosclerosis obliterans), the TEE yield would be extremely low and the examination could be omitted. Likewise, if a direct source of embolism was clearly discovered by transthoracic echocardiography, TEE could be omitted in selected cases. All other patients should have TEE for further evaluation.

SUMMARY

Transesophageal echocardiography has opened an exciting avenue of cardiac imaging. Because of its semi-invasive nature and added cost, its clinical applicability has been under great scrutiny. No aspect is more controversial than usefulness in patients referred for source of embolism. Clearly, TEE has advantages over transthoracic echocardiography in identifying potential sources of emboli. Identification becomes more sensitive the higher the degree of suspicion and the greater the likelihood of underlying cardiac disease, and the procedure probably should not be done in all patients referred for source of emboli. An even more difficult but highly pertinent question is, What impact do the increased TEE findings have on subsequent patient management? With the emphasis on cost-effectiveness and efficient use of diagnostic procedures, future studies need to be designed to answer these questions.

REFERENCES

1. Seward JB, Khandheria BK, Oh JK, et al. Transesophageal echocardiography: technique, anatomic correlations, implementation, and clinical applications. *Mayo Clin Proc* 1988;63:649–80.

2. Seward JB, Khandheria BK, Edwards WD, et al. Biplanar transesophageal echocardiography: anatomic correlations, image orientation, and clinical applications. *Mayo Clin Proc* 1990;65:1193–213.

3. Adams RD, Victor M. *Principles of Neurology,* 4th ed. New York: McGraw-Hill, 1989:617–92.

4. Cerebral Embolism Task Force. Cardiogenic brain embolism. *Arch Neurol* 1986;43:71–84.

5. Cerebral Embolism Task Force. Cardiogenic brain embolism. The second report of the Cerebral Embolism Task Force. *Arch Neurol* 1989;46:727–43.

6. Sherman DG, Dyken ML, Fisher M, et al. Cerebral embolism. *Chest* 1986;89 Suppl:82S-98S.

7. Lovett JL, Sandok BA, Giuliani ER, Nasser FN. Two-dimensional echocardiography in patients with focal cerebral ischemia. *Ann Intern Med* 1981;95:1–4.

8. Come PC, Riley MF, Bivas NK. Roles of echocardiography and arrhythmia monitoring in the evaluation of patients with suspected systemic embolism. *Ann Neurol* 1983;13:527–31.

9. Greenland P, Knopman DS, Mikell FL, et al. Echocardiography in diagnostic assessment of stroke. *Ann Intern Med* 1981;95:51–3.

10. Fanning WJ, Vaccaro PS, Satiani B, et al. The role of echocardiography in patients with acute peripheral arterial embolization. *Ann Vasc Surg* 1986;1:316–20.

11. Larson EB, Stratton JR, Pearlman AS. Selective use of two-dimensional echocardiography in stroke syndromes (editorial). *Ann Intern Med* 1981;95:112–4.

12. Rolak LA, Gilmer W, Strittmatter WJ. Low yield in the diagnostic evaluation of transient ischemic attacks. *Neurology* 1990;40:747–8.

13. DePace NL, Soulen RL, Kotler MN, Mintz GS. Two dimensional echocardiographic detection of intraatrial masses. *Am J Cardiol* 1981;48:954–60.

14. Come PC, Riley MF, Markis JE, Malagold M. Limitations of echocardiographic techniques in evaluation of left atrial masses. *Am J Cardiol* 1981;48:947–53.

15. Shrestha NK, Moreno FL, Narciso FV, et al. Two-dimensional echocardiographic diagnosis of left atrial thrombus in rheumatic heart disease: a clinicopathologic study. *Circulation* 1983;67:341–7.

16. Schweizer P, Bardos P, Erbel R, et al. Detection of left atrial thrombi by echocardiography. *Br Heart J* 1981;45:148–56.

17. Aschenberg W, Schlüter M, Kremer P, et al. Transesophageal two-dimensional echocardiography for the detection of left atrial appendage thrombus. *J Am Coll Cardiol* 1986;7:163–6.

18. Pop G, Sutherland GR, Koudstaal PJ, et al. Transesophageal echocardiography in the detection of intracardiac embolic sources in patients with transient ischemic attacks. *Stroke* 1990;21:560–5.

19. Daniel WG, Nellessen U, Schröder E, et al. Left atrial spontaneous echo contrast in mitral valve disease: an indicator for an increased thromboembolic risk. *J Am Coll Cardiol* 1988;11:1204–11.

20. Erbel R, Stern H, Ehrenthal W, et al. Detection of spontaneous echocardiographic contrast within the left atrium by transesophageal echocardiography: spontaneous echocardiographic contrast. *Clin Cardiol* 1986;9:245–52.

21. Obarski T, Klein A, Stewart W, et al. Left atrial smoke by transesophageal echocardiography: correlations with mitral valve area, atrial fibrillation, and embolic events in patients with mitral stenosis (abstract). *J Am Soc Echocardiogr* 1990;3:212.

22. Black IW, Hopkins AP, Lee LCL, Walsh WF. Left atrial spontaneous echo contrast: a clinical and echocardiographic analysis. *J Am Coll Cardiol* 1991;18:398–404.

23. Castello R, Pearson AC, Labovitz AJ. Prevalence and clinical implications of atrial spontaneous contrast in patients undergoing transesophageal echocardiography. *Am J Cardiol* 1990;65:1149–53.

24. Chan K, Cohen G, Dore S. Left atrial spontaneous contrast in mitral stenosis: a transesophageal echo study (abstract). *J Am Soc Echocardiogr* 1990;3: 212.

25. Chen Y-T, Kan M-N, Chen J-S, et al. Contributing factors to formation of left atrial spontaneous echo contrast in mitral valvular disease. *J Ultrasound Med* 1990;9:151–5.

26. Hagen PT, Scholz DG, Edwards WD. Incidence and size of patent foramen ovale during the first 10 decades of life: an autopsy study of 965 normal hearts. *Mayo Clin Proc* 1984;59:17–20.

27. Johnson BI. Paradoxical embolism. *J Clin Pathol* 1951;4:316–32.

28. Nellessen U, Daniel WG, Matheis G, et al. Impending paradoxical embolism from atrial thrombus: correct diagnosis by transesophageal echocardiography and prevention by surgery. *J Am Coll Cardiol* 1985;5:1002–4.

29. Lechat P, Mas JL, Lascault G, et al. Prevalence of patent foramen ovale in patients with stroke. *N Engl J Med* 1988;318:1148–52.

30. Mügge A, Daniel WG, Klöpper JW, Lichtlen PR. Visualization of patent foramen ovale by transesophageal color-coded Doppler echocardiography. *Am J Cardiol* 1988;62:837–8.

31. Khandheria BK, Click RL, Sinak LJ, et al. Prevalence of patent foramen ovale assessed by contrast transesophageal echocardiography (abstract). *Circulation* 1990;82 Suppl 3:III–109.

32. Stahl JA, Fisher EA, Budd JH, et al. Contrast 2-D transesophageal echo: the method of choice to detect patent foramen ovale (abstract). *Circulation* 1990;82 Suppl 3:III–109.

33. de Belder M, Tourikis L, Leech G. Patent foramen ovale—risk factor for thromboembolic events in all age groups? (abstract). *Circulation* 1990;82 Suppl 3:III–109.

34. DeCoodt P, Kacenelenbogen R, Capon A, et al. Prevalence of patent foramen ovale in patients with cerebral ischemic events assessed by contrast transesophageal echocardiography (abstract). Proceedings of the International Symposium on Transesophageal Echocardiography, Mainz, Germany, Oct. 31 to Nov. 2, 1990.

35. Zhu W-X, Khandheria BK, Click RL, et al. Patent foramen ovale detected by contrast transesophageal echo: a lack of association with systemic embolic events (abstract). *Circulation* 1991;84 Suppl 2:II–694.

36. Falk RH. PFO or UFO? The role of a patent foramen ovale in cryptogenic stroke (editorial). *Am Heart J* 1991;121:1264–6.

37. Belkin RN, Waugh RA, Kisslo J. Interatrial shunting in atrial septal aneurysm. *Am J Cardiol* 1986;57: 310–2.

38. Belkin RN, Hurwitz BJ, Kisslo J. Atrial septal aneurysm: association with cerebrovascular and peripheral embolic events. *Stroke* 1987;18:856–62.

39. Silver MD, Dorsey JS. Aneurysms of the septum primum in adults. *Arch Pathol Lab Med* 1978;102: 62–5.

40. Grosgogeat Y, Lhermitte F, Carpentier A, et al. Anévrysme de la cloison interauriculaire révélé par une embolie cérébrale. *Arch Mal Coeur* 1973;66: 169–77.

41. Gallet B, Malergue MC, Adams C, et al. Atrial septal aneurysm—a potential cause of systemic embolism: an echocardiographic study. *Br Heart J* 1985;53:292–7.

42. Schneider B, Hanrath P, Vogel P, Meinertz T. Improved morphologic characterization of atrial septal aneurysm by transesophageal echocardiography: relation to cerebrovascular events. *J Am Coll Cardiol* 1990;16:1000–9.

43. Daniel WG, Dennig K, Angermann C, et al. Clinical implications of atrial septal aneurysms: a multicenter study using transesophageal echocardiography (abstract). *Circulation* 1990;82 Suppl 3:III–246.

44. Pearson AC, Nagelhout D, Castello R, et al. Atrial septal aneurysm and stroke: a transesophageal echocardiographic study. *J Am Coll Cardiol* 1991;18: 1223–9.

45. Sanfilippo AJ, Picard MH, Newell JB, et al. Echocardiographic assessment of patients with infectious endocarditis: prediction of risk for complications. *J Am Coll Cardiol* 1991;18:1191–9.

46. Erbel R, Rohmann S, Drexler M, et al. Improved diagnostic value of echocardiography in patients with infective endocarditis by transesophageal approach. A prospective study. *Eur Heart J* 1988; 9:43–53.

47. Daniel WG, Schröder E, Mügge A, Lichtlen PR. Transesophageal echocardiography in infective endocarditis. *Am J Cardiac Imaging* 1988;2:78–85.

48. Klodas E, Edwards WD, Khandheria BK. Use of transesophageal echocardiography for improving detection of valvular vegetations in subacute bacterial endocarditis. *J Am Soc Echocardiogr* 1989;2: 386–9.

49. Shively BK, Gurule FT, Roldan CA, et al. Diagnostic value of transesophageal compared with transthoracic echocardiography in infective endocarditis. *J Am Coll Cardiol* 1991;18:391–7.

50. Espinosa RE, Click RL, Bailey KR, et al. Transesophageal echocardiography in patients with sus-

pected cardiac source of embolism (abstract). *Circulation* 1990;82 Suppl 3:III–245.

51. Karalis DG, Chandrasekaran K, Victor MF, et al. Recognition and embolic potential of intraaortic atherosclerotic debris. *J Am Coll Cardiol* 1991;17: 73–8.

52. Daniel WG, Angermann C, Engberding R, et al. Transesophageal echocardiography in patients with cerebral ischemic events and arterial embolism—a European Multicenter Study (abstract). *Circulation* 1989;80 Suppl 2:II–473.

53. Zenker G, Erbel R, Krämer G, et al. Transesophageal two-dimensional echocardiography in young patients with cerebral ischemic events. *Stroke* 1988; 19:345–8.

54. Pearson AC, Labovitz AJ, Tatineni S, Gomez CR. Superiority of transesophageal echocardiography in detecting cardiac source of embolism in patients with cerebral ischemia of uncertain etiology. *J Am Coll Cardiol* 1991;17:66–72.

55. Lee RJ, Bartzokis TC, Grogin HR, et al. Superiority of transesophageal echocardiography in detection of intracardiac sources of emboli (abstract). *Circulation* 1989;80 Suppl 2:II–403.

56. Malouf JF, Bdeir M, Stefadouros MA. Usefulness of transesophageal echocardiography (TEE) in acute non-hemorrhagic stroke (abstract). *Circulation* 1990;82 Suppl 3:III–245.

57. Jacobs NH, Whyte S, Kelleher AD, et al. Limited role of transesophageal echocardiography in unselected patients with cerebral ischemic events (abstract). *Circulation* 1990;82 Suppl 3:III–110.

58. Black IW, Hopkins AP, Lee LCL, et al. Should all patients with embolic events have transesophageal echocardiography? (abstract). *Circulation* 1990;82 Suppl 3:III–246.

59. Hofmann T, Kasper W, Meinertz T, et al. Echocardiographic evaluation of patients with clinically suspected arterial emboli. *Lancet* 1990;336:1421–4.

60. Hata JS, Biller J, Stuhlmuller JE, et al. Impact of transesophageal echocardiography on the management of patients admitted with focal cerebral ischemia (abstract). *Circulation* 1991;84 Suppl 2: II–693.

61. Bell WR, Simon TL, DeMets DL. The clinical features of submassive and massive pulmonary emboli. *Am J Med* 1977;62:355–60.

62. Stein PD, Willis PW III, DeMets DL. History and physical examination in acute pulmonary embolism in patients without preexisting cardiac or pulmonary disease. *Am J Cardiol* 1981;47:218–23.

63. Modan B, Sharon E, Jelin N. Factors contributing to the incorrect diagnosis of pulmonary embolic disease. *Chest* 1972;62:388–93.

64. Hull RD, Hirsh J, Carter CJ, et al. Pulmonary angiography, ventilation lung scanning, and venography for clinically suspected pulmonary embolism with abnormal perfusion lung scan. *Ann Intern Med* 1983;98:891–9.

65. Kasper W, Meinertz T, Henkel B, et al. Echocardiographic findings in patients with proved pulmonary embolism. *Am Heart J* 1986;112:1284–90.

66. Oh JK, Seward JB, Khandheria BK, et al. Transesophageal echocardiography in critically ill patients. *Am J Cardiol* 1990;66:1492–5.

67. Klein AL, Stewart WC, Cosgrove DM III, et al. Visualization of acute pulmonary emboli by transesophageal echocardiography. *J Am Soc Echocardiogr* 1990;3:412–5.

68. Nixdorff U, Erbel R, Drexler M, Meyer J. Detection of thromboembolus of the right pulmonary artery by transesophageal two-dimensional echocardiography. *Am J Cardiol* 1988;61:488–9.

69. Wittlich N, Erbel R, Eichler A, et al. Detection of central pulmonary artery thromboemboli by transesophageal echocardiography in patients with severe pulmonary embolism. *J Am Soc Echocardiogr* 1992;5:515–524.

16

Intraoperative Applications of Transesophageal Echocardiography

William K. Freeman • *Patrick W. O'Leary* • *Martin D. Abel*
Thomas J. Losasso • *Donald A. Muzzi*

Over the past decade, the horizons of two-dimensional and Doppler echocardiography have been vastly expanded through numerous applications in the operating room. Intraoperative echocardiography is a valuable adjunct in the evaluation of surgical procedures for primary valvular disease, hypertrophic obstructive cardiomyopathy, congenital heart disease, thoracic aortic disease, and a variety of other indications, such as neoplastic or traumatic cardiac disease. Transesophageal echocardiography (TEE) has also been implemented during a broad spectrum of noncardiac operations, most notably selected peripheral vascular, neurologic, and orthopedic surgical procedures.

TECHNIQUE AND INDICATIONS

Epicardial Approach

Before the clinical availability of TEE imaging systems, numerous investigators reported favorable experiences with epicardial intraoperative echocardiography. Although initially used as a two-dimensional technique for the evaluation of left ventricular function [1,2], this method was soon extended to the intraoperative evaluation of valvular repair by both contrast [3,4] and color Doppler [5–7] echocardiography. Concomitantly, multiple investigators described the significant impact of two-dimensional and color Doppler echocardiography on the intraoperative surgical management of congenital heart disease [8–11].

Epicardial echocardiography is generally performed with standard transthoracic imaging systems; transducers enclosed within long, sterile sleeves are introduced into the operative field. Echocardiographic imaging in this fashion has been shown to be safe and without risk of perioperative infectious complications [12]. On-heart application of the transducer is not limited by the orientation of the heart within the mediastinum, and, because of the mobility of transducer positioning, multiple high-resolution, long- and short-axis imaging planes analogous to transthoracic parasternal, subclavicular, and subcostal windows are readily obtainable [7,13]. Continuous-wave Doppler interrogation of the left ventricular outflow tract and aortic valve is possible by placement of a nonimaging transducer in the sulcus of the aorta and superior vena cava.

Epicardial echocardiography requires that either the surgeon be facile with this technique or the echocardiologist scrub in to perform the examination; either way, a second person is required to operate the ultrasound machine controls. This approach interrupts the operation, invades the sterile field, and may be cumbersome to perform. Imaging windows available may be limited by surgical exposure, cardiopulmonary bypass cannulae, pacing wires, and even coronary artery bypass grafts. A hyperdynamic heart may compromise a stable transducer position for two-dimensional imaging and introduce considerable wall motion artifact during Doppler colorflow mapping. Attempting to stabilize the transducer position on the heart by firm pressure may precipitate cardiac arrhythmias or hypotension, especially if the transducer is applied over the right ventricular outflow tract. An incomplete interface of the ultrasonic gel with the transducer enclosed within the sterile sleeve may also degrade image quality. Farfield epicardial imaging may limit delineation of posteriorly directed mitral regurgitant jets, and pulsed-wave Doppler interrogation of pulmonary venous inflow is not readily accomplished by this approach. Acoustic shadowing of the left atrium by aortic valve prostheses or calcific disease may also significantly obscure color-flow Doppler evaluation of mitral regurgitation.

Transesophageal Approach

Monoplane TEE initially opened a unique window to the heart, providing multiple high-resolution shortaxis and four-chamber imaging planes [14]. Unlike epicardial echocardiography, TEE has its transducer position limited to the esophagus and fundus of the stomach; hence, available images depend on the orientation of the heart within the mediastinum. As described in Chapters 4 and 5, monoplane TEE has been greatly supplemented by longitudinal biplanar [15] and multiplanar [16] imaging, which has facilitated a more orthogonal visualization of the heart and has provided improved imaging of various aspects of cardiovascular anatomy, particularly the ascending aorta, left and right ventricular outflow tracts, and atrial septum.

The safety of TEE in the conscious patient is well recognized (see Chapter 3). In the operative setting,

TEE can be performed with a similar minimal risk of complications, which are usually confined to benign transient arrhythmias [17–19]. Unless there is need for monitoring of left ventricular function during induction of anesthesia, the TEE probe is usually introduced after endotracheal intubation with the patient in the supine position under general anesthesia. For optimal access, it is best to insert the TEE probe before sterile draping of the patient. Digital introduction and guidance of the instrument around the endotracheal tube is most often all that is needed for esophageal intubation. Occasionally, anteflexion of the patient's neck and even mild lateral rotation of the head are required to allow passage of the TEE probe. Rarely, if these maneuvers are unsuccessful or significant resistance is encountered with probe insertion, direct laryngoscopic visualization of the esophageal orifice with the patient's head in a retroflexed position permits probe insertion in nearly all cases. Care should be taken to avoid disturbing the positions of the endotracheal tube and intravenous and hemodynamic monitoring lines. Esophageal monitoring devices, such as temperature probes, should be removed before TEE probe insertion to prevent inadvertent migration of such devices into the stomach. Insertion of a bite block for protection of the TEE endoscope is generally not necessary in patients under general anesthesia.

After probe placement, continuous TEE imaging is possible without intrusion into the sterile field or interruption of the operative procedure (Fig. 16-1). The echocardiography system is placed on one side of the anesthesia screen, and the TEE examiner likewise stands off to the side to allow the anesthesiologist unimpeded access to the patient.

Although the echocardiologist has considerably more time to perform intraoperative TEE than epicardial examinations, TEE imaging may be limited by electrocautery artifacts that are not shielded by currently available systems. After cessation of cardiopulmonary bypass, imaging on several systems may also be limited by triggering of the automatic cooling circuit on the TEE probe by intravascular rewarming to temperatures around 39°C. A few systems allow override of the automatic cooling function and reprogramming of the autocool temperature, but most require cooling before imaging can be resumed and hence interrupt the postbypass examination.

Once in place, the TEE probe is committed for as long as needed for that operative procedure; with-

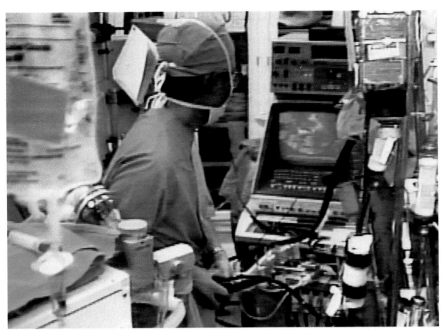

Fig. 16-1. Transesophageal echocardiography in the operating room. The TEE examination is performed without interruption of the operation or intrusion into the operative field. The imaging system is situated adjacent to the head of the operating table, permitting full access to the patient.

drawing the probe for another study, resterilizing, and attempting reinsertion under sterile draping is not practical. Prolonged intubation has not been reported to cause esophageal injury in patients undergoing intraoperative TEE, but as an added precaution, the imaging system should be turned off when not in use to avoid any potential for thermal mucosal injury. In our initial experience, transient laryngoparalysis was noted during very prolonged esophageal intubation for upright neurosurgical procedures; adopting a more neutral position for the patient's head eliminated this problem.

In a recent double-blind study of 48 patients undergoing cardiac surgery, the postoperative side effects of intraoperative TEE were examined [20]. The mean duration of intraoperative TEE examination was 5.4 ± 2.3 hours in patients randomized to TEE. On the second postoperative day, there were no significant differences in incidences of discomfort with swallowing, nausea, pharyngeal erythema, and minor oropharyngeal trauma between patients who did and those who did not have TEE. There was also no difference between groups in the time from endotracheal extubation to first oral intake in this randomized study [20]. These investigators concluded that prolonged esophageal intubation during intraoperative TEE can be performed without adverse side effects or risk to the patient, findings entirely consistent with our experience.

The size of the transducer head of the earlier TEE probes limited intraoperative evaluation of pediatric patients. In 1989, it was recommended that no patient under the age of 8 years be studied by TEE because of the size of instruments then available [21]. With the continuing development of pediatric endoscopes with maximal transducer tip dimensions of 7 to 8 mm and shaft diameters of about 6 mm, TEE is possible in patients weighing less than 15 kg and even in neonates without difficulty in probe manipulation or risk of significant complications [22–24]. Although currently available adult-sized probes are becoming more streamlined, instruments with a maximal dimension of greater than 13 mm should not be used in patients weighing 20 kg or less [23]. In our recent experience, biplane TEE probes with maximal dimensions of 10 to 12 mm have been used without problems in intraoperative study of patients with an average body weight of 15 to 20 kg. (See "Congenital Heart Disease" section, below.)

As for examination in the conscious patient, esophageal diseases such as stricture, diverticula, and carcinoma; active upper gastrointestinal bleeding; and severe cervical spine disease are relative to absolute contraindications to intraoperative TEE (Chapter 3). Not uncommonly, a large diaphragmatic hernia can significantly limit imaging from the esophageal window because transducer-mucosal apposition is incomplete. Occasionally, TEE images are considerably altered in quality if the chest is open rather than closed or if the patient is in the supine rather than the lateral decubitus position. Rarely, mural calcification of a severely enlarged left atrium, usually in patients with advanced rheumatic heart disease, can significantly compromise TEE imaging from all windows because of acoustic shadowing.

The relative advantages and disadvantages of the transesophageal over the epicardial approaches to intraoperative echocardiography are summarized in Table 16-1. Although the image quality of epicardial echocardiography initially surpassed that of TEE simply because more phased-array crystals were available in transthoracic transducers, continued advances in the miniaturization and sophistication of TEE transducers have greatly reduced this difference.

Physician Training

The general guidelines for training in TEE examination are presented in Chapter 3. In the intraoperative echocardiography practice at the Mayo Clinic, nearly all examinations, particularly those evaluating cardiac reparative procedures, are directly performed and interpreted by an attending staff echocardiologist in the operating room. Because our current practice almost exclusively involves TEE, echocardiologists are completely trained in biplane TEE before beginning intraoperative studies. The potential impact of intraoperative TEE interpretation on surgical decision-making is very significant and mandates that the examiner be fully cognizant of the capabilities and potential pitfalls of this technique. The intraoperative setting also requires the

Table 16-1. Comparison of transesophageal and epicardial intraoperative echocardiography

Transesophageal imaging	Epicardial imaging
Does not invade operative field	Invades operative field
Does not interrupt operation; increased imaging time	Interrupts operation; limited imaging time
Easy to perform; requires one examiner	Potentially cumbersome to perform; requires two examiners
Can evaluate cardiac operations and monitor noncardiac operations	Can evaluate cardiac operations only
Transducer position depends on cardiac orientation to esophagus and stomach; imaging planes increased with biplane transducer	Transducer position independent of cardiac orientation within mediastinum; multiple imaging planes available
Variable availability of steerable CW Doppler imaging; good for MV and TV, limited for AV and LVOT	CW Doppler imaging available for AV and LVOT, limited for MV, TV
Excellent PW Doppler study of MV and pulmonary veins; stable sample volume	Limited PW Doppler study of MV and pulmonary veins; potentially unstable sample volume
Potential acoustic shadowing of LVOT, apical LV, and VS by mitral prosthesis or calcific disease	Potential acoustic shadowing of LA by aortic prosthesis or calcific disease
Limited by electrocautery artifact and automatic cooling function of probe after bypass	Limited by surgical exposure, bypass cannulae, pacing wires, bypass grafts, and motion artifacts
Rarely precipitates supraventricular dysrhythmias or minor oropharyngeal injury	Uncommonly causes cardiac irritability or hemodynamic compromise with transducer pressure on heart

AV, aortic valve; CW, continuous-wave; LA, left atrium; LV, left ventricle; LVOT, left ventricular outflow tract; MV, mitral valve; PW, pulsed-wave; TV, tricuspid valve; VS, ventricular septum.

TEE examiner to be not only comprehensive with a high level of technical proficiency but also able to perform expeditious goal-directed examinations.

An increasing number of anesthesiologists are becoming involved with intraoperative TEE, and formal training guidelines remain to be set forth. At our institution, anesthesiology staff and residents rotate through the echocardiography laboratory for didactic teaching. Our impression is that the best training is obtained through a close working relationship with the echocardiologist in the operating room over a period of several months. Experienced anesthesiologists are entirely capable of introducing the TEE probe, obtaining standard imaging planes, and monitoring global and segmental left ventricular function. The echocardiologist should be present when (1) there is difficulty in performing the examination, (2) Doppler examination is required, (3) a

cardiac reparative procedure is under evaluation, (4) any unanticipated or unclarified findings are detected, and (5) the patient is not doing well and a cardiac cause is suspected. To facilitate the most complete and optimal intraoperative TEE examination, the echocardiologist must be readily available and work in close conjunction with both the anesthesiologist and the surgeon.

Indications

For the reasons discussed above, intraoperative echocardiography for both adult and pediatric patients at the Mayo Clinic is now almost exclusively performed with TEE. The indications for intraoperative TEE in our initial and subsequent experience are shown in Figure 16-2. Initially, over three-quarters of all intraoperative TEE examinations were

Fig. 16-2. Indications for intraoperative TEE at Mayo Medical Center. A. During the initial 35 months (Jan. 1, 1988, to Nov. 30, 1990) of intraoperative TEE in 317 patients, nearly one-half of all studies (48%) were for the evaluation of mitral valve repair. One-fourth (24%) of patients were evaluated during prosthetic valve replacement. B. In 959 patients studied over the following 2 years (1991 and 1992), evaluation of operations for congenital heart disease increased nearly fivefold (to 28%) because of the availability of pediatric TEE probes, becoming the second most common indication for intraoperative TEE. Evaluation of mitral valve surgery remained the most common indication (36%). Assessment of aortic valve operations (particularly homograft replacement) was performed in nearly one-fourth (23%) of patients. HOCM = hypertrophic obstructive cardiomyopathy.

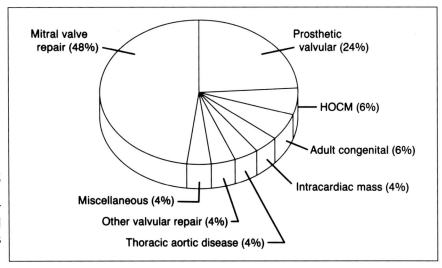

A

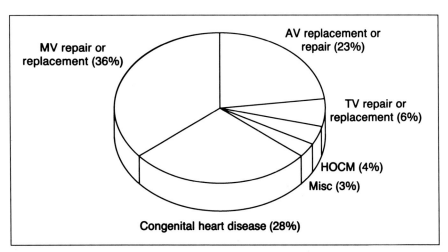

B

performed to evaluate surgical procedures for adult valvular heart disease. The most important indication for intraoperative TEE was the evaluation of mitral valve repair (48% of all patients) (see below). Nearly one-quarter of examinations were for procedures involving prosthetic valve replacement. In this group, most often TEE was performed to evaluate mitral or tricuspid regurgitation before and after aortic valve replacement for either severe stenosis or regurgitation. Evaluation of tricuspid regurgitation associated with severe mitral stenosis or regurgitation requiring mitral valve replacement was also commonly done. Also included in this subset were patients reoperated on for prosthetic valve failure in whom TEE was useful for delineation of periprosthetic regurgitation or intracardiac shunts complicating previous prosthetic valve implantation.

In our experience, intraoperative TEE was also indicated for evaluation of surgical procedures for hypertrophic obstructive cardiomyopathy, intracardiac masses, and thoracic aortic disease, such as aneurysm or dissection. Because the availability of pediatric TEE probes was limited, intraoperative study of congenital heart disease was confined primarily to adolescent and adult patients, composing only 6% of our initial experience.

Since pediatric probes have become available, and with further miniaturization of adult probes, the number of patients having TEE during congenital heart operations has increased greatly since 1991, and this indication now constitutes nearly one-third (28%) of the current intraoperative TEE practice (Fig. 16-2B) (see "Congenital Heart Disease" section, below). In our initial experience, intraoperative TEE was performed for monitoring during noncardiac surgery in approximately 2% of patients. It continues to be uncommonly used for this purpose, primarily in selected patients during vascular surgery to evaluate left ventricular segmental function and during neurosurgery to determine the potential for paradoxical air embolism.

APPLICATIONS OF INTRAOPERATIVE TEE DURING CARDIOVASCULAR SURGERY

Mitral Valve Repair

Mitral valve reconstruction is now clearly favored over prosthetic replacement for the surgical treatment of mitral regurgitation [25–28]. Mitral valve repair is associated with improved operative [27] and late [28] mortality and with minimization of potential complications associated with mitral prostheses, such as thromboembolism [28,29], infective endocarditis [30], and bleeding secondary to anticoagulant therapy [29].

Technique and Evaluation

Vital to the effectiveness of mitral valve repair is the intraoperative assessment of mitral competence after reconstructive procedures. Accordingly, several techniques of intraoperative echocardiography have been described. Such methods include left ventricular contrast echocardiography with either epicardial [3] or transesophageal [31] imaging and Doppler color-flow mapping with epicardial echocardiography [6,7,32] or TEE [17,33,34].

With the escalating surgical trend toward mitral valve repair for mitral regurgitation, this procedure has become the primary indication for intraoperative TEE in adult patients at the Mayo Clinic (Fig. 16-2). This technique [14] readily offers high resolution real-time delineation of the functional pathoanatomy of the mitral valve leaflets, annulus, and support apparatus, aiding the surgeon in planning approaches to mitral valve repair.

In contemporary practice, degenerative mitral valve disease is clearly the most common cause of mitral regurgitation requiring operative repair. As described in Chapter 9, mitral leaflet redundancy, prolapse, ruptured chordae, and flail leaflet segments caused by myxomatous degeneration of the mitral valve are readily demonstrable on TEE [35,36] (Fig. 16-3). The location and degree of mitral leaflet malcoaptation can be visualized on tomographic four-chamber and two-chamber scanning of the entirety of the valve with transverse and longitudinal TEE, respectively (Fig. 16-4). Determination of the extent of mitral annular dilatation and calcification is possible with these imaging planes. It is also important, especially in patients with ischemic heart disease, to examine the myocardial support of the mitral apparatus. The best approach is from the transgastric window. Transverse TEE short-axis imaging delineates global and regional left ventricular function. Localized myocardial dysfunction may range from segmental hypokinesis to regional thinning with infarct expansion and may have a significant effect on the technique or even feasibility of mitral valve repair in patients with ischemic mitral regurgitation. Examination of the mitral support apparatus has also been greatly supplemented by transgastric longitudi-

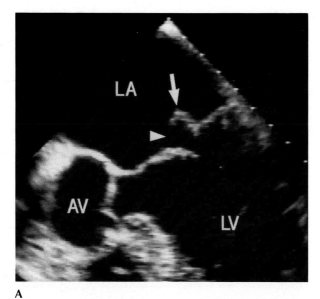

A

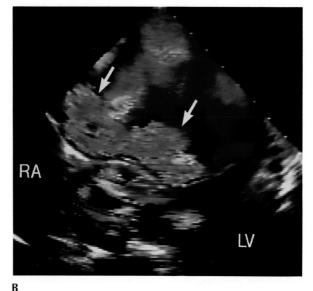

B

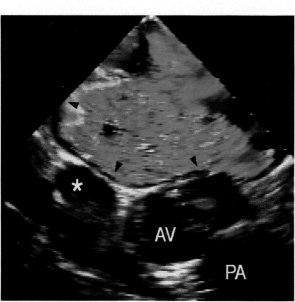

C

Fig. 16-3.   Mitral valve prolapse with flail; left ventricular outflow view in the transverse plane. A. There is prolapse of the posterior mitral leaflet, with a flail leaflet segment (*arrow*) producing a large deficiency in coaptation (arrow*head*) with the anterior leaflet. B. The mechanism of mitral regurgitation is further demonstrated on color-flow Doppler imaging by an eccentric anteromedial regurgitant jet (*arrows*), characteristic for severe myxomatous disease involving primarily the posterior leaflet. C. Basal short-axis imaging reveals a broad regurgitant jet sweeping along the entire anteromedial superior left atrium (*arrowheads*), typical of severe mitral regurgitation. (*Asterisk* = superior vena cava.)

nal long-axis imaging of the left ventricle, which allows the clearest visualization of the chordal apparatus in conjunction with both papillary muscles. Mitral chordal and leaflet retraction caused by either papillary muscle infarction (usually with underlying regional left ventricular expansion) or rheumatic subvalvular disease (which is often shadowed by mitral leaflet disease in other views) is best seen in this imaging plane. The potential for mitral valve repair of less common lesions causing mitral regurgitation (e.g., congenital cleft or infective endocarditis) can likewise be assessed by comprehensive TEE imaging in multiple long, short, and four-chamber imaging planes.

Semiquantitation of mitral regurgitation severity by TEE color Doppler imaging in which jet width at the regurgitant orifice, central jet area, and dimension ratios are compared with those of the left atrium has been shown to correlate with gradation by left ventricular angiography [37] (see Chapter 9). Assessment of residual mitral regurgitation by intraoperative TEE also agrees well with the severity of mitral regurgitation determined by contrast left ventriculography in the early postoperative period [33].

As with transthoracic examination, detailed delineation of the mitral regurgitant jet in multiple planes is necessary. Eccentric jets, typically associated with mitral valve prolapse or flail, are often sheetlike and

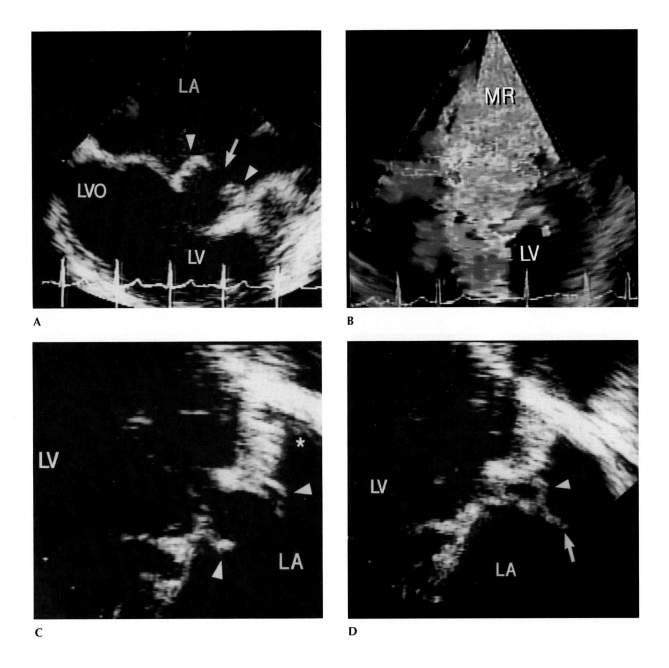

adhere to the adjacent wall of the left atrium by the Coanda effect [38]. Such jets wrap around along the circumference of the left atrium, and multiple orthogonal images are required to appreciate the full extent of the regurgitant signal (Fig. 16-5). As discussed in Chapter 9, quantitative Doppler echocardiography using analysis of the proximal isovelocity surface area (PISA) improves the accuracy of color Doppler imaging in the evaluation of severity of eccentric mitral regurgitant jets [39].

Pulsed-wave Doppler imaging of pulmonary venous inflow is a useful adjunct to color Doppler mapping of mitral regurgitation. If significant left ventricular dysfunction or atrial fibrillation is absent, the systolic component of pulmonary venous filling diminishes with increasing severity of mitral regurgitation (reflecting increasingly higher mean left atrial pressures). Reversal of systolic pulmonary venous flow has been shown to be both a highly sensitive and a specific marker for severe mitral regurgitation [40], and it resolves after successful mitral valve repair (Fig. 16-6).

Color-flow Doppler imaging supplements the two-dimensional study by further elucidating the

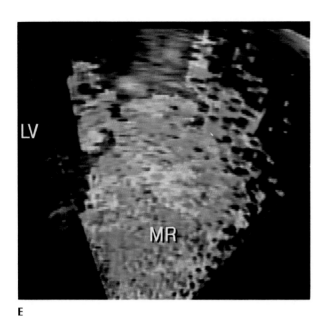

E

Fig. 16-4. Degenerative bileaflet mitral valve disease; biplane TEE. A. Because of the vertical orientation of this patient's heart, transverse imaging in the four-chamber view is markedly foreshortened. Portions of both mitral leaflets appear unsupported *(arrowheads)*, producing a central defect in coaptation *(arrow).* B. A broad jet of mitral regurgitation emanates through this malcoaptation. The central jet trajectory is typical for relatively balanced lesions of both leaflets or for annular dilatation. C. Longitudinal imaging in the left ventricular inflow plane. Flail segments of both mitral leaflets *(arrowheads)* are identified in this view. D. Further scanning in the same view reveals another severely prolapsing portion of the anterior leaflet *(arrowhead)* with an attached ruptured chordae *(arrow).* E. Torrential mitral regurgitation fills the left atrium on color Doppler imaging. *(Asterisk =* left atrial appendage.)

primary mechanism of mitral regurgitation [41], again aiding decision-making plans for repair. Posterior leaflet prolapse or flail typically propagates an eccentric regurgitant jet directed anteromedially, anterior leaflet prolapse or flail a posterolateral trajectory, and bileaflet prolapse a more central jet direction if both leaflets are involved to a similar degree. A central mitral regurgitant jet is usually seen with mitral annular dilatation, symmetrical distortion of left ventricular support, or rheumatic disease causing equal restriction of commissural closure of both leaflets. Asymmetrical restriction of leaflet closure causes leaflet override by the more mobile leaflet, producing eccentric regurgitation in the direction opposite to the overriding leaflet. Mitral leaflet perforation (see Chapter 11, Figure 11-14) can be accurately localized by color Doppler imaging with a narrow, sometimes eccentric regurgitant jet traversing the involved leaflet body; even meticulous two-dimensional scanning may not visualize tiny perforations.

After mitral valve repair and cessation of cardiopulmonary bypass, a critically important objective of repeat TEE is careful examination of the mitral leaflets for mechanisms of significant malcoaptation, such as residual prolapse, override, and incomplete coaptation secondary to annular dilatation, excessive leaflet plication, or rheumatic disease (Fig. 16-7). The finding of postrepair mitral systolic anterior motion may necessitate revision of the initial repair [42], but as discussed below, systolic anterior

motion is often due to a reversible hyperdynamic hemodynamic state. Although multiple methods of intraoperative assessment of residual mitral regurgitation have been described [43], only intraoperative echocardiography can provide visualization of the functional results of mitral repair in the contracting heart. This immediate feedback can give the surgeon valuable information in planning revision of the repair should residual mitral regurgitation be detected by any method, including composite Doppler echocardiography.

Doppler TEE examination after mitral valve repair should be performed only after a thorough two-dimensional examination has delineated the anatomic sequelae of the reparative procedure. Semiquantitation of residual mitral regurgitation should incorporate visual three-dimensional reconstruction of the color Doppler jet through use of multiple TEE imaging planes. As in the preoperative evaluation, color Doppler echocardiography can localize the site of residual mitral malcoaptation and help define the mechanism of mitral regurgitation by mapping the trajectory of the regurgitant jet. Pulsed-wave Doppler imaging of pulmonary venous inflow should routinely be repeated and compared with the prerepair spectral pattern to further aid in the exclusion or definition of hemodynamically significant residual mitral regurgitation.

The multifaceted effects of general anesthesia, vasodilator or vasopressor infusions, intravascular volume status, myocardial preservation techniques,

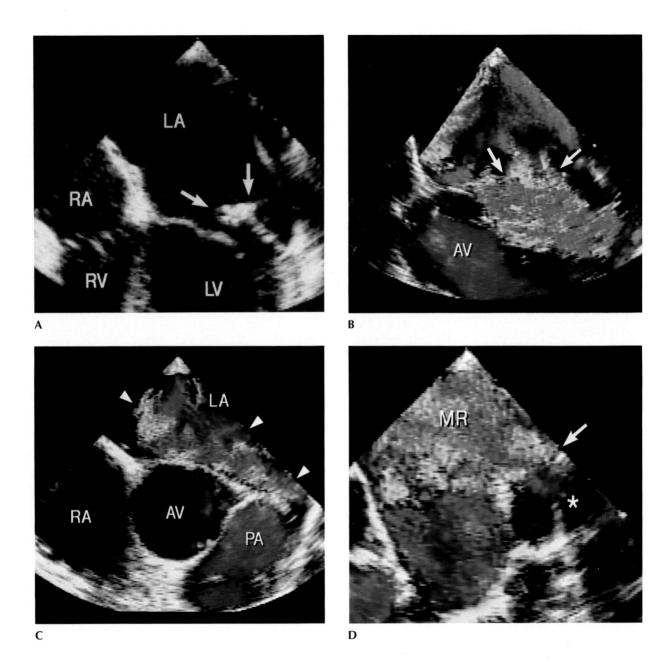

and cardiac rhythm evoke a complex intraoperative hemodynamic milieu that significantly influences myocardial and valvular function and, hence, interpretation of two-dimensional and Doppler echocardiographic findings. This complexity is discussed in detail under "Dynamic Potential Pitfalls," below.

Impact and Outcome

Previous studies with epicardial color Doppler echocardiography identified inadequate initial mitral valve repair in 8% to 17% of cases [6,7,42]. Color Doppler findings of significant residual regurgitation have correlated poorly with results of fluid fill-

ing of the arrested left ventricle and measurement of pulmonary capillary wedge v-wave pressures [32]. In a series of 309 patients studied by either epicardial echocardiography or TEE at the Cleveland Clinic, the causes of immediate failure of mitral repair in 26 patients were as follows: left ventricular outflow tract obstruction due to systolic anterior motion of the mitral valve (38%), incomplete repair (most often with residual leaflet prolapse) (38%), and suture dehiscence (23%) [42].

We subsequently reported a series of 143 patients undergoing mitral valve repair for mitral regurgitation studied by intraoperative TEE [44]. Most patients were operated on for myxomatous disease

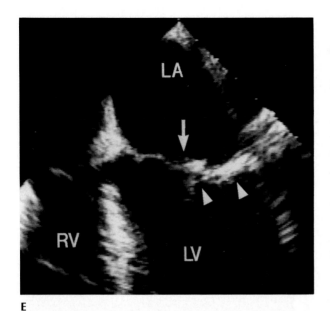

E

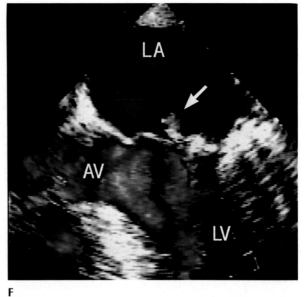

F

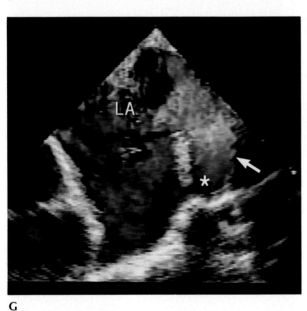

G

Fig. 16-5. Healed infective endocarditis; successful mitral valve repair. A. Transverse four-chamber view. The posterior mitral leaflet is flail with multiple chronic vegetations (*arrows*). The anterior leaflet is normal. B. Color Doppler imaging demonstrates a broad truncated anteromedial jet of mitral regurgitation (*arrows*). C. Basal short-axis imaging in the transverse plane detects an extensive sheet of mitral regurgitation (*arrowheads*) tracking along the entire anteromedial left atrium. D. The jet of mitral regurgitation wraps around to fill the dome of the left atrium in this cephalad basal short-axis view. Mitral regurgitation is also seen to reflux (*arrow*) into the left upper pulmonary vein (*asterisk*). E. After mitral valve repair, there is intact coaptation of the anterior leaflet (*arrow*) with the plicated posterior leaflet (*arrowheads*) after quadrangular resection of the flail segment. F. Trivial central mitral regurgitation (*arrow*) is identified in the left ventricular outflow view (compare with B). G. No mitral regurgitation is identified on basal short-axis imaging (compare with D) at the level of the left upper pulmonary vein; normal antegrade pulmonary venous inflow (*arrow*) is present. (A, E, and F from Freeman et al. [44]. By permission of the American College of Cardiology.)

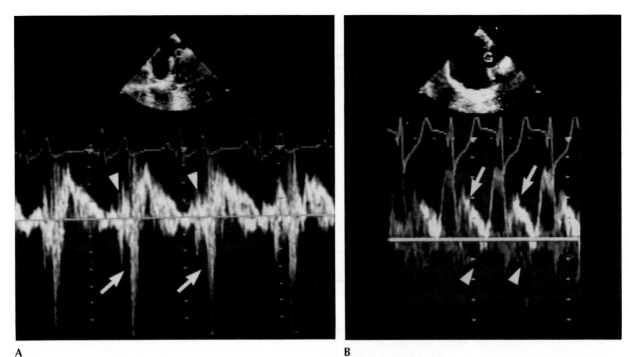

A   B

Fig. 16-6.   Pulsed-wave Doppler analysis of left upper pulmonary venous inflow; same patient as that in Figure 16-5. A. Before mitral valve repair. Turbulent systolic reversal (*arrows*) of pulmonary venous inflow, a highly sensitive finding for severe mitral regurgitation, is present (corresponding to color Doppler findings in Figure 16-5 D) with marked dimunition of antegrade systolic flow (*arrowheads*). B. After successful mitral valve repair. No systolic flow reversal remains (*arrowheads*), and laminar antegrade systolic flow (*arrows*) has returned. The systolic filling velocity is blunted because of transiently high left atrial filling pressures; trivial residual mitral regurgitation was confirmed by color Doppler imaging (Figure 16-5 F).

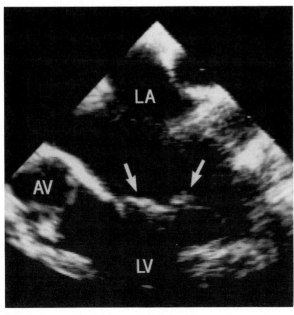

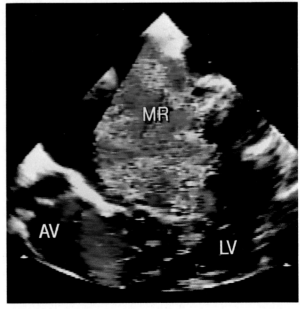

A   B

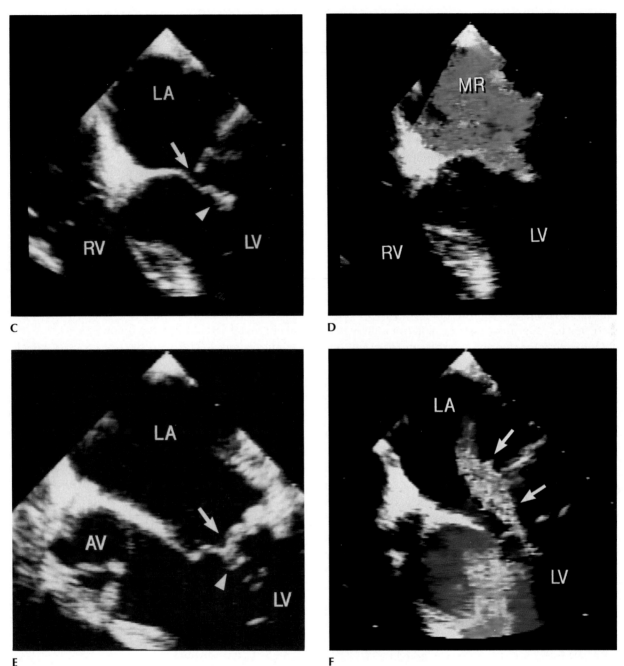

Fig. 16-7. ◄   Mitral valve repair for bileaflet mitral prolapse; transverse four-chamber and left ventricular outflow views. A. Before mitral valve repair, symmetrical redundancy and prolapse of both leaflets (*arrows*) is present. B. Severe central mitral regurgitation is detected by color Doppler imaging. C. After initial repair with bileaflet mitral plication, excessive tethering of the anterior leaflet (*arrowhead*) produces override of the posterior leaflet and malcoaptation *(arrow)*. D. Severe residual anteromedial mitral regurgitation with complete left atrial wraparound is detected on color-flow mapping. E. After a second period of cardiopulmonary bypass, partial release of the initial anterior leaflet plication and further posterior leaflet plication greatly increase the margins of leaflet coaptation (*arrowhead*); there is no residual malcoaptation (*arrow*) or prolapse. F. A narrow jet of mild central mitral regurgitation (*arrows*) was present at the time the patient left the operating room. (From Freeman et al. [44]. By permission of the American College of Cardiology.)

with or without chordal rupture (70%); other indications for operation were ischemic myocardial dysfunction (13%), congenital cleft mitral valve (6%), rheumatic disease (3%), and miscellaneous disorders (endocarditis, dilated left ventricle, and trauma) (8%). After initial repair, significant (grade ≥ III/IV) residual mitral regurgitation was detected by composite TEE Doppler study in 11 (7.7%) patients and prompted successful revision or replacement in all but 1 patient. The risk of significant residual mitral regurgitation was 1.7% in patients with isolated posterior leaflet disease (posterior leaflet prolapse with or without flail) and 22.5% in patients with anterior or bileaflet disease [44].

In our series [44], systolic anterior motion of the mitral valve caused moderate to severe residual mitral regurgitation in 13 (9.1%) patients after repair. In our early experience (the first five patients), we believed that significant systolic anterior motion was an indication for revision or replacement of the initial repair. In the remaining eight (5.6%) patients, we observed that systolic anterior motion was transient. This phenomenon resolved completely or nearly so when hyperdynamic hemodynamic status after bypass was corrected by intravascular volume repletion and cessation of inotropic therapy [44] (Fig. 16-8). All patients had grade I/IV (mild) or less mitral regurgitation without further surgical intervention before leaving the operating room.

Transthoracic echocardiography performed in 132 patients in this series [44] before hospital dismissal demonstrated excellent results in 86% with grade I/IV or less residual mitral regurgitation; only three patients (2.3%) had more than grade II/IV (moderate) mitral regurgitation. A significant discrepancy (> one grade) in the severity of mitral regurgitation between predismissal transthoracic echocardiography and intraoperative TEE was noted in 17 (13%) patients. In nearly all cases, mitral regurgitation was underestimated by intraoperative TEE, most likely because of significantly lower left ventricular afterload conditions in the operating room. However, in only three patients (2.3%) thought to have insignificant mitral regurgitation on the basis of intraoperative TEE findings was grade II/IV or greater residual mitral regurgitation detected before hospital dismissal [44].

The impact of intraoperative TEE on the operative management of ischemic mitral regurgitation was reported by Sheikh et al. [34]. They found that TEE altered plans for a mitral valve procedure in 11% of patients undergoing coronary artery bypass surgery.

Intraoperative TEE identified inadequate results in 17% of all patients undergoing mitral valve repair, prompting immediate revision or replacement. Importantly, the degree of mitral regurgitation detected by TEE after cardiopulmonary bypass was an important predictor of long-term survival and was more significant than age, ejection fraction, or postbypass left ventricular regional wall motion abnormalities in Cox regression analysis [34]. Actuarial survival in patients with grade II to III residual mitral regurgitation after coronary bypass surgery (with or without a mitral valve procedure) was nearly 50% lower than that in patients with grade I or less mitral regurgitation (approximately 45% and 90%, respectively, at 1 year). Worsening left ventricular regional wall motion detected by TEE after cardiopulmonary bypass was also associated with actuarial survival that was 25% less than that in patients with unchanged or improved left ventricular function [34].

Intraoperative TEE also has an ancillary benefit during mitral valve surgical procedures in the detection of findings unsuspected on preoperative evaluation. Such findings have directly prompted additional, unplanned surgical procedures in 3% to 8% of patients [18,34,44]. The unsuspected findings consist most often of intracardiac shunts (Fig. 16-9), occasionally of other significant valvular regurgitant lesions, and uncommonly of intracardiac masses.

Other Cardiac Valvular Procedures

In contrast to the extensive documentation in mitral valve repair, limited information has been reported in the literature on the usefulness of intraoperative TEE in the evaluation of other valvular repair or replacement operations.

Aortic Valve Disease
Intraoperative TEE has been used for evaluation in a small number of patients undergoing ultrasonic aortic valve decalcification for severe aortic stenosis [45]. After such debridement, TEE demonstrated

Fig. 16-8. Systolic anterior motion after mitral valve repair; magnified left ventricular outflow view in the transverse plane. A. Before mitral valve repair, a large flail segment (*arrow*) of the posterior leaflet due to chordal rupture (*arrowhead*) is identified. The anterior leaflet is anatomically normal. B. After posterior leaflet resection and plication with ring annuloplasty, severe systolic anterior motion of the anterior leaflet

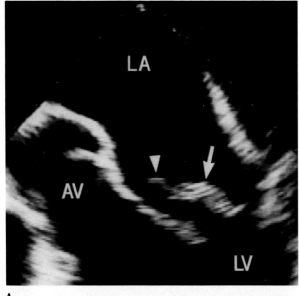

A

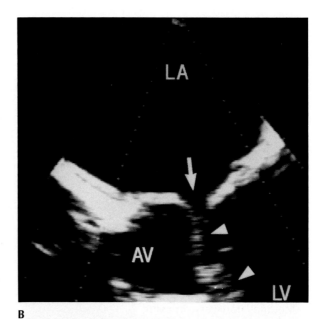

B

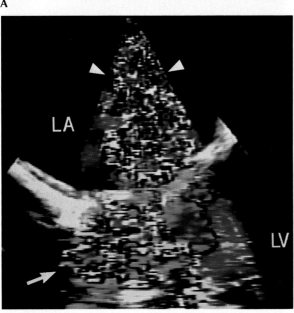

C

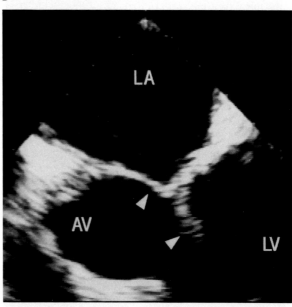

D

(*arrowheads*) causes a large deficiency in coaptation (*arrow*) with the plicated posterior leaflet. At this time, the patient was hypovolemic and receiving dopamine intravenously. C. Color-flow imaging demonstrates moderately severe residual mitral regurgitation (*arrowheads*); the posterolateral trajectory is perpendicular to the left ventricular outflow tract (*arrow*) and characteristic of a systolic anterior motion mechanism. Turbulent flow in the left ventricular outflow tract is due to obstruction caused by the mitral systolic anterior motion. D. After intravascular volume repletion and cessation of inotropic therapy, the systolic anterior motion has resolved (*arrowheads*) and leaflet coaptation is intact; no revision of the mitral repair was performed. E. Color-flow Doppler imaging reveals laminar flow in the left ventricular outflow tract (*arrow*), consistent with resolution of obstruction. No residual mitral regurgitation was present (*arrowhead*). (From Freeman et al. [44]. By permission of the American College of Cardiology.)

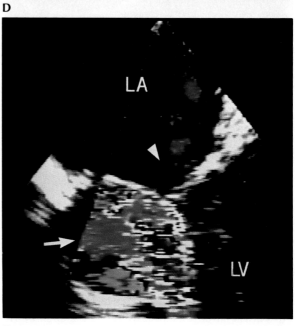

E

Fig. 16-9. Ancillary impact of intraoperative TEE during open commissurotomy for mitral stenosis; transverse four-chamber views. A. Before cardiopulmonary bypass, a secundum atrial septal defect (*arrows*) is incidentally discovered; there is severe mitral stenosis (*arrowheads*). B. A moderate left-to-right interatrial shunt (*arrows*) across this defect is confirmed by color-flow imaging. C. Modified transverse imaging of the atrial septum. After mitral commissurotomy and closure of the atrial septal defect, no residual interatrial shunt is detected on color-flow mapping (*arrow*).

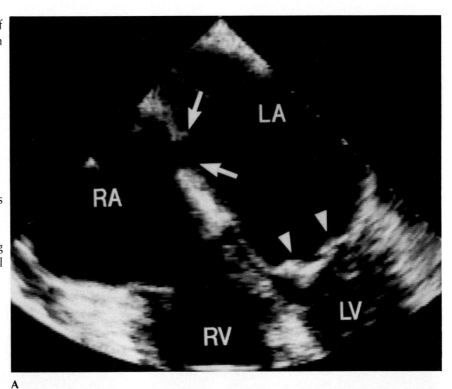

A

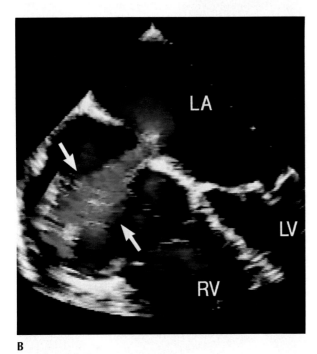

B

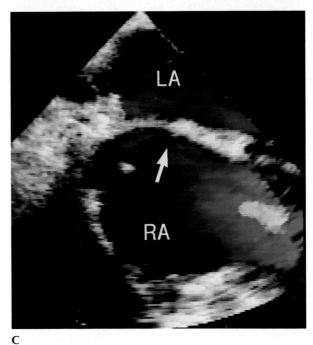

C

greatly increased aortic cusp mobility and, in some patients, elimination of aortic regurgitation due to improved cusp coaptation. Unfortunately, an unacceptable incidence of significant aortic regurgitation [45,46] and a significant trend toward restenosis [46] were noted on early transthoracic Doppler follow-up studies after this procedure. Ultrasonic aortic valve decalcification has since been abandoned as primary surgical therapy for valvular aortic stenosis.

Intraoperative epicardial echocardiography has been found to be a useful adjunct for the sizing of aortic valve allografts, minimizing delay between allograft thawing procedures and implantation. Using this technique, Bartzokis et al. [47] found that there was a good correlation ($r = 0.78$) between aortic annular dimensions determined by intraoperative echocardiography before cardiopulmonary bypass and direct annular measurement by the surgeon. Aortic valve allograft selection was guided by intraoperative echocardiographic measurements in 17 of 20 (85%) patients in this series [47].

The dimensions of the aortic valve annulus can be readily obtained by intraoperative TEE, most reliably by longitudinal long-axis imaging of the aortic valve and left ventricular outflow tract. Caution should be exercised in patients with extensive calcific disease extending into the aortic annulus. In such cases, surgical debridement of the annulus may be necessary before allograft placement, enlarging the annulus to a dimension significantly greater than that initially appreciated by echocardiography.

Intraoperative TEE for the evaluation of repair procedures is likely to become of use much more for aortic regurgitation [48] than for aortic stenosis. Intraoperative two-dimensional examination is useful for the delineation of the mechanism of aortic regurgitation, such as cusp prolapse or incomplete coaptation due to enlargement of the aortic root and annulus (see Chapter 9 and Figure 14-13). Semiquantitation of associated regurgitation should be performed by composite biplanar long- and short-axis color Doppler imaging. With central regurgitant jets, the ratio of subvalvular jet to outflow tract dimension (on long-axis imaging) and the ratio of subvalvular jet to outflow tract area (on short-axis imaging) correlate well with angiographic gradation of aortic regurgitation [49] (see Chapter 9 for details). The trajectory of the aortic regurgitant jet also aids in the clarification of the mechanism and insufficiency; defects in central coaptation cause central jets, and asymmetrical cusp malcoaptation produces eccentric jets usually directed away from the most affected cusp. Longitudinal short-axis color Doppler imaging of the aortic valve usually can pinpoint the exact site and size of the regurgitant orifice, further guiding surgical repair efforts (Fig. 16-10). Significant residual aortic regurgitation shown by intraoperative color Doppler evaluation after initial aortic valve repair was noted in 7% of patients studied by Cosgrove et al. [48], prompting immediate successful revision of the repair in all patients in this series.

Tricuspid Regurgitation

Intraoperative TEE is also useful in the evaluation of the mechanism and severity of tricuspid regurgitation, which is often associated with surgical mitral or aortic valvular disease. In a series of patients

studied by Czer et al. [5] with epicardial echocardiography, grade III to IV tricuspid regurgitation was found in 40% of patients requiring mitral valve repair or replacement. Even after successful mitral valve procedures, these investigators noted a significant (two or more grades) reduction in tricuspid regurgitation in only 14% of patients without concomitant tricuspid repair. The incidence of inadequate initial tricuspid valve repair detected by epicardial color-flow imaging was previously reported to be about 5% [5,50]. In a recent preliminary report of 195 patients studied by intraoperative epicardial or transesophageal echocardiography or both, Klein et al. [51] found that 4% of patients required revision of the initial tricuspid repair at the time of operation; however, 14% had late failure of the repair at a mean follow-up period of 109 days.

Significant tricuspid regurgitation usually results from a combination of leaflet malcoaptation and tricuspid annular dilatation, both of which can be delineated by intraoperative TEE, which guides and subsequently evaluates tricuspid repair (Fig. 16-11). We have also reported the detection of traumatic tricuspid regurgitation by intraoperative TEE in a patient after decannulation of the right side of the heart following mitral valve repair [52]. In this patient, the septal leaflet of the tricuspid valve (which was normal before cardiopulmonary bypass) was flail because of papillary muscle rupture, most likely precipitated by cannulation (Fig. 16-12). After detection by TEE, successful tricuspid repair was performed.

Other Regurgitation

Often, intraoperative TEE is performed to evaluate secondary valvular regurgitation during surgery for a primary valvular lesion. The most common situation is evaluation of mitral regurgitation during prosthetic replacement for severe aortic valve stenosis or regurgitation. Because of high left ventricular diastolic pressures, diastolic mitral regurgitation can be prominent in such patients, along with functional systolic regurgitation. If the mitral valve leaflets and support apparatus are normal or only mildly abnormal, our experience has been that significant reduction in mitral regurgitation occurs after successful aortic valve replacement, eliminating the need for a mitral valve procedure (Fig. 16-13). Often, considerable tricuspid annular enlargement exists if significant tricuspid regurgitation is associated with right ventricular pressure overload due to left-sided valvular lesions, and as noted by others [5], concomitant tricuspid annuloplasty is usually warranted.

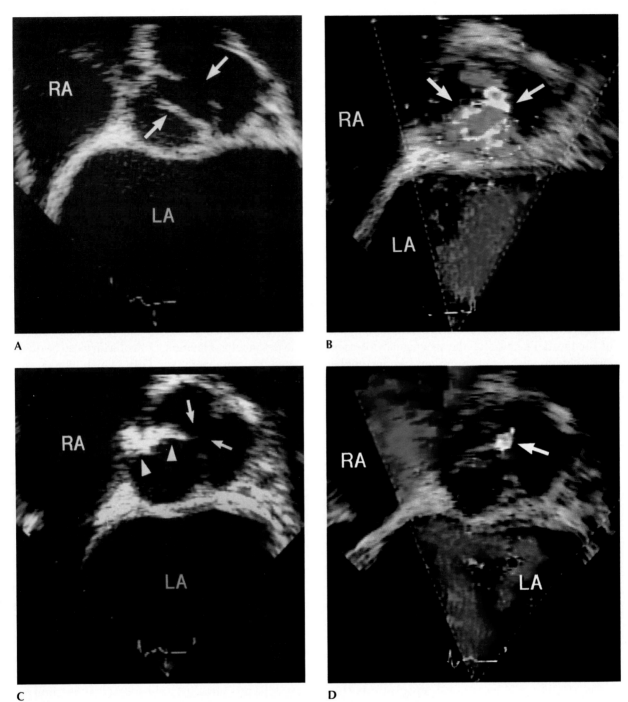

Fig. 16-10. Aortic valve repair; longitudinal short-axis imaging. A. Before repair, there is grossly incomplete diastolic coaptation of the noncoronary cusp (*arrows*). B. Severe aortic regurgitation (*arrows*) emanates from this defect on color-flow Doppler imaging. C. After aortic valve repair, the site of commissural plication (*arrowheads*) between the noncoronary cusp and right coronary cusp is visualized. There is now intact diastolic coaptation of all cusps (*arrows*). D. Trivial residual central aortic regurgitation (*arrow*) persists on color Doppler mapping.

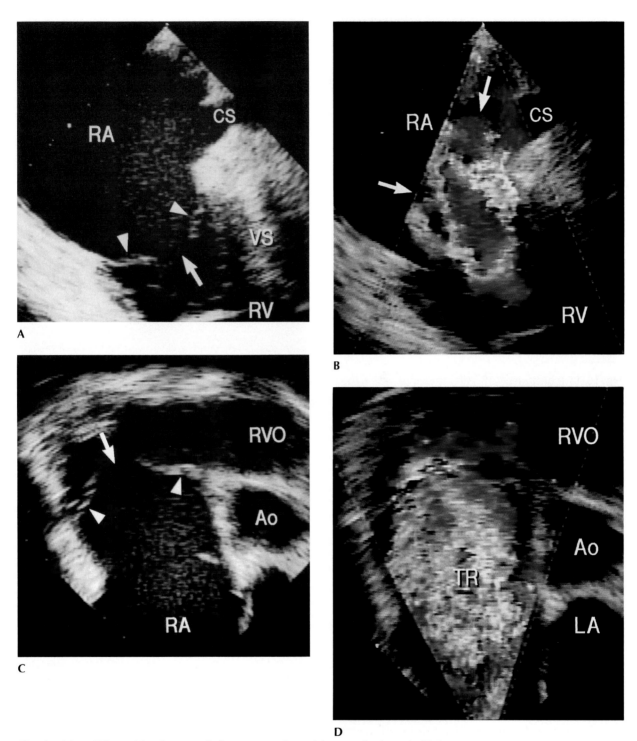

Fig. 16-11. Tricuspid valve repair for severe tricuspid regurgitation. A. Right ventricular inflow view, transverse plane. The tricuspid annulus is severely dilated, with substantial separation of the tricuspid leaflets (*arrowheads*); complete lack of central coaptation (*arrow*) is present. B. A broad central jet of tricuspid regurgitation (*arrows*) traverses this defect. The homogeneous central blue Doppler signal indicates laminar nonturbulent regurgitant flow through the large regurgitant orifice and is characteristic of free tricuspid regurgitation. C. Longitudinal short-axis imaging also delineates the expansive gap (*arrow*) between the noncoapting tricuspid leaflets (*arrowheads*). D. Color Doppler imaging confirms torrential tricuspid regurgitation, which fills the severely enlarged right atrium. (continued)

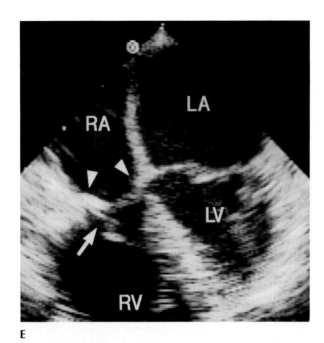

E

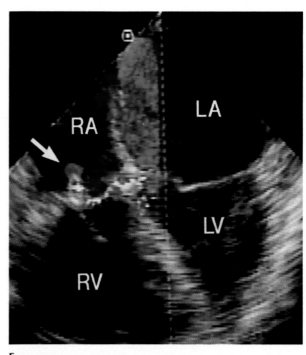

F

Fig. 16-11 (continued)   E. After tricuspid repair, the tricuspid annulus has been dramatically reduced (*arrowheads*) by tricuspid ring annuloplasty. The anterior tricuspid leaflet has been plicated (*arrow*) and leaflet coaptation is intact. F. Trivial residual tricuspid regurgitation (*arrow*) is detected on color Doppler imaging.

Hypertrophic Obstructive Cardiomyopathy

Intraoperative echocardiography has been a very useful adjunct for the evaluation of surgery for hypertrophic obstructive cardiomyopathy [53–58]. At the Mayo Clinic, we perform intraoperative TEE routinely in patients undergoing operation for hypertrophic obstructive cardiomyopathy.

Intraoperative TEE provides the surgeon with two-dimensional visualization of the structure of the hypertrophied ventricular septum and delineates the extent of myectomy. Importantly, the functional morphology of the mitral valve, degree of systolic anterior motion, and severity of associated mitral regurgitation both before and after myectomy can be readily assessed by TEE (Fig. 16-14). As noted below, significant primary mitral valve disease and regurgitation (which will not improve with myectomy alone) are identified in approximately 20% of patients undergoing surgery for hypertrophic obstructive cardiomyopathy [57]. Even with the availability of steerable continuous-wave Doppler biplane TEE systems, reliable determination of left ventricular outflow tract pressure gradients by TEE is not always possible, because of significant angles of incidence of the interrogating beam to the outflow tract from the transesophageal window. Occasionally, Doppler assessment of the left ventricular outflow tract can be achieved by transgastric longitudinal long-axis imaging, but if continuous-wave Doppler echocardiography is to be used, epicardial application of a nonimaging transducer is often necessary [56]. We currently assess left ventricular outflow tract obstruction by simultaneous needle catheterization of the left ventricle and proximal ascending aorta. After myectomy, intraoperative TEE is also valuable for the exclusion of potential complications of myectomy, such as aortic regurgitation and ventricular septal defect.

At our institution, intraoperative TEE has been performed in 36 consecutive patients undergoing septal myectomy for hypertrophic obstructive cardiomyopathy [57]. Systolic anterior motion of an otherwise normal mitral valve was the mechanism of mitral regurgitation in 25 (70%) patients. Eight (22%) patients had various degrees of mitral valve prolapse (three patients with a posterior leaflet flail

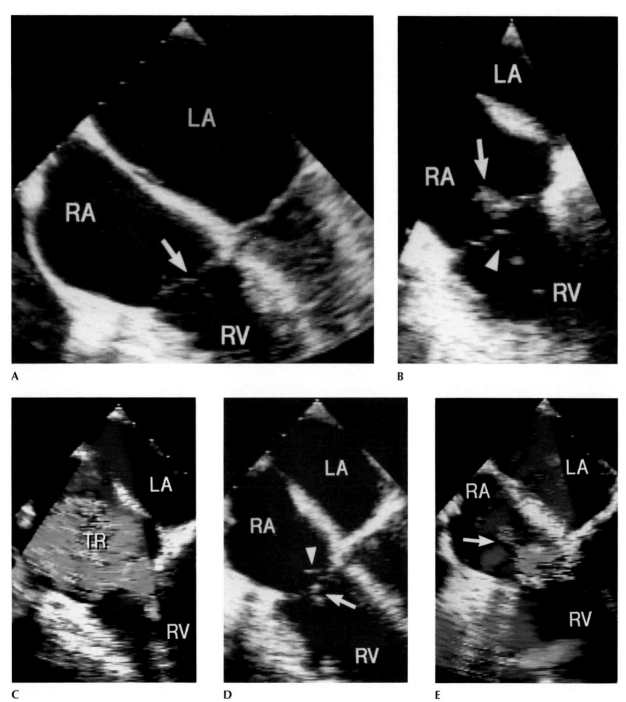

A   B   C   D   E

Fig. 16-12.   Tricuspid valve trauma associated with cannulation of the right side of the heart during cardiopulmonary bypass for mitral valve repair; transverse four-chamber views. A. Before cannulation, the tricuspid valve (*arrow*) was normal; there was no significant tricuspid regurgitation. Surgical repair of a flail posterior mitral leaflet (not seen in this view) was successfully performed. B. Immediately after decannulation, a ruptured papillary muscle (*arrow*) attached to a now flail septal leaflet is identified; the anterior leaflet (*arrowhead*) was not traumatized. C. Acute, severe tricuspid regurgitation is detected by color Doppler imaging. D. After tricuspid valve repair, the flail segment has been resected and the plicated septal leaflet (*arrow*) coapts normally; a suture (*arrowhead*) is visualized along the atrial aspect of the repair. E. Mild residual central tricuspid regurgitation (*arrow*) is detected by color-flow imaging. (A–C from Johnston et al. [52]. By permission of the American Society of Echocardiography.)

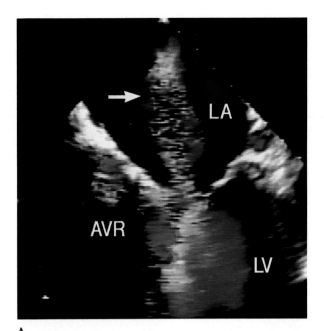

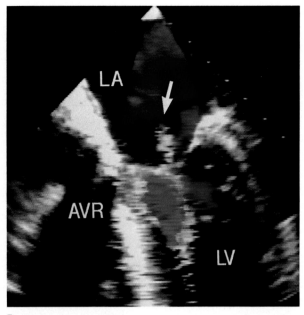

A

B

Fig. 16-13. Evaluation of mitral regurgitation during surgical replacement of a severely regurgitant aortic valve prosthesis; transverse four-chamber view. A. Before repeat aortic valve replacement, mild to moderate central mitral regurgitation (*arrow*) is detected. The mitral annulus was only mildly dilated, and the mitral leaflets were normal for the patient's age. B. After rereplacement of the aortic valve, only trivial residual mitral regurgitation (*arrow*) is present. Concomitant mitral valve exploration and repair were not done because of the findings on TEE.

segment) in addition to systolic anterior motion. Three (8%) patients had severe calcific mitral sclerotic disease without systolic anterior motion as the cause of mitral regurgitation [57]. Mitral valve repair or replacement, performed in seven (19%) patients, was prompted in two by intraoperative TEE after initial myectomy. Intraoperative TEE detected grade III to IV residual mitral regurgitation in three (8%) patients, prompting revision of the myectomy or a mitral valve procedure (or both) during a second period of cardiopulmonary bypass (Fig. 16-15). Another patient was found to have a postmyectomy ventricular septal defect, which was successfully repaired. Hence, intraoperative TEE had a significant effect on the surgical management of 11% of patients undergoing operation for hypertrophic obstructive cardiomyopathy and confirmed satisfactory results in the remainder [57]. The degree of residual mitral regurgitation as assessed by intraoperative TEE was generally mild (grade 1.3 ± 0.9 on a scale of 1 [I] mild, to 4 [IV] severe) before patients left the operating room and agreed closely with the mean grade of mitral regurgitation (grade

1.0 ± 0.6) determined before hospital dismissal by transthoracic Doppler evaluation at similar left ventricular outflow pressure gradients [57].

In a recent report of 32 patients undergoing myectomy, Grigg et al. [58] found that intraoperative TEE was useful in both clarifying the mechanisms of mitral systolic anterior motion and measuring ventricular septal and left ventricular outflow tract dimensions before and after myectomy. After myectomy, the mean basal ventricular septal thickness decreased from 23 to 11 mm and the mean outflow tract dimension increased from 15 to 24 mm. Complete resolution of mitral systolic anterior motion accompanied by significant reduction in mitral regurgitation was noted by intraoperative TEE in 84% of patients after myectomy; all but two (6%) patients had adequate resolution of left ventricular outflow tract obstruction in this series [58].

Congenital Heart Disease

The intraoperative use of echocardiography during the repair of congenital heart defects began in the

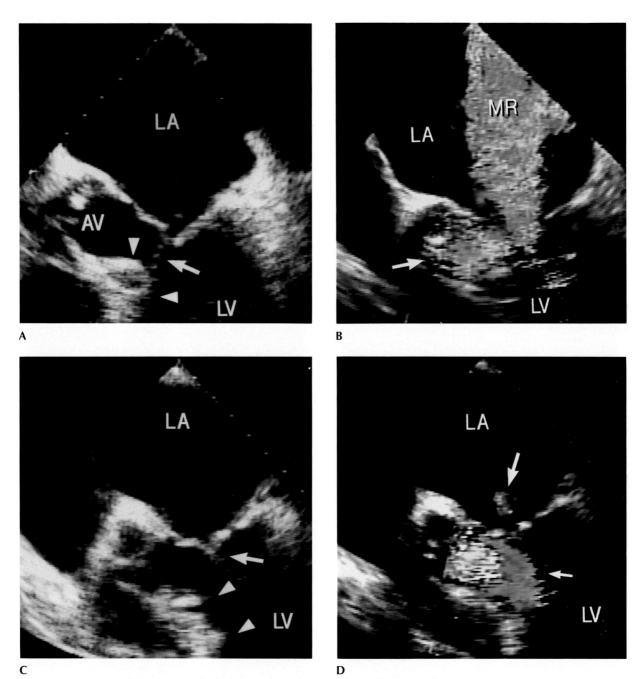

Fig. 16-14. Septal myectomy for hypertrophic obstructive cardiomyopathy; left ventricular outflow view in the transverse plane. A. Before cardiopulmonary bypass, prominent systolic anterior motion of the anterior mitral leaflet (*arrow*) abuts the severely hypertrophied basal ventricular septum (*arrowheads*) throughout systole. B. Color-flow Doppler imaging reveals turbulent left ventricular outflow (*arrow*) due to subvalvular obstruction; grade III/IV mitral regurgitation in a trajectory perpendicular to the left ventricular outflow tract is typical for regurgitation due to systolic anterior motion of the mitral valve. C. After septal myectomy (*arrowheads*), mitral valve leaflet coaptation is normal (*arrow*); there is no residual systolic anterior motion. D. Laminar left ventricular outflow (*small arrow*) is now seen on color Doppler imaging; nonturbulent central aliasing (yellow) is consistent with absence of obstruction. Trivial residual mitral regurgitation (*large arrow*) is detected; a mitral valve procedure was not done.

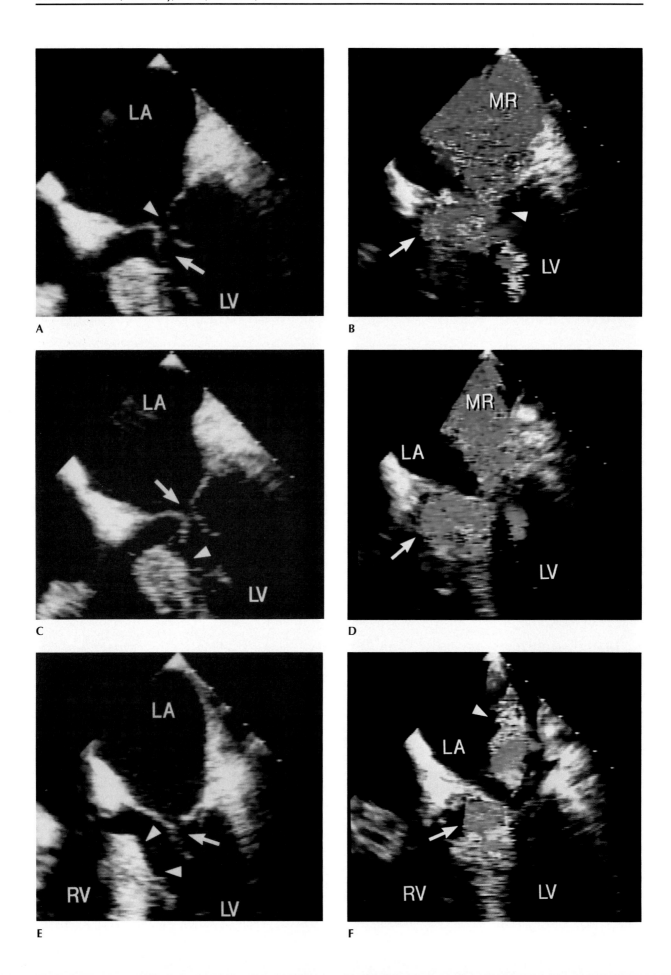

◀ **Fig. 16-15.** Septal myectomy for hypertrophic obstructive cardiomyopathy; left ventricular outflow view in the transverse plane. A. Before myectomy, severe systolic anterior motion of the anterior mitral leaflet (*arrow*) results in inadequate coaptation (*arrowhead*) with the posterior leaflet. B. Severe posterolateral mitral regurgitation issues from the site of malcoaptation (*arrowhead*); turbulent flow within the left ventricular outflow tract (*arrow*) due to obstruction is present. C. After the initial septal myectomy (*arrowhead*), significant persistent systolic anterior motion still causes incomplete mitral leaflet coaptation (*arrow*). D. Color Doppler imaging is consistent with persistent left ventricular outflow obstruction (*arrow*); moderately severe mitral regurgitation remains. E. A second period of cardiopulmonary bypass and a more extensive septal myectomy (*arrowheads*) was prompted by the above initial results. Systolic anterior motion of the anterior leaflet has largely resolved (*arrow*). F. Less color Doppler turbulence is noted in the left ventricular outflow tract (*arrow*); only mild residual mitral regurgitation (*arrowhead*) is now detected.

mid-1980s. Initially, intraoperative imaging was limited to use of transthoracic probes in sterile sheaths. This combination was placed on the epicardial surface for the examination. Using this technique, several investigators found that epicardial echocardiography contributed significantly to the perioperative management of patients with congenital heart disease [8–10]. The studies by Hagler et al. [9] and Ungerleider et al. [10] demonstrated a significant improvement in study quality and diagnostic value when color-flow Doppler imaging was used.

Ungerleider et al. [10] found that besides the obvious advantage of confirming the status of the surgical repair while the patient was still in the operating room, intraoperative echocardiography detected significant residual lesions that placed patients at greater risk for subsequent reoperation. These investigators observed a 42% reoperation rate for patients with residual lesions and only a 3% rate for those without. Furthermore, early mortality (death within 30 days of operation) was greater in the group with significant residual abnormalities. The early mortality was 29% for those with unsatisfactory results identified by intraoperative echocardiography compared with 10% for those without significant residual abnormalities [10].

Despite the documented clinical usefulness of epicardial echocardiography, several disadvantages

have limited its use (see Table 16-1). Pediatric patients also may not tolerate epicardial probe manipulation, most frequently because of ventricular ectopy and occasionally because of transient hypotension due to transducer pressure. The limitations of epicardial echocardiography have prompted congenital cardiologists and cardiac surgeons to seek an alternative method for performing intraoperative echocardiography. As in acquired cardiac disease, a shift in technique has occurred favoring TEE. The transesophageal approach has become the most widely used method for intraoperative echocardiography in congenital heart disease in the past few years.

The first reports of intraoperative TEE for congenital heart disease appeared in 1990. Stümper et al. [22] reported use of monoplane intraoperative TEE during atrial septal defect closure in three teenaged patients. Cyran et al. [59] demonstrated that with an appropriately sized probe, patients as young as 2 years could undergo intraoperative TEE monitoring. Lam et al. [23] subsequently described guidelines for transducer size in smaller patients. They recommended that transesophageal probes with tip diameters of 13 mm or more be used only in patients weighing more than 17 kg. Probes with a tip diameter of 11 mm were thought to be safe in patients between 12 and 17 kg in weight. The smallest probe available, with a 7-mm tip diameter, was used in patients between 4 and 12 kg. Our guidelines follow these closely. We use 12- or 13-mm probes in patients who weigh 15 kg or more. A 10-mm probe is used for patients between 7 and 15 kg and a 7-mm monoplane probe is used for those who weigh between 4 and 7 kg. A 5-mm monoplane probe is used for neonates. Occasionally in patients at the lower limits of these ranges, the probe chosen does not enter the esophagus easily. In these instances, a slightly smaller probe is used.

More recent studies have focused on the clinical value of intraoperative TEE. Several authors [23,60–63] have now published reports of relatively large series in which intraoperative TEE had a significant positive influence on both the intraoperative and the perioperative management of patients with congenital heart disease. All of these studies have shown that intraoperative TEE can make accurate diagnoses and is quite sensitive in detecting residual lesions.

In these studies, rates of positive preoperative impact are between 9% and 31% [23,60–63]. Prebypass intraoperative TEE has been most useful for delineating more posterior anatomy, such as the pulmonary veins and the structure, attachments, and function of the atrioventricular valves. Transesophageal echocardiography has also been important for the intraoperative evaluation of left ventricular outflow obstruction (Fig. 16-16) and atrial septal defects (Fig. 16-17). After cardiopulmonary bypass, the reported rates of immediate reoperation based on intraoperative TEE findings range from 4% to 13% [23,61,63]. Intraoperative TEE is valuable for assessing residual obstruction and regurgitation, evaluating the integrity of the atrial and ventricular septa (Figs. 16-17 and 16-18), confirming the patency of anastomoses (such as with modified Fontan procedures or right ventricular to pulmonary artery conduits) (Fig. 16-19), and evaluating ventricular function. Intraoperative TEE has also been shown to detect important functional or hemodynamic derangements that may not require reoperation but have nevertheless changed postoperative medical management in 6% to 10% of patients studied [23,61,63]. In addition, our experience suggests that intraoperative TEE becomes more valuable as the congenital defect and surgical repair increase in complexity [63].

In the largest study to date of the smallest patients (mean age, 3.1 years, and mean weight, 13.2 kg), Ritter [61] reported no significant complications of TEE during 157 studies performed in 127 patients. Intraoperative TEE was able to identify structures or define hemodynamics that were not apparent by transthoracic echocardiography in 56% of the studies performed, representing 40% of the patients in the entire surgical group. In 48 of the 155 (31%) studies performed prior to cardiopulmonary bypass, TEE refined the preoperative transthoracic echocardiographic diagnosis. Significant residual abnormalities detected by TEE after cardiopulmonary bypass led to a second operative procedure in 4% of patients [61].

In the same study, Ritter also noted the value of biplane TEE imaging in congenital heart disease. Twenty-six biplane examinations were performed, and in 20 of these studies (77%), the addition of the longitudinal plane images provided information that significantly affected clinical management and was unavailable from transverse monoplane images. It was found that the longitudinal imaging provided unique information on left atrioventricular valve regurgitation, both the right and the left ventricular outflow tracts, the proximal great arteries, and residual ventricular septal defects [61]

Our recent experience [63] with 104 biplane intraoperative TEE examinations for congenital heart disease (mean age, 8 years, and mean weight, 24 kg) confirms Ritter's observations. Preoperative biplane TEE revealed new information that altered the surgical procedure in 12% of the patients. These TEE findings were considered "new" only if they were not identified by any other test in the patient's preoperative evaluation (including transthoracic echocardiography, cardiac catheterization, and magnetic resonance imaging when these studies had been performed). Another 4% of this group had intraoperative TEE findings that were different from those of the preoperative evaluation and appropriately altered surgical management. After the initial surgical procedure, significant residual defects detected by biplane TEE led to immediate reoperation in 9% of the patients. An additional 16% of the group had residual defects or functional derangements that were not amenable to further repair or were thought not to be severe enough to warrant reoperation. However, the information gained by postoperative TEE altered the medical management of each of these patients [63].

We concur with Ritter's conclusion that biplane TEE is clearly superior in the examination of patients with congenital heart defects. We found that the availability of orthogonal imaging planes improved our diagnostic ability in nearly every case. The longitudinal plane provided superior delineation of the ventricular outflow tracts, great arteries and veins, and cavopulmonary anastomoses. The transverse imaging plane is superior in visualizing two-dimensional anatomy at the crux of the heart, in imaging the right pulmonary artery, and in assessing ventricular function [63]. In contrast to the observation from Ritter's series [61], we found that the longitudinal plane did not have a major advantage over the transverse plane for assessment of atrioventricular valve regurgitation but instead was complementary.

Both Ritter's report [61] and our series [63] noted the relative advantages and disadvantages of the transverse and the longitudinal imaging planes. Is monoplane TEE imaging adequate in any clinical situation? Given the high frequency of added diagnostic information available from the biplanar examinations in both series [61,63], we believe that a composite biplanar examination is generally the most useful and accurate method for the full delineation of any cardiac structure or malformation. We currently limit monoplane TEE to patients who

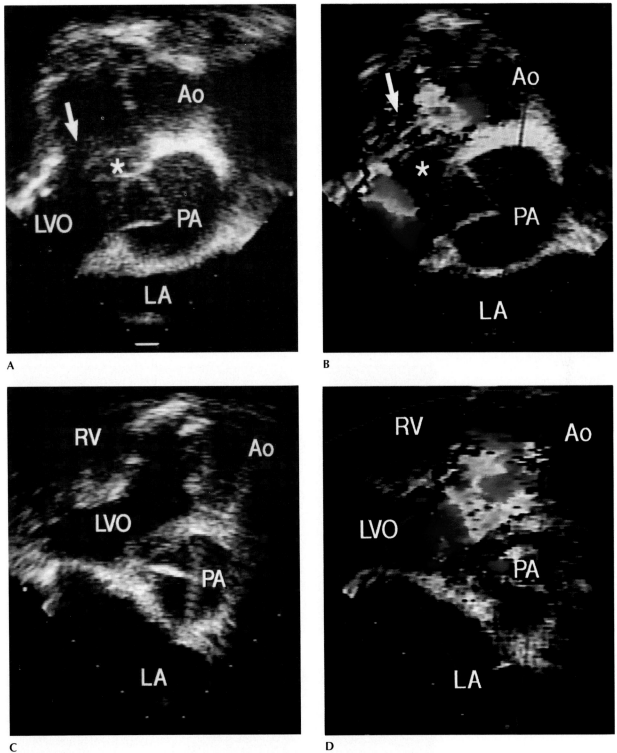

Fig. 16-16. Subaortic obstruction after prior repair of complex congenital heart disease; modified left ventricular outflow views in the longitudinal plane. A. Before cardiopulmonary bypass, a prominent subaortic conus muscle *(asterisk)* causes severe obstruction *(arrow)* of the left ventricular outflow tract. Preoperative transthoracic echocardiography and angiography erroneously suggested that the subaortic obstruction was caused by encroachment from a previous ventricular septal patch graft repair. B. Color Doppler imaging reveals normal laminar flow (orange-red) below the conus muscle and turbulent (yellow-green mosaic) flow distal to the obstruction *(arrow)*. C. After resection of the obstructive conus muscle, imaging after cardiopulmonary bypass demonstrates that the left ventricular outflow tract is widely patent. D. A much broader color-flow signal, which is laminar with central aliasing (orange) is now visualized in the left ventricular outflow tract; no turbulence is identified to suggest residual obstruction. (Ao = proximal ascending aorta; PA = stump of previously ligated main pulmonary artery.)

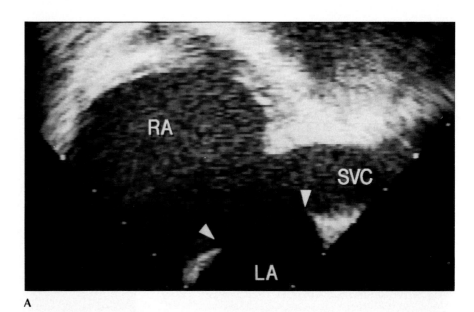

A

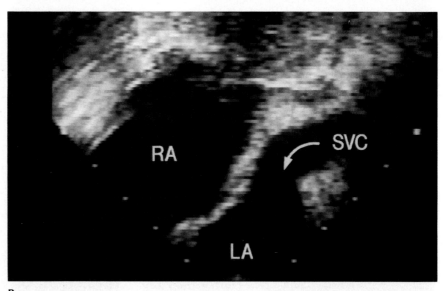

B

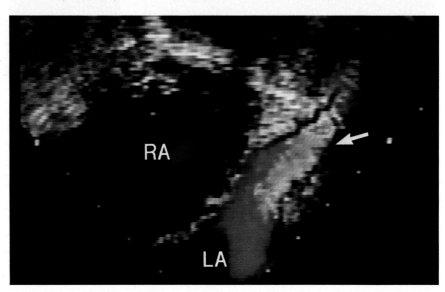

C

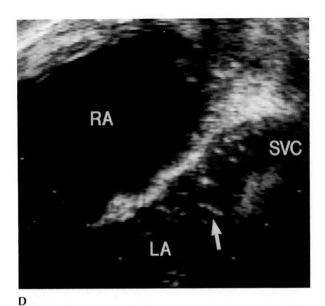

D

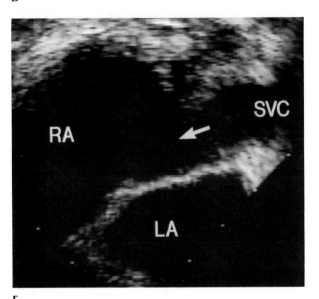

E

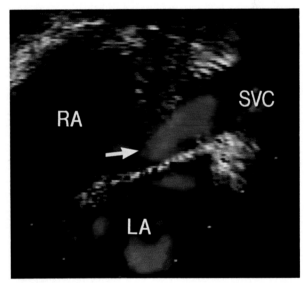

F

Fig. 16-17.   Repair of sinus venosus atrial septal defect; longitudinal long-axis imaging planes. A. Before cardiopulmonary bypass, a large sinus venosus atrial septal defect (*arrowheads*), measuring approximately 2.3 cm in this view, is seen. Pulmonary venous drainage (not shown) was normal. B. Imaging after cardiopulmonary bypass revealed that the atrial septal patch graft repair directed the orifice of the superior vena cava (*curved arrow*) into the left atrium. C. Color Doppler imaging demonstrates caval flow (*arrow*) into the left atrium.
D. Systemic venous shunting into the left atrium is also confirmed by contrast echocardiography. Agitated saline was injected into an internal jugular venous catheter, with microbubbles (*arrow*) entering the left atrium through the superior vena cava; there was no normal appearance of contrast medium in the right atrium. E. Cardiopulmonary bypass was reinstituted and the atrial septal patch repair revised; there is now correct communication (*arrow*) of the superior vena cava to the right atrium. F. Normal superior vena caval inflow (*arrow*) is detected on color-flow imaging.

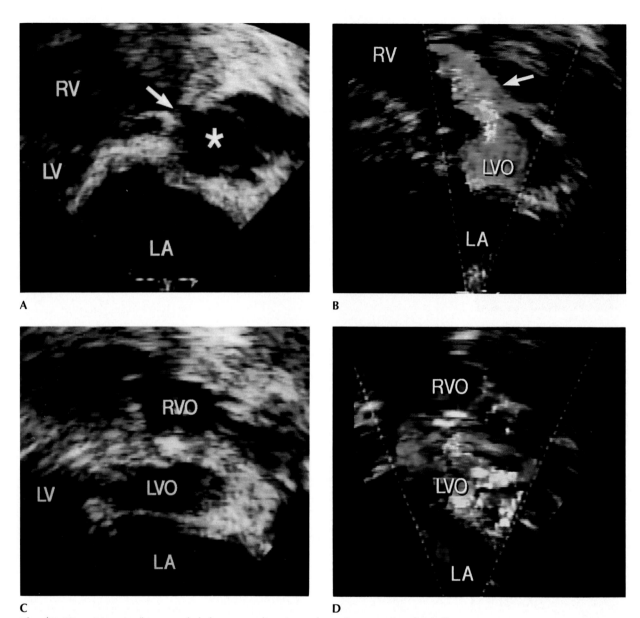

Fig. 16-18.   Ventricular septal defect complicating subaortic resection for left ventricular outflow obstruction; modified longitudinal left ventricular outflow views. A. Off-axis imaging. Immediately after cardiopulmonary bypass, a ventricular septal defect *(arrow)* is identified at the site of subaortic resection *(asterisk)*. B. Color-flow imaging demonstrates a moderate left-to-right interventricular shunt *(arrow)* exiting the left ventricular outflow tract and entering the right ventricular outflow tract. C. After a second period of cardiopulmonary bypass and repair of this defect, repeat imaging shows that the ventricular septum between the right ventricular outflow tract and the left ventricular outflow tract is intact. D. Color-flow Doppler imaging reveals no residual shunt into the right ventricular outflow tract.

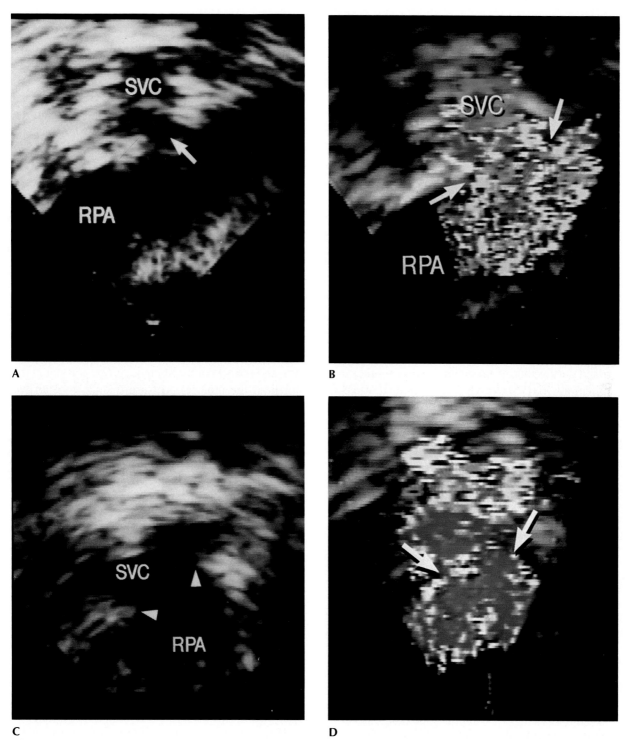

Fig. 16-19. Modified Fontan anastomosis for tricuspid atresia; apex-down basal short-axis imaging in the transverse plane. A. After the initial surgical procedure and cardiopulmonary bypass, imaging demonstrates that the anastomosis (*arrow*) between the superior vena cava and the right pulmonary artery is quite narrow. B. The laminar flow signal of the superior vena cava (blue) becomes highly turbulent (yellow-green mosaic) as it crosses the anastomosis (*arrows*) and enters the right pulmonary artery, consistent with obstruction. Zero-shifted, pulsed-wave Doppler imaging revealed a maximal velocity of 2 m/sec in this location, confirming significant obstruction of the anastomosis. These findings were confirmed by direct hemodynamic measurements, and cardiopulmonary bypass was reinstituted. C. After revision of the stenotic anastomosis, repeat imaging shows a much larger connection (*arrowheads*) between the superior vena cava and the right pulmonary artery. D. Color Doppler study reveals a laminar flow pattern across the anastomosis (*arrows*), consistent with normal, unobstructed function of the revised Fontan connection.

weigh less than 7 kg or who are unable to tolerate even the smallest biplane probe available. In a recent preliminary report of 42 operations for adult congenital heart disease, 90% of which were evaluated by biplane intraoperative TEE, Marelli et al. [64] found that TEE clarified or detected unsuspected lesions in 36% of studies; surgical management was altered in 12% as a result of TEE.

Although intraoperative TEE provides a large amount of highly accurate information, it has some limitations. Structures anterior to either the left main stem bronchus or prosthetic material (such as valves, conduits, and patches) are difficult to fully examine because these structures impede ultrasound transmission. We also found that real-time intraoperative TEE did not consistently detect very small (< 3 mm) residual ventricular septal defects (VSDs) demonstrated during routine predismissal transthoracic examinations [63]. Six of 18 (33%) residual VSDs in our series that were less than 3 mm in diameter were undetected by intraoperative TEE. All 43 septal defects (native or residual) of larger diameter were accurately defined.

The experience of Wienecke et al. [24] suggests that TEE may detect residual VSDs with as much sensitivity as epicardial echocardiography. Their series is relatively small (18 patients and seven residual VSDs). Furthermore, to achieve accuracy comparable with that of the epicardial examination, the TEE studies had to be retrospectively reviewed in a frame-by-frame analysis. After examining the information from these two series, we suspect that with current technology, epicardial echocardiography is likely superior to TEE for detection of very small residual VSDs. However, TEE was able to detect all of the clinically important VSDs in both studies. Therefore, when indicated, intraoperative TEE should be the initial investigation performed and epicardial echocardiography should be reserved for situations in which the TEE examination is inadequate or inconclusive.

Unusual abnormalities of visceral and cardiac position can provide unique challenges to the transesophageal echocardiographer. We studied two patients with visceral situs inversus and levocardia. In these patients, the esophagus and stomach were oriented to the right and the heart was primarily in the left chest. Image quality was suboptimal (particularly the transgastric views) as a result of the increased distance between the transducer and the heart.

The literature describing intraoperative TEE for congenital heart disease is remarkably free from reports of complications. Lam et al. [23] reported minor esophageal bleeding after insertion of a 14-mm probe in a 20-kg patient. The only clinical manifestation of this complication was a small amount of blood on the probe tip; further intervention was not required. This patient had received heparin before probe insertion, and the anticoagulation may have contributed to the development of esophageal bleeding. Gilbert et al. [65] reported that left main stem bronchus obstruction developed in a 15-kg child after insertion of a 14-mm probe. The obstruction was relieved by removal of the probe. We have seen descending aortic compression in a 7-kg child during use of a 10-mm probe [9]. Femoral arterial blood pressure was decreased during posterior rotation and retroflexion. When the probe was not in this position, the femoral pressure tracing was normal. Another child (17 kg) in our series had a transient rise in the inspiratory pressure required for ventilation during esophageal intubation with a 13-mm probe. After the initial insertion, ventilatory pressures returned to baseline, and the child tolerated the examination well.

These cases point out the need for caution and careful patient monitoring when TEE is performed in pediatric patients. We recommend that the transesophageal probe be placed before heparinization and remain in the esophagus throughout the surgical procedure. We routinely advance the transducer tip into the stomach when preoperative imaging is completed. With this maneuver, the smallest diameter of the probe is in the esophagus during cardiopulmonary bypass. The echocardiographic system is routinely turned off during cardiopulmonary bypass to eliminate any chance of thermal injury to the esophagus.

How can the current limitations of intraoperative TEE be overcome? The most pressing need is for the development of high-resolution, small-diameter, low-profile biplane and multiplane transesophageal probes that could be accommodated by all patients, including neonates. In addition, one must not forget that epicardial and contrast echocardiography are still useful. Many of the limitations of TEE are related to limited ability to image far anterior structures, especially with interposed prosthetic material. Imaging anterior structures is one of the strengths of epicardial echocardiography. Furthermore, when color-flow imaging is difficult to interpret, as with multiple jets and prosthetic shadowing, the addition of contrast echocardiography (using either the transesophageal or the epicardial approach) contributes to definitive diagnosis.

We suggest that most intraoperative echocardiography procedures be done from the transesophageal window, because the examination does not interfere with the surgical procedure. However, when there are findings of concern or areas that cannot be imaged adequately by TEE, epicardial echocardiography or contrast echocardiography (or both) should be used to obtain the information unavailable from the routine transesophageal examination.

Intraoperative TEE has had a significant positive effect on the care of patients with congenital heart disease. Complications from TEE examinations performed in the operating room have been extremely rare. There is a need for further product development so that state-of-the-art intraoperative monitoring can be provided for even the smallest (neonatal) patients. Ideally, all available diagnostic modalities, including transesophageal, epicardial, and contrast echocardiography, should be used in complementary fashion as indicated to optimize the intraoperative and perioperative care of patients with congenital heart disease.

Miscellaneous Applications In Cardiovascular Surgery

Mass Lesions
The evaluation of intracardiac neoplasms by TEE is discussed in detail in Chapter 12. Intraoperative TEE provides valuable information to the surgeon both before and after tumor resection.

As has been reported during surgery for intracardiac myxoma [66–68], TEE can precisely localize tumor attachment, define the tumor's effect on and potential invasion of surrounding anatomic structures, and identify multifocal tumors within the heart. After tumor resection, TEE is useful to confirm complete removal, to detect residual valvular regurgitation caused by trauma from either the tumor or surgical excision, and to exclude a possible intracardiac communication precipitated by surgical resection.

Intraoperative TEE has also been used to delineate the nature and extent of secondary neoplastic invasion of the heart, particularly in patients with renal cell carcinoma [69,70] (see Chapter 12, Figure 12–22). Treiger et al. [69] found that TEE provided

highly accurate definition of intracaval neoplastic extension of renal cell carcinoma into the right heart; images were superior to characterization by preoperative computed tomography, magnetic resonance imaging, or inferior venacavography in three of five patients studied. After tumor resection, absence of tumor embolization, residual tumor, and inferior vena caval obstruction has been reliably confirmed by TEE in such cases [69,70] (Fig. 16-20). We have also used intraoperative TEE to evaluate intracaval extension of other genitourinary neoplasms, such as uterine sarcoma.

Other mass lesions have also been evaluated by both TEE and epicardial echocardiography in the operating room. Use of TEE for diagnosis of massive pulmonary thromboembolism and subsequent guidance of pulmonary embolectomy without cardiopulmonary bypass has been reported [71]. Localization of bullet fragments and identification of residual intracardiac trauma due to gunshot wounds have been described [72–74]. Intraoperative echocardiography has also been used to locate an embolized disc from a fractured tilting disc mitral prosthesis [75].

Circulatory Assist Devices
Transesophageal echocardiography has been reported to be quite useful in the intraoperative evaluation of circulatory assist devices. Simon et al. [76] found TEE to be very useful in several aspects of mechanically assisted circulation. By delineation of left or right ventricular performance and failure, TEE guides selection of the appropriate assist device. Echocardiographic evaluation of cannulae position and ventricular response to various pump flow functions aids in optimization of assist device hemodynamic support. Recovery of ventricular function and response to weaning of the assist device can likewise be assessed by TEE [76,77].

Thoracic Aortic Disease
The usefulness of TEE in the investigation of various diseases of the thoracic aorta is discussed in Chapter 14. In aortic dissection, TEE is valuable for the intraoperative characterization of the extent of intimal flap formation, location of intimal tears, involvement of the aortic root and valve, and presence of complications such as aortic rupture, cardiac tamponade, and saccular aneurysm formation [78–80]. Intraluminal thoracic aortic thrombus complicating repair of coarctation has been identified by intraoperative TEE, prompting reoperation for removal [81].

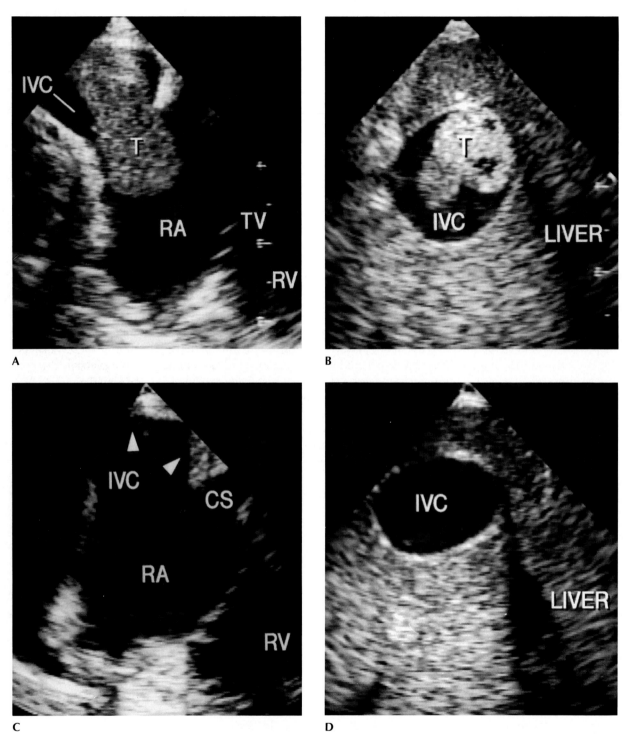

Fig. 16-20. Intracaval extension of metastatic renal cell carcinoma.
A. Modified right ventricular inflow view in the transverse plane. Before surgical
resection, a large tumor *(T)* protrudes from the inferior vena cava into the right
atrium. B. Transgastric short-axis imaging of the inferior vena cava demonstrates
intracaval tumor. C. After nephrectomy and removal of intracaval metastasis,
intraoperative TEE confirms the absence of residual tumor within the right
atrium; the orifice of the inferior vena cava (*arrowheads*) is widely patent. D.
Transgastric short-axis imaging of the inferior vena cava reveals no residual
tumor, irregularities of the lumen, or obstruction.

Extensive atheromatous disease of the ascending and transverse arch portions of the thoracic aorta is a risk factor for perioperative cerebrovascular accident complicating cardiac surgery with cardiopulmonary bypass. Such disease can be readily detected by TEE; complex, protruding, and even mobile atheromatous debris has been found in about 20% of patients undergoing coronary artery bypass grafting or valvular surgery [82,83]. Ribakove et al. [82], finding that intraoperative palpation of the aorta was a very insensitive means of detection of even gross intraluminal disease, reported that TEE was valuable not only for guiding placement of aortic cannulae but also for prompting total hypothermic circulatory arrest for aortic exploration and endarterectomy before cardiopulmonary bypass. In a recently published report on a series of 130 patients undergoing cardiac surgery with cardiopulmonary bypass, Katz et al. [83] noted detection of protruding atheromas within the ascending aorta and arch in 23 (18%) patients. In 19 (83%) of these patients, no significant abnormalities were palpated by the surgeon before aortic cannulation. Five (4%) patients had a perioperative stroke. Logistic regression analysis identified intraluminal aortic atheroma as the only predictor of perioperative stroke, whereas a carotid bruit, history of cerebrovascular disease, aortic calcification, or duration of cardiopulmonary bypass did not [83]. Using epicardial ultrasonography with a 7-MHz transducer, Kouchoukos [84] detected atheromatous disease severe enough to warrant modification of surgical approach in 14% of patients older than 60 years. These same investigators noted proximal aortic disease so extensive that femoral cannulation, hypothermic circulatory arrest, and replacement of portions of the ascending aorta and arch were necessary in 2.5% of patients before the planned cardiac operation under cardiopulmonary bypass could be pursued [84].

Aortic complications of prior cardiopulmonary bypass procedures, such as localized dissection, may rarely be encountered. We have observed disruption of an aortic cannulation site repair from a prior surgical procedure manifested by perforation of the ascending aorta at this site and contained by a massive mediastinal hematoma (Fig.16-21). The patient was undergoing reoperation for a failed aortic valve prosthesis; after discovery of this complication by intraoperative TEE, femoral-femoral extracorporeal bypass was performed to avoid exsanguination during sternotomy.

MONITORING FOR INTRAOPERATIVE EMBOLISM

Cardiac Surgery

Intracardiac air is routinely encountered in patients after cardiac operations, such as valvular or congenital heart surgery, in which the chambers of the heart are opened to air [85,86]. At the end of the cardiac surgical procedure, maneuvers are undertaken to ensure that intracardiac air has been eliminated. These procedures include placement of the patient in the Trendelenburg position, transient carotid artery compression, and prolonged venting of the left ventricle.

Transesophageal echocardiography is an exquisitely sensitive monitor of intracardiac air and should be used to detect intracardiac air before cardiopulmonary bypass is discontinued (Fig. 16-22). Significant amounts of air necessitate prolonged venting maneuvers to avoid potential arterial air embolism. It is often very difficult to eliminate completely all intracardiac air microbubbles that may be trapped in the ventricular trabeculations or pulmonary circulation. The clinical significance of small amounts of microscopic intracardiac air after open heart surgery is uncertain. In one study of 82 patients undergoing cardiac surgery, left ventricular intracavitary microbubbles were found more often in valvular surgery (75%) than in coronary revascularization (10%) [86]. Mechanical attempts to eradicate the microbubbles were usually unsuccessful. Despite this failure to eliminate all microbubbles, no new focal neurologic deficits were found postoperatively. Thus, it was concluded that although intracavitary left ventricular microbubbles were often detected during "open" cardiac operations, their presence was not predictive of postoperative neurologic complications [86].

Orthopedic Surgery

During surgery for total hip arthroplasty, significant hemodynamic deterioration occasionally develops during reaming of the femoral shaft or at the time of insertion of methyl methacrylate cement. Preliminary studies have suggested that embolization of air, fat, or cement occurs at these times or later with manipulation of the joint [87–90]. Because cemented total hip arthroplasty is associated with a significantly greater degree of embolism than is the

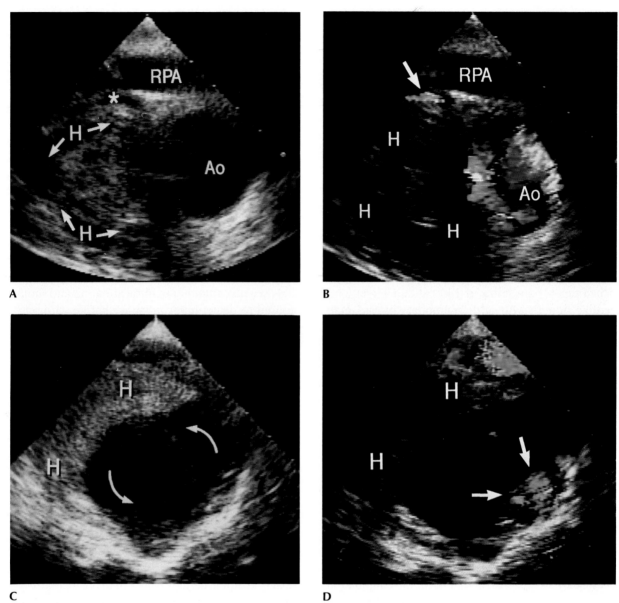

Fig. 16-21.   Contained rupture of a previous ascending aortic cannulation site with periaortic hematoma formation; basal short-axis imaging in the transverse plane. A. A large periaortic hematoma *(arrows)* is discovered shortly after anesthetic induction during reoperation for a failed aortic prosthesis implanted 1 year earlier. The superior vena cava *(asterisk)* is compressed at this level just anterior to the right pulmonary artery. B. Color-flow Doppler imaging reveals high-velocity flow signals within the slit-like lumen of the superior vena cava *(arrow)*, consistent with extrinsic obstruction due to the hematoma, normal flow signals are present in the ascending aorta. C. Scanning in a more cephalad plane revealed swirling spontaneous echocontrast *(curved arrows)* within the laminated hematoma on real-time examination, a finding highly suspicious for a communication with the systemic circulation. D. Color Doppler imaging confirms pulsatile flow *(arrows)* into this periaortic cavity. Normal flow within the right pulmonary artery is seen near the apex of the sector. With these findings, femoral-femoral extracorporeal bypass was instituted before repeat sternotomy to avoid the risk of massive hemorrhage.

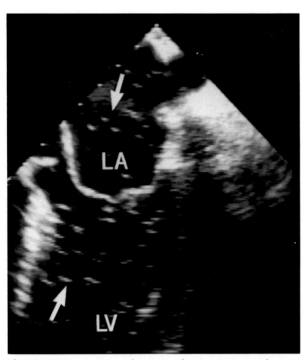

Fig. 16-22.   Intracardiac air after cessation of cardiopulmonary bypass; modified transverse imaging plane. Numerous microcavitations (*arrows*) representing microscopic air are seen within both the left atrium and the left ventricle. Such microbubbles, which may be seen entering the left side of the heart through the pulmonary veins (particularly after open heart operations), support the hypothesis that pulmonary venous air is entrapped during extracorporeal circulation.

noncemented operation, the increases in intramedullary pressure that occur with cementing may be the cause of embolism [89]. In a recent report of 24 patients undergoing surgery for long bone fractures, the fat embolism syndrome developed in 75% of patients noted on intraoperative TEE to have large quantities of echogenic material within the right heart during the orthopedic procedure [91]. This embolic material consisted of numerous small masses of 1 to 10 mm in diameter and also of larger discrete emboli of 1 to 8 cm. Only 17% of the patients had such findings on TEE; the fat embolism syndrome did not develop in patients without these findings [91]. These studies suggest that TEE may have a role in monitoring selected patients undergoing major orthopedic operations; TEE is also useful for the detection of other causes of hypotension, such as venous thromboembolism and hypovolemia.

Liver Surgery

In 16 adult patients, TEE was used to help elucidate the mechanism of myocardial dysfunction that accompanies liver transplantation [92]. Occasionally, isolated right ventricular failure could account for some of the hemodynamic instability seen during liver transplantation. More often, venous, pulmonary, and paradoxical embolization of air and thrombi contributed to right ventricular failure. Air embolism during liver transplantation occurs particularly at the time of vein-to-vein bypass, and TEE is the ideal tool for recognizing this [93]. Risk of disrupting esophageal varices in patients with portal hypertension is minimal but does exist. Hence, the potential benefit of TEE monitoring for air embolism in patients undergoing liver surgery must be weighed against the risks of variceal bleeding.

Neurosurgery

Transesophageal echocardiography has several intraoperative applications in neuroanesthesia and neurosurgery. Specifically, TEE can be used as a monitor of venous air embolism (VAE) and paradoxical air embolism (PAE) and may be useful in verifying the correct placement of ventriculoatrial shunts intraoperatively.

Venous air embolism is a well-recognized complication of neurosurgical procedures in patients who are in the sitting position. Previous studies indicate that the incidence of VAE is between 8% and 24% during cervical laminectomy and between 41% and 45% during posterior fossa surgery that is performed with patients in the sitting position. In addition, in patients undergoing posterior fossa surgery in nonsitting positions (i.e., supine, prone, "park bench," and lateral), the incidence of VAE is approximately 12% [94]. The most important factors that limit morbidity and mortality from VAE are early diagnosis and prompt treatment. At present, the most sensitive monitors for intraoperative detection of VAE are transthoracic Doppler and TEE two-dimensional imaging. In a dog model of VAE, audible changes in Doppler signals and the appearance of echogenic densities in the right atrium on TEE occurred almost simultaneously during episodes of VAE [95]. In these experiments, there was no difference in the volume of infused air when VAE was first detected by Doppler and TEE imaging [96].

In a human study comparing the sensitivity of the transthoracic Doppler, TEE two-dimensional imaging, and transesophageal Doppler examinations to detect air microbubbles injected through a right atrial catheter, both the TEE imaging and the transesophageal Doppler studies were more sensitive than the transthoracic Doppler procedure in detecting VAE [97]. The increased sensitivity of transesophageal Doppler imaging compared with transthoracic Doppler imaging is related to its ability to remove chest wall configuration and lung volumes as confounding factors in the transmission of an ultrasonic signal.

Paradoxical air embolism is a rare complication in patients undergoing neurosurgical procedures, but when it occurs, the results can be devastating [98]. It has been postulated that a patent foramen ovale (PFO) predisposes patients to development of PAE during episodes of VAE. Venous air entering the pulmonary circulation results in an increase in pulmonary artery pressure secondary to obstruction of pulmonary arterial blood flow and, possibly, reflex vasoconstriction. The resultant pulmonary hypertension may yield increases in right atrial and ventricular pressures relative to left-sided pressures. Thus, a right-to-left atrial pressure gradient may occur that predisposes to development of PAE if a PFO exists.

Transesophageal echocardiography may be used preoperatively to identify patients with a PFO and thus alert the clinician to the potential increased risk of PAE (see Chapter 15). In autopsy studies, a probe-patent foramen ovale was present in 25% to 35% of patients with no history of cardiac disease [99,100]. In studies of transthoracic echocardiography with peripheral venous injection of contrast material, the incidence of PFO ranged from 10% to 18% [101,102]. Preoperative transthoracic echocardiography in the evaluation of patients undergoing neurosurgical procedures in the sitting position revealed a detection rate of 6% to 10% [103,104]. In another series in which TEE with contrast enhancement and pulsed-wave Doppler imaging was used, a PFO was detected in 26% of the patients [105].

Intraoperative TEE with provocative maneuvers may be used after induction of anesthesia to detect a PFO. Our current practice is to induce anesthesia and then place a multiorifice catheter in the superior aspect of the right atrium. The intra-atrial septum is then imaged with TEE, and 20 cm of positive end-expiratory pressure is applied for 10 to 15 seconds. Immediately after the positive end-expiratory pres-

sure is removed, right atrial pressure transiently exceeds left atrial pressure [106]. Simultaneous with the release of positive end-expiratory pressure, 10 ml of agitated saline is injected into the right atrial catheter, opacifying the right atrium. If the microbubbles are observed in the left atrium within two to three cardiac cycles, a PFO is present.

When a PFO is identified before the surgical procedure begins, one may choose to perform the operation in a position associated with a lower incidence of VAE than the sitting position. Performing the operation in this alternative position with lower risk of VAE might, theoretically, lower the risk of PAE. In addition, appropriate clinical decisions can be made if PAE is diagnosed during an episode of VAE that occurs during the surgical procedure. Failure to detect a PFO either preoperatively or intraoperatively by use of provocative maneuvers does not entirely eliminate the risk of PAE [107]. However, the sensitivity of TEE to detect PAE during episodes of VAE is very high, and hence the likelihood of clinically significant PAE occurring intraoperatively that is undetected by TEE is remote.

Accurate placement of the distal end of a ventriculoatrial shunt catheter near the junction of the superior vena cava and right atrium, a commonly used treatment of hydrocephalus, is important for long-term shunt function and for avoiding cardiac arrhythmias, thrombus formation, and damage to myocardial tissue [108]. Standard methods of intraoperative localization, including chest radiography, pressure measurements, and electrocardiographic recording, can be inaccurate or unreliable. Intraoperatively, TEE can be used to readily localize the distal end of the catheter near the cavoatrial junction [109].

INTRAOPERATIVE MONITORING OF LEFT VENTRICULAR FUNCTION

Normal Wall Motion

The evaluation of left ventricular (LV) function by TEE is discussed in Chapter 7. During systole, the normal LV wall thickens and the endocardium moves inward, greatly reducing the size of the LV cavity. In the normal left ventricle, contraction measured by systolic wall thickening or inward endocardial motion increases from base to apex, resulting in a fractional area change that is about 20% greater at the apex than at the base. The stroke volume of the left ventricle, however, is derived primarily from basal and midcavity contraction, because the absolute change in area is much greater at the base than at the apex. There are also normal variations in regional LV performance. Intraoperatively, global LV function may be assessed by estimating or calculating the fractional area change of the left ventricle from the following formula:

$$FAC \ (\%) = \frac{EDA - ESA}{EDA} \times 100$$

in which FAC is fractional area change, which is equivalent to the area ejection fraction, EDA is end-diastolic area, and ESA is end-systolic area [110]. This measurement is obtained by imaging the heart in the transgastric short-axis view at the LV midcavity (papillary muscle level). The FAC overestimates LV function if regional wall motion abnormalities (RWMA) exist at the base or apex of the left ventricle, because they are not taken into account in the calculation. In addition, alterations in loading conditions of the left ventricle (e.g., mitral regurgitation and aortic stenosis) influence FAC. Therefore, it is important to keep in mind that the FAC, like the ejection fraction measurement, is a load-dependent index of LV performance and that loading conditions must be considered when this measurement is used. Nevertheless, the FAC can be used in patients to make clinical decisions. For example, in a patient with hyperdynamic LV function and a small LV EDA, hypovolemia is the most likely cause. In a patient with decreased FAC and increased LV EDA, the most likely cause is diminished LV contractility, suggesting that inotropic therapy would be helpful.

Automated Edge Detection

A major problem encountered by anesthesiologists using TEE to monitor global LV function is quantifying the changes that occur over time. Outlining the endocardium is a laborious and time-consuming procedure. When it is performed off-line, intraobserver and interobserver variability is low. When it is attempted on-line, however, real-time analysis, except when done by very experienced persons, is not as reproducible. This lack of reproducibility reduces the specificity and sensitivity of echocardiographic monitoring of left ventricular function. An automated quantification method should be able to measure ESA and EDA and detect RWMA. Previous

attempts to digitize the endocardial and epicardial LV borders have met with limited success despite complex mathematical modeling [111,112]. A new technique that uses acoustic quantification technology (Hewlett-Packard, Andover, MA) can differentiate myocardium from the blood pool blood and thereby measure changes in LV cavity size (blood area) within a user-defined zone [113–115]. The changes in LV area can be displayed graphically in real time. In fact, any area-based measurement of cardiac function can be displayed (e.g., FAC compared with time or as a derivative of time, EDA, or ESA). Continuing measurement of EDA may be used to follow preload, and the ESA can be used to assess changes in contractility [116].

Monitoring for Myocardial Ischemia

Segmental LV regional wall motion analysis is reviewed in Chapters 7 and 8. Ideally, complete evaluation of regional LV performance requires that multiple views of the left ventricle be obtained, e.g., at the base, midcavity, and apex. A qualitative impression of LV contraction is obtained by evaluating LV wall thickening and endocardial motion. Although attempts are being made to use computer-assisted edge detection techniques to quantify regional LV function, this technology is not available clinically. As previously described, however, recent advances in acoustic quantification allow a real-time display of FAC, and it is likely that in the near future adaptations will allow quantification of RWMA. Qualitative schemes describe regional wall motion as normal, hypokinetic, akinetic, or dyskinetic. Regional wall motion is normal if there are obvious systolic wall thickening and inward endocardial motion. *Hypokinesia* refers to abnormal systolic wall thickening or inward endocardial motion and may be graded as mild, moderate, or severe. Because mild degrees of hypokinesia are difficult to detect, more sophisticated techniques of diagnosis than simple visual assessment may be required. *Akinesia* refers to the absence of systolic wall thickening or inward endocardial motion. *Dyskinesia* refers to paradoxical motion in which a portion of the wall moves in the opposite direction to the rest of the left ventricle and may even become thinner rather than thicker during systole. This is a pattern typical of transmural myocardial infarction and LV aneurysm. A scoring system based on regional systolic function can be readily applied to this schema (see Chapter 7).

Myocardial Perfusion and LV Regional Wall Motion

It has been well documented that a new RWMA is an early and sensitive indicator of acute myocardial ischemia that precedes any electrocardiographic evidence of ischemia [117,118]. Although the sensitivity of echocardiography in detecting ischemia is beyond dispute, its specificity has recently been questioned [119,120]. Most studies have equated a transient new RWMA with myocardial ischemia and persistent changes in regional wall motion with acute myocardial infarction, but these assumptions may be incorrect for the following reasons. First, large changes in LV loading conditions, such as institution of cardiopulmonary bypass, may also alter LV systolic function. Second, the area of dysfunctional myocardium is invariably larger than the ischemic or infarcted zone [121]. The exact cause for RWMA in nonischemic areas is unknown, but it may be due to a mechanical tethering effect of noncontracting and contracting muscle [122]. Finally, RWMA may persist for a time after alleviation of the ischemic insult ("stunned" myocardium) [123]. In certain nonacute circumstances causing down-regulation of myocardial function, RWMA may occur with diminished coronary perfusion without the loss of myocardial muscle viability ("hibernating" myocardium) [124].

Clinical Studies

Smith et al. [125] demonstrated that in patients undergoing either vascular surgery or coronary artery bypass grafting, new RWMA were both a more sensitive and an earlier marker of intraoperative ischemia than surface electrocardiographic findings (Table 16-2). In addition, the persistence of RWMA was strongly correlated with perioperative myocardial infarction. In this study, data were recorded intraoperatively for subsequent analysis. It is unlikely that the diagnostic sensitivity of TEE would have been as good if the analysis had been performed on-line in the operating room. In a preliminary study of regional LV function in which real-time analysis in the operating room was compared with analysis of video recordings, there was total agreement on regional wall motion score in approximately 66% of epochs [126]. In 5% of epochs, however, there was disagreement by more than two grades. Leung et al. [127] confirmed that in patients undergoing coronary artery bypass grafting, ischemia (new RWMA) diagnosed by echocardiography occurred more frequently than ischemia (ST segment changes) diagnosed by electrocardiography. Surprisingly, the relative incidence of new RWMA was greater after cardiopulmonary bypass when the myocardium had been revascularized than before bypass. Although this finding raises additional questions about the specificity of TEE for ischemia detection, postbypass new RWMA were related to an adverse clinical outcome. London et al. [128] evaluated the "natural history" of RWMA in 156 high-risk patients undergoing noncardiac surgery. They found that 40% of all new RWMA occurred in the absence of any hemodynamic changes. There was also a significant discordance between electrocardiographic and TEE findings of ischemia. More importantly, they found a poor correlation between new intraoperative RWMA and postoperative cardiac complications. In the multivariate analysis of 285 patients undergoing noncardiac surgery, the Study of Perioperative Ischemia Research Group found that when compared with preoperative clinical risk

Table 16-2. Comparison of transesophageal echocardiography and electrocardiography for intraoperative detection of myocardial ischemia

Two-dimensional echocardiography	Electrocardiography
More sensitive (4 times)	Insensitive to subendocardial ischemia
Provides earlier warning	Relatively late indicator of ischemia
Persistent RWMA may predict MI	May miss MI
Can be used with rhythm disorders	Cannot be interpreted with BBB or pacing
Cannot be used during induction	Can be used during induction
Risk of esophageal trauma (rare)	Noninvasive
Qualitative, subjective diagnosis	Quantifiable, objective diagnosis
Computerized edge detection (investigational)	Computerized ST segment analysis (available)

BBB, bundle-branch block; MI, myocardial infarction; RWMA, regional wall motion abnormalities.
Modified from Smith et al. [125].

stratification, both intraoperative TEE and 12-lead electrocardiographic monitoring had little incremental value in identifying patients at high risk for perioperative ischemic events [129].

The above observations indicate that the use of TEE to reduce perioperative cardiac morbidity in patients with ischemic heart disease has met with mixed results. Intraoperative TEE appears to be a fair predictor of adverse outcome in patients having coronary bypass surgery and far less predictive of ischemic events in patients having noncardiac surgery [128,129] than initially suspected [125]. Additionally, because all of the TEE analyses were performed off-line in these studies, more investigation using real-time on-line quantitative analyses is necessary before definitive clinical recommendations can be made.

Limitations in the Use of TEE to Diagnose Myocardial Ischemia

Errors in the interpretation of RWMA are often due to images of poor quality or to operator inexperience. Poor quality may be caused by inappropriate settings on the ultrasonograph or dropout in the lateral segments of the sector arc. Occasionally, a true short-axis view of the left ventricle cannot be obtained. Oblique views may produce a false impression of RWMA. Misinterpretation of regional wall motion may be related to translational or rotational changes in cardiac position throughout the cardiac or respiratory cycle that can be amplified after pericardiotomy. Omission of short-axis views at the base and apex of the left ventricle may overlook RWMA present only in these cross sections. Temporal heterogeneity of LV contraction due to abnormal LV activation (bundle-branch block or paced rhythm) may lead to a false interpretation of regional systolic function, because even though all the ventricular wall segments may contract normally, they do so at slightly different times, so that the impression given is regional dysfunction within segments with delayed electrical activation. There is also increasing uncertainty about the specificity of transient RWMA as a marker of myocardial ischemia. Intermittent myocardial ischemia can produce areas of postischemic ("stunned") myocardium. In a canine study, Buffington and Coyle [119] showed that the postischemic myocardium responds differently to alterations in loading conditions than does the normal myocardium and that this difference must be taken into account in clinical studies in which regional contraction is used to monitor the heart for ischemia.

In an accompanying editorial, Lowenstein et al. [120] emphasized that the clinical usefulness of TEE to detect ischemia is critically dependent on the specificity of RWMA as a marker of ischemia. This specificity is most in question after cardiopulmonary bypass during which the heart was made ischemic by a period of aortic cross-clamping. Thus, the diagnosis of new RWMA after relief of ischemia may not necessarily correlate with continuing ischemia (or infarction) and therefore may result in erroneous clinical decisions. In addition to the above considerations, TEE is usually not routinely used during critical periods of anesthesia, namely, induction and emergence, when the highest percentage of ischemic events may occur.

These limitations will be offset, however, with improvements in the use of future technologic advances. For example, biplane imaging will likely improve the sensitivity of TEE to detect RWMA [130]. With cine-loop technology, selected images can be maintained in computer memory and subsequently displayed, either in a split-screen or in a quad-screen format. Thus, one can make a side-by-side comparison of images of LV segmental wall motion obtained at different times. This technology is likely to lead to significant improvements in interobserver variability and minimize subjective interpretation.

Although all methods have some limitations, TEE has provided a unique opportunity for further elucidation of the complex interactions of the heart in response to anesthesia and surgery. This section has deliberately emphasized the limitations of TEE in the intraoperative evaluation and monitoring of LV function in an attempt to present a balanced appreciation of this intriguing technology and to note that further investigation is needed to define its applications within the operating room.

DYNAMIC POTENTIAL PITFALLS

A labile hemodynamic milieu exists within the operating room, especially during operations in which cardiopulmonary bypass procedures are used. The multiple effects of general anesthesia are inescapable, and depending on the agents used, various degrees of peripheral vasodilation and myocardial depression are inevitable. Left ventricular preload is highly dependent on intravascular volume status, which may vary widely from gross hypovolemia to volume overload throughout the surgical procedure, particularly after cessation of extracorporeal circulation. Vasodilator infusions of agents such as nitroprusside can cause major reductions in left ventricular afterload and preload. Conversely, vasopressor and, less so, inotropic agents may precipitate significant increases in left ventricular afterload.

The recovery of myocardial function after systemic hypothermia, cardioplegic arrest, and coronary bypass grafting also varies considerably. Apparent segmental and global myocardial function may also be influenced by a host of intraoperative arrhythmias, most often atrial tachydysrhythmias and paced rhythms.

The evaluation of valvular regurgitant lesions by TEE color Doppler imaging depends on existing preload and afterload conditions, which are in turn related to a dynamic interplay of actions among intravascular volume status, vasodilator or vasopressor infusions, myocardial function, and the effects of general anesthesia. Vasodilator infusions with or without intravascular volume depletion may cause significant underestimation of valvular regurgitation, especially mitral regurgitation (Fig. 16-23). Hypovolemia and excessive catecholamine infusion are often responsible for systolic anterior motion after cardiopulmonary bypass for mitral repair. This phenomenon, which may be accompanied by severe residual mitral regurgitation, is potentially reversible with volume repletion and withdrawal of inotropic agents [44] (see Fig. 16-8). The magnitude of this phenomenon is often amplified during operations for hypertrophic obstructive cardiomyopathy. Multifactorial reduction in afterload may cause significant underestimation not only of valvular regurgitation by TEE color-flow Doppler mapping but also of intracardiac shunts assessed by this technique.

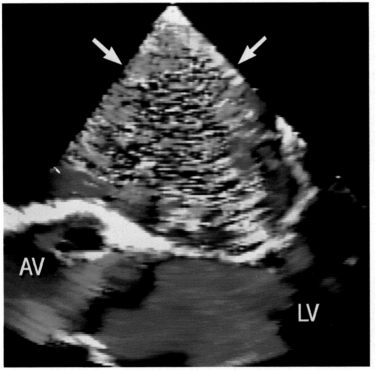

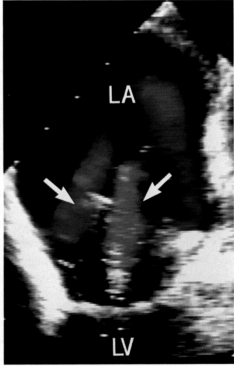

A   B

Fig. 16-23.   Impact of afterload reduction therapy on the assessment of mitral regurgitation during intraoperative TEE; transverse imaging planes. A. Without intravenous nitroprusside infusion, severe central mitral regurgitation (*arrows*) was detected by color Doppler imaging while the systolic blood pressure was 140 mm Hg. B. During administration of nitroprusside at a moderate dosage, only trivial mitral regurgitation (*arrows*) could be appreciated in this magnified view of the left atrium. At this time, the systolic blood pressure was in the range of 80 to 90 mm Hg. Such a labile intraoperative hemodynamic milieu often has a major impact on the severity of regurgitant lesions and must always be taken into account during evaluation by TEE (see text).

Changes in preload and afterload also affect interpretation of regional and global left ventricular function during both cardiac and, less dramatically so, noncardiac operations.

The intraoperative echocardiographer must be cognizant of these multiple hemodynamic influences while recognizing the inability to control a significant portion of them. In general, and if possible, it is best to perform intraoperative TEE, and especially color-flow imaging, during a "physiologic" hemodynamic state, one resembling the patient's preoperative status (if stable at that time). The patient's blood pressure should be monitored throughout TEE evaluation, ideally supplemented by information on left ventricular filling pressure if hemodynamic monitoring is being performed. Before TEE evaluation, volume infusion should be given if filling pressures are low and infusion of an alpha-agonist, such as phenylephrine, should be considered if the blood pressure remains inappropriately depressed without other evident cause.

The cardiac dysrhythmias, especially after cardiopulmonary bypass, may confound interpretation of both the two-dimensional and the color Doppler examinations. Color Doppler evaluation of regurgitant or shunt lesions may be seriously compromised if rapid atrial dysrhythmias are present. Temporary ventricular pacing with atrioventricular dissociation or frequent ectopy may also cause intermittent dyschronism between valve closure and myocardial contraction, significantly increasing the degree of apparent atrioventricular valvular regurgitation on color Doppler TEE.

SUMMARY

Transesophageal echocardiography has become a valuable adjunct in the intraoperative evaluation of a wide spectrum of surgical procedures for congenital and acquired heart disease. The role of intraoperative TEE monitoring during noncardiac surgery is currently far less well defined. The echocardiologist must recognize the multiple factors affecting the dynamic intraoperative hemodynamic environment and interpret TEE findings accordingly. Continuing advances in both instrumentation and experience should further refine and broaden both research and clinical applications of TEE in the operating room.

REFERENCES

1. Likoff M, Reichek N, St. John Sutton M, et al. Epicardial mapping of segmental myocardial function: an echocardiographic method applicable in man. *Circulation* 1982;66:1050–8.
2. Dubroff JM, Clark MB, Wong CYH, et al. Left ventricular ejection fraction during cardiac surgery: a two-dimensional echocardiographic study. *Circulation* 1983;68:95–103.
3. Goldman ME, Mindich BP, Teichholz LE, et al. Intraoperative contrast echocardiography to evaluate mitral valve operations. *J Am Coll Cardiol* 1984;4:1035–40.
4. Goldman ME, Guarino T, Fuster V, Mindich B. The necessity for tricuspid valve repair can be determined intraoperatively by two-dimensional echocardiography. *J Thorac Cardiovasc Surg* 1987;94:542–50.
5. Czer LSC, Maurer G, Bolger A, et al. Tricuspid valve repair: operative and follow-up evaluation by Doppler color flow mapping. *J Thorac Cardiovasc Surg* 1989;98:101–11.
6. Maurer G, Czer LSC, Chaux A, et al. Intraoperative Doppler color flow mapping for assessment of valve repair for mitral regurgitation. *Am J Cardiol* 1987;60:333–7.
7. Stewart WJ, Currie PJ, Salcedo EE, et al. Intraoperative Doppler color flow mapping for decision-making in valve repair for mitral regurgitation: technique and results in 100 patients. *Circulation* 1990;81:556–66.
8. Gussenhoven EJ, van Herweden LA, Roelandt J, et al. Intraoperative two-dimensional echocardiography in congenital heart disease. *J Am Coll Cardiol* 1987;9:565–72.
9. Hagler DJ, Tajik AJ, Seward JB, et al. Intraoperative two-dimensional Doppler echocardiography. A preliminary study for congenital heart disease. *J Thorac Cardiovasc Surg* 1988;95:516–22.
10. Ungerleider RM, Greeley WJ, Sheikh KH, et al. The use of intraoperative echo with Doppler color flow imaging to predict outcome after repair of congenital cardiac defects. *Ann Surg* 1989;210:526–34.
11. Ungerleider RM, Greeley WJ, Sheikh KH, et al. Routine use of intraoperative epicardial echocardiography and Doppler color flow imaging to guide and evaluate repair of congenital heart lesions. *J Thorac Cardiovasc Surg* 1990;100:297–309.
12. Goldman ME, Mindich BP. Intraoperative two-dimensional echocardiography: new application of an old technique. *J Am Coll Cardiol* 1986;7:374–82.

13. Currie PJ, Stewart WJ. Intraoperative echocardiography in mitral valve repair for mitral regurgitation. *Am J Card Imaging* 1990;4:192–206.

14. Seward JB, Khandheria BK, Oh JK, et al. Transesophageal echocardiography: technique, anatomic correlations, implementation and clinical applications. *Mayo Clin Proc* 1988;63:649–80.

15. Seward JB, Khandheria BK, Edwards WD, et al. Biplanar transesophageal echocardiography: anatomic correlations, image orientation, and clinical applications. *Mayo Clin Proc* 1990;65:1193–213.

16. Seward JB, Khandheria BK, Freeman WK, et al. Multiplane transesophageal echocardiography: image orientation, examination technique, anatomic correlations, and clinical applications. *Mayo Clin Proc* 1993;68:523–51.

17. Shintani H, Nakano S, Matsuda H, et al. Efficacy of transesophageal echocardiography as a perioperative monitor in patients undergoing cardiovascular surgery: analysis of 149 consecutive studies. *J Cardiovasc Surg* 1990;31:564–70.

18. Sheikh KH, de Bruijn NP, Rankin JS, et al. The utility of transesophageal echocardiography and Doppler color flow imaging in patients undergoing cardiac valve surgery. *J Am Coll Cardiol* 1990;15:363–72.

19. Daniel WG, Erbel R, Kasper W, et al. Safety of transesophageal echocardiography: a multicenter survey of 10,419 examinations. *Circulation* 1991;83:817–21.

20. Öwall A, Ståhl L, Settergren G. Incidence of sore throat and patient complaints after intraoperative transesophageal echocardiography during cardiac surgery. *J Cardiothorac Vasc Anesth* 1992;6:15–6.

21. Sutherland GR, van Daele ME, Stümper OF, et al. Epicardial and transesophageal echocardiography during surgery for congenital heart disease. *Int J Card Imaging* 1989;4:37–40.

22. Stümper OFW, Elzenga NJ, Hess J, Sutherland GR. Transesophageal echocardiography in children with congenital heart disease: an initial experience. *J Am Coll Cardiol* 1990;16:433–41.

23. Lam J, Neirotti RA, Nijveld A, et al. Transesophageal echocardiography in pediatric patients: preliminary results. *J Am Soc Echocardiogr* 1991;4:43–50.

24. Wienecke M, Fyfe DA, Kline CH, et al. Comparison of intraoperative transesophageal echocardiography to epicardial imaging in children undergoing ventricular septal defect repair. *J Am Soc Echocardiogr* 1991;4:607–14.

25. Carpentier A, Chauvaud S, Fabiani JN, et al. Reconstructive surgery of mitral valve incompetence: ten-year appraisal. *J Thorac Cardiovasc Surg* 1980;79:338–48.

26. Galloway AC, Colvin SB, Baumann FG, et al. Current concepts of mitral valve reconstruction for mitral insufficiency. *Circulation* 1988;78:1087–98.

27. Cosgrove DM, Chavez AM, Lytle BW, et al. Results of mitral valve reconstruction. *Circulation* 1986;74 Suppl l:I–82-I–7.

28. Orszulak TA, Schaff HV, Danielson GD, et al. Mitral regurgitation due to ruptured chordae tendineae: early and late results of valve repair. *J Thorac Cardiovasc Surg* 1985;89:491–8.

29. Galloway AC, Colvin SB, Baumann FG, et al. Long-term results of mitral valve reconstruction with Carpentier techniques in 148 patients with mitral insufficiency. *Circulation* 1988;78 Suppl l:I–97-I–105.

30. Sand ME, Naftel DC, Blackstone EH, et al. A comparison of repair and replacement for mitral valve incompetence. *J Thorac Cardiovasc Surg* 1987;94:208–19.

31. Dahm M, Iversen S, Schmid FX, et al. Intraoperative evaluation of reconstruction of the atrioventricular valves by transesophageal echocardiography. *Thorac Cardiovasc Surg* 1987;35:140–2.

32. Czer LSC, Maurer G, Bolger AF, et al. Intraoperative evaluation of mitral regurgitation by Doppler color flow mapping. *Circulation* 1987;76 Suppl 3:III–108-III–16.

33. Reichert SL, Visser CA, Moulijn AC, et al. Intraoperative transesophageal color-coded Doppler echocardiography for evaluation of residual regurgitation after mitral valve repair. *J Thorac Cardiovasc Surg* 1990;100:756–61.

34. Sheikh KH, Bengtson JR, Rankin JS, et al. Intraoperative transesophageal Doppler color flow imaging used to guide patient selection and operative treatment of ischemic mitral regurgitation. *Circulation* 1991;84:594–604.

35. Hozumi T, Yoshikawa J, Yoshida K, et al. Direct visualization of ruptured chordae tendineae by transesophageal two-dimensional echocardiography. *J Am Coll Cardiol* 1990;16:1315–9.

36. Himelman RB, Kusumoto F, Oken K, et al. The flail mitral valve: echocardiographic findings by precordial and transesophageal imaging and Doppler color flow mapping. *J Am Coll Cardiol* 1991;17:272–9.

37. Kamp O, Dijkstra J-W, Huitink H, et al. Transesophageal color flow mapping in the assessment of native mitral valvular regurgitation: comparison with left ventricular angiography. *J Am Soc Echocardiogr* 1991;4:598–606.

38. Chen C, Thomas JD, Anconina J, et al. Impact of impinging wall jet on color Doppler quantification of mitral regurgitation. *Circulation* 1991; 84:712–20.

39. Chen C, Koschyk D, Brockhoff C, et al. Noninvasive estimation of regurgitant flow rate and volume in patients with mitral regurgitation by Doppler color mapping of accelerating flow field. *J Am Coll Cardiol* 1993;21:374–83.

40. Klein AL, Obarski TP, Stewart WJ, et al. Transesophageal Doppler echocardiography of pulmonary venous flow: a new marker of mitral regurgitation severity. *J Am Coll Cardiol* 1991;18:518–26.

41. Stewart WJ, Currie PJ, Salcedo EE, et al. Jet direction by color flow mapping accurately depicts the mechanism of mitral regurgitation (abstract). *Circulation* 1988;78 Suppl 2:II–434.

42. Marwick TH, Stewart WJ, Currie PJ, Cosgrove DM. Mechanisms of failure of mitral valve repair: an echocardiographic study. *Am Heart J* 1991;122:149–56.

43. Pluth JR. Mitral valve reconstruction versus prosthetic valve replacement. *Cardiovasc Clin* 1982;12 no. 3:117–26.

44. Freeman WK, Schaff HV, Khandheria BK, et al. Intraoperative evaluation of mitral valve regurgitation and repair by transesophageal echocardiography: incidence and significance of systolic anterior motion. *J Am Coll Cardiol* 1992;20:599–609.

45. Craver JM. Aortic valve debridement by ultrasonic surgical aspirator: a word of caution. *Ann Thorac Surg* 1990;49:746–53.

46. Freeman WK, Schaff HV, Orszulak TA, Tajik AJ. Ultrasonic aortic valve decalcification: serial Doppler echocardiographic follow-up. *J Am Coll Cardiol* 1990;16:623–30.

47. Bartzokis T, St. Goar F, DiBiase A, et al. Freehand allograft aortic valve replacement and aortic root replacement. Utility of intraoperative echocardiography and Doppler color flow mapping. *J Thorac Cardiovasc Surg* 1991;101:545–54.

48. Cosgrove DM, Rosenkranz ER, Hendren WG, et al. Valvuloplasty for aortic insufficiency. *J Thorac Cardiovasc Surg* 1991;102:571–7.

49. Rafferty T, Durkin MA, Sittig D, et al. Transesophageal color flow Doppler imaging for aortic insufficiency in patients having cardiac operations. *J Thorac Cardiovasc Surg* 1992;104:521–5.

50. Klein AL, Stewart WJ, Salcedo EE, et al. The role of intraoperative echocardiography in tricuspid valve repair (abstract). *J Am Coll Cardiol* 1990;15:61A.

51. Klein AL, Azzam SJ, Stewart WJ, et al. Does intraoperative echocardiography prevent the development of tricuspid regurgitation during long-term follow-up for tricuspid repair surgery? (Abstract.) *J Am Coll Cardiol* 1993;21:320A.

52. Johnston SR, Freeman WK, Schaff HV, Tajik AJ. Severe tricuspid regurgitation after mitral valve repair: diagnosis by intraoperative transesophageal echocardiography. *J Am Soc Echocardiogr* 1990;3:416–9.

53. Stanley TE III, Rankin JS. Idiopathic hypertrophic subaortic stenosis and ischemic mitral regurgitation: the value of intraoperative transesophageal echocardiography and Doppler color flow imaging in guiding operative therapy. *Anesthesiology* 1990;72:1083–5.

54. Eng J, Nair UR, Scott PJ, Walker DR. Intraoperative transesophageal echocardiography for hypertrophic cardiomyopathy (letter to the editor). *Ann Thorac Surg* 1990;50:513–4.

55. Widimsky P, Ten Cate FJ, Vletter W, van Herwerden L. Potential applications for transesophageal echocardiography in hypertrophic cardiomyopathies. *J Am Soc Echocardiogr* 1992;5:163–7.

56. Stewart WJ, Schiavone WA, Salcedo EE, et al. Intraoperative Doppler echocardiography in hypertrophic cardiomyopathy: correlations with the obstructive gradient. *J Am Coll Cardiol* 1987;10:327–35.

57. Freeman WK, Schaff HV, Oh JK, Danielson GK. Evaluation of hypertrophic cardiomyopathy by intraoperative transesophageal echocardiography (abstract). *J Am Coll Cardiol* 1993;21:321A.

58. Grigg LE, Wigle ED, Williams WG, et al. Transesophageal Doppler echocardiography in obstructive hypertrophic cardiomyopathy: clarification of pathophysiology and importance in intraoperative decision making. *J Am Coll Cardiol* 1992;20:42–52.

59. Cyran SE, Myers JL, Gleason MM, et al. Application of intraoperative transesophageal echocardiography in infants and small children. *J Cardiovasc Surg* 1991;32:318–21.

60. Roberson DA, Muhiudeen IA, Silverman NH, et al. Intraoperative transesophageal echocardiography of atrioventricular septal defect. *J Am Coll Cardiol* 1991;18:537–45.

61. Ritter SB. Transesophageal real-time echocardiography in infants and children with congenital heart disease. *J Am Coll Cardiol* 1991;18:569–80.

62. Stümper O, Kaulitz R, Elzenga NJ, et al. The value of transesophageal echocardiography in children with congenital heart disease. *J Am Soc Echocardiogr* 1991;4:164–76.

63. O'Leary PW, Hagler DJ, Seward JB, et al. Biplane intraoperative transesophageal echocardiography in congenital heart disease. *J Am Coll Cardiol* (submitted for publication).

64. Marelli AJ, Child JS, Sangwan S, Laks H. The usefulness of intraoperative transesophageal echocardiography in adult congenital heart disease (abstract). *J Am Coll Cardiol* 1993;21:320A.

65. Gilbert TB, Panico FG, McGill WA, et al. Bronchial obstruction by transesophageal echocardiography probe in a pediatric cardiac patient. *Anesth Analg* 1992;74:156–8.

66. Milano A, Dan M, Bortolotti U. Left atrial myxoma: excision guided by transesophageal cross-sectional echocardiography. *Int J Cardiol* 1990;27:125–7.

67. Smith ST, Hautamaki K, Lewis JW Jr, et al. Transthoracic and transesophageal echocardiography in the diagnosis and surgical management of right atrial myxoma. *Chest* 1991;100:575–6.

68. Lebovic S, Koorn R, Reich DL. Role of two-dimensional transoesophageal echocardiography in the management of right ventricular tumour. *Can J Anaesth* 1991;38:1050–4.

69. Treiger BF, Humphrey LS, Peterson CV Jr, et al. Transesophageal echocardiography in renal cell carcinoma: an accurate diagnostic technique for intracaval neoplastic extension. *J Urol* 1991;145:1138–40.

70. Allen G, Klingman R, Ferraris VA, et al. Transesophageal echocardiography in the surgical management of renal cell carcinoma with intracardiac extension. *J Cardiovasc Surg* 1991;32:833–6.

71. Deleuze Ph, Saada M, DePaulis R, et al. Intraoperative transesophageal echocardiography for pulmonary embolectomy without cardiopulmonary bypass. *Ann Thorac Surg* 1991;52:137–8.

72. Stolf NAG, Fernandes PM, Pomerantzeff PMA, et al. Bullet in the intraventricular septum: report of surgical removal in two cases. *Thorac Cardiovasc Surg* 1988;36:51–3.

73. Brathwaite CEM, Weiss RL, Baldino WA, et al. Multichamber gunshot wounds of the heart: the utility of transesophageal echocardiography. *Chest* 1992;101:287–8.

74. Sheikh K, Cilley J, O'Connor W, DelRossi AJ. Intra-operative echocardiography: a useful tool in the localization of small intracardiac foreign bodies. *J Cardiovasc Surg* 1989;30:42–3.

75. Tanaka M, Abe T, Takeuchi E, et al. Intraoperative echocardiography of a dislodged Björk-Shiley mitral valve disc. *Ann Thorac Surg* 1991;51:315–6.

76. Simon P, Owen AN, Moritz A, et al. Transesophageal echocardiographic evaluation in mechanically assisted circulation. *Eur J Cardiothorac Surg* 1991;5:492–7.

77. Savage RM, Duffy CI, Thomas JD, et al. Transesophageal echocardiography (TEE) is indicated in the placement of the implantable left ventricular assist device (abstract). *J Am Coll Cardiol* 1993;21:321A.

78. Kyo S, Takamoto S, Adachi H, et al. Intraoperative evaluation of repair of aortic dissection: surgical decision making. *Int J Card Imaging* 1989;4:49–50.

79. Schippers OA, Gussenhoven WJ, van Herwerden LA, et al. The role of intraoperative two-dimensional echocardiography in the assessment of thoracic aorta pathology. *Thorac Cardiovasc Surg* 1988;36:208–13.

80. Ballal RS, Nanda NC, Gatewood R, et al. Usefulness of transesophageal echocardiography in assessment of aortic dissection. *Circulation* 1991;84:1903–14.

81. Thwaites BK, Stamatos JM, Crowl FD, et al. Transesophageal echocardiographic diagnosis of intraaortic thrombus during coarctation repair. *Anesthesiology* 1992;76:638–9.

82. Ribakove GH, Katz ES, Galloway AC, et al. Surgical implications of transesophageal echocardiography to grade the atheromatous aortic arch. *Ann Thorac Surg* 1992;53:758-61.

83. Katz ES, Tunick PA, Rusinek H, et al. Protruding aortic atheromas predict stroke in elderly patients undergoing cardiopulmonary bypass: experience with intraoperative transesophageal echocardiography. *J Am Coll Cardiol* 1992;20:70–7.

84. Kouchoukos NT. Discussion. *Ann Thorac Surg* 1992;53:762–3.

85. Oka Y, Moriwaki KM, Hong Y, et al. Detection of air emboli in the left heart by M-mode transesophageal echocardiography following cardiopulmonary bypass. *Anesthesiology* 1985;63:109–13.

86. Topol EJ, Humphrey LS, Borkon AM, et al. Value of intraoperative left ventricular microbubbles detected by transesophageal two-dimensional echocardiography in predicting neurologic outcome after cardiac operations. *Am J Cardiol* 1985;56:773–5.

87. Wenda K, Henrichs KJ, Biegler M, Erbel R. Nachweis von Markembolien während Oberschenkelmarknagelungen mittels transösophagealer Echokardiographie. *Unfallchirurgie* 1989;15:73–6.

88. Ereth MH, Abel MD, Lennon RL, Rehder K. Ventilation-perfusion ($\dot{V}_A/\dot{Q}$) relationship in patients

undergoing total hip arthroplasty (abstract). *Anesth Analg* 1990;70:S99.

89. Ereth MH, Lennon RL, Rose SH, Lewallen DG. Hemodynamic changes in patients undergoing total hip arthroplasty: cemented vs. noncemented (abstract). *Anesthesiology* 1990;73:A110.

90. Weber JG, Ereth MH, Abel MD. Greater embolic echogenesis in cemented vs. noncemented total hip arthroplasty (abstract). *Anesthesiology* 1991; 75:A390.

91. Pell ACH, Keating JF, Christie J, Sutherland GR. Use of transesophageal echocardiography to predict patients at risk of the fat embolism syndrome following traumatic injuries (abstract). *J Am Coll Cardiol* 1993;21:264A.

92. Ellis JE, Lichtor JL, Feinstein SB, et al. Right heart dysfunction, pulmonary embolism, and paradoxical embolization during liver transplantation: a transesophageal two-dimensional echocardiographic study. *Anesth Analg* 1989;68:777–82.

93. Prager MC, Gregory GA, Ascher NL, Roberts JP. Massive venous air embolism during orthotopic liver transplantation. *Anesthesiology* 1990; 72:198–200.

94. Black S, Ockert DB, Oliver WC Jr, Cucchiara RF. Outcome following posterior fossa craniectomy in patients in the sitting or horizontal positions. *Anesthesiology* 1988;69:49–56.

95. Glenski JA, Cucchiara RF, Michenfelder JD. Transesophageal echocardiography and transcutaneous O_2 and CO_2 monitoring for detection of venous air embolism. *Anesthesiology* 1986; 64:541–5.

96. Losasso TJ, Black S, Muzzi DA, Cucchiara RF. Detection and hemodynamic consequences of venous air embolism: does N_2O make a difference? (Abstract.) *Anesthesiology* 1989;71:A620.

97. Muzzi DA, Losasso TJ, Black S, Nishimura R. Comparison of a transesophageal and precordial ultrasonic Doppler sensor in the detection of venous air embolism. *Anesth Analg* 1990;70:103–4.

98. Gronert GA, Messick JM Jr, Cucchiara RF, Michenfelder JD. Paradoxical air embolism from a patent foramen ovale. *Anesthesiology* 1979; 50:548–9.

99. Thompson T, Evans W. Paradoxical embolism. *Q J Med* 1930;23:135–50.

100. Hagen PT, Scholz DG, Edwards WD. Incidence and size of patent foramen ovale during the first 10 decades of life: an autopsy study of 965 normal hearts. *Mayo Clin Proc* 1984;59:17–20.

101. Lechat P, Mas JL, Lascault G, et al. Prevalence of patent foramen ovale in patients with stroke. *N Engl J Med* 1988;318:1148–52.

102. Lynch JJ, Schuchard GH, Gross CM, Wann LS. Prevalence of right-to-left atrial shunting in a healthy population: detection by Valsalva maneuver contrast echocardiography. *Am J Cardiol* 1984;53:1478–80.

103. Guggiari M, Lechat Ph, Garen-Colonne C, et al. Early detection of patent foramen ovale by two-dimensional contrast echocardiography for prevention of paradoxical air embolism during the sitting position. *Anesth Analg* 1988;67:192–4.

104. Black S, Muzzi DA, Nishimura RA, Cucchiara RF. Preoperative and intraoperative echocardiography to detect right-to-left shunt in patients undergoing neurosurgical procedures in the sitting position. *Anesthesiology* 1990;72:436–8.

105. Konstadt SN, Louie EK, Black S, et al. Intraoperative detection of patent foramen ovale by transesophageal echocardiography. *Anesthesiology* 1991;74:212–6.

106. Black S, Cucchiara RF, Nishimura RA, Michenfelder JD. Parameters affecting occurrence of paradoxical air embolism. *Anesthesiology* 1989; 71:235–41.

107. Cucchiara RF, Nishimura RA, Black S. Failure of preoperative echo testing to prevent paradoxical air embolism: report of the two cases. *Anesthesiology* 1989;71:604–7.

108. Illingworth RD, Logue V, Symon L, Uemura K. The ventriculocaval shunt in the treatment of adult hydrocephalus: results and complications in 101 patients. *J Neurosurg* 1971;35:681–5.

109. McGrail KM, Muzzi DA, Losasso TJ, Meyer FB. Ventriculoatrial shunt distal catheter placement using transesophageal echocardiography: technical note. *Neurosurgery* 1992;30:747–9.

110. Abel MD, Nishimura RA, Callahan MJ, et al. Evaluation of intraoperative transesophageal two-dimensional echocardiography. *Anesthesiology* 1987;66:64–8.

111. Thomas JD, Hagege AA, Choong CY, et al. Improved accuracy of echocardiographic endocardial borders by spatiotemporal filtered Fourier reconstruction: description of the method and optimization of filter cutoffs. *Circulation* 1988;77:415–28.

112. Geiser EA, Conetta DA, Limacher MC, et al. A second-generation computer-based edge detection algorithm for short-axis, two-dimensional echocardiographic images: accuracy and improvement in interobserver variability. *J Am Soc Echocardiogr* 1990;3:79–90.

113. Cahalan MK, Ionescu P, Melton H. Automated real-time analysis of transesophageal echocardiograms (abstract). *Anesthesiology* 1991;75 Suppl:A385.

114. Klein SC, Waggoner AD, Holland MR, et al. Echocardiographic on-line measurement and display of left ventricular (LV) cavity areas and function: reproducibility and normal values in control subjects (abstract). *Circulation* 1991;84 Suppl 2:II–584.

115. Pinto FJ, Siegel LC, Kreitzman TR, et al. On-line estimation of cardiac output with a new automated edge detection system using transesophageal echocardiography: comparison with thermodilution (abstract). *Circulation* 1991;84 Suppl 2:II–585.

116. O'Kelly BF, Tubau JF, Knight AA, et al. Measurement of left ventricular contractility using transesophageal echocardiography in patients undergoing coronary artery bypass grafting. *Am Heart J* 1991;122:1041–9.

117. Tennant R, Wiggers CJ. The effect of coronary occlusion on myocardial contraction. *Am J Physiol* 1935;112:351–61.

118. Alam M, Khaja F, Brymer J, et al. Echocardiographic evaluation of left ventricular function during coronary artery angioplasty. *Am J Cardiol* 1986;57:20–5.

119. Buffington CW, Coyle RJ. Altered load dependence of postischemic myocardium. *Anesthesiology* 1991;75:464–74.

120. Lowenstein E, Haering JM, Douglas PS. Acute ventricular wall motion heterogeneity. A valuable but imperfect index of myocardial ischemia (editorial). *Anesthesiology* 1991;75:385–7.

121. Lima JAC, Becker LC, Melin JA, et al. Impaired thickening of nonischemic myocardium during acute regional ischemia in the dog. *Circulation* 1985;71:1048–59.

122. Force T, Kemper A, Perkins L, et al. Overestimation of infarct size by quantitative two-dimensional echocardiography: the role of tethering and of analytic procedures. Circulation 1986;73:1360–8.

123. Heyndrickx GR, Millard RW, McRitchie RJ, et al. Regional myocardial functional and electrophysiological alterations after brief coronary artery occlusion in conscious dogs. *J Clin Invest* 1975;56:978–85.

124. Rahimtoola SH. The hibernating myocardium. *Am Heart J* 1989;117:211–21.

125. Smith JS, Cahalan MK, Benefiel DJ, et al. Intraoperative detection of myocardial ischemia in high-risk patients: electrocardiography versus two-dimensional transesophageal echocardiography. *Circulation* 1985;72:1015–21.

126. Villamaria FJ, Abel MD, Nishimura RA. Can transesophageal echocardiography provide useful information in real time in the operating room? (Abstract.) *Anesth Analg* 1988;67:S246.

127. Leung JM, O'Kelly B, Browner WS, et al. Prognostic importance of postbypass regional wall-motion abnormalities in patients undergoing coronary artery bypass graft surgery. *Anesthesiology* 1989;71:16–25.

128. London MJ, Tubau JF, Wong MG, et al. The "natural history" of segmental wall motion abnormalities in patients undergoing noncardiac surgery. *Anesthesiology* 1990;73:644–55.

129. Eisenberg MJ, London MJ, Leung JM, et al. Monitoring for myocardial ischemia during noncardiac surgery. A technology assessment of transesophageal echocardiography and 12-lead electrocardiography. The Study of Perioperative Ischemia Research Group. *JAMA* 1992;268:210–6.

130. Shah PM, Kyo S, Matsumura M, Omoto R. Utility of biplane transesophageal echocardiography in left ventricular wall motion analysis. *J Cardiothorac Vasc Anesth* 1991;5:316–9.

17

Transesophageal Echocardiography in Critically Ill Patients

Jae K. Oh • *William K. Freeman*

Critically ill patients require urgent and expeditious evaluation so that potentially lifesaving medical or surgical therapeutic intervention can be instituted. Most often, the clinical condition of such patients requires management in an intensive care unit with multiple intravenous infusions, hemodynamic monitoring catheters, mechanical ventilation, and, less commonly, hemodynamic support devices. Transportation of these patients to diagnostic procedure areas for evaluation is not only cumbersome but also potentially dangerous because of cardiopulmonary instability. In this situation, the ideal diagnostic procedure should be transportable to the patient's bedside, rapid, and highly sensitive to multiple diagnostic possibilities that may account for the patient's condition.

The advent of transthoracic two-dimensional and Doppler echocardiography initially afforded such a modality in the assessment of the critically ill patient [1–9]. The ability of this approach to provide structural, functional, and hemodynamic data in the elucidation of serious cardiovascular disease makes echocardiography an excellent diagnostic tool in the evaluation of critically ill patients. Unfortunately, the transthoracic approach is frequently limited in the postoperative or post-traumatic period by moni-

toring equipment, life support interventions (particularly mechanical ventilation), and bandages, wounds, and drainage tubes. A patient's body habitus, pulmonary disease, or even simple confinement to the supine position may further restrict the capabilities of transthoracic echocardiography in the delineation of potentially life-threatening problems.

Transesophageal echocardiography (TEE) offers an alternative acoustic window that overcomes the vast majority of limitations of transthoracic echocardiography while yielding detailed, high-resolution two-dimensional and Doppler information in nearly all patients in critical condition [10–13]. In this chapter, the procedure, indications, and impact of TEE in the critically ill patient are discussed.

TECHNIQUE

The procedural aspects of TEE examination in the clinically stable outpatient or inpatient are fully described in Chapters 2 and 3. Modification of these previously described approaches is commonly necessary in the critically ill patient.

In contrast to the clinically stable patient, the critically ill patient frequently has an impaired sensorium and cannot cooperate during the TEE procedure. Such patients may be mildly agitated to grossly combative, placing both themselves and the operator at risk for potential injury. It is important to obtain hemodynamic and respiratory stability as much as possible before TEE in such patients. If the patient has marginal or clearly deteriorating respiratory function, it is best to proceed with endotracheal intubation and mechanical ventilation before TEE. All monitoring and life support devices should be secured and repeatedly observed for proper function. In complicated situations it is advisable to always have the patient's nurse present during TEE for this purpose and also for helping the TEE assistant with premedication and patient attention.

Premedication for TEE in the critically ill patient is guided by clinical judgment of the individual's situation. In patients with significantly depressed central nervous system function, sedation is generally not needed and is often contraindicated. Local anesthetic spray of the oropharynx is also not necessary and could increase the likelihood of aspiration in patients with a gag reflex already impaired from a cerebrovascular accident or general central nervous system depression. Provided that there are no contraindications, secretion control with an antisialogogue such as glycopyrrolate (see Chapter 3) is advisable in all critically ill patients. The mildly agitated patient may be adequately sedated with standard intravenous doses of benzodiazepines, such as midazolam or diazepam, supplemented with low intravenous doses of narcotics, such as meperidine or morphine. The severely agitated or combative patient requires high doses of a preferably short-acting benzodiazepine, namely, midazolam, often with moderate doses of a narcotic given intravenously as needed. Occasionally, extremely agitated patients receiving mechanical ventilation may not be adequately controlled with these premedications, and additional paralyzation with an agent such as vecuronium is indicated. In selected cases, administration of an ultra-short-acting anesthetic induction hypnotic, such as propofol, can greatly facilitate the TEE examination without undue hemodynamic instability. At all times, premedication for TEE must be titrated in accordance with the patient's hemodynamic and respiratory stability and tolerance. The patient's blood pressure, heart rate, respiration, and peripheral oxygen saturation must be carefully and continuously monitored.

The various techniques for introduction of the TEE probe are reviewed in Chapter 3. Quite often, TEE is performed in critically ill patients who are receiving mechanical ventilation. In such patients, the probe should be introduced digitally. One finger or even two are used to guide the TEE probe to the midline of the oropharynx, posterior to the endotracheal tube, while the probe is advanced into the esophagus (Fig. 17-1). The endotracheal tube must be secured before TEE begins and its position constantly monitored during probe introduction and manipulation to prevent inadvertent migration of the tube down the right mainstem bronchus or partial withdrawal from the trachea. The TEE examination may be performed with the patient in a partial left lateral decubitus position, even if intubated. Not uncommonly, especially in patients with mechanical hemodynamic support devices or in the early period after cardiac surgery, the examination needs to be performed while the patient is confined to the supine position. In the supine position, gentle anteflexion of the patient's head, occasionally with some lateral rotation toward the examiner, facilitates introduction of the probe. A gentle jaw thrust maneuver or placing the head in a "sniffing" position may also be attempted. In trauma patients the head must not be manipulated until cervical spine instability has been excluded. Rarely is probe introduction under direct laryngoscopic visualization necessary. A nasogastric tube need not be removed unless, in conjunction with an endotracheal tube, it crowds the oropharynx and prevents easy passage of the TEE probe. The nasogastric tube may even help guide the probe into the esophagus and usually does not interfere with TEE imaging.

SAFETY AND FEASIBILITY

Transesophageal echocardiography is now generally accepted as a very safe imaging procedure. It is feasible in over 98% of the general population in whom it is attempted, and the incidence of complications (which are generally minor) is usually less than 0.5% [14–18]. However, because TEE is semi-invasive, there was initial concern that it was not safe to be used in critically ill patients. Investigators from several institutions have subsequently demonstrated that TEE is definitely feasible and safe in the critical care patient population [10–13]. In four

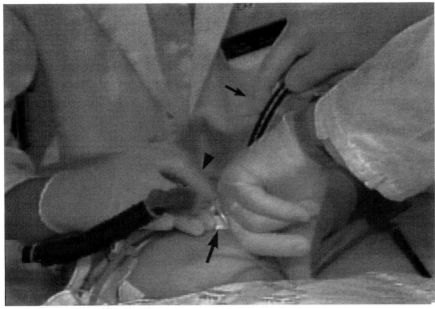

A

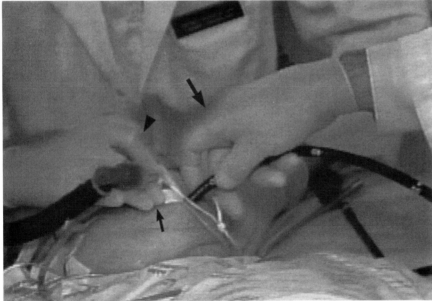

B

Fig. 17-1. Introduction of the TEE probe in a critically ill patient receiving mechanical ventilation. A. The probe is introduced by the examiner's right hand (*small arrow*) as the tip is guided to the midline of the oropharynx posterior to the endotracheal tube by the deep digital approach with the left index finger (*large arrow*). The TEE assistant has secured the endotracheal tube (*arrowhead*). B. The TEE probe is advanced (*large arrow*) with the endotracheal tube situated to the right of the patient's mouth (*small arrow*) to facilitate probe manipulation. The position of the endotracheal tube is continuously monitored throughout the TEE examination (*arrowhead*).

studies [10–13] reporting a cumulative total of 308 TEE examinations in critically ill patients, 5 (1.6%) potentially serious complications occurred during TEE. Oh et al. [11] reported worsening respiratory failure and hypoxemia complicating TEE in two patients with preexisting severe left ventricular dysfunction; in both, the baseline state returned immediately after probe withdrawal. Vomiting of gastric contents, sedative-induced severe hypotension, and generalized seizure (in a patient with a history of seizures) were reported in one patient each in the series of Pearson et al. [10]. To date, no deaths have been reported to be associated with TEE in critically ill patients.

Blood pressure and heart rate may increase mildly during TEE, usually because of agitation and discomfort in inadequately sedated patients. Such changes, even when small, may produce deleterious effects in critically ill patients with tenuous hemodynamic reserve. The same patient response should also be avoided in patients with acute aortic dissection [19], even though TEE in such cases generally has been found to be safe by numerous investigators (see Chapter 14). Hence, our practice is to ensure adequate but not excessive sedation to minimize any sympathetic autonomic nervous system reactivity that may compromise marginally compensated patients during TEE. Once again, premedication for TEE must be individualized and carefully titrated (especially in patients not mechanically ventilated) according to the patient's cardiorespiratory response. Echocardiologists performing TEE in this subgroup of patients should be prepared to manage cardiopulmonary emergencies should they occur during the procedure.

INDICATIONS AND IMPACT: MAYO CLINIC EXPERIENCE

General Experience

Of 5,441 TEE procedures performed at the Mayo Medical Center over a 5-year period, 7% were performed outside the echocardiography laboratory in the intensive care setting (Fig. 17-2); 6% took place in a medical or surgical intensive care unit, 0.5% in the emergency room, and 0.5% in the cardiac

catheterization laboratory. Of the patients examined, 3% were clinically unstable or critically ill. The primary indication for TEE in critically ill patients in our practice has been hemodynamic instability, ranging from systemic hypotension to pulmonary edema to shock [11]. Other indications have been infective endocarditis and complications thereof, aortic dissection, traumatic cardiac disease, and cardiac donor evaluation.

In our experience, the greatest clinical impact of TEE in critically ill patients has been in the evaluation of shock syndromes. In an initial analysis of 44 patients with shock [20], we found that transthoracic echocardiography was only partially diagnostic in 48% of them and inadequate for interpretation in the remaining 52%. All patients in this series were receiving inotropic support, and all but one were mechanically ventilated during the time of echocardiographic evaluation. Transesophageal echocardiography revealed diagnostic images in all 44 patients. There were no significant complications during TEE except for transient worsening of hypoxemia in one patient with right ventricular infarction and right-to-left interatrial shunting through a patent foramen ovale.

The findings of TEE in this patient population are shown in Table 17-1. Crucially important cardiovascular findings responsible for the patient's hemo-

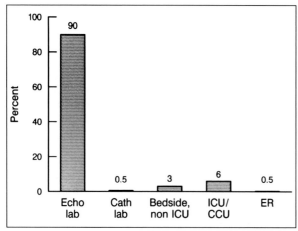

Fig. 17-2. Location of 5,441 TEE studies performed at the Mayo Medical Center over a 5-year period. Of the 10% of TEE procedures done outside the echocardiography laboratory, 6% were in a medical or surgical intensive care unit or the coronary care unit, 3% at the bedside in a nonintensive-care setting, 0.5% in the cardiac catheterization laboratory, and 0.5% in the emergency room. Intraoperative TEE procedures are not included in this analysis.

Table 17-1. Findings on transesophageal echocardiography in patients with shock syndromes

	No. of patients
Mitral regurgitation	9
Severe	4
Moderate	3
Papillary muscle rupture	2
Right ventricular infarction or dysfunction	7
Right-to-left shunt via PFO	2
Severe left ventricular dysfunction	7
Hypovolemia	5
LVOT obstruction also present	2
Cardiac tamponade	4
Myocardial free-wall rupture	1
Postinfarction ventricular septal rupture	2
Aorta-left atrium shunt	1
Aortic rupture	1
Miscellaneous	4
Normal examination	4

Data from Oh et al. [11, 20].

dynamic compromise were obtained in 30 (68%) of the 44 patients. Life-threatening structural complications of myocardial infarction, surgical procedures, or trauma were found in 20% of cases. A small, volume-contracted left ventricle with hyperdynamic function was noted in 11% of patients, and in the absence of any other cardiac abnormalities on TEE, this finding was consistent with severe intravascular volume depletion as the cause of the hypotensive state. Only four patients (9%) had entirely normal TEE examination results in this clinical situation, and a noncardiovascular cause for hemodynamic compromise was found by other investigation in each patient.

On the basis of TEE findings in this series [20], 13 patients (30%) underwent urgent cardiac surgery: mitral valve replacement or repair in five, exploration and relief of tamponade in four, repair of postinfarction ventricular septal rupture in two, repair of aortic rupture in one, and closure of patent foramen ovale to correct severe hypoxemia due to right-to-left shunting after right ventricular infarction in one.

Illustrative Cases

The following patient vignettes from our practice demonstrate the impact of TEE in the evaluation of critically ill patients.

Precipitous pulmonary edema and hypotension complicated the course of a 71-year-old man 4 days after an acute inferior myocardial infarction. Transthoracic echocardiography showed localized inferior left ventricular akinesis and otherwise hyperdynamic global left ventricular systolic function. The patient's rapid deterioration required mechanical ventilation, which compromised both the auscultatory and the transthoracic Doppler echocardiographic examinations. Transesophageal echocardiography readily revealed that the posteromedial papillary muscle had ruptured, resulting in a flail posterior mitral leaflet and acute severe mitral regurgitation (Fig. 17-3). The patient was taken to the cardiac catheterization laboratory for intra-aortic balloon pump insertion and coronary angiography only, and from there he underwent successful emergency mitral valve replacement with coronary bypass.

Two days after intravenous adminstration of streptokinase for an anteroseptal myocardial infarction, a new systolic murmur was audible across the precordium in a 64-year-old man, who subsequently suffered rapid cardiovascular collapse. Transtho-racic echocardiography revealed no pericardial effusion and suggested an interventricular shunt on technically difficult color Doppler imaging. Antero-septal ventricular septal rupture with left-to-right interventricular shunting was detected on TEE (Fig. 17-4). As in the preceding patient, cardiac surgery was performed without further diagnostic imaging except for coronary angiography. Evaluation of the complications of ischemic heart disease is discussed in detail in Chapter 8.

Immediately on admission to the surgical intensive care unit after aortic valve replacement for severe aortic stenosis, an elderly woman was found to be persistently hypotensive, with profound hypoxemia and peripheral oxygen desaturation despite maximal ventilatory support. Transthoracic echocardiography was ordered to rule out cardiac tamponade; no pericardial effusion was noted, but the right-sided cardiac chambers appeared enlarged, with indeterminate right ventricular function. Transesophageal echocardiography was performed for further evaluation. The right ventricle was severely enlarged, with akinesis of all but the anterior segments, and there was inferoseptal left ventricular akinesis. The findings were consistent with an inferior myocardial infarction with extensive right ventricular involvement, presumably due to right coronary artery embolization at the time of aortic valve replacement. Right and left ventricular function were normal on the preoperative echocardiogram during evaluation of the severe aortic stenosis, and preoperative coronary angiography did not reveal significant occlusive disease. On TEE, the right atrium also was enlarged, with bulging of the atrial septum toward the left atrium, consistent with severely increased right atrial filling pressures (Fig. 17-5). Imaging in the longitudinal plane revealed a persistently patent foramen ovale through which a significant and continuous right-to-left interatrial shunt passed. On the basis of the TEE findings, the patent foramen ovale was surgically closed to correct the patient's refractory severe hypoxemia.

TEE has rarely been used in our practice to guide balloon-tipped catheter occlusion of a patent foramen ovale to temporarily interrupt right-to-left interatrial shunting causing severe systemic oxygen desaturation in patients with extensive right ventricular infarction. In the patient shown in Figure 17-6, balloon-tipped catheter occlusion of patent foramen ovale shunting increased the peripheral oxygen saturation from 80% to 96%. The degree of right-to-left interatrial shunting in this clinical situation can also

Fig. 17-3. Papillary muscle rupture complicating acute inferior myocardial infarction; magnified transverse four-chamber view. A. The ruptured head of the posteromedial papillary muscle (*arrow*) prolapses freely into the left atrium; the posterior mitral valve leaflet (*arrowhead*) is flail. B. A broad jet of severe anteromedial mitral regurgitation (*arrow*) is detected on color Doppler imaging.

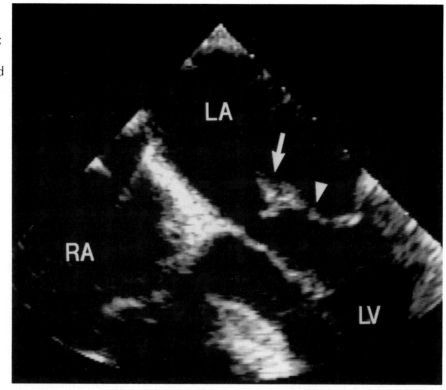

A

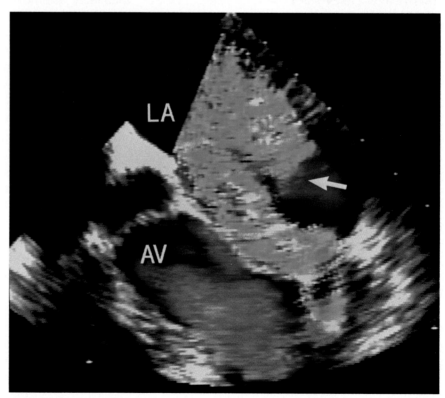

B

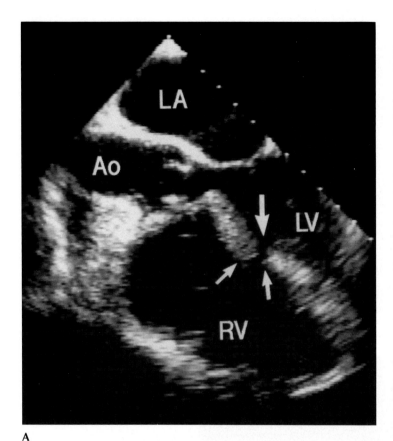
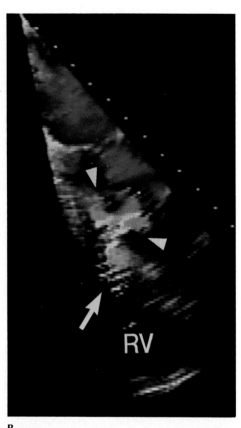

A   B

Fig. 17-4.   Ventricular septal rupture complicating acute anteroseptal myocardial infarction; left ventricular outflow view in the transverse plane. A. Myocardial rupture has caused disruption of the mid-anteroseptum (*large arrow*); discontinuity of the right ventricular margins of the septum (*small arrows*) is evident in this systolic frame. B. Color-flow imaging during systole reveals left ventricular flow entrained into the site of septal rupture (*arrowheads*), and a turbulent left-to-right interventricular shunt (*large arrow*) enters the moderately enlarged right ventricle.

be readily assessed by intravenous injection of an agitated contrast agent (see Chapter 8, Figure 8-9).

An obese 64-year-old woman became severely hypotensive in the surgical intensive care unit 10 hours after coronary artery bypass surgery. Transthoracic echocardiography in search of cardiac tamponade was technically very difficult and yielded no useful information. Transesophageal echocardiography revealed a large pericardial effusion with a partially congealed appearance consistent with organizing intrapericardial hematoma (Fig. 17-7). This hemorrhagic collection caused severe extrinsic compression of the left atrium and extended along the posterior aspects of both ventricles and laterally to the right atrium. Pulsed-wave Doppler imaging of mitral and pulmonary venous inflow demonstrated

nearly complete absence of antegrade diastolic inflow during inspiration, consistent with the hemodynamics of cardiac tamponade [21]. The attending cardiac surgeon, on viewing the images during TEE, proceeded immediately with open pericardial exploration and evacuation of the hemorrhagic effusion and hematoma at the bedside, restoring stable hemodynamics thereafter.

Hypotension developed in a 73-year-old man after perioperative insertion of a pulmonary artery hemodynamic monitoring catheter during aortic aneurysm surgery. Transesophageal two-dimensional echocardiography demonstrated a large pericardial effusion and a small, hyperdynamic left ventricle (Fig. 17-8). On transgastric imaging, mobile tissue fragments were visualized along the inferior right ventricular

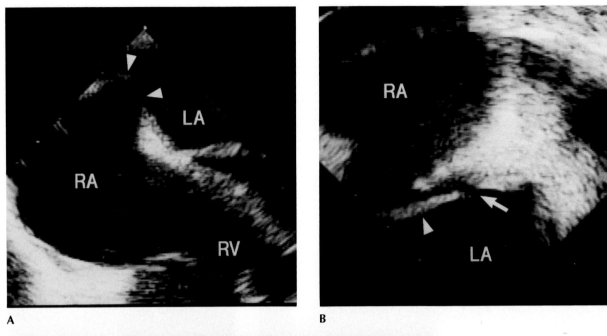

A

B

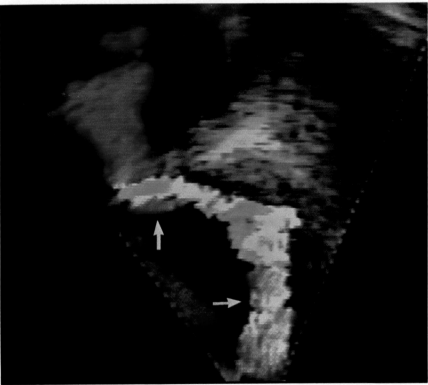

C

Fig. 17-5. Right ventricular infarction complicating aortic valve replacement; magnified transverse four-chamber view focusing on the right atrium. A. The right ventricle and right atrium are severely enlarged; the fossa ovalis membrane (*arrowheads*) bulges far into the left atrium, consistent with significantly increased mean right atrial pressures. B. Longitudinal imaging of the atrial septum. The fossa ovalis membrane (*arrowhead*) is displaced toward the left atrium, and a large patent foramen ovale (*arrow*) is visualized. C. Prominent right-to-left interatrial shunting (*arrows*) traversing the patent foramen ovale is detected by color Doppler imaging. Because right atrial pressure was severely increased, this shunt was continuous throughout both the respiratory and the cardiac cycles.

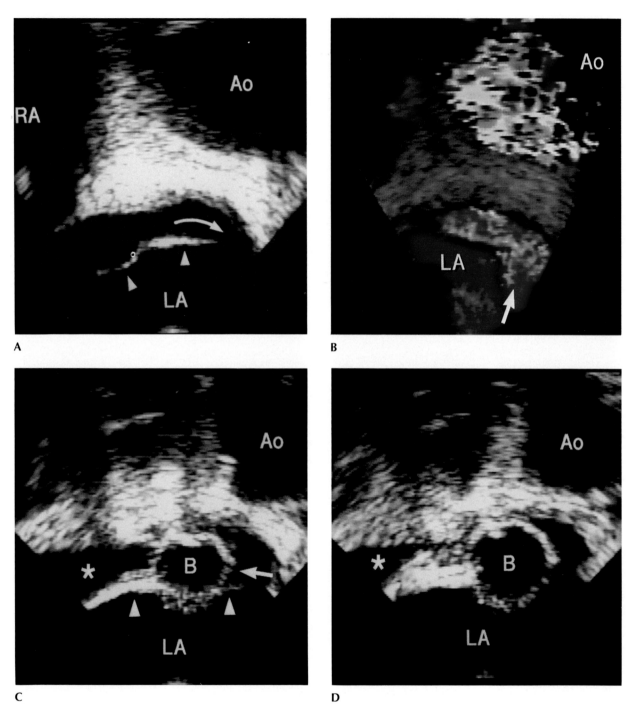

Fig. 17-6. Interatrial shunting complicating right ventricular infarction; balloon-tipped catheter occlusion of a patent foramen ovale; magnified longitudinal long-axis views. A. The fossa ovalis membrane (*arrowheads*) is markedly displaced in the left atrium, and a large patent foramen ovale (*curved arrow*) is present. B. On color-flow mapping, nonturbulent and laminar shunt flow (*arrow*) enters the left atrium via the patent foramen ovale. C. A partially inflated balloon (*B*) on the tip of a catheter is situated in the distal portion (*arrow*) of the patent foramen ovale (*asterisk*), partially expanding the fossa ovalis membrane (*arrowheads*). D. The fully inflated balloon has been passed into the left atrium and pulled back to occlude the foramen ovale.

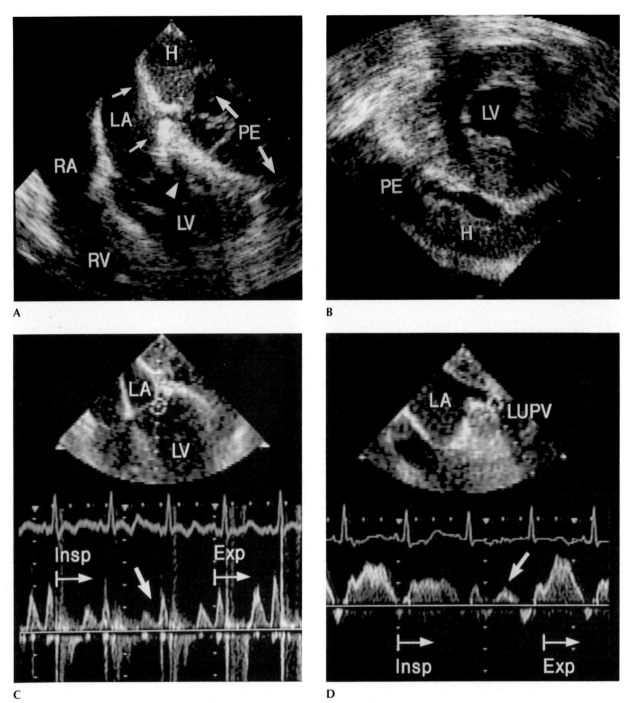

Fig. 17-7. Cardiac tamponade causing severe hemodynamic compromise after coronary bypass surgery. A. Four-chamber view in the transverse plane. A large, loculated hemorrhagic pericardial effusion (*PE, large arrows*) with partial hematoma formation causes severe extrinsic compression of the posterolateral left atrial free wall (*small arrows*) and less severe compression of the left ventricle (*arrowhead*). B. Transgastric short-axis imaging in the transverse plane; apex-down orientation. Partial hematoma formation is seen within the posterior pericardial effusion. C. Pulsed-wave Doppler imaging reveals marked dimunition of mitral inflow velocities (*large arrow*) during inspiration, increasing with expiration, consistent with dissociation of intracardiac and intrathoracic pressures due to tamponade physiology [21]. D. Pulsed-wave Doppler study of the left upper pulmonary vein reveals corresponding severe reduction of inflow (*large arrow*) during inspiration and increase with expiration.

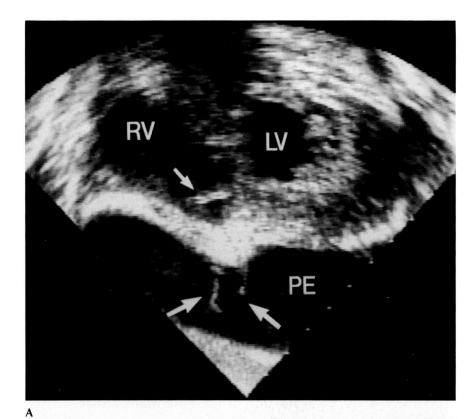

A

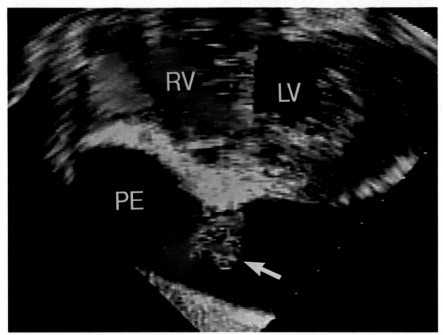

B

Fig. 17-8. Perforation of the right ventricle complicating insertion of a hemodynamic monitoring catheter; transgastric short-axis imaging in the transverse plane, apex-down orientation. A. Tissue fragments (*large arrows*) are detected adjacent to the posteromedial right ventricular free wall, which is also struck by the hemodynamic monitoring catheter (*small arrow*) within the right ventricle. There is a large posterior pericardial effusion. B. Color-flow Doppler imaging demonstrates low-velocity blood flow (*arrow*) extravasating into the pericardial effusion *(PE)* from this site, confirming right ventricular perforation in this location (which was not visible on two-dimensional examination).

free wall. Color-flow Doppler imaging detected flow extravasating from this region into the pericardial effusion, identifying rupture of the right ventricular free wall. Emergency surgical exploration found disruption of the right ventricle in this location caused by trauma at the time of hemodynamic line placement.

A 58-year-old man was found to have refractory severe hypotension and anemia during emergency exploratory laparotomy for multiple visceral injuries sustained during a motor vehicle accident. Intraoperative TEE, done for further evaluation of the patient's unstable hemodynamics, revealed partial transection of the proximal descending thoracic aorta (Fig. 17-9), a lesion associated with severe deceleration trauma [22,23]. Immediate aortic repair was prompted by this finding on TEE. In this case, as in most patients (without previous significant left ventricular dysfunction) who have severe depletion of intravascular volume from any cause, the left ventricle was found to be significantly contracted in size and to have hyperdynamic function (Fig. 17-10).

Precipitate onset of severe retrosternal and interscapular back pain prompted a need for TEE in an elderly woman. Within minutes of introduction of the TEE probe, the cause of the patient's problem was found to be acute aortic dissection (Fig. 17-11). The utility of TEE in the evaluation of patients with suspected aortic dissection is discussed further in Chapter 14.

As with hemodynamically significant mitral regurgitation complicating ischemic heart disease (Fig. 17-3), TEE has been very useful in the identification of severe mitral regurgitation of other origins causing rapid clinical deterioration. We recently described a small group of patients with hypertrophic obstructive cardiomyopathy who presented with symptoms ranging from accelerating left ventricular failure to fulminant acute pulmonary edema and hemodynamic collapse due to severe mitral regurgitation caused by ruptured chordae tendineae [24] (Fig. 17-12). Because of accompanying murmurs of left outflow tract obstruction and extremis of the patient, such mitral regurgitation was not always evident on physical examination. Not uncommonly, transthoracic echocardiography failed to detect the flail mitral leaflet segment; accurate determination of the severity of associated mitral regurgitation was hindered by the eccentricity of the regurgitant jets

and occasionally by acoustic shadowing of the left atrium by mitral annular calcification. In these patients, TEE expeditiously made the correct diagnosis, prompted surgical intervention, and also aided in the intraoperative assessment of mitral valve repair [24].

The essential role of TEE in the echocardiographic evaluation of prosthetic mitral regurgitation is reviewed in Chapter 10. This is exemplified in a patient we studied who had recurrent acute pulmonary edema after bileaflet St. Jude mitral valve replacement. In this patient, cardiac catheterization was unrevealing and left ventriculography did not detect prosthetic mitral regurgitation. Transesophageal echocardiography, performed in the catheterization laboratory for further evaluation, demonstrated intermittent sticking of one prosthetic leaflet in the open position, which precipitated acute severe mitral regurgitation (Fig. 17-13). Partial thrombosis of the tilting mechanism of this sticking prosthetic leaflet was found at the time of repeat surgery.

Evaluation of the Potential Cardiac Donor

We have also found TEE to be valuable for the evaluation of potential cardiac transplantation donors. Because a significant proportion of donor candidates are victims of motor vehicle accidents, it is important to exclude potentially serious cardiac trauma resulting from chest injuries before organ procurement. Such traumatic lesions may include right or, rarely, left ventricular contusion (with or without apical thrombus), tricuspid valve disruption (such as flail or perforated leaflet) with tricuspid regurgitation, coronary thrombus manifested by regional wall motion abnormalities, rupture of the aorta, and pericardial effusion [9,23]. Transthoracic echocardiography may be severely limited because of both chest trauma and the need for mechanical ventilation in such brain-dead donor candidates. Even major abnormalities, such as extensive right ventricular contusion with a flail tricuspid valve, that are readily obvious on TEE (Fig. 17-14) may be difficult to delineate on a technically difficult transthoracic study. Our preliminary experience has shown that fewer than half of potentially significant cardiac abnormalities detected by TEE are appreciated by transthoracic echocardiography in potential cardiac donor candidates. In our practice, therefore,

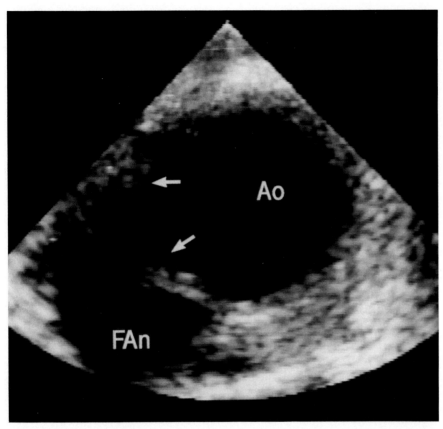

A

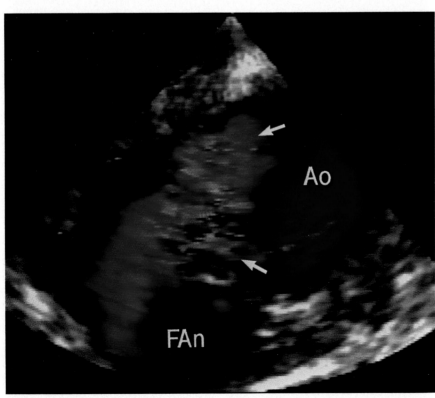

B

Fig. 17-9. Traumatic partial transection of the descending thoracic aorta; transverse short-axis imaging. A. A large rent (*arrows*) in the descending thoracic aorta is present, with the aortic rupture contained by a false aneurysm (*FAn*) in the paraaortic space. B. Color Doppler imaging reveals free communication of blood flow (*arrows*) into the false aneurysm.

Fig. 17-10. Hemodynamically significant hypovolemia; transgastric short-axis imaging in the transverse plane with apex-down orientation.
A. During end-diastole, the left ventricular cavity is severely contracted because of lack of filling volume. B. Nearly complete left ventricular cavity obliteration (*asterisk*) is noted during systole.

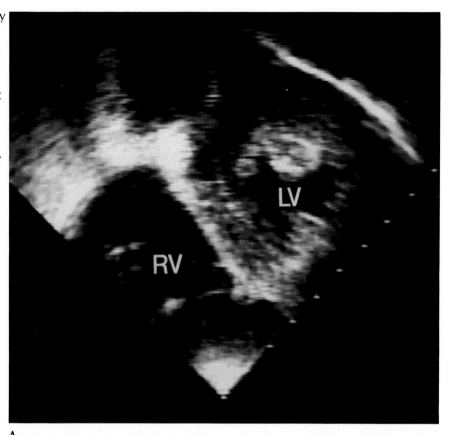

A

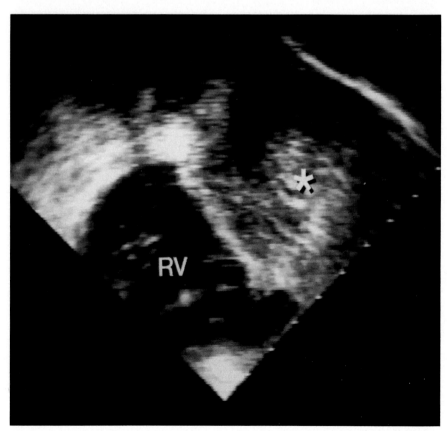

B

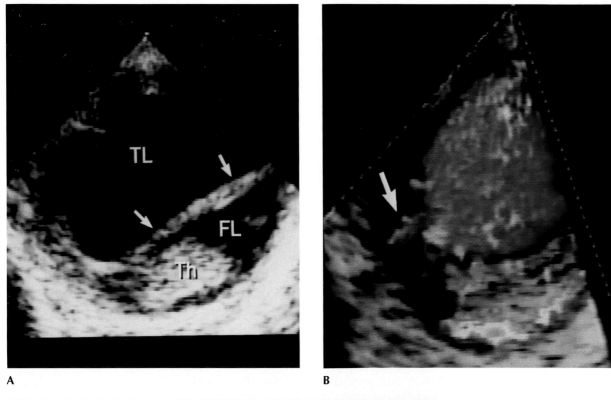

A   B

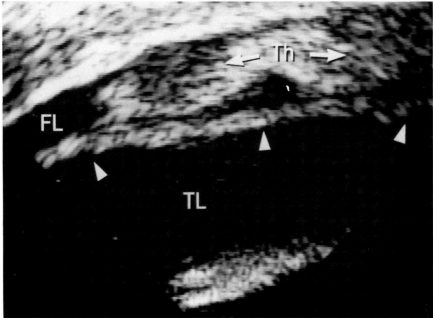

C

Fig. 17-11.   Aortic dissection. A. Short-axis imaging of the descending thoracic aorta in the transverse plane. An intimal flap (*arrows*) separates the true lumen from the false lumen. The false lumen is partially thrombosed (*Th*). B. Color Doppler imaging demonstrates laminar flow (orange) within the true lumen and turbulent flow (yellow-green mosaic) in the smaller false lumen. A small communication (*arrow*) between the two channels is also seen at this level. C. Longitudinal long-axis plane. The linear intimal flap (*arrowheads*) that partitions the true and false lumens is clearly seen. The thrombus (*arrows*) within the false lumen was mobile on real-time examination.

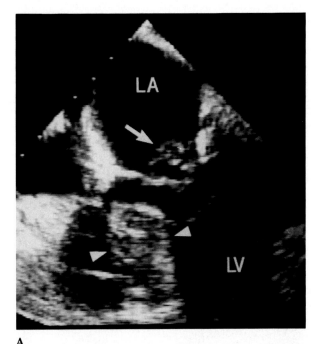

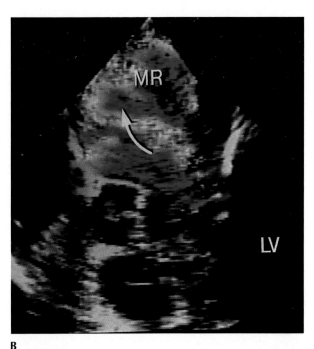

A   B

Fig. 17-12. Severe mitral regurgitation causing hemodynamic decompensation in a patient with hypertrophic obstructive cardiomyopathy; transverse four-chamber imaging. A. A large flail segment of the posterior mitral leaflet (*arrow*), not detected on transthoracic imaging, is visualized. Severe asymmetrical ventricular septal hypertrophy (*arrowheads*), measuring 25 mm, is also evident. B. Severe anteromedial mitral regurgitation (*curved arrow*), also not appreciated by the transthoracic approach, is detected on color-flow imaging. Because of progressive hemodynamic collapse, this patient underwent emergency mitral valve repair and septal myectomy immediately after TEE.

all patients initially hospitalized at our institution undergo TEE before potential cardiac donor status is established.

Stringent exclusion criteria for cardiac donor candidacy based on echocardiographic findings have yet to be established. Such criteria at our institution are currently individualized and take into account the nature and extent of the cardiac abnormality on TEE, status of global right and left ventricular function, potential surgical repairability of detected lesions if the heart is transplanted, and urgency of need for the potential donor heart.

Transesophageal Echocardiography During Cardiopulmonary Resuscitation

In our experience TEE has rarely been performed in patients undergoing cardiopulmonary resuscitation in a desperate attempt to identify a potentially correctable cause for the patient's arrest. The yield of TEE in this situation and the effect on overall patient outcome have been disappointingly minimal. Routine performance of TEE during cardiopulmonary arrest is not warranted, especially if transthoracic echocardiography is adequate to exclude a hemodynamically significant pericardial effusion.

However, interesting observations on the potential mechanism of closed-chest cardiopulmonary resuscitation have been noted on TEE. Two general mechanisms have been proposed based on the "cardiac pump" theory or the "thoracic pump" theory [25]. In the "cardiac pump" theory, the heart is compressed between the sternum and paraspinal structures, with lateral motion limited by pericardial restraints. The compression phase forces an ejection volume from the heart against a closed mitral valve, and the release phase allows cardiac filling with opening of the mitral valve. The "thoracic pump" theory states that external compression causes a generalized increase in intrathoracic pressure, which is then transmitted to all cardiac chambers and great vessels. Because of systemic venous valves at the thoracic outlet, this pressure cannot be conveyed to

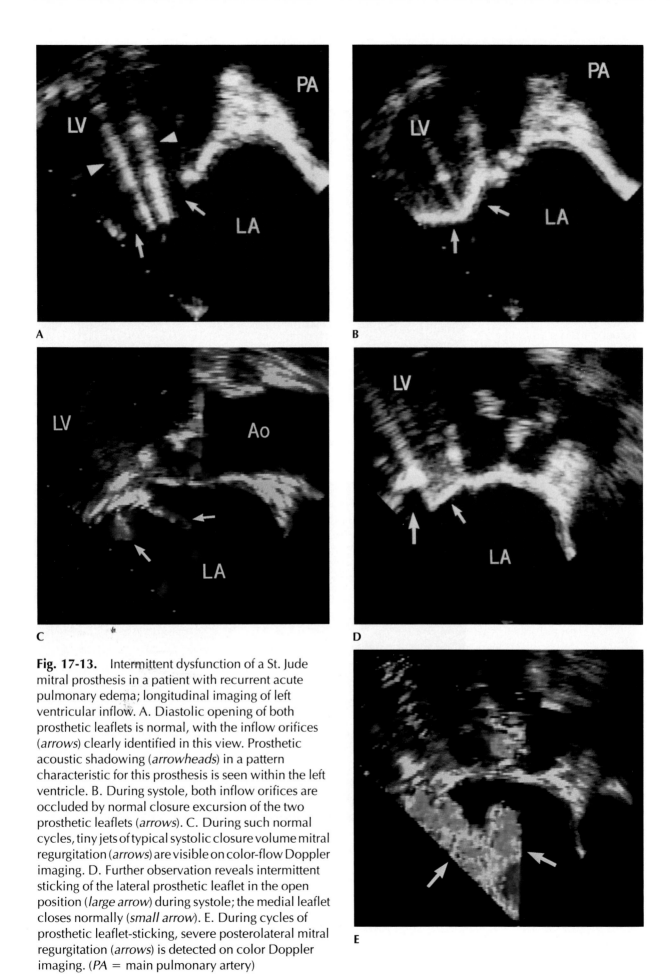

Fig. 17-13. Intermittent dysfunction of a St. Jude mitral prosthesis in a patient with recurrent acute pulmonary edema; longitudinal imaging of left ventricular inflow. A. Diastolic opening of both prosthetic leaflets is normal, with the inflow orifices (*arrows*) clearly identified in this view. Prosthetic acoustic shadowing (*arrowheads*) in a pattern characteristic for this prosthesis is seen within the left ventricle. B. During systole, both inflow orifices are occluded by normal closure excursion of the two prosthetic leaflets (*arrows*). C. During such normal cycles, tiny jets of typical systolic closure volume mitral regurgitation (*arrows*) are visible on color-flow Doppler imaging. D. Further observation reveals intermittent sticking of the lateral prosthetic leaflet in the open position (*large arrow*) during systole; the medial leaflet closes normally (*small arrow*). E. During cycles of prosthetic leaflet-sticking, severe posterolateral mitral regurgitation (*arrows*) is detected on color Doppler imaging. (*PA* = main pulmonary artery)

Fig. 17-14. Traumatic right ventricular contusion and tricuspid valve disruption; modified right ventricular inflow view at 0 degrees multiplane imaging. A. The right ventricle is markedly enlarged and was nearly akinetic on real-time examination. The anterior tricuspid leaflet (*large arrow*) is unsupported and flail; both the anterior and the septal (*small arrow*) leaflets are dwarfed by profound tricuspid annular dilatation, which is responsible for an expansive gap between the noncoapting leaflets. B. Free tricuspid regurgitation (*arrows*) is demonstrated by color-flow Doppler imaging.

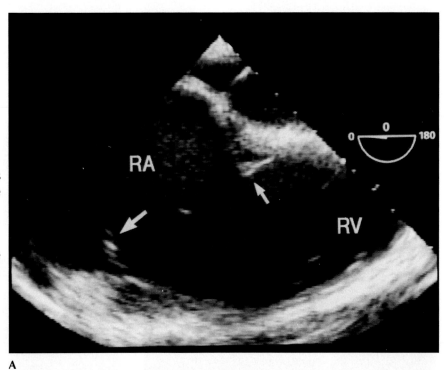

A

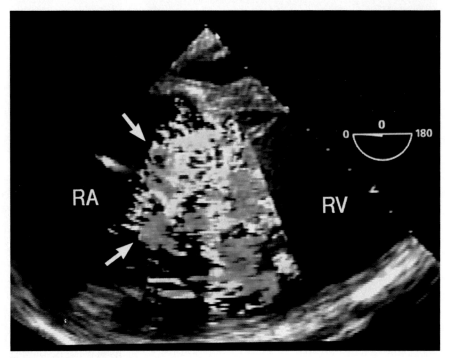

B

the more peripheral venous circulation, and hence an arteriovenous pressure gradient is generated, resulting in antegrade distal systemic perfusion. In the "thoracic pump" theory, the heart acts as a passive conduit, with both the mitral and the aortic valves open during the compression phase, allowing intrathoracic blood to be ejected directly into the systemic circulation.

When performing TEE during cardiopulmonary resuscitation (Fig. 17-15), we have observed significant compression of the right ventricle and, to a lesser degree, the left ventricle during external chest compression. With compression, the mitral valve closed, the aortic valve opened, and mitral regurgitation was generated, indicative of a positive left ventricular to left atrial pressure gradient favoring flow into the left atrium [25]. During the release phase, there was mitral valve opening, with left ventricular filling detected on color Doppler mapping. These TEE findings are consistent with the "cardiac pump" theory of cardiopulmonary resuscitation. The "thoracic pump" theory would necessitate a positive left atrial to left ventricular gradient favoring flow into the left ventricle through an open mitral valve during chest compression, events that are incompatible with TEE findings.

Our observations were recently confirmed in a larger series of 18 patients studied with TEE during cardiopulmonary resuscitation [26]. In this study, antegrade flow was detected only in the aorta and pulmonary artery during chest compression, whereas pulmonary venous and mitral inflow occurred only during the relaxation phase, findings again in keeping with the "cardiac pump" theory and not the "thoracic pump" model.

INDICATIONS AND IMPACT: OTHER REPORTED EXPERIENCE

Investigators from several other institutions have likewise reported a very favorable experience with TEE in the critically ill patient, and the vital role of TEE in the evaluation of such patients is becoming increasingly well established [10,12,13].

Pearson et al. [10] reported the results of 62 TEE studies in 61 patients referred most commonly for clinically suspected thoracic aortic dissection (29%), source of embolus (26%), or complications after myocardial infarction (10%). In this series, TEE provided clinically important information not obtainable with transthoracic echocardiography in 27 patients (44%).

In comparing 112 transthoracic and transesophageal echocardiographic studies in 104 critically ill patients, Font et al. [12] found that 131 significant findings were detected by TEE, whereas only 95 such findings (73%) were evident on transthoracic study. The primary indications for TEE in this study were suspected infective endocarditis (46%), native or prosthetic valve dysfunction (43%), and assessment of left ventricular function (19%).

Foster and Schiller [13] recently described the findings of 83 TEE examinations performed in 69 critically ill patients. The leading indications for TEE in this group were suspected infective endocarditis (43%), source of embolus (13%), hypotension (10%), and evaluation of mitral regurgitation (10%). Unexpected findings were detected in 21 (25%) of the 83 TEE studies, prompting a change in clinical management in 17%. On the basis of TEE findings, 19% of the 69 patients had surgical intervention without further investigation; another 22% were further evaluated by cardiac catheterization or angiography.

Postoperative Cardiac Surgery

The crucial role of TEE in the assessment of hemodynamically unstable patients in the perioperative period after cardiac surgery is well recognized [10–13,18,27–31]. Perhaps in no other subgroup of critically ill patients are the transthoracic echocardiographic windows so compromised by surgical wounds, bandages, chest drains, mechanical ventilation with positive end-expiratory pressure, and residual air interfacing with mediastinal structures in the immediate postoperative state.

Reichert et al. [29] reported the utility of TEE in 60 consecutive patients with hypotension refractory to inotropic infusion (and in nearly half, mechanical hemodynamic support) early after a variety of cardiac operations. In this series, the following diagnoses were made by TEE as primary causes of postoperative hypotension: left ventricular failure (27%), hypovolemia (23%), right ventricular failure (18%), biventricular failure (13%), and cardiac tamponade (10%). Transesophageal echocardiography was inconclusive in determining the cause of hypotension in 9% of patients. Comparison of the TEE

Fig. 17-15. Transesophageal echocardiography during closed-chest cardiopulmonary resuscitation. A. During chest compression, the right ventricular free wall is compressed (*small arrows*) with antegrade blood flow, and dense spontaneous echocontrast (*curved arrows*) exits the open aortic valve (*large arrow*). The mitral valve leaflets (*arrowheads*) are in a closed position. B. Central mitral regurgitation (*large arrow*) is detected by color-flow Doppler imaging during the compression phase; the right ventricular free wall is compressed (*small arrows*).

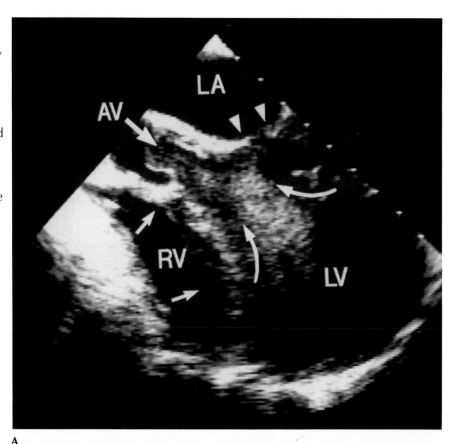

A

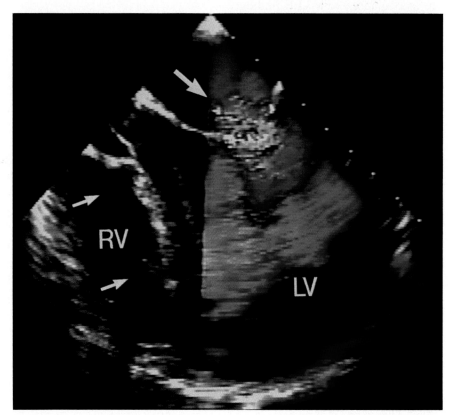

B

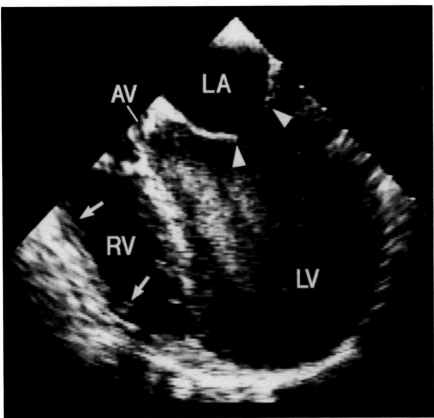

C

Fig. 17-15 (continued).
C. During the release phase, the right ventricular free wall expands (*arrows*), the aortic valve is closed, and the mitral leaflets (*arrowheads*) are partially open. D. Antegrade mitral inflow (*large arrow*) is detected on color Doppler imaging, coursing through the partially open mitral leaflets (*arrowheads*). The right ventricle is expanded (*small arrows*) during the release phase.

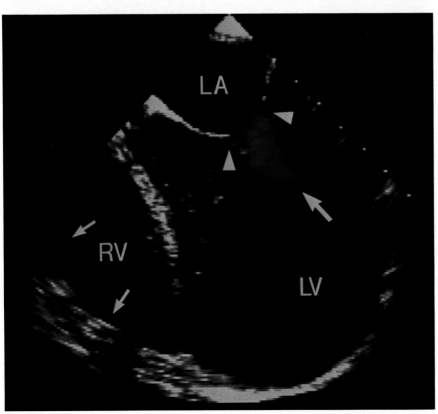

D

impressions with hemodynamic monitoring data revealed agreement on the diagnosis in 30 patients (50%). Six of the remaining patients had increased left ventricular filling pressures (likely spuriously); however, TEE findings were consistent with hypovolemia, and volume repletion resulted in increased blood pressure in all patients. Five patients had hemodynamics suggestive of tamponade; however, no evidence of tamponade or a compressive intrapericardial hematoma was found on TEE, so that unnecessary surgical reexploration was avoided. In two other patients, a large loculated intrapericardial hematoma was found on TEE, whereas hemodynamic measurements did not suggest tamponade. Postoperative right ventricular and biventricular failure were associated with very high mortality, as these investigators noted in a separate report [30].

Several investigators have demonstrated that TEE is an outstanding modality for the bedside diagnosis of intrapericardial hematoma causing localized tamponade and hemodynamic instability in patients after cardiac surgery [27,28,31]. Previous transthoracic

echocardiographic studies showed that postoperative pericardial effusions are localized in nearly two-thirds of cases, and in less than one-third of such patients are there clinically evident signs (e.g., pulsus paradoxus) and diastolic pressure equalization on hemodynamic measurements to suggest tamponade [8]. Intrapericardial hematoma generally organizes adjacent to the right atrium and, less frequently, the right ventricle [27,28,31], with extrinsic compression of these chambers resulting in a low cardiac output state and hypotension (Fig. 17-16). However, as noted in Figure 17-7, localized postoperative tamponade may also compromise left-sided cardiac chambers. Because of far-field imaging and acoustic appearances similar to surrounding tissue, completely organized intrapericardial hematoma is often very difficult to recognize by transthoracic echocardiography. In one report, such hematomas were undetected by the transthoracic approach in all cases in which they were readily identified by TEE [28].

Other postoperative applications of TEE in the cardiac patient have included two-dimensional and

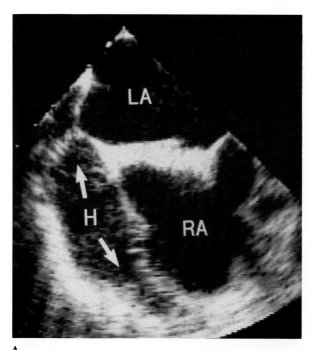
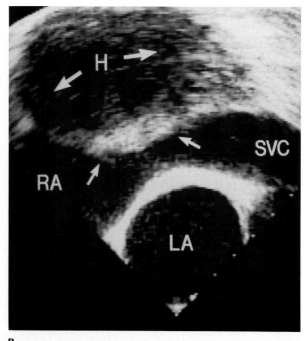

A   B

Fig. 17-16.   Localized intrapericardial hematoma causing low cardiac output shortly after cardiac surgery. A. Modified basal short-axis imaging in the transverse plane. A large, loculated intrapericardial hematoma (*arrows*) is compressing the right atrium. B. Longitudinal long-axis imaging demonstrates significant compression and compromise of the lumen of the superior vena cava at its junction with the right atrium (*small arrows*) caused by the hematoma (*large arrows*).

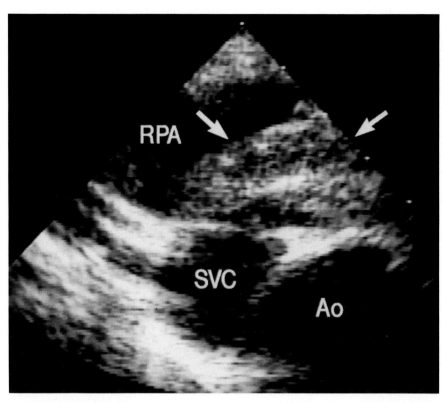

Fig. 17-17. Central pulmonary artery thromboembolism; magnified high basal short-axis imaging in the transverse plane. A large tubular thromboembolus (*arrows*) is coiled within the proximal right pulmonary artery; the thrombus was nonadherent and mobile during real-time examination, consistent with a subacute event. This patient presented with dyspnea, severe hypoxemia, and systemic hypotension.

pulsed-wave Doppler assessment of the hemodynamics of positive pressure ventilation [32] and of intra-aortic balloon counterpulsation [33].

Intrathoracic Trauma

Limited information is available on the usefulness of TEE in the evaluation of the patient with suspected cardiovascular injury due to chest trauma.

Transesophageal echocardiography was performed in 58 patients with thoracic trauma in a series recently reported by Brooks et al. [23]. Among 50 patients also studied with transthoracic echocardiography, cardiac contusion was evident in 6 (12%), whereas TEE detected contusion in 26 patients (52%). In almost all cases, myocardial contusion was noted as segmental hypokinesis of the right ventricle or the ventricular septum or both. Twenty-one patients in the same study population had a widened mediastinum on the chest radiograph at admission. Thoracic aortic disruption was detected in three patients (14%), confirmed in each case by aortography. Negative results of TEE were also confirmed by aortography or anatomically in the remaining 18 patients.

Other investigators have likewise acknowledged the usefulness of TEE in facilitating rapid diagnosis of the life-threatening lesion of traumatic aortic rupture [22,34]. Contained intimal disruption with intraluminal thrombus formation has also been detected by TEE as a traumatic aortic lesion [35]. Transesophageal echocardiography has been performed to evaluate penetrating chest trauma, such as gunshot wounds of the heart [36].

Other Applications

Transesophageal echocardiography has been used to delineate many other disease entities and complications thereof commonly included in the differential diagnosis of critically ill patients with or without hemodynamic instability.

Complications of acute myocardial infarction, such as ventricular septal rupture [37] or papillary muscle rupture [38], are readily diagnosed by two-dimensional and Doppler TEE. Contained left ventricular free-wall rupture, however, may be more difficult to delineate by TEE, particularly if there has been no significant pseudoaneurysm formation or if the far left ventricular apex is involved [39]. The role of TEE in the evaluation of complications of ischemic heart disease is reviewed in Chapter 8.

Multiple reports have described the detection of pulmonary artery thromboembolism by TEE in

Fig. 17-18. Deep venous thromboembolism associated with paradoxical embolism; modified four-chamber imaging in the transverse plane. A. A large, serpiginous thromboembolism-in-transit (*small arrows*) is present in the right side of the heart; the atrial septum (*arrowheads*) bulges far into the left atrium, consistent with right atrial pressure overload. A thrombus (*large arrows*) is also seen prolapsing across the mitral valve. B. Off-axis transverse plane imaging reveals paradoxical embolism in transit with thrombus (*large arrows*) traversing the atrial septum (*asterisk*) through a large patent foramen ovale (*arrowheads*). This patient presented with a large pulmonary embolism and simultaneous acute thromboembolic occlusion of the left common femoral artery several days after total hip arthroplasty.

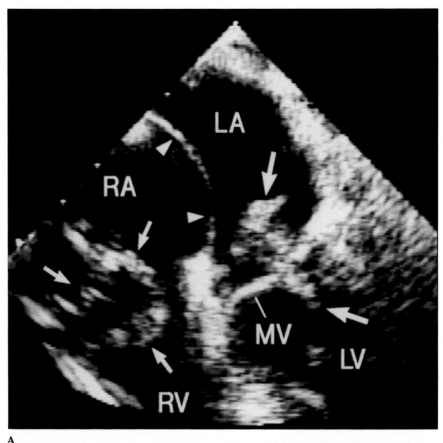

A

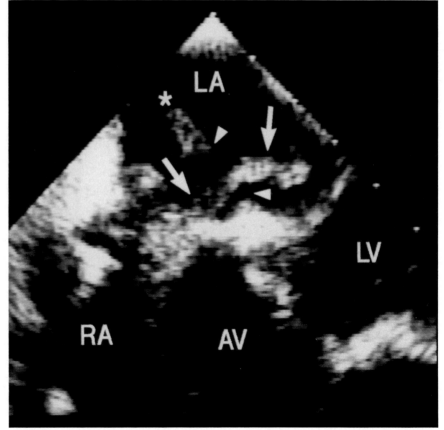

B

patients with a broad spectrum of clinical presentations, including acute cardiopulmonary decompensation [40–44] (Fig. 17-17). Although generally not helpful in hemodynamically insignificant, more peripheral pulmonary thromboembolism, TEE may provide a sensitive means of detection of central thromboembolism associated with hemodynamic compromise. Among 60 patients with echocardiographic signs of right ventricular pressure overload caused by pulmonary thromboembolism, TEE detected central pulmonary artery emboli in 35 (58%); accompanying right atrial thrombus was present in 6 patients (10%) [43]. Transthoracic echocardiography detected central pulmonary thromboembolism in only 11% of these patients, and right atrial thrombus was noted in just two of the six patients in whom it was present. Compared with reference standards of pulmonary angiography (36 patients), digital subtraction pulmonary angiography (16 patients), surgical exploration (15 patients), computed tomography (13 patients), and necropsy (5 patients), the overall sensitivity of TEE in the detection of central pulmonary artery thromboembolism was 97% and the specificity was 88%.

Transesophageal echocardiography has also been used to assess the efficacy of both standard anticoagulation [44] and thrombolytic [42] therapeutic interventions for central pulmonary thromboembolism. Failure of another therapeutic intervention, that is, an inferior vena caval filter, to prevent pulmonary embolism has also been detected by TEE [45]. In this case, the filter had migrated from its intended position in the inferior vena cava and on TEE was discovered to be in the proximal right pulmonary artery.

Analogous to the pathophysiology of right ventricular infarction, acute right ventricular pressure overload associated with extensive pulmonary embolism may promote right-to-left interatrial shunting through a patent foramen ovale, exacerbating systemic hypoxemia. Such shunting, precipitated by significant increases in right ventricular filling pressures, may occur in 40% of patients with hemodynamically significant pulmonary embolism [46] and can easily be detected by intravenous injection of contrast medium and color-flow Doppler mapping during TEE. Associated paradoxical systemic embolism manifested by an acute neurologic deficit or peripheral vascular occlusion may occur in nearly 60% of such cases (Fig. 17-18). Marked right-to-

left interatrial shunting mimicking the presentation of pulmonary embolism has also been reported to complicate occult cardiac tamponade; both problems were ultimately defined by TEE [47].

The role of TEE in the expeditious diagnosis of aortic dissection is discussed in detail in Chapter 14. When critically compared with magnetic resonance imaging or contrast-enhanced computed tomography, TEE remains a very highly sensitive means of diagnosis; for hemodynamically unstable patients in whom rapid bedside diagnosis is imperative, it is the imaging procedure of choice [48].

As presented in Chapter 11, TEE has become the definitive imaging technique for the diagnosis of infective endocarditis and its complications [49,50].

SUMMARY

Prompt identification of the cause of the critically ill patient's condition is mandatory if potentially lifesaving medical and often surgical therapeutic interventions are to be instituted. Transesophageal echocardiography is the ideal imaging modality for immediate bedside detection or exclusion of a broad spectrum of differential diagnostic possibilities. Perhaps in no other circumstance in the practice of TEE is the diagnostic yield higher or the impact on clinical decision-making greater than in the evaluation of the critically ill patient.

REFERENCES

1. Mintz GS, Victor MF, Kotler MN, et al. Two-dimensional echocardiographic identification of surgically correctable complications of acute myocardial infarction. *Circulation* 1981;64:91–6.

2. Nishimura RA, Tajik AJ, Shub C, et al. Role of two-dimensional echocardiography in the prediction of in-hospital complications after acute myocardial infarction. *J Am Coll Cardiol* 1984;4:1080–7.

3. Sutherland GR, Smyllie JH, Roelandt JRTC. Advantages of colour flow imaging in the diagnosis of left ventricular pseudoaneurysm. *Br Heart J* 1989;61:59–64.

4. Smyllie JH, Sutherland GR, Geuskens R, et al. Doppler color flow mapping in the diagnosis of ventricular septal rupture and acute mitral regurgitation after myocardial infarction. *J Am Coll Cardiol* 1990;15:1449–55.

5. Sanfilippo AJ, Weyman AE. The role of echocardiography in managing critically ill patients. Part 2: Specific clinical applications. *J Crit Illness* 1988 May;3:27–44.

6. Parker MM, Cunnion RE, Parrillo JE. Echocardiography and nuclear cardiac imaging in the critical care unit. *JAMA* 1985;254:2935–9.

7. Khandheria BK, Tajik AJ, Taylor CL, et al. Aortic dissection: review of value and limitations of two-dimensional echocardiography in a six-year experience. *J Am Soc Echocardiogr* 1989;2:17–24.

8. D'Cruz IA, Kensey K, Campbell C, et al. Two-dimensional echocardiography in cardiac tamponade occurring after cardiac surgery. *J Am Coll Cardiol* 1985;5:1250–2.

9. Miller FA Jr, Seward JB, Gersh BJ, et al. Two-dimensional echocardiographic findings in cardiac trauma. *Am J Cardiol* 1982;50:1022–7.

10. Pearson AC, Castello R, Labovitz AJ. Safety and utility of transesophageal echocardiography in the critically ill patient. *Am Heart J* 1990;119:1083–9.

11. Oh JK, Seward JB, Khandheria BK, et al. Transesophageal echocardiography in critically ill patients. *Am J Cardiol* 1990;66:1492–5.

12. Font VE, Obarski TP, Klein AL, et al. Transesophageal echocardiography in the critical care unit. *Cleve Clin J Med* 1991;58:315–22.

13. Foster E, Schiller NB. The role of transesophageal echocardiography in critical care: UCSF experience. *J Am Soc Echocardiogr* 1992;5:368–74.

14. Seward JB, Khandheria BK, Oh JK, et al. Transesophageal echocardiography: technique, anatomic correlations, implementation, and clinical applications. *Mayo Clin Proc* 1988;63:649–80.

15. Matsuzaki M, Toma Y, Kusukawa R. Clinical applications of transesophageal echocardiography. *Circulation* 1990;82:709–22.

16. Daniel WG, Erbel R, Kasper W, et al. Safety of transesophageal echocardiography: a multicenter survey of 10,410 examinations. *Circulation* 1991;83:817–21.

17. Chan K-L, Cohen GI, Sochowski RA, Baird RG. Complications of transesophageal echocardiography in ambulatory adult patients: analysis of 1500 consecutive examinations. *J Am Soc Echocardiogr* 1991;4:577–82.

18. Ansari A. Transesophageal two-dimensional echocardiography: current perspectives. *Prog Cardiovasc Dis* 1993;35:349–97.

19. Silvey SV, Stoughton TL, Pearl W, et al. Rupture of the outer partition of aortic dissection during transesophageal echocardiography. *Am J Cardiol* 1991;68:286–7.

20. Oh JK, Sinak LJ, Freeman WK, et al. Transesophageal echocardiography in patients with shock syndrome (abstract). *Circulation* 1991;84 Suppl 2:II–127.

21. Appleton CP, Hatle LK, Popp RL. Cardiac tamponade and pericardial effusion: respiratory variation in transvalvular flow velocities studied by Doppler echocardiography. *J Am Coll Cardiol* 1988;11:1020–30.

22. Snow CC, Appelbe AF, Martin TD, Martin RP. Diagnosis of aortic transection of transesophageal echocardiography. *J Am Soc Echocardiogr* 1992;5:100–2.

23. Brooks SW, Young JC, Cmolik B, et al. The use of transesophageal echocardiography in the evaluation of chest trauma. *J Trauma* 1992,32:761–6.

24. Zhu W-X, Oh JK, Kopecky SL, et al. Mitral regurgitation due to ruptured chordae tendineae in patients with hypertrophic obstructive cardiomyopathy. *J Am Coll Cardiol* 1992;20:242–7.

25. Higano ST, Oh JK, Ewy GA, Seward JB. The mechanism of blood flow during closed chest cardiac massage in humans: transesophageal echocardiographic observations. *Mayo Clin Proc* 1990;65:1432–40.

26. Pell ACH, Bloomfield P, Robertson CE, et al. Direct cardiac compression generates systemic blood flow during cardiopulmonary resuscitation: evidence against the thoracic pump (abstract). *J Am Coll Cardiol* 1993;21 Suppl A:147A.

27. Chan K-L. Transesophageal echocardiography for assessing cause of hypotension after cardiac surgery. *Am J Cardiol* 1988;62:1142–3.

28. Kochar GS, Jacobs LE, Kotler MN. Right atrial compression in postoperative cardiac patients: detection by transesophageal echocardiography. *J Am Coll Cardiol* 1990;16:511–6.

29. Reichert CLA, Visser CA, Koolen JJ, et al. Transesophageal echocardiography in hypotensive patients after cardiac operations: comparison with hemodynamic parameters. *J Thorac Cardiovasc Surg* 1992;104:321–6.

30. Reichert CL, Visser CA, van den Brink RB, et al. Prognostic value of biventricular function in hypotensive patients after cardiac surgery as assessed by transesophageal echocardiography. *J Cardiothorac Vasc Anesth* 1992;6:429–32.

31. Beppu S, Tanaka N, Nakatani S, et al. Pericardial clot after open heart surgery: its specific localization and haemodynamics. *Eur Heart J* 1993;14:230–4.

32. Poelaert JI, Reichert CL, Koolen JJ, et al. Transesophageal echo-Doppler evaluation of the hemodynamic effects of positive-pressure ventilation

after coronary artery surgery. *J Cardiothorac Vasc Anesth* 1992;6:438–43.

33. Katz ES, Tunick PA, Kronzon I. Observations of coronary flow augmentation and balloon function during intraaortic balloon counterpulsation using transesophageal echocardiography. *Am J Cardiol* 1992;69:1635–9.

34. Sparks MB, Burchard KW, Marrin CAS, et al. Transesophageal echocardiography: preliminary results in patients with traumatic aortic rupture. *Arch Surg* 1991;126:711–4.

35. Davis GA, Sauerisen S, Chandrasekaran K, et al. Subclinical traumatic aortic injury diagnosed by transesophageal echocardiography. *Am Heart J* 1992;123:534–6.

36. Brathwaite CEM, Weiss RL, Baldino WA, et al. Multichamber gunshot wounds of the heart: the utility of transesophageal echocardiography. *Chest* 1992;101:287–8.

37. Ballal RS, Sanyal RS, Nanda NC, Mahan EF III. Usefulness of transesophageal echocardiography in the diagnosis of ventricular septal rupture secondary to acute myocardial infarction. *Am J Cardiol* 1993;71:367–70.

38. Patel AM, Miller FA Jr, Khandheria BK, et al. Role of transesophageal echocardiography in the diagnosis of papillary muscle rupture secondary to myocardial infarction. *Am Heart J* 1989;118:1330–3.

39. Stoddard MF, Dawkins PR, Longaker RA, et al. Transesophageal echocardiography in the detection of left ventricular pseudoaneurysm. *Am Heart J* 1993;125:534–9.

40. Nixdorff U, Erbel R, Drexler M, Meyer J. Detection of thromboembolus of the right pulmonary artery by transesophageal two-dimensional echocardiography. *Am J Cardiol* 1988;61:488–9.

41. Klein AL, Stewart WC, Cosgrove DM III, et al. Visualization of acute pulmonary emboli by transesophageal echocardiography. *J Am Soc Echocardiogr* 1990;3:412–5.

42. Dall'Aglio V, Nicolosi GL, Zanuttini D. Transthoracic and transesophageal echocardiographic documentation of disappearance of massive right atrial and pulmonary artery thromboemboli after fibrinolytic therapy and normalization of left ventricular dimensions and function. *Eur Heart J* 1990;11:863–5.

43. Wittlich N, Erbel R, Eichler A, et al. Detection of central pulmonary artery thromboemboli by transesophageal echocardiography in patients with severe pulmonary embolism. *J Am Soc Echocardiogr* 1992;5:515–24.

44. Cerel A, Burger AJ. The diagnosis of a pulmonary artery thrombus by transesophageal echocardiography. *Chest* 1993;103:944–5.

45. Rao KM, Simons AJ, Hare CL, Smulyan H. Migration of a Kimray-Greenfield filter into the pulmonary artery: localization by transesophageal echocardiography. *Am Heart J* 1993;125:543–4.

46. Kasper W, Geibel A, Tiede N, Just H. Patent foramen ovale in patients with hemodynamically significant pulmonary embolism. *Lancet* 1992;340:561–4.

47. Thompson RC, Finck SJ, Leventhal JP, Safford RE. Right-to-left shunt across a patent foramen ovale caused by cardiac tamponade: diagnosis by transesophageal echocardiography. *Mayo Clin Proc* 1991;66:391–4.

48. Nienaber CA, von Kodolitsch Y, Nicolas V, et al. The diagnosis of thoracic aortic dissection by noninvasive imaging procedures. *N Engl J Med* 1993;328:1–9.

49. Mügge A, Daniel WG, Frank G, Lichtlen PR. Echocardiography in infective endocarditis: reassessment of prognostic implications of vegetation size determined by the transthoracic and the transesophageal approach. *J Am Coll Cardiol* 1989;14:631–8.

50. Daniel WG, Mügge A, Martin RP, et al. Improvement in the diagnosis of abscesses associated with endocarditis by transesophageal echocardiography. *N Engl J Med* 1991;324:795–800.

18

Three-Dimensional Reconstruction by Transesophageal Echocardiography

James B. Seward • *Marek Belohlavek*
David A. Foley • *James F. Greenleaf*

Three-dimensional (3-D) reconstruction of ultrasound images has been an elusive challenge. Although a number of investigators have successfully produced 3-D ultrasound images, there has been little success in developing clinically usable reconstruction techniques. Limited ultrasound windows to the heart and limited access to high-speed digital computer capability have been practical problems. The ultimate objective of 3-D reconstruction imaging is to electronically extract the heart from the body of a living patient and, with 3-D rendering of the image, noninvasively assess anatomy, function, and histology.

Two simultaneous events have brought 3-D ultrasound reconstruction to a point where it appears to be the next advance in clinical echocardiography. First, computer technology has made significant advances in memory and digital manipulation. Affordable digital image acquisition and computer manipulation will soon allow conventional echocardiographic equipment to process images into a 3-D format. Second, with the advent of invasive ultrasound, in particular transesophageal echocardiography (TEE), a predictable, high-quality ultrasound window is available for collection of tomographic images suitable for volumetric reconstruction. New transducer technology, in particular multiplane TEE, incorporates a motor-driven step function for the incremental rotation of the transducer. Electrocardiographic and respiratory gaiting may also be necessary. It is predicted that these two technologic advances (computer technology and image acquisition through invasive echocardiography) will permit clinical 3-D reconstruction of cardiac anatomy in the near future. The discussion that follows briefly explains the process of 3-D reconstruction using conventional TEE and illustrates some of the newest clinical applications.

IMAGE ACQUISITION METHODS

Although TEE serves as an excellent window to the heart, it is nevertheless limited. Two scan techniques, linear [1–4] and rotational [5–9], are currently the most practical means of acquiring sequential series of tomographic two-dimensional (2-D) images of the heart (Fig. 18-1). Investigational volumetric scanning techniques show great promise but are far from clinical usefulness at this time [10–13].

Linear Scan

This technique involves moving a TEE transducer in discrete steps perpendicular to the imaging plane (see Fig. 18-1A) [1,2]. Resultant sequential parallel 2-D images are stored and then digitally combined to create a 3-D image [3]. This method is often referred to as "breadloafing." Clinically, this method has most commonly been used to obtain intravascular 3-D ultrasound images [14–16]. Another innovative system uses a TEE probe, made rigid after esophageal intubation, that moves a transverse ultrasound transducer longitudinally, collecting sequential cross-sectional 2-D images perpendicular to the long axis of the probe [4]. These data are then used for 3-D and four-dimensional (4-D) reconstruction of the heart.

Rotational Scan

Because the ultrasound window to the heart is frequently too small to permit "breadloafing," rotational scanning techniques (see Fig. 18-1B) have been used to obtain sequential images from a discrete window. Rotational scans are obtained in two ways. In the first method, a longitudinal scan plane is rotated in discrete increments, producing a fanlike or pyramidal data volume [5,6]. This fanlike method requires an external stepper device that rotates the endoscope at fixed degrees of rotation. Such stepper devices are not now clinically available. The second rotational method is a circular rotation technique that produces a conical volume [7]. This method uses incremental rotation of a multiplane transducer. Multiplane TEE transducers suitable for collection of a conical data set should be available in the near future.

Volumetric Scan

Another novel approach to 3-D ultrasound imaging is a transducer that generates a pyramidal burst of ultrasound (see Fig. 18-1C) [10,11]. The resulting signals are used to create a 3-D image in real time (4-D imaging). This technique requires extensive processing of computer data and rapid formation of electronic beams, which limit image resolution. This system, although extremely promising, will require a few more years to bring to clinical application.

THREE-DIMENSIONAL IMAGE RENDERING

After an image acquisition technique is selected, the rendering of an interpretable 3-D reconstruction is the greatest challenge. About five steps are required to process stored analog video images into a 3-D image suitable for display and interpretation.

Step 1: Region of Interest Defined

The ultrasound image contains more information than is required for 3-D reconstruction. When only the areas of interest are defined, the computer memory required for reconstruction is considerably reduced.

Step 2: Digitization

Currently, most images are acquired and stored in analog video. For accomplishment of 3-D reconstruction, the defined image must be digitized into a numerical matrix.

Step 3: Conversion, Reregistration, and Interpolation

Depending on the method of acquisition, the digital images must be reformatted into a rectangular matrix. Thus, pyramidal or conical acquisition requires a *conversion* step. *Reregistration* is a process of realigning borders of sequential images, which may be out of alignment because of motion during acquisition. *Interpolation* completes the volume matrix by filling in missing data between acquired tomographic views. For example, a conical acquisition has dense data at the apex of the scan cone and fewer data points in the far field. Statistical logic is used to fill in data between the image slices by interpolation.

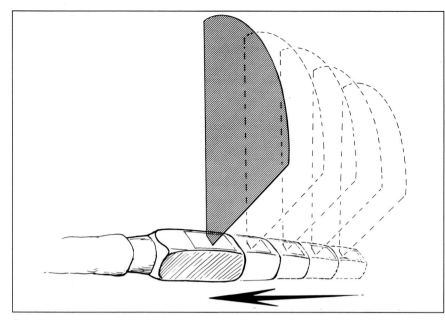

Fig. 18-1. Image acquisition methods. A. Linear ("breadloaf") scan. The esophageal transducer is moved linearly to scan the heart or aorta in predefined increments. Multiple parallel 2-D images are stacked together to create the 3-D image. B. "Fanlike" scan. The longitudinal imaging array is swept across the object by rotation of the transducer shaft, so that a pyramidal volume is scanned. C. "Propeller-like" scan. The ultrasound imaging array is rotated in incremental steps to scan a conical volume.

A

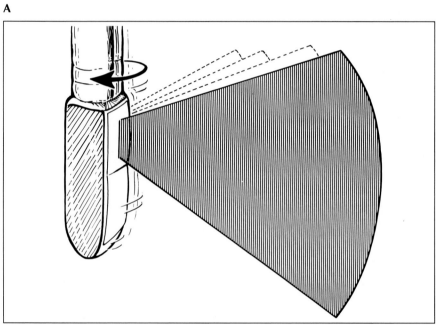

B

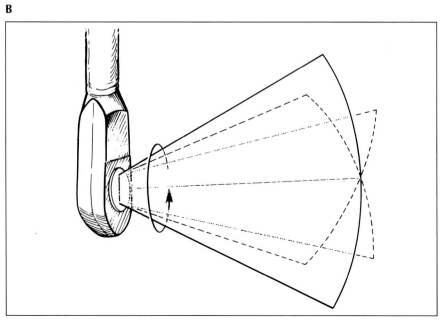

C

579

Step 4: Enhancement

Ultrasound images are inherently noisy, and various enhancement techniques are used to improve the image and reduce artifacts.

Step 5: Segmentation

At this point, the 3-D data volume is available, but the area or organ of interest is embedded within a rectangular reconstruction matrix. Segmentation is an interactive process that allows one to separate the organ or area of interest from the surrounding nonessential data.

THREE-DIMENSIONAL IMAGE DISPLAY

A number of methods for displaying 3-D images in an understandable manner have been developed [17].

Tomographic Displays

Orthogonal Tomographic Display

The 3-D reconstructed volume can be simultaneously cut and displayed in three orthogonal tomographic planes [17] (Fig. 18-2A). The three tomographic planes can be randomly moved to show a 3-D tomographic perspective.

Interactive Tomographic Display

The 3-D volume image can be cut in any manner or direction by a tomographic knife [1,2,18] (Fig. 18-2B). The operator can virtually "fly" through the object, cutting it in any conceivable manner.

Three-Dimensional Displays

Wire-Frame Display

Wire-frame display [9,19] (Fig. 18-3A) is the simplest method, which defines boundaries of interest by points interconnected by lines. The completed

Fig. 18-2. Tomographic 3-D image displays. A. Interactive orthogonal tomographic display. Three orthogonal sections, simultaneously derived from the 3-D-rendered image, allow visualization of the heart in three orthogonal perspectives. The level of each section can be interactively modified by repositioning the plane of any section (*arrow*). Top left. Volume of human heart rendered in vitro. Top right. Four-chamber view. Bottom left. Long-axis sagittal view. Bottom right. Short-axis view. B. Interactive oblique tomographic display. The image plane can be interactively positioned anywhere in the image. The observer can "fly" through the 3-D image volume while cutting the heart into unique tomographic planes. Navigational terms (boxed) were once used to describe the maneuver.

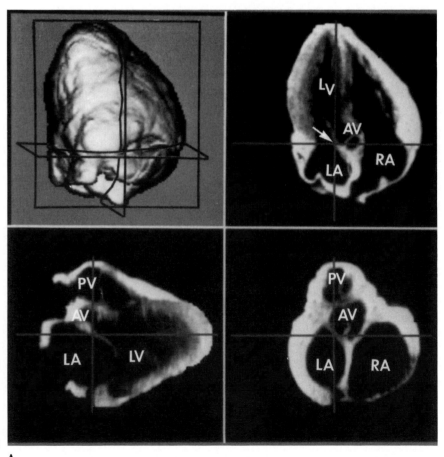

A

image gives the illusion of a "wire frame." This reconstruction technique is useful for the measurement of volume and assessment of motion dynamics.

Surface Rendering

The surface of the segmented (extracted) 3-D object can be displayed by shadowing techniques that provide a 3-D perspective [20–22] (Fig. 18-3B). Pairs of images created with a slight offset can be projected to give a visual 3-D presentation of the object. With surface rendering, the internal contents of the object are all set to one density and not displayed.

Volume Rendering

The most complex 3-D display is based on ray tracing. Volume rendering maintains the internal structure of the object [23] (Fig. 18-3C). A cut surface reveals ultrasound texture. This display attempts to accurately depict all the ultrasound texture and motion of the heart and most closely realizes the concept of "computer vivisection" of reconstructed 3-D anatomy.

APPLICATIONS OF THREE-DIMENSIONAL TEE

Current applications of ultrasound 3-D reconstruction remain exploratory and are not generally available. However, as noted above, TEE currently is the most logical approach to image acquisition. Computer technology is available that can produce 3-D images for the acquisition of serial images. Clinical 3-D reconstruction using TEE is expected to be available within 1 to 3 years.

At present, three primary applications of 3-D image reconstruction appear to have clinical utility (Fig. 18-4): (1) assessment of volume and function through 3-D rendering of the cardiac chamber size, volume, and global and regional function [6,19,24,25]; (2) assessment of 3-D time motion of valves or other dynamic processes, such as color-flow Doppler jets [26,27]; and (3) dissection of the heart into areas of interest, such as the atrial septum, for the study of normal and abnormal anatomy. Other applications, such as electronic surgical repair, will follow.

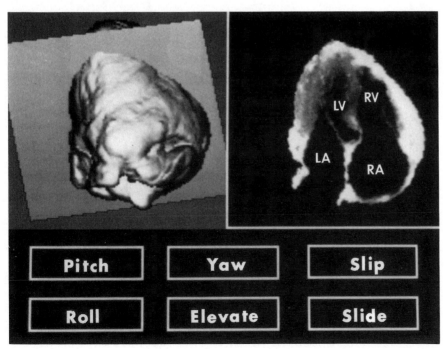

B

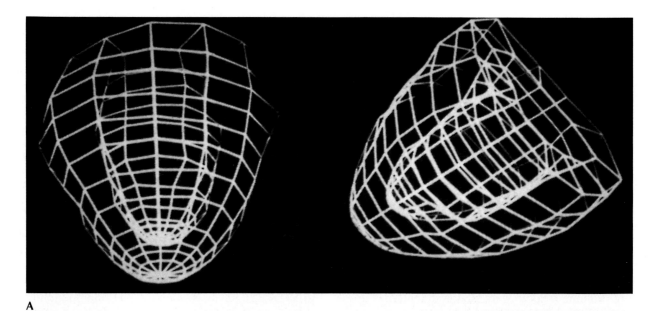

A

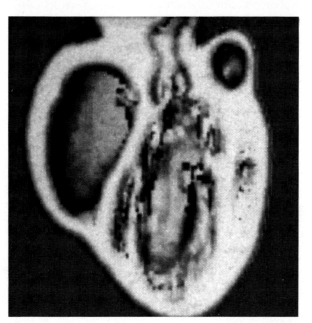

B

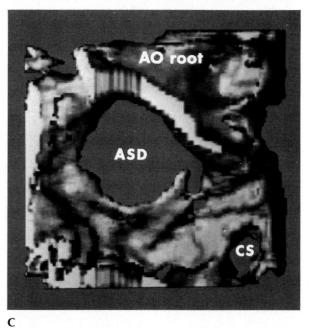

C

Fig. 18-3.   Three-dimensional displays. A. "Wire-frame" 3-D reconstruction of a human left ventricle at end-systole. This display permits a gross description of ventricular shape, size, and wall thickness. (From The American Society of Echocardiography, Subcommittee on Digital Image Processing, Skorton DJ, Collins SM, Garcia E, et al. Digital signal and image processing in echocardiography. *Am Heart J* 1985;110:1266–83. By permission of Mosby-Year Book.) B. Shaded display of the endocardial surface of a canine heart. The sectioned image demonstrates details of valve cusps, papillary muscles, and wall trabeculation. (From McCann et al. [8]. By permission of the Institute of Electrical and Electronic Engineers.) C. Volume rendering of secundum atrial septal defect. A 3-D reconstruction is created from a transesophageal "fanlike" rotational scan. The atrial septum is viewed from the right atrial surface. A large secundum atrial septal defect is visualized. Surrounding anatomic structures include the orifice of the coronary sinus and the atrial surface of the aortic root.

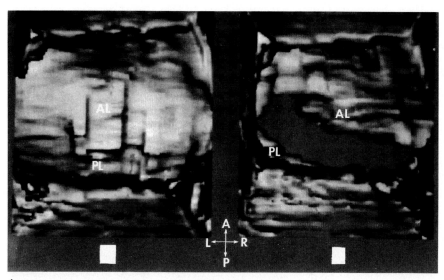

A

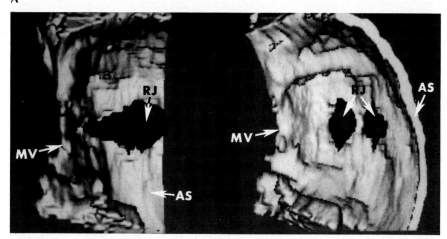

B

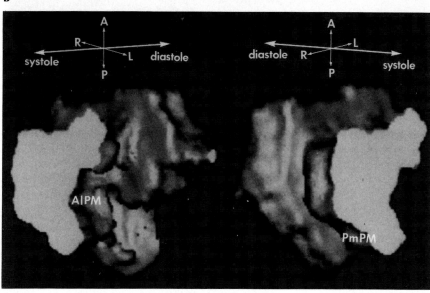

C

Fig. 18-4. Applications of 3-D reconstruction. A. Normal mitral valve. A dynamic 3-D scan (i.e., 4-D reconstruction) is produced from a TEE "fanlike" scan. The mitral leaflets are viewed from the left atrium looking toward the orifice of the mitral valve. Left. Systole. Right. Diastole. B. Color-flow images (shown in black and white) of mild mitral valve regurgitation reconstructions of the mitral valve and mitral regurgitation jets (*RJ*). Left. Viewing across the atrial surface of the mitral valve toward the atrial septum. Right. Looking toward the mitral valve leaflets parallel to the atrial septum. Now two small jets (*arrows*) are visible. C. Functional 3-D display of the left ventricle. A time series of 15 cross-sectional images of the left ventricle at the level of the papillary muscles was used to create a left ventricular cast demonstrating global and regional contractile function. Left. Lateral left ventricular cavity. Note the indentation due to the anterolateral papillary muscle (*AlPM*). Right. Septal left ventricular cavity. The smaller posteromedial papillary muscle (*PmPM*) indentation is visible. This reconstruction is displayed as a contracting (undulating) tube of varying dimensions depending on global and regional wall motion.

Fig. 18-4 (continued).
D. Electronic vivisection. Top. Stenotic mitral valve by 3-D rendering has been electronically extracted from its annulus. Bottom. The potential of 3-D electronic surgery is illustrated by positioning a sized valvular prosthesis into the mitral valve annulus to simulate surgical replacement. Electronic "vivisection" is envisioned as a means of extracting body parts from a living patient and then performing reconstructive surgery or other therapy in anticipation of the actual procedure. (*AL* = anterior leaflet; *L* = left; *PL* = posterior leaflet.)

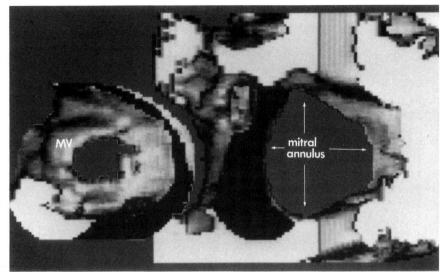

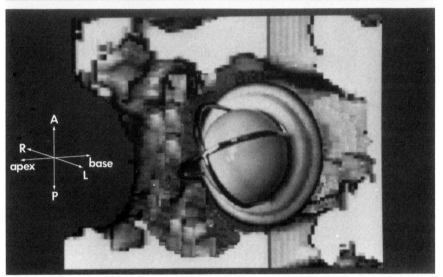

D

SUMMARY

The ultimate goal of 3-D reconstruction is electronic extraction of a body structure (e.g., the heart) and dissection of various structural, functional, and histologic pieces of information. Because the ultrasound windows are limited, invasive procedures, such as TEE, are most suited to this challenge.

REFERENCES

1. Robinson DE. Display of three-dimensional ultrasonic data for medical diagnosis. *J Acoust Soc Am* 1972;52:673–87.

2. Matsumoto M, Matsuo H, Kitabatake A, et al. Three-dimensional echocardiograms and two-dimensional echocardiographic images at desired planes by a computerized system. *Ultrasound Med Biol* 1977;3:163–78.

3. Kuroda T, Kinter TM, Seward JB, et al. Accuracy of three-dimensional volume measurement using biplane transesophageal echocardiographic probe: in vitro experiment. *J Am Soc Echocardiogr* 1991;4:475–84.

4. Wollschläger H, Zeiher AM, Klein HP, et al. Transesophageal echo computer tomography (ECHO-CT): a new method for perspective views of the beating heart (abstract). *Circulation* 1990;82 Suppl 3:III–670.

5. Fine DG, Sapoznikov D, Mosseri M, Gostman MS. Three dimensional echocardiographic reconstruction: qualitative and quantitative evaluation of ventricular function. *Comput Methods Programs Biomed* 1988;26:33–43.

6. Zoghbi WA, Buckey JC, Massey MA, Blomqvist CG. Determination of left ventricular volumes with use of a new nongeometric echocardiographic method: clinical validation and potential application. *J Am Coll Cardiol* 1990;15:610–7.

7. Nixon JV, Saffer SI, Lipscomb K, Blomqvist CG. Three-dimensional echoventriculography. *Am Heart J* 1983;106:435–43.

8. McCann HA, Sharp JC, Kinter TM, et al. Multidimensional ultrasonic imaging for cardiology. *Proc IEEE* 1988;76:1063–73.

9. Fazzalari NL, Goldblatt E, Adams APS. A composite three-dimensional echocardiographic technique for left ventricular volume estimation in children: comparison with angiography and established echographic methods. *J Clin Ultrasound* 1986; 14:663–74.

10. von Ramm OT, Pavy HA, Smith SW, Kisslo J. Real-time, three-dimensional echocardiography: the first human images (abstract). *Circulation* 1991;84 Suppl 2:II–685.

11. Shattuck DP, Weinshenker MD, Smith SW, von Ramm OT. Explososcan: a parallel processing technique for high speed ultrasound imaging with linear phased arrays. *J Acoust Soc Am* 1984;75:1273–82.

12. Smith WS, Pavy HG, von Ramm OT. High-speed ultrasound volumetric imaging system. Part 1: transducer design and beam steering. *IEEE Trans Ultrason Ferroelec Freq Contr* 1991;38:101–108.

13. von Ramm OT, Smith WS, Pavy HG. High-speed ultrasound volumetric imaging system. Part II: parallel processing and image display. *IEEE Trans Ultrason Ferroelec Freq Contr* 1991;38:109–15.

14. Kitney RI, Moura L, Straughan K. 3-D visualization of arterial structures using ultrasound and Voxel modelling. *Int J Card Imaging* 1989;4 (no. 1):135–43.

15. Chandrasekaran K, Porter T, D'Adamo A, et al. Three-dimensional volumetric imaging of pulmonary arteries in humans by intravascular ultrasound: feasibility and clinical potential (abstract). *Circulation* 1991;84 Suppl 2:II–685.

16. Rosenfield K, Losordo DW, Ramaswamy K, et al. Three-dimensional reconstruction of human coronary and peripheral arteries from images recorded during two-dimensional intravascular ultrasound examination. *Circulation* 1991;84:1938–56.

17. Robb RA, Barillot C. Interactive display and analysis of 3-D medical images. *IEEE Trans Med Imaging* 1989;8:217–26.

18. Greenleaf JF. Three-dimensional imaging in ultrasound. *J Med Syst* 1982;6:579–89.

19. Geiser EA, Ariet M, Conetta DA, et al. Dynamic three-dimensional echocardiographic reconstruction of the intact human left ventricle: technique and initial observations in patients. *Am Heart J* 1982;103:1056–65.

20. Heffernan PB, Robb RA. A new method for shaded surface display of biological and medical images. *IEEE Trans Med Imaging* 1985;MI-4:26–38.

21. Greenleaf JF, Tu JS, Wood EH. Computer generated three-dimensional oscilloscopic images and associated techniques for display and study of the spatial distribution of pulmonary blood flow. *IEEE Trans Nucl Sci* 1970;NS-17:353–9.

22. Coulam CM, Greenleaf JF, Tsakiris AG, Wood EH. Three-dimensional computerized display of physiologic models and data. *Comput Biomed Res* 1972;5:166–79.

23. Ney DR, Fishman EK, Magid D, Drebin RA. Volumetric rendering of computed tomography data: principles and techniques. *IEEE Comput Graphics Applications* 1990:24–32.

24. Martin RW, Bashein G. Measurement of stroke volume with three-dimensional transesophageal ultrasonic scanning: comparison with thermodilution measurement. *Anesthesiology* 1989;70:470–6.

25. Fazzalari NL, Davidson JA, Mazumdar J, et al. Three dimensional reconstruction of the left ventricle from four anatomically defined apical two-dimensional echocardiographic views. *Acta Cardiol* 1984;39:409–35.

26. Levine RA, Handschumacher MD, Sanfilippo AJ, et al. Three-dimensional echocardiographic reconstruction of the mitral valve, with implications for the diagnosis of mitral valve prolapse. *Circulation* 1989;80:589–98.

27. Handschumacher MD, Sanfilippo AJ, Harrigan P, et al. A new three-dimensional echocardiographic method for quantitating mitral valve prolapse (abstract). *J Am Coll Cardiol* 1989;13:227A.

This text is based on, and all illustrations unless noted in legend are from, Belohlavek M, Foley DA, Gerber TC, Kinter TM, Greenleaf JF, Seward JB. Three- and four-dimensional cardiovascular ultrasound imaging: a new era for echocardiography. Mayo Clin Proc 1993;68:221–40.

Index

Note: Page numbers followed by *f* indicate figures; those followed by *t* indicate tables.